T0298693

The Science of Mental Health

Volume 3
Schizophrenia

Series Content

The Science
of Mental Health

Volume 3
Schizophrenia

Edited with introductions by

Steven Hyman
National Institute of Mental Health

ROUTLEDGE
New York/London

Published in 2001 by

Routledge
711 Third Avenue
New York, NY 10017

Published in Great Britain by
Routledge
2 Park Square, Milton Park
Abingdon, Oxon OX14 4RN

Routledge is an Imprint of Taylor & Francis Books, Inc.
Copyright © 2001 by Routledge

Library of Congress Cataloging-in-Publication Data

The science of mental health / edited with introductions by Steven Hyman.
    p. cm.
Includes bibliographical references.
 ISBN 0-8153-3743-4 (set)
 1. Mental health. I. Hyman, Steven E.
RA790 .S435 2002
616.89--dc21
                        2001048491

POD ISBN: 9780415532525
Set ISBN: 9780815337430
Vol 1:   9780815337447
Vol 2:   9780815337454
Vol 3:   9780815337461
Vol 4:   9780815337478
Vol 5:   9780815337485
Vol 6:   9780815337492
Vol 7:   9780815337508
Vol 8:   9780815337515
Vol 9:   9780815337522
Vol 10:   9780815337539

Contents

Introduction

Schizophrenia is a chronic, disabling disorder of the brain that is manifest in severe behavioral symptoms. Schizophrenia affects approximately 1 person in 100 worldwide (Kendler et al., 1996; Bromet and Fennig, 1999) and is a leading cause of disability in both developed and developing countries. This volume contains articles that provide a broad background to understanding this severe mental disorder. The introduction gives a brief review of symptoms. Several overview papers present hypotheses explaining the etiology and the causes of symptoms. These papers demonstrate that there is still much to learn about schizophrenia and not all experts are in full agreement. Entries are also included that describe epidemiology and genetics, with the epidemiologic articles presenting not only incidence and prevalence of the illness but also possible environmental risk factors that might interact with genetic factors to produce the disease.

Schizophrenia is now understood to result from a complex interaction between genetics and environment. As he or she must in many developing fields, the reader will have to do some of the work of integration. For example, Mortensen et al. (1999) have identified possible environmental factors that increase the risk of schizophrenia but do not provide a sophisticated understanding of how these risks might operate in conjunction with genetic risk factors.

Given the hypothesis that schizophrenia represents a disorder of brain development (Weinberger, 1987), there is a section on recent evidence from neuroimaging studies that bear on possible developmental abnormalities. This section is followed by ones on neurobiology and on treatment.

Schizophrenia generally announces itself in the late teen years or early twenties, although there may be earlier prodromal symptoms. Very rarely, schizophrenia begins in childhood or the early teen years. These early-onset cases are generally very severe, and they have provided valuable information about brain development (Rapoport et al., 1999). According to current diagnostic criteria, the defining characteristics of schizophrenia are psychotic symptoms and a chronic course. Psychotic symptoms include disturbances in perception— hallucinations and illusions— and abnormalities in the form and content of thought. (Hallucinations are false perceptions that occur in the absence of a sensory stimulus; illusions represent misinterpretations of sensory stimuli that are present.) The hallucinations that characterize schizophrenia are most often auditory and are generally composed of voices, noises, or even music. Hallucinations may also occur in other sensory modalities but are less common. Abnormalities in the content of thought include delusions, which are fixed, culturally inappropriate beliefs that are held despite all reasonable evidence to the contrary, and inaccurate ideas of reference, beliefs that ordinary events have special significance for the individual (for example, the belief that a license plate on a passing automobile is meant to convey a signal to the individual). Abnormalities in the form of thought include disorganized or illogical speech consisting of ideas that have no clear connection to one another, often described as "loosening of associations." Schizophrenia is also characterized by disturbances of emotion. For example, individuals with schizophrenia may be unresponsive to emotional stimuli that would affect a normal person ("blunting of affect") or may exhibit inappropriate affect, for example, giggling in response to sad or somber events.

For many individuals with schizophrenia, the disabling symptoms are what have often been called negative or deficit symptoms, especially deficits in cognitive functioning. There may be an impoverishment of ideas and of speech and difficulties with working memory— the ability to hold information in consciousness so that it can be usefully manipulated. People with schizophrenia often exhibit lack of motivation, which also has profound effects on functioning. Overall, people with schizophrenia exhibit marked impairment in social and occupation roles, with deterioration in their level of functioning prior to the onset of full-blown illness.

Schizophrenia is characterized typically by a prodromal period that may be marked by difficulties in socializing and abnormal patterns of thinking, but the full-blown illness generally begins with an episode of florid psychosis. Subsequently, schizophrenia is characterized by periods of active psychotic symptoms followed by at least partial remissions (Robinson et al., 1999). During these remissions, however, negative or deficit symptoms often continue and contribute to long-term disability. Suicide is an all-too-common outcome of schizophrenia, resulting in death for perhaps 10 to 15 percent of those afflicted with the illness. Social and cognitive functioning generally deteriorates in the early years of illness and then stabilizes (Heaton et al., 2001). Approximately 80 percent of people with schizophrenia have poor outcomes as measured by the frequency and severity of relapses, unremitting symptoms, or poor overall social and occupational functioning.

There is no longer any doubt that schizophrenia is a profound disorder affecting the structure and function of the brain and that it has strong genetic risk factors that interact with nongenetic risks. Earlier notions that schizophrenia might represent an extreme form of eccentricity or that it might result from poor parenting or malignant social forces have long been put to rest. One of the critical breakthroughs in the reconceptualization of schizophrenia as a medical illness came from the work of Seymour Kety et al. (1968), who began to demonstrate a genetic risk by comparing the prevalence of the illness in the biological versus adopted relatives of adoptees with schizophrenia. By studying individuals adopted early in life, one can begin to separate genetic and environmental risk factors (although this design is not perfect, because the relevant environmental factors may begin before birth). This classic study is complemented by a reanalysis by Kendler and Gruenberg (1984) that uses more modern diagnostic methods. Significantly, the existence of genetic risk factors holds up in this later study.

As is the case for all mental disorders, the genetic risks for schizophrenia are not straightforward. Although genes are important in the aggregate, there does not appear to be any one gene that causes schizophrenia. This important point emerges from the reviews by Baron (2001) and from the entry by Egan et al. (2001). The general understanding of genetics in society and indeed among health professionals has lagged behind the extraordinary advances of the 1990s. The common understanding of hereditary factors is often limited to traits caused by single genes, often described as Mendelian traits, after the founder of modern genetics, the Austrian monk Gregor Mendel.

In the nineteenth century Mendel wrote about traits of pea plants that resulted from the actions of single genes. Well-known single-gene or Mendelian disorders include such illnesses as Huntington's chorea and cystic fibrosis. Mendelian traits can be further characterized as either dominant, as is the case for Huntington's chorea, or recessive, as is the case for cystic fibrosis. A dominant disorder often occurs when a mutation in a critical gene results in a protein that has a novel and harmful function. In the case of Huntington's disease, a mutated protein literally becomes a toxic agent, causing the death of nerve cells in several critical brain regions. The most common cause of a recessive trait is a mutation that inactivates a critical gene. Because humans, like all animals, inherit two copies of each gene, one copy from their father and one from their mother, a single harmful mutation may not produce an observable trait (phenotype) if the second, normal copy can compensate. Recessive disorders occur when a person inherits defective copies of a gene from both father and mother. While there are other mechanisms by which single-gene traits can occur, the upshot is that for Mendelian disorders a genetic mutation causes the disorder. In mental disorders such as schizophrenia, the role of genes is quite different. A single gene does not cause the illness; rather, multiple genes interact with each other to create risk for the illness. Nongenetic factors that convert risk into illness must also be present. This is exemplified by the situation that may occur with identical (monozygotic) twins, who share 100 percent of their DNA sequences. If one twin has schizophrenia, the other has a 50 percent chance of developing schizophrenia as well. This is an enormous increase over the general population risk of 1 percent. This finding corroborates the findings from Kety et al., and from many subsequent investigators, that genes play a major role in risk of schizophrenia. At the same time, the risk for the unaffected twin is only 50 percent, not 100 percent. Therefore, nongenetic factors, developmental and environmental, must play a role in converting genetic risk into illness.

To make matters more complex, not only is it likely that multiple genes are involved in creating risk but there may be different genetic pathways to the illness. Put another way, no one gene may be either necessary or sufficient. This complexity has created substantial obstacles for gene hunters, but it is important that they eventually succeed. Finding genes that produce risk is not simply a matter of idle curiosity, because genes encode the protein building blocks of cells; thus, finding versions of genes that produce risk will give us important insights into what goes wrong in the brain in schizophrenia. Moreover, by pointing us toward important biochemical pathways, risk genes will likely suggest novel therapies. A novel approach to finding risk genes is illustrated in the paper by Egan et al. (2001), who have found a version of a gene that influences brain function in general that may also affect the risk of schizophrenia.

Studies of the course of disease, often described as the natural history of disease, are important as backgrounds against which to think about pathogenesis and judge the success or failure of treatments. One important line of thought is that schizophrenia is a disorder of brain development. To date, there has been little direct evidence for this hypothesis. Until recently, the major evidence for the developmental hypothesis has been the typical age of onset of schizophrenia in late teens and early twenties, an important period of brain development during which neural connections (synapses) are winnowed, brain and behavior change under the influence of gonadal steroids (sex hormones), and myelination of certain brain regions occurs. Other arguments for this hypothesis have been based on negative evidence: the failure to find markers of inflammation or neurodegeneration (Arnold et al., 1998) on postmortem examination of the brains of people with schizophrenia. The existing postmortem studies (reviewed in Harrison, 1999) are too few in number and have involved too few brains to provide certainty. There is far more to do in this regard. Recent indirect evidence that brain development is altered in schizophrenia comes from the use of noninvasive neuroimaging in childhood-onset cases of schizophrenia. Two articles from the team of Rapoport and colleagues, based at the National Institute of Mental Health, demonstrate progressive changes in the brain that deviate from expected patterns of brain development in people with early-onset schizophrenia (Rapoport et al., 1999). Magnetic resonance imaging and advanced methods of data analysis reveal striking patterns of abnormal gray-matter development in young people with schizophrenia. Much still needs to be learned, however, about the relationship of schizophrenia and brain development.

Recent years have seen a profusion of studies of brain abnormalities that occur in schizophrenia. Articles included in this volume involve multiple disciplines, including cognitive science, neuroimaging, pharmacology, systems-level neuroscience, and molecular biology. It is gratifying that some observations are convergent, but many still are not. One important set of observations derived from the postmortem study of the brains of people with schizophrenia reveals abnormalities of brain structure. Normal brains contain nerve cells with a rich protrusion of processes (neuropil) of which the dendrites form the most important information-receiving structures. There is evidence from several groups (Rajkowska, 1998; Selemon and Goldman-Rakic, 1999; Glantz and Lewis, 2000) that schizophrenia is characterized by decreased neuropil without cell loss (leading to an increased packing density of nerve cells). Similar findings have been described in autism. Such cellular abnormalities may underlie well-characterized changes in the large-scale structure of the brain in schizophrenia. Certain brain regions appear to be abnormally small in schizophrenia, with the most replicated findings focused on the prefrontal cortex, the temporal lobes, and the thalamus, a critical structure that controls information going to the cerebral cortex.

This apparent loss of tissue in schizophrenia (perhaps decreased neuropil) results in enlargement of the fluid-filled ventricles of the brain. This ventricular enlargement was the first well-corroborated evidence for brain abnormalities in schizophrenia. A difficulty in proving this is the marked diversity of ventricular size in normal populations. An interesting early study (Suddath et al., 1990) that addressed the question compared the brains of identical twins in which one suffered from schizophrenia and the other did not. These "discordant" twins permitted ideal conditions for comparison; in almost every case the ventricles were larger in the twin with schizophrenia. Structural studies of brain abnormalities have been supplemented by cognitive neuroscience in combination with functional imaging. Here we see early attempts to correlate psychotic symptoms or cognitive deficits with altered activity in brain activation (Barch et al., 2001). The most consistent findings are of decreased activity of the dorsal prefrontal cortex correlated with deficits in working memory or other aspects of frontal lobe function.

Superimposed on the abnormal structural brain anatomy of people with schizophrenia appear to be abnormalities of the chemical communication systems of the brain. Because most pharmacologic treatments block the action of the neurotransmitter dopamine, this neurotransmitter and its receptors in the brain have been an important focus of research. Laruelle et al. (1996) provided evidence that the release mechanisms for dopamine may be in schizophrenia. Other research has implicated additional neurotransmitters in treatment, if not pathogenesis, including glutamate (Goff and Coyle, 2001) and serotonin. However, the ways in which posited neurochemical abnormalities and documented anatomic abnormalities might occur and how they might interact remains an important frontier of research.

The treatment and course of schizophrenia have improved markedly since the introduction of antipsychotic drugs in the 1950s. A second wave of improvement came in the late 1980s and the 1990s with the widespread introduction of a new generation of antipsychotic drugs with fewer motor side effects and possibly greater efficacy against negative symptoms (Kane et al., 1988). In addition, a variety of psychological and social interventions have been shown to make a substantial difference in the ability of people with schizophrenia to avoid relapse and to be maintained in a community setting (Bustillo et al., 2001). It is important to recognize that pharmacologic and psychosocial treatments do not represent an either-or situation, but truly complement each other.

Schizophrenia is one of the most devastating illnesses that confronts humanity. Over the past decades our very conception of this illness has been revolutionized. We are now deeply involved in understanding the details of risk, pathogenesis, and treatment and look forward to the day when treatments are safer and more effective and when we can begin to think deeply about prevention.

Neuron, Vol. 28, 325–334, November, 2000, Copyright ©2000 by Cell Press

Catching Up on Schizophrenia: Natural History and Neurobiology

Review

David A. Lewis*‡ and Jeffrey A. Lieberman†‡
*Departments of Psychiatry and Neuroscience
University of Pittsburgh School of Medicine
†Departments of Psychiatry, Pharmacology,
and Radiology
University of North Carolina School of Medicine

Introduction

Schizophrenia is a brain disorder that is expressed in the form of abnormal mental functions and disturbed behavior. These manifestations characteristically appear in the late second and third decades of life as a heterogeneous constellation of three classes of clinical features. Positive symptoms include delusions (false beliefs), hallucinations (false perceptions), and thought disorganization. Negative symptoms refer to the loss of motivation and emotional vibrancy. Disturbances in basic cognitive functions, such as attention, executive functions, and specific forms of memory (particularly working memory), are also consistently observed in patients and are now thought to be central to the behavioral disturbances and functional disability of schizophrenia. In addition, many patients have concomitant mood symptoms including depression and anxiety that may contribute to the 10% lifetime incidence of suicide in schizophrenia.

Etiology

Vulnerability to schizophrenia is clearly related to genetic factors (Tsuang, 2000). Family, twin, and adoption studies have demonstrated that the morbid risk of schizophrenia in relatives correlates with the degree of shared genes. In contrast to the 1% incidence of schizophrenia in the general population, the incidence of schizophrenia is ∼2% in third degree relatives (e.g., first cousins) of an individual with schizophrenia, 2%–6% in second degree relatives (e.g., nieces/nephews), and 6%–17% in first degree relatives (e.g., parents, siblings or children) (Gottesman, 1991). Among twins, the incidence of schizophrenia is ∼17% in dizygotic twins of affected individuals, and nearly 50% in monozygotic twins (Gottesman, 1991). Finally, adoption studies have demonstrated that the risk of schizophrenia is related to the presence of the disorder in biological parents but not in the adoptive parents (Gottesman and Shields, 1982).

Regions on a number of chromosomes (e.g., 1, 6, 8, 10, 13, and 22) have been implicated as sites of potential vulnerability genes (Pulver, 2000). For example, 22q11–13 has shown suggestive findings in a number of linkage studies. Interestingly, deletions at this chromosomal region are associated with velo-cardio-facial syndrome (a congenital disorder characterized by cleft palate, car-

diac malformations, and a distinctive facial appearance), which carries a substantially increased risk of schizophrenia, although the incidence of bipolar disorder in this syndrome is increased as well. Recently, chromosome 1q21–22 was identified as the location of a major vulnerability locus for familial schizophrenia with sufficient power to permit positional cloning of the underlying gene(s) (Brzustowicz et al., 2000).

Environmental factors (including exposure to infectious, autoimmune, toxic, or traumatic insults and stress during gestation or childhood) also may play a role in the pathogenesis of schizophrenia, perhaps via subtle alterations of neurodevelopment (Marcelis et al., 1998). Moreover, maturational processes including apoptosis, synaptic pruning, and myelination, occurring in the postnatal period through adolescence, may unmask the genetic vulnerability to schizophrenia (Lewis, 1997; Jarskog et al., 2000; Raedler et al., 2000). Thus, the etiology of schizophrenia has been conceptualized as involving multiple hits (consisting of genes conferring vulnerability and environmental insults), which are revealed in the context of developmental maturation of brain circuitry. However, unlike other genetic neurodevelopmental disorders (e.g., Down's syndrome or Fragile X syndrome), or severe gestational and birth traumas (e.g., fetal hypoxia or kernicterus), there are no immediate overt manifestations of schizophrenia. Rather, most individuals appear to function normally until they enter the greatest period of risk in late adolescence and early adulthood.

The 1% lifetime incidence of schizophrenia is fairly consistent across cultures, countries, racial groups, and genders (Bromet and Fennig, 1999). There are, however, some notable exceptions that support the involvement of the hypothesized etiologic factors previously described. Studies in both the northern and summer hemispheres have found that persons with schizophrenia show a modest excess of births in the winter and spring months, although similar observations have been made for depressive disorders (Torrey et al., 1997). Individuals with schizophrenia also tend to inhabit lower socioeconomic strata and to be more numerous in urban and selected immigrant populations (Mortensen et al., 1999). In addition, although equal numbers of males and females are affected, some data suggest that males may have more severe manifestations of the disorder, including an earlier age of onset (by 2–4 years), more marked neuropathological abnormalities, poorer response to treatment, and less favorable outcome (Szymanski et al., 1995; Hafner et al., 1998).

Thus, schizophrenia appears to be a polygenic disorder and to be associated with environmental and developmental vulnerability factors. The complexity of these potential interactions clearly complicates research on the underlying disease mechanisms. The clinical syndrome recognized as schizophrenia may be a unitary disease process with a range of severity and clinical manifestations across individuals, perhaps depending upon the degree to which different brain regions or circuits are affected. Alternatively, the clinical heterogeneity could reflect the possibility that what is recognized

‡To whom correspondence should be addressed (e-mail: lewisda@msx.upmc.edu [D. A. L.], jlieberman@css.unc.edu [J. A. L.]).

1

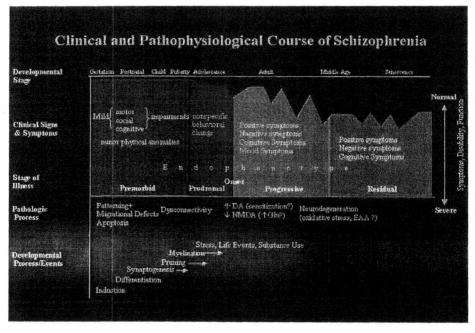

Figure 1. Clinical and Pathophysiological Course of Schizophrenia

The diagram attempts to integrate and schematically depict the clinical and pathophysiologcal course of schizophrenia in its various clinical stages. To orient the reader starting from the top row: "Developmental Stage" describes the stage of life during which the various events and phenomena occur; "Clinical Signs and Symptoms" refers to the mental and behavioral manifestations of the illness; "Stage of Illness" describes all premorbid and morbid phases of the illness; "Pathologic Process" refers to the hypothesized pathogenic and pathophysiologic mechanisms that underlie and are causal to the clinical manifestations of the disorder; "Developmental Process and Events" indicates the neurobiological maturational processes and environmental events that may unmask or destabilize the neural circuits made vulnerable by etiologic and pathogenic factors. The following abbreviations are DA, dopamine; NMDA, N-methyl D-aspartate; Glu, glutamate.

as schizophrenia represents a constellation of diseases that share some phenotypic features. Differentiating among these possibilities will require the definitive identification of specific causal factor(s).

Course of Schizophrenia

The time course of schizophrenia follows the fairly stereotyped pattern depicted in Figure 1. High-risk and longitudinal birth cohort studies have identified mild deficits in social, motor, and cognitive functions during childhood and adolescence that may represent premorbid features of the illness (Jones, 1997). For example, subtle motor abnormalities during infancy (Walker and Lewine, 1990) and deficits in social functioning, organizational ability, and intellectual functioning at ages 16–17 have both been reported to be associated with the later appearance of schizophrenia (Davidson et al., 1999). In addition, a number of minor physical anomalies, such as variations in limb length and angle and finger-print patterns, are present in a subgroup of patients and can also be detected in populations with increased genetic risk. All of these features, however, are mild in severity and have low predictive validity as individual markers.

Prodromal symptoms and behaviors (i.e., those that herald the approaching onset of the illness) may include attenuated positive symptoms (e.g., illusions, ideas of reference, magical thinking, superstitiousness), mood symptoms (e.g., anxiety, dysphoria, irritability), cognitive symptoms (e.g., distractibility, concentration difficulties), social withdrawal, or obsessive behaviors to name a few (McGlashan, 1996; Yung and McGorry, 1996). Because many of these prodromal phenomena extensively overlap with the range of mental experiences and behaviors of persons in the ages of risk who do not subsequently develop schizophrenia, they cannot be considered diagnostic. In the vast majority of cases, these prodromal manifestations, and subsequently positive and negative symptoms by which the diagnosis is made, develop gradually over a period of weeks, months or even years beginning some time in the mid second through the third decade of life. The environmental events that typically occur during this developmental epoch (e.g., entering college, the military or the workforce, exposure to drug abuse) may act as stressors on vulnerable neural circuits that exceed their adaptive capacity, thereby producing the behavioral symptoms that signal the onset of the illness (Lieberman et al.,

1997). In contrast, schizophrenia rarely has its onset before puberty or after age 40.

The evidence that schizophrenia is a genetically mediated, neurodevelopmental disorder bred the belief that affected individuals were "doomed from the womb" and thus had a pessimistic prognosis. In contrast, recent studies have shown that, if treated properly early in the course of their illness, most patients experience a substantial reduction and even remission of psychotic symptoms following an initial episode, although associated negative and cognitive symptoms can persist (Lieberman et al., 1993; Sheitman et al., 1997; Robinson et al., 1999a). However, following recovery, the majority of patients eventually discontinue medication and then subsequently experience a relapse of psychotic symptoms. In the context of subsequent psychotic episodes, they may not respond to treatment as well as in prior episodes and fail to achieve symptom remission (Lieberman et al., 1996; Robinson et al., 1999b). Through this process of repeated exacerbations and relative remissions, most patients sustain the clinical deterioration that is the hallmark of schizophrenia and that leads to an end-stage of the illness in which severely affected patients exhibit persistent symptoms and profound functional disability (Figure 1). Interestingly, this pattern of clinical deterioration is most pronounced in the early stages of the illness (first 5–10 years) and then reaches a plateau (although the most severe variants may continue to decline into senescence [Harvey et al., 1999]).

Pathogenesis and Pathophysiology
A major challenge in schizophrenia research has been to understand how a genetically mediated, neurodevelopmental disorder is not expressed clinically until 1.5–3 decades postnatally, but then proceeds to progressively disable its victims. It is hypothesized that the interaction of a genetic diathesis and early neurodevelopmental insults result in defective connectivity between a number of brain regions, including the midbrain, nucleus accumbens, thalamus, temporo-limbic, and prefrontal cortices (Selemon and Goldman-Rakic, 1999). This defective neural circuitry is then vulnerable to dysfunction when unmasked by the developmental processes and events of adolescence (myelination, synaptic pruning, and hormonal effects of puberty on CNS) and exposure to stressors as the individual moves through the age of risk (Lieberman et al., 1997; Raedler et al., 2000) (Figure 1).

These factors have prompted speculation about which neurochemical systems might mediate the progressive changes seen during the early phases of schizophrenia (Lieberman, 1999). Such speculation has centered on the dopamine and glutamate systems (Figure 2). An overactivity of dopamine neurotransmission in the mesencephalic projections to the limbic striatum has long been suspected in schizophrenia. However, the evidence supporting the involvement of dopamine had, until recently, been predominantly indirect. This included the positive correlation between the clinical potency and D_2 binding affinity of antipsychotic drugs, on one hand, and the ability of indirect dopamine agonists to induce psychosis in healthy volunteers and provoke psychotic symptoms at very low doses in patients

with schizophrenia, on the other (Carlsson 1988). Although both postmortem and PET studies had found increased levels of D_2 receptors in the brains of schizophrenia patients, antipsychotic drug treatment as the cause could not be ruled out (Wong et al., 1986; Farde et al., 1990). More recently, direct evidence of dopamine hyperactivity has emerged from both preclinical and clinical studies, implicating dysfunctions in presynaptic storage, release, reuptake, and metabolic mechanisms in dopamine meso-limbic systems (Giros et al., 1996; Laruelle et al., 1996; Breier et al., 1997). These studies suggest that abnormalities in dopamine storage, vesicular transport, release, or reuptake by the presynaptic neuron may be the proximal cause of psychotic symptoms (Laruelle et al., 1999) and may contribute to the risk for schizophrenia (Egan et al., 2000). It has been further hypothesized that disturbances in the presynaptic regulation of dopamine could lead to enduring consequences through the induction of sensitization and/or oxidative stress (Lieberman et al., 1997; Laruelle, 2000). In contrast, the functional activity of dopamine may be decreased in the neocortex in schizophrenia (Davis et al., 1991; Okuba et al., 1997; Akil et al., 1999).

Glutamate has also been implicated in schizophrenia by studies of behavioral effects of NMDA receptor antagonists (e.g., PCP, MK-801, ketamine) and in the context of the NMDA receptor hypofunction hypothesis (Javitt and Zukin, 1991; Olney and Farber, 1995; Jentsch and Roth, 1999). Acute administration produces psychotic symptoms and cognitive dysfunction in healthy subjects (Krystal et al., 1994) and exacerbates psychotic, negative, and cognitive symptoms in patients with schizophrenia (Lahti et al., 1995). NMDA receptor hypofunction induced by the administration of NMDA antagonists results in decreased corticofugal inhibition of subcortical dopamine neurons and consequent increased mesolimbic dopamine release (Breier et al., 1998; Kegeles et al., 2000), while chronic administration produces decreased release, or hypoactivity, of dopamine in the prefrontal cortex (Jentsch and Roth, 1999). It has also been suggested that hypofunctioning NMDA receptors can cause an excess compensatory release of glutamate that can overactivate other glutamate receptor subtypes that are not being antagonized and are functionally active (Moghaddam and Adams, 1998; Duncan et al., 2000). Finally, NMDA receptor hypofunction may also produce disturbances in neuroplasticity of neurons by altering synaptic connectivity.

Structural Pathology
Structural brain abnormalities have also been extensively documented in individuals with schizophrenia (McCarley et al., 1999). These include enlargement of the lateral and third ventricles and reduced volume of the cortical gray matter and related structures. The latter changes do not appear to represent a uniform abnormality, but rather to effect preferentially certain association cortices including those located in the superior temporal gyrus, the dorsal prefrontal cortex (PFC), and limbic areas such as the hippocampal formation and anterior cingulate cortex (Goldstein et al., 1999; McCarley et al., 1999) (Figure 2). Many of these structural abnormalities are evident in first-episode, never-medicated subjects

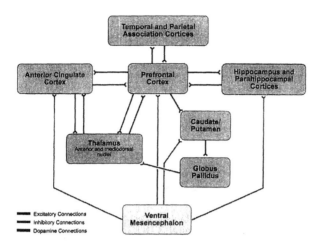

Figure 2. Affected Brain Regions in Sc
zophrenia
Schematic diagram summarizing some of th
brain regions that have most consistentl
been implicated in the pathophysiology c
schizophrenia. The nature of the pathophys
ological changes appears to differ across re
gions with a reduction in neuronal numbe
reported in some nuclei of the thalamus, de
creases in markers of synaptic connectivit
in the prefrontal cortex and hippocampal for
mation, and evidence of either a function
excess or deficit of dopamine neurotransmis
sion in the striatum and prefrontal cortex, re
spectively.

with schizophrenia, and may be present prior to the clinical onset of illness, suggesting that they reflect the primary disease process and are not a secondary consequence of the illness or of its treatment. In addition, longitudinal neuroimaging studies have shown apparent neuropathological progression in the form of gray matter volume decreases and fluid compartment increases (in lateral and third ventricles and subarachnoid space) over the course of the illness (Davis et al., 1998; Gur et al., 1998a; Rapoport et al., 1999). The fact that postmortem studies have not found evidence of gliosis is consistent with an emphasis on the hypothesized role of neurodevelopmental factors in the pathogenesis and pathophysiology of schizophrenia (Harrison, 1999). However, recent evidence also suggests the possible involvement of apoptotic mechanisms (Jarskog et al., 2000).

Circuitry-Based Pathological Changes
Understanding the pathophysiological significance of these structural brain abnormalities requires knowledge of which specific neural elements are affected and how the disturbances in different brain regions may be related. To date, these questions have been most extensively explored for the neural circuitry of the hippocampal formation and the dorsal PFC.

Multiple imaging and postmortem studies over the past 2 decades have documented a slight bilateral reduction in the volume of the hippocampal formation (Harrison, 1999; McCarley et al., 1999), an observation supported by more recent in vivo proton spectroscopy findings of reduced hippocampal N-acetyl aspartate, a putative marker of neuronal pathology, in both unmedicated adult and childhood onset subjects with schizophrenia (Bertolino et al., 1998). In addition, positron emission tomography studies have provided evidence of hippocampal dysfunction during episodic memory retrieval in subjects with schizophrenia (Heckers et al., 1998). Initial reports of hippocampal neuron disarray or misplaced neurons in the superficial layers of the adjacent entorhinal cortex have been widely cited, but these observations have not been replicated in most

subsequent studies (Harrison, 1999). Reduced hippo campal volume also does not appear to be attributabl to decreased neuronal number, but several independen studies have found reductions in neuronal cell body siz in various subregions of the hippocampus proper (Bene et al., 1991; Arnold et al., 1995; Zaidel et al., 1997). I addition, there are consistent reports of reductions ii the gene products for synaptophysin and related pre synaptic markers and in dendritic markers, such as mi crotubule-associated protein, in certain subdivisions o the hippocampus (see Weinberger, 1999, for review) Although these findings are limited in a number of re spects, they have given rise to testable models postulat ing that genes involved in the formation and mainte nance of hippocampal circuitry play a role in diseas vulnerability (Weinberger, 1999).

In general, the magnitude and consistency of gra matter reduction in the PFC is not as robust as in th hippocampal formation. However, multiple studies o the PFC have been motivated by the observation tha subjects with schizophrenia consistently perform poorl on certain cognitive tasks, such as those requiring work ing memory, that are subserved by circuitry involving th dorsal PFC (Goldman-Rakic, 1994). In addition, thes subjects fail to show normal activation of the dorsa lateral PFC (e.g., Brodmann area 46) when attemptin to perform the Wisconsin Card Sort Task, N-back task or other tasks that require working memory (Weinberge et al., 1986; Taylor, 1996). Since the long-term prognosi for individuals with schizophrenia appears to be bes predicted, not by the severity of positive symptoms, bu by the degree of cognitive impairment (Green, 1996 Weinberger and Gallhofer, 1997), understanding the na ture of PFC brain abnormalities may be particularly im portant for improving clinical outcome.

Many, but not all, postmortem studies have reported a 5%–10% reduction in cortical thickness, with a corre sponding increase in cell packing density, but no chang in total neuron number, in the dorsal PFC of subject with schizophrenia (Selemon and Goldman-Rakic, 1999) Although the size of some PFC neuronal populations particularly pyramidal neurons in deep layer 3, is smaller in schizophrenic subjects (Rajkowska et al., 1998), these findings are also likely to reflect a decrease in the number of axon terminals, distal dendrites, and dendritic spines that represent the principal components of cortical synapses. Consistent with this interpretation, levels of synaptophysin, a presynaptic terminal protein, have been found to be decreased in the PFC of subjects with schizophrenia in multiple studies (Perrone-Bizzozero et al., 1996; Glantz and Lewis, 1997; Karson et al., 1999; Honer et al., 1999). Furthermore, as in the hippocampus, levels of N-acetyl aspartate, a marker of axonal and/or neuronal integrity, are reduced in the PFC of subjects with schizophrenia (Bertolino et al., 2000).

The reason for this reduction in synaptic connectivity in the PFC is not fully known. One contributing factor may be fewer projections from the thalamus. Indeed, enlargement of the third ventricle (whose lateral boundaries are formed by the thalamus) appears to reflect a reduction in size of the thalamus (Andreasen et al., 1994; Buchsbaum et al., 1996; Frazier et al., 1996; Gur et al., 1998b). Moreover, thalamic volume has been correlated with prefrontal white matter volume in subjects with schizophrenia, suggesting that a reduction in thalamic volume is associated with fewer axonal projections to the PFC (Portas et al., 1998). Consistent with these observations, several postmortem studies have revealed a 30% reduction in the total number of neurons in both the mediodorsal thalamic nucleus (MD), the principal source of thalamic projections to the PFC, and in the anterior nuclei, which project to the PFC and anterior cingulate cortex, but not in at least some other thalamic nuclei (Pakkenberg, 1990; Popken et al., 2000; Young et al., 2000). However, the small sample sizes and limited assessment of potential confounds in these studies indicate that additional investigations in this area are required.

Despite these limitations, the potential importance of these findings is strengthened by the convergence of other lines of evidence that support the hypothesis that schizophrenia is associated with abnormalities in thalamo-prefrontal connectivity (Figure 3). For example, a putative marker of MD axon terminals appear to be reduced in the PFC of subjects with schizophrenia (Lewis, 2000). In addition, basilar dendritic spines on PFC deep layer 3 pyramidal neurons, a principal synaptic target of the excitatory projections from the MD, have been reported to be decreased by ~25% in subjects with schizophrenia (Garey et al., 1998; Glantz and Lewis, 2000). In contrast, pyramidal neurons in at least some other cortical layers or regions of the same subjects, and in individuals with major depressive disorder, appear to lack or to exhibit less marked changes in spine density. Since the elimination of presynaptic axon terminals typically leads to resorption of the postsynaptic dendritic spine, these observations are consistent with a reduced number of afferents from the MD in schizophrenia.

In the primate visual system, monocular deprivation, which leads to reduced cortical inputs from the thalamus, has been associated with a decline in markers of activity in cortical γ-aminobutyric acid (GABA) neurons (Hendry and Jones, 1988), including the expression of the mRNA for glutamic acid decarboxylase (GAD_{67}), the synthesizing enzyme for GABA. If these findings in the visual system hold for MD-PFC connectivity, then a similar reduction in GAD_{67} mRNA expression would be expected in the PFC of subjects with schizophrenia. Consistent with this prediction, GAD_{67} mRNA and protein levels have been reported to be reduced in the PFC of subjects with schizophrenia (Akbarian et al., 1995; Costa et al., 2000; Volk et al., 2000). Furthermore, it appears that a subset of GABA neurons (~25%) is primarily affected. For example, the density of GABA transporter-immunoreactive axon cartridges (the distinctive, vertically arrayed axon terminals of GABAergic chandelier neurons, which synapse exclusively on the axon initial segment of pyramidal neurons), is selectively decreased in the dorsal PFC of subjects with schizophrenia (but not in individuals with other psychiatric disorders) with the reduction most evident in the middle cortical layers (Pierri et al., 1999).

Thus, correlative evidence across a range of observations suggests that schizophrenia is associated with impaired MD-PFC connectivity. Given the dependence of working memory tasks on the integrity of this circuitry, it would not be surprising if such an impairment could account for working memory dysfunction in schizophrenia. The relationship of this impairment to the positive and negative symptoms of schizophrenia is less obvious. Nor is it clear that MD-PFC connections are the primary site of pathogenesis. For example, experimental studies in rodents suggest that dysfunction of the PFC may appear postpubertally following perinatal lesions of the hippocampus (Weinberger and Lipska, 1995). Finally, the apparent deficits in PFC function are also likely to reflect disturbances in both intrinsic and cortico-cortical connections (Goldman-Rakic and Selemon, 1997; Mirnics et al., 2000).

Treatment of Schizophrenia

Much remains to be learned about the etiology and pathophysiology of schizophrenia, but the efficacy of treatments for this disorder has been clearly demonstrated (see Table 1). Although all available treatments have limitations in their effectiveness and are associated with adverse side effects, it is an established fact that antipsychotic medications can alleviate the psychotic symptoms of the disorder and prevent their recurrence (Kane, 1996). Moreover, in doing so, antipsychotic drug treatment, strategically used, appears to reduce the degree of clinical deterioration that occurs from progression of the illness. This has led to the hypothesis that the early identification and treatment of schizophrenia (before or soon after symptom onset) may reduce, or even prevent, the cumulative morbidity of the illness (McGlashan, 1996). Although pharmacotherapy provides the foundation for the treatment of schizophrenia, various psychosocial therapies can be useful adjuncts to drug treatment (Kane, 1996).

Until recently, most pharmacological treatments for schizophrenia were based on synaptic modulation of dopamine neuronal systems mainly by antagonism of postsynaptic D_2 receptors. With the advent of the so-called atypical antipsychotic drugs, this focus has now broadened to include other neurotransmitters such as serotonin, norepinephrine, acetylcholine, histamine, and glutamate, as well as various neuropeptides and neu-

5

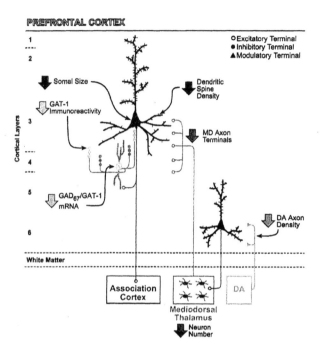

PREFRONTAL CORTEX

○ Excitatory Terminal
● Inhibitory Terminal
▲ Modulatory Terminal

Somal Size
GAT-1 Immunoreactivity
Dendritic Spine Density
MD Axon Terminals
GAD₆₇/GAT-1 mRNA
DA Axon Density

White Matter

Association Cortex

Mediodorsal Thalamus
Neuron Number

Figure 3. Cortical Circuitry in Schizophrenia

Schematic diagram summarizing disturbances in the connectivity between the mediodorsal (MD) thalamic nucleus and the dorsal prefrontal cortex (PFC) in schizophrenia. Postmortem studies have reported that subjects with schizophrenia have (1) decreased number of neurons in the mediodorsal thalamic nucleus; (2) diminished density of parvalbumin-positive varicosities, a putative marker of thalamic axon terminals, selectively in deep layers 3–4, the termination zone of MD projections to the PFC; (3) preferential reduction in spine density on the basilar dendrites of deep layer 3 pyramidal neurons, a principal synaptic target of the excitatory projections from the MD; (4) reduced expression of the mRNA for glutamic acid decarboxylase (GAD₆₇), the synthesizing enzyme for GABA, in a subset of PFC GABA neurons; (5) decreased density of GABA transporter (GAT-1)-immunoreactive axon cartridges, the distinctive, vertically arrayed axon terminals of GABAergic chandelier neurons, which synapse exclusively on the axon initial segment of pyramidal neurons; and (6) decreased dopamine innervation of layer 6, the principal location of pyramidal neurons that provide corticothalamic feedback projections (see Lewis, 2000, for additional details and references).

rosteroids (Kinon and Lieberman, 1996). These compounds have either low ratios of affinities for the D_2 and 5-HT_{2a} receptors (called D_2/5-HT_2 antagonists [e.g., risperidone]) or possess affinities for some combination of multiple neuroreceptors and reuptake sites including $D_{1,2,3,4}$, 5-$HT_{1a,b, 2a,c, 3, 6, 7}$, $NE\alpha_{1, 2}$, $MACH_{1, 4}$, $H_{1,2}$, DAT, NET, ST (called multi-neuroreceptor antagonists [e.g., clozapine]). At present, all effective treatments appear to possess some threshold level of D_2 receptor antagonism, though selective nondopamine antagonists have attempted to challenge this concept (Kapur et al., 2000). At the same time, there is clearly no pharmacologic "magic bullet" for the different pathologic dimensions of schizophrenia. This is reflected by the common practice of using multiple drugs in combination when treating patients with schizophrenia. Whereas, the psychotic symptoms appear to be mediated primarily by dopamine overactivity in mesolimbic circuits and negative symptoms by dopamine underactivity in prefrontal cortical neurons (thus can be exacerbated by classical antipsychotics with high D_2 affinity), the cognitive impairment appears to also involve disturbances in glutamate activity. Interestingly, the second generation or atypical antipsychotic drugs, which are thought to have a broader range of therapeutic effects including reducing cognitive impairment, have been found to block the cellular and behavioral effects of NMDA antagonists, despite the fact that they lack affinities for any of the ionotropic or metabotropic glutamate receptors (Mohn et al., 1999; Duncan et al., 2000). It is therefore assumed that atypical antipsychotic drugs must be acting more directly through dopamine receptors (S. Miyamoto et al., submitted) or

other neuroreceptors (e.g., 5-HT, noradrenergic, etc. [Duncan et al., 2000]) in modifying glutamate mediated function and behavior.

Schizophrenia researchers have historically used pharmacology in a bootstrap approach to simultaneously develop treatments and pathophysiological disease models (as previously described). This productive process of cross-fertilization continues as we see experimental treatments and drug development strategies derive from the results of the emerging neuroscience of schizophrenia (Miyamoto et al., 2001).

Future Directions

These research findings provide new opportunities and new challenges to understanding and treating schizophrenia. Certainly, a major challenge is to determine the genetic susceptibilities and pathogenetic mechanisms that can produce the complex clinical phenotype of schizophrenia. The identification of pathways of dysfunction, such as thalamo-prefrontal circuitry or the connections linking other cortical, subcortical, and cerebellar regions implicated in schizophrenia, permits studies of the relationships among the various alterations in a circuit and the elucidation of a putative endophenotype. For example, does a given abnormality represent a primary brain disturbance due to a causal factor of the disorder, or does it reflect a downstream pathologic consequence of the primary brain disturbance or an adaptive response that attempts to normalize the function of the circuit?

Answers to these types of questions may create new opportunities for research at the intersection between

Table 1. Treatment of Schizophrenia

Interventions	Advantages	Disadvantages
Pharmacological		
Antipsychotic Drugs (APDS)		
CLASSICAL: High-affinity D_2 antagonists	Reduces and prevents recurrence of psychotic symptoms.	Limited efficacy against negative and cognitive symptoms. High rates of extrapyramidal symptoms (EPS) and tardive dyskinesia (TD).
ATYPICAL: Mixed neuroreceptor antagonists; low-affinity D_2 high affinity $5HT_{2A}$ (e.g., clozapine, risperidone, olanzapine, quetiapine, ziprasidone)	Reduces and prevents psychotic symptoms; broader efficacy against negative mood and cognitive symptoms; may prevent illness progression. Less EPS and TD.	Various side effects including blood dyscrasias, weight gain, increased glucose, and triglycerides; more expensive.
Adjunctive Treatements of APDS		
Benzodiazepines	Control agitation.	Limited potency and duration of action.
Mood stabilizers Anticonvulsants Lithium	Augment antipsychotic effects; control mood symptoms and hostility.	Few studies; limited efficacy.
Antidepressants	Reduce depressive and negative symptoms.	Limited efficacy against negative symptoms.
Anticholinergics	Reduce EPS.	Side effects (dry mouth, constipation, memory impairment).
Dopamine agonists	Reduce negative symptoms.	Possible exacerbation of psychotic symptoms.
Experimental Treatments		
Dopamine partial agonists (e.g., aripripazole)	May reduce psychotic and negative symptoms; few side effects.	Few clinically available compounds; few studies.
5-HT agents (e.g., M100907, ritanserin)	May improve negative symptoms; few side effects.	No proof of concept as monotherapeutic agent. Weak effect as adjunct; few clinically available compounds.
Cholinergic agonists (muscarinic/nicotinic)	?	No proof of concept.
Glutamatergic agents		
Allosteric modulators (e.g., glycine, serine, D-cycloserine)	Reduce negative symptoms; may improve cognition, prevent illness progression.	Weak to moderate effect; few studies and clinically available compounds.
Glycine uptake inhibitors	?	No proof of concept.
Glutamate release-inhibiting drugs (e.g., LY-293558)	?	No proof of concept.
AMPA/kainate receptor agonists (e.g., CX516)	May improve congnition.	Very few studies.
Protein kinase C inhibitors (e.g., tamoxifen)	?	No proof of concept.
Steroidal agents (e.g., estrogen, dihydroepiandrosterone)	May reduce negative symptoms; improve cognition; prevent illness progression.	Few studies.
Phsopholipid compounds (e.g., 3-omega fatty	May improve cognition; prevent illness progression.	No proof of concept.
Psychosocial		
Psychoeducation	Increases awareness and insight of patient family.	Few studies; must be combined with drug R_x.
Psychotherapies	May be useful adjunct.	Limited to problem-oriented and supportive therapies; must be combined with drug R_x.
Assertive community treatment	Improves R_x compliance.	Underutilized more labor intensive.
Cognitive behavioral therapy	May reduce positive symptoms.	Few studies; must be combined with drug R_x.

systems level investigations and genetic approaches. Current views hold that schizophrenia is probably a consequence of multiple interacting genes; individually, these genes may have relatively little independent influence, and they may not all be involved in every individual who meets diagnostic criteria for the illness. Thus, assessment of the patterns of altered gene expression in the affected brain circuits of subjects with schizophrenia (using cDNA microarray technology or related tech-

niques), and comparison of the chromosomal locations of these genes with regions implicated in schizophrenia through linkage studies (Pulver, 2000), may provide convergent approaches to the identification of specific vulnerability genes. For example, a recent study of gene expression profiling in the dorsal PFC of subjects with schizophrenia revealed that, of over 250 gene groups, the group of genes encoding proteins involved in the regulation of presynaptic function were most consistently altered (Mirnics et al., 2000). Although the subjects with schizophrenia appeared to share a common abnormality in the control of synaptic transmission, the specific combinations of genes involved in presynaptic function that showed reduced expression differed among them. Interestingly, a number of the chromosomal loci that have been implicated in schizophrenia contain genes encoding proteins related to presynaptic function (Mirnics et al., 2000).

Recent research suggests that the heterogeneous phenotype of schizophrenia may be the result of multiple pathophysiological processes occurring at different stages of the illness (Lieberman, 1999). These can be further characterized using multiple investigative approaches including in vivo neuroimaging, genetics, molecular neuropathology, and the development of animal models. Although animal models can only approximate the complex clinical phenotype of schizophrenia, they are essential to understand the molecular and cellular mechanisms that underlie the pathogenesis and pathophysiology of schizophrenia and can be used to test predictions from direct investigations of the illness. For example, conditional knockouts can be used to assess the consequences, at different stages of development, of the deficient expression of genes observed in subjects with schizophrenia. Therapeutic strategies based on this knowledge offer the promise of more effective interventions (including secondary and tertiary prevention), reduced morbidity, and better outcomes for patients.

Thus, it should be apparent that although great progress has been made in catching up on schizophrenia, much remains to be done.

References

Akbarian, S., Kim, J.J., Potkin, S.G., Hagman, J.O., Tafazzoli, A., Bunney, W.E., Jr., and Jones, E.G. (1995). Gene expression for glutamic acid decarboxylase is reduced without loss of neurons in prefrontal cortex of schizophrenics. Arch. Gen. Psychiatry 52, 258–266.

Akil, M., Pierri, J.N., Whitehead, R.E., Edgar, C.L., Mohila, C., and Lewis, D.A. (1999). Lamina-specific alteration in the dopamine innervation of the prefrontal cortex in schizophrenic subjects. Am. J. Psychiatry 156, 1580–1589.

Andreasen, N.C., Arndt, S., Swayze, V., II, Cizaldo, T., Flaum, M., O'Leary, D., Ehrhardt, J.C., and Yuh, W.T.C. (1994). Thalamic abnormalities in schizophrenia visualized through magnetic resonance image averaging. Science 266, 294–298.

Arnold, S.E., Franz, B.R., Ruben, B.A., Gur, C., Gur, R.E., Shapiro, R.M., Moberg, P.J., and Trojanowski, J.Q. (1995). Smaller neuron size in schizophrenia in hippocampal subfields that mediate cortical-hippocampal interactions. Am. J. Psychiatry 152, 738–748.

Benes, F.M., Sorensen, I., and Bird, E.D. (1991). Reduced neuronal size in posterior hippocampus of schizophrenic patients. Schizophr. Bull. 17, 597–608.

Bertolino, A., Kumra, S., Callicott, J.H., Mattay, V.S., Lestz, R.M., Jacobsen, L., Barnett, I.S., Duyn, J.H., Frank, J.A., Rapoport, J.L., and Weinberger, D.R. (1998). Common pattern of cortical pathology in childhood-onset and adult-onset schizophrenia as identified by proton magnetic resonance spectroscopic imaging. Am. J. Psychiatry 155, 1376–1383.

Bertolino, A., Esposito, G., Callicott, J.H., Mattay, V.S., Van Horn, J.D., Frank, J.A., Berman, K.F., and Weinberger, D.R. (2000). Specific relationship between prefrontal neuronal N-acetylaspartate and activation of the working memory cortical network in schizophrenia. Am. J. Psychiatry 157, 26–33.

Breier, A., Su, T.P., Saunders, R., Carson, R.E., Kolachana, B.A., de Bartolomeis, A., Weinberger, D.R., Weisenfeld, N., Malhotra, A.K., Eckelman, W.C., and Pickar, D. (1997). Schizophrenia is associated with elevated amphetamine-induced synaptic dopamine concentrations: evidence from a novel positron emission tomography method. Proc. Natl. Acad. Sci. USA 94, 2569–2574.

Breier, A., Adler, C.M., Weisenfeld, N., Su, T.P., Elman, I., Picken, L., Malhotra, A.K., and Pickar, D. (1998). Effects of NMDA antagonism on striatal dopamine release in healthy subjects: application of a novel PET approach. Synapse 29, 142–147.

Bromet, E.J., and Fennig, S. (1999). Epidemiology and natural history of schizophrenia. Biol. Psychiatry 46, 871–881.

Brzustowicz, L.M., Hodgkinson, K.A., Chow, E.W.C., Honer, W.G., and Bassett, A.S. (2000). Location of a major vulnerability locus for familial schizophrenia on chromosome 1q21-q22. Science 288, 678–682.

Buchsbaum, M.S., Someya, T., Teng, C.Y., Abel, L., Chin, S., Najafi, A., Haier, R.J., Wu, J., and Bunney, W.E., Jr. (1996). PET and MRI of the thalamus in never-medicated patients with schizophrenia. Am. J. Psychiatry 153, 191–199.

Carlsson, A. (1988). The current status of the dopamine hypothesis of schizophrenia. Neuropsychopharmacology 1, 179–186.

Costa, E., Pesold, C., Auta, J., Caruncho, H., Davis, J.M., Davidkova, G., Dwivedi, Y., Grayson, D.R., Rodriguez, M., Uzunov, D.P., and Guidotti, A. (2000). Reelin and GAD₆₇ downregulation and psychosis vulnerability. Biol. Psychiatry 47, 68S.

Davidson, M., Reichenberg, A., Rabinowitz, J., Weiser, M., Kaplan, Z., and Mark, M. (1999). Behavioral and intellectual markers for schizophrenia in apparently healthy male adolescents. Am. J. Psychiatry 156, 1328–1335.

Davis, K.L., Kahn, R.S., Ko, G., and Davidson, M. (1991). Dopamine in schizophrenia: a review and reconceptualization. Am. J. Psychiatry 148, 1474–1486.

Davis, K.L., Buchsbaum, M.S., Shihabuddin, L., Spiegel-Cohen, J., Metzger, M., Frecska, E., Keefe, R.S., and Powchik, P. (1998). Ventricular enlargement in poor-outcome schizophrenia. Biol. Psychiatry 43, 783–793.

Duncan, G.E., Miyamoto, S., Leipzig, J.N., and Lieberman, J.A. (2000). Comparison of the effects of clozapine, risperidone, olanzapine on ketamine-induced alterations in regional brain metabolism. J. Pharmacol. Exper. Therapeutics 293, 8–14.

Egan, M., Goldberg, T., Kolachana, B., Callicott, J., Mazanti, C., Goldman, D., and Weinberger, D. (2000). Effect of COMT108/158 Met genotype on frontal lobe function and risk for schizophrenia. Proc. Natl. Acad. Sci. USA, in press.

Farde, L., Wiesel, F.-A., Stone-Elander, S., Halldin, C., Nordstrom, A.-L., Hall, H., and Sedvall, G. (1990). D2 dopamine receptors in neuroleptic-naive schizophrenic patients, Arch. Gen. Psychiatry, 47 213–219.

Frazier, J.A., Giedd, J.N., Hamburger, S.D., Albus, K.E., Kaysen, D., Vaituzis, A.C., Rajapakse, J.C., Lenane, M.C., McKenna, K., Jacobsen, L.K., et al. (1996). Brain anatomic magnetic resonance imaging in childhood-onset schizophrenia. Arch. Gen. Psychiatry 53, 617–624.

Garey, L.J., Ong, W.Y., Patel, T.S., Kanani, M., Davis, A., Mortimer, A.M., Barnes, T.R.E., and Hirsch, S.R. (1998). Reduced dendritic spine density on cerebral cortical pyramidal neurons in schizophrenia. J. Neurol. Neurosurg. Psychiatry 65, 446–453.

Giros, B., Jaber, M., Jones, S.R., Wightman, R.M., and Caron, M.G. (1996). Hyperlocomotion and indifference to cocaine and amphetamine in mice lacking the dopamine transporter. Nature 379, 606–612.

Glantz, L.A., and Lewis, D.A. (1997). Reduction of synaptophysin immunoreactivity in the prefrontal cortex of subjects with schizophrenia: regional and diagnostic specificity. Arch. Gen. Psychiatry 54, 943–952.

Glantz, L.A., and Lewis, D.A. (2000). Decreased dendritic spine denity on prefrontal cortical pyramidal neurons in schizophrenia. Arch. Gen. Psychiatry 57, 65–73.

Goldman-Rakic, P.S. (1994). Working memory dysfunction in schizophrenia. J. Neuropsychiatry 6, 348–357.

Goldman-Rakic, P.S., and Selemon, L.D. (1997). Functional and anatomical aspects of prefrontal pathology in schizophrenia. Schizophr. Bull. 23, 437–458.

Goldstein, J.M., Goodman, J.M., Seidman, L.J., Kennedy, D.N., Makris, N., Lee, H., Tourville, J., Caviness, V.S., Faraone, S.V., and Tsuang, M.T. (1999). Cortical abnormalities in schizophrenia identified by structural magnetic resonance imaging. Arch. Gen. Psychiatry 56, 537–547.

Gottesman, I.I. (1991). Schizophrenia Genesis: The Origins of Madness (New York: Freeman).

Gottesman, I.I., and Shields, J. (1982). Schizophrenia: The Epigenetic Puzzle (Cambridge, UK: Cambridge University Press).

Green, M.F. (1996). What are the functional consequences of neurocognitive deficits in schizophrenia? Am. J. Psychiatry 153, 321–330.

Gur, R.E., Cowell, P., Turetsky, B.I., Gallacher, F., Cannon, T., Bilker, W., and Gur, R.C. (1998a). A follow-up magnetic resonance imaging study of schizophrenia. Arch. Gen. Psychiatry 55, 145–152.

Gur, R.E., Maany, V., Mozley, P.D., Swanson, C., Bilker, W., and Gur, R.C. (1998b). Subcortical MRI volumes in neuroleptic-naive and treated patients with schizophrenia. Am. J. Psychiatry 155, 1711–1717.

Hafner, H., Hambrecht, M., Loffler, W., Munk-Jorgenson, P., and Reicher-Rossler, A. (1998). Causes and consequences of the gender difference in age of onset of schizophrenia. Schizophrenia Bull. 24, 99–113.

Harrison, P.J. (1999). The neuropathology of schizophrenia: a critical review of the data and their interpretation. Brain 122, 593–624.

Harvey, P.D., Silverman, J.M., Mohs, R.C., Parrella, M., White, L., Powchik, P., Davidson, M., and Davis, K.L. (1999). Cognitive decline in late-life schizophrenia: a longitudinal study of geriatric, chronically hospitalized patients. Biol. Psychiatry 45, 32–40.

Heckers, S., Rauch, S.L., Goff, D., Savage, C.R., Schacter, D.L., Fischman, A.J., and Alpert, N.M. (1998). Impaired recruitment of the hippocampus during conscious recollection in schizophrenia. Nat. Neurosci. 1, 318–323.

Hendry, S.H.C., and Jones, E.G. (1988). Activity-dependent regulation of GABA expression in the visual cortex of adult monkeys. Neuron 1, 701–712.

Honer, W.G., Falkai, P., Chen, C., Arango, V., Mann, J.J., and Dwork, A.J. (1999). Synaptic and plasticity-associated proteins in anterior frontal cortex in severe mental illness. Neuroscience 91, 1247–1255.

Jarskog, L.F., Gilmore, J.H., Selinger, E.S., and Lieberman, J.A. (2000). Cortical BCL-2 protein expression and apoptotic regulation in schizophrenia. Biol. Psychiatry 48, 641–651.

Javitt, D.C., and Zukin, S.R. (1991). Recent advances in the phencyclidine model of schizophrenia. Am. J. Psychiatry 148, 1301–1308.

Jentsch, J.D., and Roth, R.H. (1999). The neuropsychopharmacology of phencyclidine: from NMDA receptor hypofunction to the dopamine hypothesis of schizophrenia. Neuropsychopharm. 20, 201–225.

Kane, J.M. (1996). Drug therapy. Schizophrenia. N. Engl. J. Med. 34, 34–41.

Jones, P. (1997). The early origins of schizophrenia. Brit. Med. Bull. 3, 135–155.

Kapur, S., Zipursky, R.B., Jones, C., Remington, G., and Houle, . (2000). Relationship between dopamine D2 occupancy, clinical response, and side effects: a double-blind PET study of first-episode schizophrenia. Am. J. Psychiatry 157, 514–520.

Karson, C.N., Mrak, R.E., Schluterman, K.O., Sturner, W.Q., Sheng, J.G., and Griffin, W.S.T. (1999). Alterations in synaptic proteins and their encoding mRNAs in prefrontal cortex in schizophrenia: a possible neurochemical basis for "hypofrontality." Mol. Psychiatry 4, 39–45.

Kegeles, L.S., Abi-Dargham, A., Zea-Ponce, Y., Rodenhiser-Hill, J., Mann, J.J., Van Heertum, R.L., Cooper, T., Carlsson, A., and Laruelle,

M. (2000). Modulation of amphetamine-induced striatal dopamine release by ketamine in humans: implications for schizophrenia. Biol. Psychiatry 48, 627–640.

Kinon, B.J., and Lieberman, J.A. (1996). Mechanisms of action of atypical antipsychotic drugs: a critical analysis. Psychopharmacology 124, 2–34.

Krystal, J.H., Karper, L.P., Seibyl, J.P., Freeman, G.K., Delaney, R., Bremner, J.D., Heninger, G.R., Bowers, M.B.J., and Charney, D.S. (1994). Subanesthetic effects of the noncompetitive NMDA antagonist, ketamine, in humans. Psychotomimetic, perceptual, cognitive, and neuroendocrine responses. Arch. Gen. Psychiatry 51, 199–214.

Lahti, A.C., Koffel, B., LaPorte, D., and Tamminga, C.A. (1995). Subanesthetic doses of ketamine stimulate psychosis in schizophrenia. Neuropsychopharmacology 13, 9–19.

Laruelle, M. (2000). The role of endogenous sensitization in the pathophysiology of schizophrenia. Brain Res. Reviews 31, 371–384.

Laruelle, M., Abi-Dargham, A., van Dyck, C.H., Gil, R., D'Souza, C.D., Erdos, J., McCance, E., Rosenblatt, W., Fingado, C., Zoghbi, S.S., et al. (1996). Single photon emission computerized tomography imaging of amphetamine-induced release in drug-free schizophrenic subjects. Proc. Natl. Acad. Sci. USA 93, 9235–9240.

Laruelle, M., Abi-Dargham, A., Gil, R., Kegeles, L., and Innis, R. (1999). Increased dopamine transmission in schizophrenia: relationship to illness phase. Biol. Psych. 46, 56–72.

Lewis, D.A. (1997). Development of the prefrontal cortex during adolescence: insights into vulnerable neural circuits in schizophrenia. Neuropsychopharmacology 16, 385–398.

Lewis, D.A. (2000). Is there a neuropathology of schizophrenia? The Neuroscientist 6, 208–218.

Lieberman, J.A. (1999). Is schizophrenia a neurodegenerative disorder? Biol. Psychiatry 46, 729–739.

Lieberman, J., Jody, D., Geisler, S., Alvir, J., Loebel, A., Szymanski, S., Woerner, M., and Borenstein, M. (1993). Time course and biological correlates of treatment response in first episode schizophrenia. Arch. Gen. Psychiatry 50, 369–376.

Lieberman, J.A., Alvir, J.M., Koreen, A., Geisler, S., Chakos, M., Sheitman, B., and Woerner, M. (1996). Psychobiologic correlates of treatment response in schizophrenia. Neuropsychopharmacology 14, 13S–21S.

Lieberman, J.A., Sheitman, B.B., and Kinon, B.J. (1997). Neurochemical sensitization in the pathophysiology of schizophrenia: deficits and dysfunction in neuronal regulation and plasticity. Neuropsychopharmacology 17, 205–229.

Marcelis, M., van Os, J., Sham, P., Jones, P., Gilvarry, C., Cannon, M., McKenzie, K., and Murray, R. (1998). Obstetric complications and familial morbid risk of psychiatric disorders. Am. J. Med. Genetics 81, 29–36.

McCarley, R.W., Wible, C.G., Frumin, M., Hirayasu, Y., Levitt, J.J., Fischer, I.A., and Shenton, M.E. (1999). MRI anatomy of schizophrenia. Biol. Psychiatry 45, 1099–1119.

McGlashan, T.H. (1996). Early detection and intervention in schizophrenia research. Schizophr. Bull. 22, 327–345.

Mimics, K., Middleton, F.A., Marquez, A., Lewis, D.A., and Levitt, P. (2000). Molecular characterization of schizophrenia viewed by microarray analysis of gene expression in prefrontal cortex. Neuron 28, 33–67.

Miyamoto, S., Duncan, G., Goff, D., and Lieberman, J. (2001). Therapeutics of Schizophrenia in Neuropsychopharmacology: The Fifth Generation of Progress (New York: Raven Press), in press.

Moghaddam, B., and Adams, B.W. (1998). Reversal of phencyclidine effects by a group II metabotropic glutamate receptor agonist in rats. Science 281, 1349–1352.

Mohn, A.R., Gainetdinov, R.R., Caron, M.G., and Koller, B.H. (1999). Mice with reduced NMDA receptor expression display behaviors related to schizophrenia. Cell 98, 427–436.

Mortensen, P.B., Pedersen, C.B., Westegaard, T., Wohlfahrt, J., Ewald, H., Mors, O., Andersen, P.K., and Melbye, M. (1999). Effects of family history and place and season of birth on the risk of schizophrenia. N. Engl. J. Med. 340, 603–608.

Okuba, Y., Suhara, T., Suzuki, K., Kobayashi, K., Inoue, O., Terasaki, O., Someya, Y., Sassa, T., Sudo, Y., Matsushima, E., et al. (1997). Decreased prefrontal dopamine D1 receptors in schizophrenia revealed by PET. Nature 385, 634–636.

Olney, J.W., and Farber, N.B. (1995). Glutamate receptor dysfunction and schizophrenia. Arch. Gen. Psychiatry 52, 998–1007.

Pakkenberg, B. (1990). Pronounced reduction of total neuron number in mediodorsal thalamic nucleus and nucleus accumbens in schizophrenics. Arch. Gen. Psychiatry 47, 1023–1028.

Perrone-Bizzozero, N.I., Sower, A.C., Bird, E.D., Benowitz, L.I., Ivins, K.J., and Neve, R.L. (1996). Levels of the growth-associated protein GAP-43 are selectively increased in association cortices in schizophrenia. Proc. Natl. Acad. Sci. USA 93, 14182–14187.

Pierri, J.N., Chaudry, A.S., Woo, T.-U., and Lewis, D.A. (1999). Alterations in chandelier neuron axon terminals in the prefrontal cortex of schizophrenic subjects. Am. J. Psychiatry 156, 1709–1719.

Popken, G.J., Bunney, W.E., Jr., Potkin, S.G., and Jones, E.G. (2000). Subnucleus-specific loss of neurons in medial thalamus of schizophrenics. Proc. Natl. Acad. Sci. USA 97, 9276–9280.

Portas, C.M., Goldstein, J.M., Shenton, M.E., Hokama, H.H., Wible, C.G., Fischer, I., Kikinis, R., Donnino, R., Jolesz, F.A., and McCarley, R.W. (1998). Volumetric evaluation of the thalamus in schizophrenic male patients using magnetic resonance imaging. Biol. Psychiatry 43, 649–659.

Pulver, A.E. (2000). Search for schizophrenia vulnerability genes. Biol. Psychiatry 47, 221–230.

Raedler, T.J., Knable, M.B., and Weinberger, D.R. (2000). Schizophrenia as a developmental disorder of the cerebral cortex. Curr. Opin. Neurobiol. 8, 157–161.

Rajkowska, G., Selemon, L.D., and Goldman-Rakic, P.S. (1998). Neuronal and glial somal size in the prefrontal cortex: a postmortem morphometric study of schizophrenia and Huntington disease. Arch. Gen. Psychiatry 55, 215–224.

Rapoport, J.L., Giedd, J.N., Blumenthal, J., Hamburger, S., Jeffries, N., Fernandez, T., Nicolson, R., Bedwell, J., Lenane, M., Zijdenbos, A., et al. (1999). Progressive cortical change during adolescence in childhood-onset schizophrenia: a longitudinal magnetic resonance imaging study. Arch. Gen. Psychiatry 56, 649–654.

Robinson, D., Woerner, M., Alvir, J., Bilder, R., Goldman, R., Geisler, S., Koreen, A., Sheitman, B., Chakos, M., Mayerhoff, D., and Lieberman, J.A. (1999a). Predictors of treatment response from a first episode of schizophrenia or schizoaffective disorder. Am. J. Psychiatry 156, 544–549.

Robinson, D., Woerner, M.G., Alvir, J.M., Bilder, R., Goldman, R., Geisler, S., Koreen, A., Sheitman, B., Chakos, M., Mayerhoff, D., and Lieberman, J.A. (1999b). Predictors of relapse following from a first episode of schizophrenia or schizoaffective disorder. Arch. Gen. Psychiatry 56, 241–247.

Selemon, L.D., and Goldman-Rakic, P.S. (1999). The reduced neuropil hypothesis: a circuit based model of schizophrenia. Biol. Psychiatry 45, 17–25.

Sheitman, B.B., Lee, H., Strous, R., and Lieberman, J.A. (1997). The evaluation and treatment of first episode psychoses. Schizophr. Bull. 23, 653–661.

Szymanski, S., Lieberman, J.A., Alvir, J.M., Mayerhoff, D., Loebel, A., Geisler, S., Chakos, M., Koreen, A., Jody, D., Kane, J., et al. (1995). Gender differences in onset of illness, treatment response, course, and biological indexes in first-episode schizophrenic patients. Am. J. Psychiatry 152, 698–703.

Taylor, S.F. (1996). Cerebral blood flow activation and functional lesions in schizophrenia. Schizophr. Res. 19, 129–140.

Torrey, E.F., Miller, J., Rawlings, R., and Yolken, R.H. (1997). Seasonality of births in schizophrenia and bipolar disorder: A review of the literature. Schizophr. Res. 28, 1–38.

Tsuang, M. (2000). Schizophrenia: genes and environment. Biol. Psychiatry 47, 210–220.

Volk, D.W., Austin, M.C., Pierri, J.N., Sampson, A.R., and Lewis, D.A. (2000). Decreased GAD_{67} mRNA expression in a subset of prefrontal cortical GABA neurons in subjects with schizophrenia. Arch. Gen. Psychiatry 57, 237–245.

Walker, E., and Lewine, R.J. (1990). Prediction of adult onset schizophrenia from childhood home movies. Am. J. Psychiatry 147, 1052–1056.

Weinberger, D.R. (1999). Cell biology of the hippocampal formation in schizophrenia. Biol. Psychiatry 45, 395–402.

Weinberger, D.R., and Gallhofer, B. (1997). Cognitive dysfunction in schizophrenia. Int. Clin. Psychopharmacol. 12S, 29–36.

Weinberger, D.R., Berman, K.F., and Zec, R.F. (1986). Physiologic dysfunction of dorsolateral prefrontal cortex in schizophrenia. Arch. Gen. Psychiatry 43, 114–124.

Weinberger, D.R., and Lipska, B.K. (1995). Cortical maldevelopment, anti-psychotic drugs, and schizophrenia: a search for common ground. Schizophr. Res. 16, 87–110.

Wong, D.F., Wagner, H.N., Tune, L.E., Dannals, R.F., Pearlsson, G.D., Links, J.M., Tamminga, C.A., Broussolle, E.P., Ravert, H.T., Wilson, A.A., et al. (1986). Positron emission tomography reveals elevated D2 dopamine receptors in drug-naive schizophrenics. Science 234, 1558–1563.

Young, K.A., Manaye, K.F., Liang, C.-L., Hicks, P.B., and German, D.C. (2000). Reduced number of mediodorsal and anterior thalamic neurons in schizophrenia. Biol. Psychiatry 47, 944–953.

Yung, A.R., and McGorry, P.D. (1996). The prodromal phase of first episode schizophrenia: past and current conceptualization. Schizophr. Bull. 22, 353–370.

Zaidel, D.W., Esiri, M.M., and Harrison, P.J. (1997). Size, shape, and orientation of neurons in the left and right hippocampus: Investigation of normal asymmetries and alterations in schizophrenia. Am. J. Psychiatry 154, 812–818.

A Unitary Model of Schizophrenia

Bleuler's "Fragmented Phrene" as Schizencephaly

Nancy C. Andreasen, MD, PhD

Finding a unifying concept behind the diversity of signs and symptoms in schizophrenia is a central challenge to contemporary research. A neo-Bleulerian unitary model is described, which defines the illness as a neurodevelopmentally derived "misconnection syndrome," involving connections between cortical regions and the cerebellum mediated through the thalamus (the cortico-cerebellar-thalamic-cortical circuit [CCTCC]). An abnormality in this circuitry, normally used to coordinate both motor and mental activity, leads to misconnections in many aspects of mental activity, or "cognitive dysmetria." As Bleuler originally proposed, "thought disorder" is the primary defining feature of schizophrenia, rather than the more obvious signs and symptoms such as delusions and hallucinations. Cognitive dysmetria, or a disorder in the CCTCC, may provide a heuristic theoretical framework for strategies to explore etiology, pathophysiology, intervention, or prevention. *Arch Gen Psychiatry. 1999;56:781-787*

At present the most important problem in schizophrenia research is not finding the gene or localizing it in the brain and understanding its neural circuits. Our most important problem is identifying the correct target at which to aim our powerful new scientific weapons. Our most pressing problem is at the clinical level: defining what schizophrenia is.

See also page 791

This overview reviews the original definition of schizophrenia, as formulated by Euger Bleuler, and proposes a model for updating it within the context of contemporary neuroscience. It derives from the need to reconceptualize the phenotype of the illness for contemporary translational research that moves from the clinical to the basic and back to the clinical again; eg, the informed choice of candidate genes, the development of animal models for this most human of diseases, or the identification of the neural circuits that improved treatments might modify. This overview argues that, for these purposes, the definition of schizophrenia

should be based on a basic cognitive disturbance rather than on phenomenology. Phenomenology (after the Greek φαινωμενον [phenomenon]: a thing that shows or is apparent) refers to objectively assessed signs and symptoms. Lathomenology (after the Greek λαθειν [lathein]: to lie hidden or be unapparent on the surface)[1] refers to the underlying process that produces the outward appearance. Thus, this overview proposes a reconceptualization of the definition of schizophrenia that emphasizes a lathomenology rather than a phenomenology. It presents reasons why the apparently heterogeneous phenotype of schizophrenia may best be defined by a basic unifying concept: a fundamental cognitive deficit that arises from abnormalities in neural circuits.

On the surface, schizophrenia seems to be heterogeneous; explaining its diverse symptoms in a coherent way has been a challenging task in clinical research. At

From the University of Iowa Hospitals and Clinics, Mental Health Clinical Research Center, Iowa City.

11

one extreme is the affect-laden paraphrenic, who can clearly describe a complex delusional system, who suffers intensely from tormenting beliefs, who occasionally hears voices ordering retaliation, and who is cognitively intact enough to formulate a plan to act on those delusions. At the opposite extreme is the patient whose thinking is so impoverished or disorganized that it is difficult to take a history, who spends most of the day (in the late 20th century) sitting in front of a TV and smoking, and who seems almost devoid of emotion. If asked, this patient cannot describe in detail the contents of the last TV program watched. Both these patients are said to have schizophrenia, although they share no symptoms in common. Between them, as exemplars of what we call schizophrenia, they exhibit symptoms that represent abnormalities in almost all aspects of human mental activity: inferential thinking, perception, language, motor and social behavior, volition, emotional expression, and hedonic capacity. Do both of these patients really have schizophrenia? How can we explain the fact that they are so different? That their symptoms are so diverse? What mechanism or explanation can unite them and explain the fact that most clinicians readily identify both as having schizophrenia, often without even taking note of the fact that they share no symptoms in common? (Bright medical students notice this all the time and are perplexed as a consequence.)

BLEULER'S UNITARY
MODEL UPDATED:
THE "FRAGMENTED PHRENE"
AS SCHIZENCEPHALY

Although Bleuler subtitled his book on dementia praecox "The Group of Schizophrenias,"[2] his major argument was that the concept of schizophrenia was unified by a single defining feature that was present in all patients who suffered from the illness that he was the first to call "schizophrenia." What was that feature? What exactly did he mean by that name? Why did he choose it?

Because he was classically educated, Bleuler would have been well aware that Greek had 3 different words to refer to mental phenomena that he could have used to rename Emil Kraepelin's recently defined disorder, dementia praecox. They are ενκεφαλον (encephalon, or brain); φρηνη (phrene, or mind); and ψυχη (psyche, or soul). While psychiatrists are literally healers (ιατροσ [iatros]) of the soul, Bleuler chose a term from the middle road for this serious and tragic disease. He apparently wished to highlight the fact that patients who developed this illness suffered a pervasive disruption of their mental processes—a fragmented phrene. He wished to emphasize that the illness did not lead inevitably to the same kind of intellectual deterioration observed in dementia in the elderly, and that the illness was nonetheless also a "neurocognitive disorder." He chose the name schizophrenia because it meant literally "a mind that is torn asunder."

Bleuler chose this name to emphasize that the illness was not a neurodegenerative disorder of adolescents (ie, dementia praecox), but rather a disorder that could begin any time between childhood and middle age, that could have a stable outcome or even improvement after onset, and that was best defined by an underlying cognitive process that was present in all patients with the disorder and that provided a unifying theme to the illness. Even Kraepelin ultimately agreed. It is time to update this unitary Bleulerian model and to use it to define a phenotype of schizophrenia that will be useful for the impending era when the human genome and the human brain have been well mapped.

A proposed updating of Bleuler's unitary approach redefines "loosening of associations" in 21st-century terms as a "misconnection syndrome" that reflects a disorder in neural circuits. It identifies a basic cognitive process that could explain the clinical diversity of schizophrenia and yet be shared by all patients whom we consider to have the illness.[3-5] (The word "cognitive" is used broadly and refers to both "rational" and "emotional" components of mental activity.) It posits that schizophrenia is a single illness with a single phenotype and that the phenotype is defined by a

fundamental cognitive abnormality rather than the diversity of symptoms with which patients present. The underlying disruption in functional neural circuitry is presumed to be a final common pathway produced by the convergence of multiple etiological and pathophysiological factors: eg, inherited DNA, regulation of gene expression, or the influence of "environmental factors" (ranging from viruses to amphetamine-induced dopamine upregulation to academic failures) on a plastic brain. The multiple factors impinge on brain development and maturation from the time of conception through early adulthood, and if a sufficient quantity of "schizophrenogenic" factors accumulates, the illness we refer to as schizophrenia is expressed—the neural dysfunction occurs, the cognitive phenotype is present, and ultimately the person begins to have symptoms. The symptoms may wax and wane, and they may vary from one person to another. Symptoms, therefore, should not be used to identify the phenotype. Instead it must be defined by the more fundamental disruption in mental processes occurring as a consequence of a disruption in neural circuitry: a schizophrenia that is due to a "schizencephaly."

Figure 1 summarizes a general conceptual framework for this unitary model. Many components of this model, such as the importance of neurodevelopmental mechanisms,[6-12] are embraced by other investigators and are not original in this summary. The general model has an hourglass shape. Rather than attempting to link a single etiology to a single outcome, as has occurred so often in schizophrenia research, it assumes that multiple etiologies flow in at the "entry level" and that multiple symptoms occur at the "output level," but that in the middle levels there is a single process that unifies the concept of the illness. This model is very similar to the way we think about cancer, for which the defining feature is abnormal regulation of cell growth and death. Cancer has multiple etiologies. It occurs as a consequence of multiple "hits," and the phenotype appears clinically when a sufficient quantity of additive risks accumu-

12

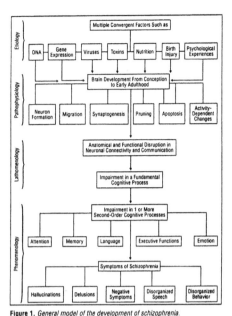

Figure 1. *General model of the development of schizophrenia.*

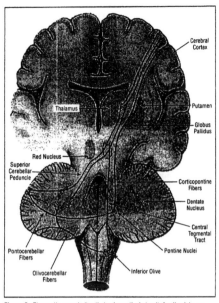

Figure 2. *The cortico-cerebellar-thalamic-cortical circuit: feedback loops between the cortex and the cerebellum.*

lates (eg, exposure to environmental toxins such as tobacco or radiation, suppression of the immune system, viral infections, or DNA-based predispositions). Likewise, cancer has multiple forms that vary depending on the organ in which it arises, which leads to a heterogeneity of symptoms, course, and severity. Yet all forms of cancer share a common fundamental mechanism: abnormal regulation of cell proliferation and destruction.

The general model shown in Figure 1 assumes cumulative negative gene-environment interactions as the etiology and resultant abnormalities in brain development (defined as continuing into early adulthood) as the pathophysiology. The principal virtues of this model are descriptive validity at the level of etiology and phenomenology combined with parsimony at the level of lathomenology. Most evidence to date suggests that a single etiology for schizophrenia is unlikely and that the disorder is clinically heterogeneous: these observations are relatively unforgiving. Yet there is room for parsimony at the

middle levels, where an abnormality in brain development leads to abnormalities in circuitry and cognition. If this general model is correct, it will give substantial leverage to research into etiology, since investigators can study a single phenotype, defined on the basis of a "neurocognitive marker." At present we do not have a well-defined and agreed-on marker, but several investigators have defined likely candidates, such as defects in eye tracking, sensory gating, working memory, or other measures of information processing or neurophysiology.[13-19]

SCHIZOPHRENIA: THE FRAGMENTED PHRENE REDEFINED AS COGNITIVE DYSMETRIA

As recently reviewed,[4] several research teams have proposed "candidate cognitive processes" to identify the unifying concept that defines its phenotype: eg, Goldman-Rakic and representationally guided behavior,[18] Frith and the inability to think in metarepresentations,[19] Braff and

abnormalities in information processing,[14,20] or our own proposal of cognitive dysmetria.[4,5,21-23] A more accurate understanding of schizophrenia at all levels will emerge as several independent groups explore such competing models.

"Synchrony," or fluidly coordinating sequences of motor activity and thought, occurs as a consequence of very rapid on-line feedback between the cerebral cortex and the cerebellum, mediated through the thalamus. The substrate of synchrony is the corticocerebellar-thalamic-cortical circuit (CCTCC). (See **Figure 2** for a schematic summary of the pattern of feedback loops that create the CCTCC.) The importance of the motor and somatosensory components of this circuit have been recognized for many years and are believed to permit individuals to perform the very rapid adjustments that are required for complex motor acts, such as hitting a tennis ball.[24] An impairment in this feedback loop leads to various types of dysmetria, such as poor tandem gait or past-pointing.[25] More re-

13

cently, however, substantial theoretical and empirical evidence has accumulated for the importance of the CCTCC in human cognition.[26-35]

Cognitive dysmetria—the hypothesized fundamental deficit in schizophrenia—is a disruption of the fluid, coordinated sequences of thought and action that are the hallmark of normal cognition. The "poor coordination" results from a defect in the timing or sequencing component of mental activity. This defect cuts across most of the traditionally defined cognitive systems (eg, memory, attention) and affects the efficiency and accuracy of their related subprocesses (eg, memory retrieval, inhibition). In a sense, therefore, the function that is disturbed might be considered to be a "metasystem" or a "metaprocess." The term *synchrony* is used to refer to the normal process and *dysmetria* to refer to its disturbance.

SCHIZENCEPHALY: ABNORMALITIES IN THE CCTCC

Cognitive dysmetria occurs as a consequence of disruptions in neural circuitry: a schizencephaly presumed to result from multiple hits occurring during the process of brain development. Three nodes in the CCTCC may be particularly important in both normal cognition and in schizophrenia: the prefrontal cortex, the cerebellum, and the thalamus. The dysfunctions that occur in schizophrenia are almost certainly not limited to these 3 nodes; other cortical regions that form feedback loops with the thalamus and cerebellum are also important (eg, hippocampus and temporal lobes). But these 3 regions are especially important for both theoretical and empirical reasons. They are all difficult regions to study well—the prefrontal cortex because of its enormous expanse and complexity, the thalamus because of its compactness and dense interconnectivity, and the cerebellum because of its fascinating architecture, relatively large size, and largely uncharted nature. This is not a case of "looking where the light is." It is a case of looking where both theory and preexisting data compel us to look.

Both the cerebellum and the prefrontal cortex are one third larger in the human brain than in chimpanzees,[36,37] suggesting that these regions may be the neural substrates for complex mental activities that are specifically human, such as complex language or episodic memory. There is substantial evidence supporting a possible abnormality in the prefrontal cortex in schizophrenia both from our group and from others. Our studies to date, using magnetic resonance imaging and positron emission tomography (PET), have increasingly converged to suggest that the prefrontal cortex is dysfunctional and that this dysfunction is present at the time of onset. Three of our 4 magnetic resonance imaging studies have shown a decrease in overall size.[8,38-40] We have observed frontal size to be decreased in first-episode patients studied very shortly after onset.[40] While some other studies of patients with more chronic disease have been negative,[41] these findings have been confirmed by others,[42] and they are supported by basic neuropathological studies.[43] Many functional imaging studies have also implicated the frontal cortex in schizophrenia,[44-51] including our own,[21-23,52,53] as have animal models.[54-56] Again, our functional imaging studies have shown that "hypofrontality" is present in first-episode patients using both single-photon emission computed tomography[52] and PET.[53] In the latter study we examined drug-naive patients and thereby ruled out medication effects as a cause of impaired frontal function.

The cerebellum possesses a unique cellular architecture that makes it particularly appropriate for coordinating rapid on-line processing,[26,27] especially for performing a timing function,[57] in cooperation with the cerebral cortex. This architecture includes a high density of granular cells (10^{11}, more than occur in the entire cerebral cortex). The granular cells have dendrites that form unusually long bifurcated branches (parallel fibers) in the molecular layer (a pattern natural for detecting temporal sequences of neuronal firing). The Purkinje cells have an unusual regular alignment and extensive branching and synapse formation in the molecular layer with the granular dendrites. This unusual architecture is modulated by differential patterns of input from the mossy and climbing fibers. The somatotopy of the cerebral cortex is closely mapped in the cerebellum; the vermis seems to be specialized to coordinate sensory and motor input and output, while the cerebrocerebellum is specialized to coordinate planning. Tract-tracing studies have steadily amassed evidence indicating that feedback/feedforward loops provide connections between cortical and cerebellar regions.[31,58,59]

Increasing evidence supports the importance of the cerebellum in schizophrenia. In a first-episode and early-onset sample, we have found that decreased cerebellar size is the strongest predictor of poor long-term outcome.[60] Our PET studies[61-66] and those of others[67-69] have supported a cognitive function for the cerebellum that is independent of motor function, as have several functional magnetic resonance imaging studies.[70,71] As our PET paradigms used to study normal cognition have been applied to the study of patients suffering from schizophrenia, the evidence for cerebellar abnormalities has been compelling. Cerebellar flow is abnormal in a variety of tasks, including recall of complex narratives, episodic memory, memory for word lists, or random episodic silent thought.[21-23,52,72] Most of these studies identify consistent abnormalities in the entire CCTCC, including the thalamus and prefrontal cortex. Our studies of neuroleptic medication effects,[73,74] as well as those of others,[75,76] indicate that neuroleptics also affect cerebellar blood flow, via a mechanism that is as yet not clearly understood. Our study of first-episode neuroleptic-naive patients has also indicated cerebellar flow abnormalities, which are increases rather than decreases; the implications of this finding require further explanation.[53]

The thalamus is of great theoretical importance for schizophrenia because of its crucial central placement, its dense interconnectivity, and its potential role as a "filter" or "gate."[77] Postmortem stud-

14

ies provided the earliest empirical evidence for thalamic abnormalities in schizophrenia.[78-81] Magnetic resonance imaging studies have given additional support,[82,83] as have PET studies.[21,46,84] We have recently confirmed that the changes in thalamic shape/size observed in patients with chronic disease via image subtraction[82] are complemented by findings from functional imaging, including abnormalities in the CCTCC seen in both patients with chronic disease and drug-naive first-episode patients studied with PET.[21-23,52,84]

COGNITIVE DYSMETRIA AND THE CLINICAL PRESENTATION OF SCHIZOPHRENIA

Just as there is no obvious neuropathology that is shared by all patients suffering from schizophrenia, so too there is no set of symptoms that defines the illness in the sense that they are shared by all patients. This fact contains an important clue. Perhaps the illness should not be defined by phenomenology, but rather should be defined by a lathomenology that can account for the diverse symptoms. Cognitive dysmetria is an attractive candidate for the lathomenology.

The concept of cognitive dysmetria suggests that patients suffering from schizophrenia have a misconnection syndrome that leads them to make abnormal associations between mental representations and to lack the ability to distinguish between the self and not-self or the important and the trivial. The multiple stimuli that bombard our consciousness cannot be normally suppressed, and the important cannot be distinguished from the unimportant. Therefore, internal representations may be attributed to the external world, leading to hallucinations. Perceptions or other information will be misconnected with inappropriate associations, leading to delusional misinterpretations. On-line monitoring of language or thoughts will be impaired or mistimed, leading to both disorganized speech and disorganized thinking. Behavior will not be adequately monitored, leading to so-

cial awkwardness, excessive aggressiveness or shyness, or other abnormalities in behavioral activities. The inability to monitor may also lead either to the "freezing" of catatonic immobility or a failure to inhibit that is expressed as catatonic excitement. Difficulties in inhibiting or prioritizing may also lead to the various negative symptoms, such as avolition or anhedonia, much as a computer locks when it cannot match signals sent at an incorrect rate or to an incorrect place.

The concept of cognitive dysmetria provides an explanation for the diverse symptoms of schizophrenia. It also explains why patients suffering from schizophrenia have an increased rate of soft signs that seems to be independent of extrapyramidal adverse effects due to neuroleptic treatment, since these were originally described by Kraepelin in the preneuroleptic era and are also seen in neuroleptic-naive first-episode patients.[85,86] Further, a general impairment in a fundamental aspect of cognitive processing also accounts for the generalized cognitive deficits that have been observed in schizophrenia.[87-89]

CAN THIS UNITARY MODEL BE FALSIFIED?

In a pivotal attack on both logical positivism and psychoanalytic theory, which both seemed able to explain everything in a frustratingly irrefutable way, Karl Popper presented the falsification tenet that forms the foundation for his philosophy of critical rationalism: the test of a good model or theory is its falsifiability—it should make predictions that can be tested through critical experiments and be disproved.[90] Although general, this proposed unitary model is also falsifiable.

The model postulates that schizophrenia is defined by a deficit in a fundamental cognitive function, cognitive dysmetria, which explains the generalized cognitive deficit and the diversity of symptoms. The nodes in the network that produce dysmetria have been specified: specialized cortical regions, the thalamus, and the cerebellum. It is conceivable that a lesion in only one

region could interfere with the functioning of the entire circuit; therefore, a definitive falsification of the hypothesis would require that abnormalities be absent in all regions, while an abnormality even in one would support the hypothesis. The distributed nature of the circuitry makes the model difficult to falsify (a problem inherent in all contemporary systems-level research operating within circuit models of the brain). However, because of the specific role of the cerebellum in timing, coordination, and sequencing, measures of cerebellar anatomy or tasks that "stress" the cerebellum constitute the "critical experiment" that can falsify this particular model. Such tasks include time perception, time production, and eye blink conditioning. If neither functional nor anatomical abnormalities are found in the cerebellum in patients with schizophrenia, then dysmetria and a dysfunctional CCTCC cannot be invoked to explain the phenomenology of schizophrenia.

HOW CAN THIS MODEL BE TRANSLATED TO THE BASIC AND CLINICAL LEVELS?

This updated Bleulerian unitary model, which conceptualizes schizophrenia as defined by a dysmetria of thought secondary to a dysfunctional CCTCC, was formulated because it defines a phenotype for schizophrenia that may be particularly useful for translational research. It translates "down" to the basic science research on molecular and genetic mechanisms, and it also translates "up" to clinical research seeking to design improved treatments.

The model assumes that the dysfunctional CCTC circuitry occurs as a consequence of a disruption of 1 or more of the processes that shape brain development, particularly in regions such as the cerebellum or the midline.[91-93] It therefore may inform the search for the developmental mechanisms of the illness by pointing toward specific candidate genes that regulate the neurodevelopment of the CCTCC. Further, the model hypothesizes that the deficit is in a metasystem that is

15

relatively basic. It therefore can be used to develop better animal models, using simple concepts such as synchrony or dysmetria to identify mechanisms that may form the basis for "higher" cognitive processes such as consciousness or language, which are disrupted in schizophrenia. Although the distance from mice to men may seem great, the identification of a very basic process, which is the substrate for more complex human phenomena such as language or consciousness, may permit us to translate the modeling of complex human mental processes to simpler animals that can be disrupted using knockout or other strategies. Examples are mutant mice that have abnormalities affecting cerebellar development, such as the leaner, lurcher, or swaying mouse.[94-96]

Conceptualizing schizophrenia in terms of a basic process that can be modeled in animals can also assist in the screening of new treatments. The current animal models used to test for drug development are relatively crude (eg, catalepsy, amphetamine-induced stereotypies). This new unitary model provides a possibility of developing cognitive tests that can be used to screen drugs in animals using processes known from existing research to be mediated by the CCTCC (eg, time discrimination).[97]

Schizophrenia research has made substantial advances during the past 2 decades, facilitated by the application of imaging tools to understand brain mechanisms. Progress on the clinical level has been slower, however. This proposed model was developed in the hope that it will provide a catalyst for other novel ideas. The proposed neo-Bleulerian model may serve the heuristic purpose of suggesting the value of more abstract cognitive models, which are not symptom-based, for defining the phenotype of schizophrenia.

Accepted for publication March 11, 1999.

This research was supported in part by grants MH31593, MH40856, and MHCRC43271 and Research Scientist Award MH00625 from the National Institute of Mental Health,

Rockville, Md; and an Established Investigator Award from the National Alliance for Research on Schizophrenia and Depression, Great Neck, NY,

Reprints: Nancy C. Andreasen, MD, PhD, University of Iowa Hospitals and Clinics, Mental Health Clinical Research Center, 2911 JPP, 200 Hawkins Dr, Iowa City, IA 52242-1057.

REFERENCES

1. Tulving E. Elements of Episodic Memory. New York, NY: Oxford University Press; 1983:123.
2. Bleuler E. Dementia Praecox or the Group of Schizophrenias. Zinkin J, trans. New York, NY: International Universities Press; 1950.
3. Andreasen NC. The role of the thalamus in schizophrenia. Can J Psychiatry. 1997;42:27-33.
4. Andreasen NC. Linking mind and brain in the study of mental illness: a project for a scientific psychopathology. Science. 1997;275:1586-1593.
5. Andreasen NC, Paradiso S, O'Leary DS. Cognitive dysmetria as an integrative theory of schizophrenia: a dysfunction in cortical-cerebellar circuitry? Schizophr Bull. 1998;24:203-218.
6. Fish B. Neurobiological antecedents of schizophrenia in children: evidence for an inherited, congenital neurointegrative defect. Arch Gen Psychiatry. 1977;125:1-24.
7. Feinberg I. Schizophrenia: caused by a fault in programmed synaptic elimination during adolescence? J Psychiatr Res. 1982;17:319-334.
8. Andreasen NC, Nasrallah HA, Dunn VD, Olson SC, Grove WM, Ehrhardt JC, Coffman JA. Structural abnormalities in the frontal system in schizophrenia: a magnetic resonance imaging study. Arch Gen Psychiatry. 1986;43:136-144.
9. Weinberger D. Implications of normal brain development for the pathogenesis of schizophrenia. Arch Gen Psychiatry. 1987;44:660-669.
10. Bloom F. Advancing a neurodevelopmental origin for schizophrenia. Arch Gen Psychiatry. 1993; 50:224-227.
11. Murray RM, Lewis SW. Is schizophrenia a neurodevelopmental disorder? BMJ. 1987;295: 681-682.
12. Murray RM, O'Callaghan E, Castle DJ, Lewis SW. A neurodevelopmental approach to the classification of schizophrenia. Schizophr Bull. 1992;18: 319-332.
13. Holzman PS, Levy DL, Proctor LR. Smooth pursuit eye movements, attention, and schizophrenia. Arch Gen Psychiatry. 1976;45:641-647.
14. Braff DL, Geyer MA. Sensorimotor gating and schizophrenia: human and animal model studies. Arch Gen Psychiatry. 1990;47:181-188.
15. Freedman R, Adler LE, Waldo MC, Pachtman E, Franks RD. Neurophysiological evidence for a defect in inhibitory pathways in schizophrenia: comparison of medicated and drug-free patients. Biol Psychiatry. 1983;18:537-551.
16. McCarley RW, Faux SF, Shenton ME, Nestor PG, Adams J. Event-related potentials in schizophrenia: their biological and clinical correlates and a new model of schizophrenic pathophysiology. Schizophr Res. 1991;4:209-231.
17. Nuechterlein KH, Dawson ME. Information processing and attentional function in the developmental course of schizophrenic disorders. Schizophr Bull. 1984;10:160-203.
18. Goldman-Rakic PS. Working memory dysfunction in schizophrenia. J Neuropsychiatry Clin Neurosci. 1994;6:348-357.
19. Frith CD. The Cognitive Neuropsychology of Schizophrenia. East Sussex, England: Lawrence A Erlbaum Associates; 1992.
20. Braff DL. Information processing and attention dysfunctions in schizophrenia. Schizophr Bull. 1993;19:233-259.

21. Andreasen NC, O'Leary DS, Cizadlo T, Arndt S, Rezai K, Ponto LLB, Watkins GL, Hichwa RD. Schizophrenia and cognitive dysmetria: a positron-emission tomography study of dysfunctional prefrontal-thalamic-cerebellar circuitry. Proc Natl Acad Sci U S A. 1996;93:9985-9990.
22. Crespo Facorro B, Paradiso S, Andreasen NC, O'Leary DS. Recalling word list reveals cognitive dysmetria in schizophrenia patients: a PET study. Am J Psychiatry. 1999;156:386-392.
23. Wiser AK, Andreasen NC, O'Leary DS, Watkins GL, Ponto LLB, Hichwa RD. Dysfunctional cortico-cerebellar circuits cause "cognitive dysmetria" in schizophrenia. Neuroreport. 1998;9:1895-1899.
24. Kandel ER, Schwartz JH, Jessell TM. Principles of Neural Science. 3rd ed. New York, NY: Elsevier Science Inc; 1991.
25. Holmes G. The cerebellum of man. Brain. 1939; 62:1-30.
26. Leiner HC, Leiner AL, Dow RS. Cognitive and language functions of the human cerebellum. Trend Neurosci. 1993;16:444-447.
27. Schmahmann JD. An emerging concept: the cerebellar contribution to higher function. Arch Neurol. 1991;48:1178-1187.
28. Ito M. The Cerebellum and Neural Control. New York, NY: Raven Press; 1984.
29. Ito M. Neural systems controlling movements. Trend Neurosci. 1986;9:515-518.
30. Ito M, ed. How Does the Cerebellum Facilitate Thought? New York, NY: Oxford University Press; 1993.
31. Middleton F, Strick P. Dentate output channels: motor and cognitive components. Prog Brain Res. 1997;114:553-566.
32. Gao J-H, Parsons LM, Bower JM, Xiong J, Li J, Fox PT. Cerebellum implicated in sensory acquisition and discrimination rather than motor control. Science. 1996;272:545-547.
33. Houk JC. On the role of the cerebellum and basal ganglia in cognitive signal processing. Prog Brain Res. 1997;114:543-552.
34. Bower JM. Is the cerebellum sensory for motor's sake, or motor for sensory's sake? the view from the whiskers of a rat. Prog Brain Res. 1997; 114:463-486.
35. Edelman GM. The Remembered Present: A Biological Theory of Consciousness. New York, NY: Basic Books Inc Publishers; 1989.
36. Fuster JM. The Prefrontal Cortex: Anatomy, Physiology, and Neuropsychology of the Prefrontal Cortex. New York, NY: Raven Press; 1989.
37. Passingham RE. Changes in the size and organization of the brain in man and his ancestors. Brain Behav Evol. 1975;11:73-90.
38. Andreasen NC, Flashman L, Flaum M, Arndt S, Swayze V, O'Leary D, Ehrhardt J, Yuh WTC. Regional brain abnormalities in schizophrenia measured with magnetic resonance imaging. JAMA. 1994;272:1763-1769.
39. Flaum M, Andreasen NC. Brain morphology in schizotypal personality as assessed by magnetic resonance imaging. In: Raine A, Lencz T, Mednick S, eds. Schizotypal Personality. New York, NY: Cambridge Publishing; 1995:385-405.
40. Andreasen NC, Ehrhardt JC, Swayze VW, Alliger RJ, Yuh WTC, Cohen G, Ziebell S. Magnetic resonance imaging of the brain in schizophrenia: the pathophysiological significance of structural abnormalities. Arch Gen Psychiatry. 1990;47:35-44.
41. Nopoulos P, Torres I, Flaum M, Andreasen NC, Ehrhardt JC, Yuh WTC. Brain morphology in first-episode schizophrenia. Am J Psychiatry. 1995; 152:1721-1724.
42. Wible CG, Shenton ME, Hokama H, Kikinis R, Joiesz FA, Metcalf D, McCarley RW. Prefrontal cortex and schizophrenia: a quantitative magnetic resonance imaging study. Arch Gen Psychiatry. 1995;52:279-288.
43. Breier A, Buchanan RW, Elkashef A, Munson RC, Kirkpatrick B, Gellad F. Brain morphology and schizophrenia: a magnetic resonance imaging study of limbic, prefrontal cortex, and caudate structures. Arch Gen Psychiatry. 1992;49:921-926.
44. Selemon LD, Rajkowska G, Goldman-Rakic PS.

16

Abnormally high neuronal density in the schizophrenic cortex: a morphometric analysis of prefrontal area 9 and occipital area 17. *Arch Gen Psychiatry.* 1995;52:805-818.

45. Buchsbaum MS, Ingvar DH, Kessler R, Waters RN, Capelletti J, Kammen DP, King C. Cerebral glucography with positron tomography. *Arch Gen Psychiatry.* 1982;39:251-259.

46. Buchsbaum MS. The frontal lobes, basal ganglia, and temporal lobes as sites for schizophrenia. *Schizophr Bull.* 1990;16:379-384.

47. Buchsbaum MS, Someya T, Teng CY, Abel L, Najafi A, Haier RJ, Wu J. PET and MRI of the thalamus in never-medicated patients with schizophrenia. *Am J Psychiatry.* 1996;153:191-199.

48. Weinberger DR, Berman KF, Zec RF. Physiological dysfunction of dorsolateral prefrontal cortex in schizophrenia: regional cerebral blood flow (rCBF) evidence. *Arch Gen Psychiatry.* 1986;43:114-124.

49. Weinberger DR, Berman KF, Illowsky BP. Physiological dysfunction of dorsolateral prefrontal cortex in schizophrenia, III: a new cohort and evidence for a monoaminergic mechanism. *Arch Gen Psychiatry.* 1988;45:609-615.

50. Berman KF, Illowsky BP, Weinberger DR. Physiological dysfunction of dorsolateral prefrontal cortex in schizophrenia, IV: further evidence for regional and behavioral specificity. *Arch Gen Psychiatry.* 1988;45:616-622.

51. Liddle PF, Friston KJ, Frith CD, Hirsch SR, Jones T, Frackowiak RSJ. Patterns of cerebral blood flow in schizophrenia. *Br J Psychiatry.* 1992;60:179-186.

52. Andreasen NC, Rezai K, Alliger R, Swayze VW, Flaum M, Kirchner P, Cohen G. Hypofrontality in neuroleptic-naive and chronic schizophrenic patients: assessment with xenon-133 single-photon emission computed tomography and the Tower of London. *Arch Gen Psychiatry.* 1992;49:943-958.

53. Andreasen NC, O'Leary DS, Flaum M, Nopoulos P, Watkins GL, Ponto LLB, Hichwa RD. "Hypofrontality" in schizophrenia: distributed dysfunctional circuits in neuroleptic naive patients. *Lancet.* 1997;349:1730-1734.

54. Goldman-Rakic PS. Topography of cognition: parallel distributed networks in primate association cortex. *Ann Rev Neurosci.* 1988;11:137-156.

55. Goldman-Rakic PS. Cellular and circuit basis of working memory in prefrontal cortex of nonhuman primates. In: Uylings HBM, Van Eden CG, De Bruin JPC, Corner MA, Feenstra MGP, eds. *Progress in Brain Research: The Prefrontal Cortex—Its Structure, Function, and Pathology.* New York, NY: Elsevier Science Publishers; 1990:325-335.

56. Swerdlow NR, Lipska BK, Weinberger DR, Braff DL, Jaskiw GE, Geyer MA. Increased sensitivity to the sensorimotor gating-disruptive effects of apomorphine after lesions of medial prefrontal cortex or ventral hippocampus in adult rats. *Psychopharmacology.* 1995;122:27-34.

57. Ivry RB, Keele SW. Timing functions of the cerebellum. *J Cog Neurosci.* 1989;1:136-152.

58. Middleton FA, Strick PL. Anatomical evidence for cerebellar and basal ganglia involvement in higher cognitive function. *Science.* 1994;266:458-461.

59. Schmahmann JD, Pandya DN. Prefrontal cortex projections to the basilar pons: implications for the cerebellar contribution to higher function. *Neurosci Lett.* 1995;199:175-178.

60. Wassink TH, Andreasen NC, Nopoulos P, Flaum M. Brain morphology as a predictor of symptoms and psychosocial outcome in schizophrenia. *Biol Psychiatry.* In press.

61. Andreasen NC, O'Leary DS, Arndt S, Cizadlo T, Hurtig R, Rezai K, Watkins GL, Ponto LLB, Hichwa R. Short-term and long-term verbal memory: a positron emission tomography study. *Proc Natl Acad Sci U S A.* 1995;92:5111-5115.

62. Andreasen NC, O'Leary DS, Arndt S, Cizadlo T, Rezai K, Watkins GL, Ponto LLB, Hichwa R. I. PET studies of memory: novel and practiced free recall of complex narratives. *Neuroimage.* 1995;2:284-295.

63. Andreasen NC, O'Leary DS, Cizadlo T, Arndt S, Rezai K, Watkins GL, Ponto LLB, Hichwa R. II. PET studies of memory: novel versus practiced free recall of word lists. *Neuroimage.* 1995;2:296-305.

64. Andreasen NC, O'Leary DS, Cizadlo T, Arndt S, Rezai K, Watkins GL, Ponto LLB, Hichwa R. Remembering the past: two facets of episodic memory explored with positron emission tomography. *Am J Psychiatry.* 1995;152:1576-1585.

65. Andreasen NC, O'Leary DS, Arndt S, Cizadlo T, Hurtig R, Rezai K, Watkins GL, Ponto LLB, Hichwa FD. Neural substrates of facial recognition. *J Neuropsychiatry Clin Neurosci.* 1996;8:139-146.

66. Paradiso S, Crespo Facorro B, Andreasen NC, O'Leary DS, Watkins LG, Ponto LLB, Hichwa RD. Brain activity assessed with PET during recall of word lists and narratives. *Neuroreport.* 1997;8:3091-3096.

67. Buckner RL, Bandettini PA, O'Craven KM, Savoy RL, Petersen SE, Raichle ME, Rosen BR. Detection of cortical activation during averaged single trials of a cognitive task using functional magnetic resonance imaging. *Proc Natl Acad Sci U S A.* 1996;93:14878-14883.

68. Raichle ME. Images of the mind: studies with modern imaging techniques. *Ann Rev Psychol.* 1994; 45:333-356.

69. Paulignan Y, Jenkins IH, Brooks DJ, Frackowiak RSJ, Passingham RE. The sensory guidance of movement: a comparison of the cerebellum and basal ganglia. *Exp Brain Res.* 1996;112:462-474.

70. Kim S-G, Ugurbil K, Strick PL. Activation of a cerebellar output nucleus during cognitive processing. *Science.* 1994;265:949-951.

71. Allen G, Buxton RB, Wong EC, Courchesne E. Attentional activation of the cerebellum independent of motor involvement. *Science.* 1997;275:1940-1943.

72. O'Leary DS, Andreasen NC, Kesler M, Ponto LLB, Watkins GL, Hichwa RD. Auditory and visual attention in patients with schizophrenia: a PET study. *Soc Neurosci Abstr.* 1997;23:1406.

73. Miller DD, Andreasen NC, O'Leary DS, Rezai K, Watkins GL, Ponto LLB, Hichwa RD. Effects of antipsychotics on regional cerebral blood flow measured with positron emission tomography (PET). *Neuropsychopharmacology.* 1997;17:230-240.

74. Miller D, Rezai K, Alliger R, Andreasen NC. The effect of antipsychotic medication on regional blood flow in schizophrenia: assessment with TC-99m HMPAO SPECT. *Biol Psychiatry.* 1997;41:550-559.

75. Holcomb HH, Cascella NG, Thaker GK, Medoff DR, Dannals RF, Tamminga CA. Functional sites of neuroleptic drug action in the human brain: PET/FDG studies with and without haloperidol. *Am J Psychiatry.* 1996;153:41-48.

76. Volkow ND, Levy A, Brodie JD, Wolf AP, Cancro R, Van Gelder P, Henn F. Low cerebellar metabolism in medicated patients with chronic schizophrenia. *Am J Psychiatry.* 1992;149:686-688.

77. Carlsson M, Carlsson A. Schizophrenia: a subcortical neurotransmitter imbalance syndrome? *Schizophr Bull.* 1990;16:425-432.

78. Bogerts B. Recent advances in the neuropathology of schizophrenia. *Schizophr Bull.* 1993;19:431-445.

79. Pakkenberg B. Pronounced reduction of total neuron number in mediodorsal thalamic nucleus and nucleus accumens in schizophrenics. *Arch Gen Psychiatry.* 1990;47:1023-1028.

80. Pakkenberg B. Stereological quantitation of human brains from normal and schizophrenic individuals. *Acta Neurol Scand.* 1992;137:20-33.

81. Stevens JR. Neuropathology of schizophrenia. *Arch Gen Psychiatry.* 1982;39:1131-1139.

82. Andreasen NC, Arndt S, Swayze V, Cizadlo T, Flaum M, O'Leary D, Ehrhardt J, Yuh WTC. Thalamic abnormalities in schizophrenia visualized through magnetic resonance image averaging. *Science.* 1994;266:294-298.

83. Flaum M, Andreasen NC. Brain morphology in schizotypal personality as assessed by magnetic resonance imaging. In: Raine A, Lencz T, Mednick S, eds. *Schizotypal Personality.* New York, NY: Cambridge Publishing; 1995:385-405.

84. Silbersweig DA, Stern E, Frith C, Cahill C, Holmes A, Grootoonk S, Seaward J et al. A functional neuroanatomy of hallucinations in schizophrenia. *Nature.* 1995;378:176-179.

85. Kraepelin E, Barclay RM, Robertson GM. *Dementia Praecox and Paraphrenia.* Edinburgh, Scotland: E&S Livingstone; 1919.

86. Gupta S, Andreasen NC, Arndt S, Flaum M, Schultz SK, Hubbard WC, Smith M. Neurological soft signs in neuroleptic-naive and neuroleptic-treated schizophrenic patients and in normal comparison subjects. *Am J Psychiatry.* 1995;152:191-196.

87. Chapman LJ, Chapman JP. Problems in the measurement of cognitive deficit. *Psychol Bull.* 1973;79:380-385.

88. Saykin AJ, Shtasel DL, Gur GE, Kester DB, Mozley LH, Stafiniak P, Gur RC. Neuropsychological deficits in neuroleptic naive patients with first-episode schizophrenia. *Arch Gen Psychiatry.* 1994;51:124-131.

89. Gold S, Arndt S, Nopoulos P, O'Leary D, Andreasen NC. A longitudinal study of cognitive function in first episode and recent onset schizophrenia. *Am J Psychiatry.* In press.

90. Popper K. *The Logic of Scientific Discovery.* New York, NY: Basic Books Inc Publishers; 1959.

91. Hatten ME, Alder J, Zimmerman K, Heintz N. Genes involved in cerebellar cell specification and differentiation. *Curr Opin Neurobiol.* 1997;7:40-47.

92. Zecevic N, Rakic P. Differentiation of purkinje cells and their relationship to other components of developing cerebellar cortex in man. *J Comp Neurol.* 1976;167:27-48.

93. Rakic P, Sidman RL. Histogenesis of cortical layers in human cerebellum, particularly the lamina dissecans. *J Comp Neurol.* 1970;139:473-500.

94. Herrup K, Wilczynski SL. Cerebellar cell degeneration in the leaner mutant mouse. *Neuroscience.* 1982;7:2185-2196.

95. Tano D, Napieralski JA, Eisenman LM, Messer A, Plummer J, Hawkes R. Novel developmental boundary in the cerebellum revealed by zebrin expression in the leaner (La/+) mutant mouse. *J Comp Neurol.* 1992;323:128-13.

96. Nusse, Roes, Varmus HE. *Wnt* genes. *Cell.* 1992; 66:1073-1087.

97. Keele SW, Ivry R. Does the cerebellum provide a common computation for diverse tasks? a timing hypothesis. *Ann N Y Acad Sci.* 1990;608:179-207.

17

Implications of Normal Brain Development for the Pathogenesis of Schizophrenia

Daniel R. Weinberger, MD

● Recent research on schizophrenia has demonstrated that in this disorder the brain is not, strictly speaking, normal. The findings suggest that nonspecific histopathology exists in the limbic system, diencephalon, and prefrontal cortex, that the pathology occurs early in development, and that the causative process is inactive long before the diagnosis is made. If these findings are valid and not epiphenomena, then the pathogenesis of schizophrenia does not appear to fit either traditional metabolic, posttraumatic, or neurodegenerative models of adult mental illness. The data are more consistent with a neurodevelopmental model in which a fixed "lesion" from early in life interacts with normal brain maturational events that occur much later. Based on neuro-ontological principles and insights from animal research about normal brain development, it is proposed that the appearance of diagnostic symptoms is linked to the normal maturation of brain areas affected by the early developmental pathology, particularly the dorsolateral prefrontal cortex. The course of the illness and the importance of stress may be related to normal maturational aspects of dopaminergic neural systems, particularly those innervating prefrontal cortex. Some implications for future research and treatment are considered.

(Arch Gen Psychiatry 1987;44:660-669)

There are three inescapable clinical "facts" about schizophrenia that should be taken into account by any effort to explain it: first, the very high probability that it will become clinically apparent in late adolescence or early adulthood; second, the role of "stress" in onset and relapse; and third, the therapeutic efficacy of neuroleptic drugs. Neurobiologic theories have tended to address only selected features of the disorder or perhaps a research finding associated with it. For example, biochemical hypotheses such as the dopamine hypothesis[1] are, for the most part, based on the third clinical fact. As valuable as biochemical

theories have been in spawning neurochemical and neuropharmacologic research, they have provided little insight into the first two inescapable facts about schizophrenia.

During the past decade, new developments in schizophrenia research have led to increasingly vigorous speculation that this illness is a primary brain disease. While compelling evidence that schizophrenia is associated with structural and physiological pathology of the brain has emerged,[1] the data have also suggested that the pathology is in the form of a fixed structural defect that occurs long before the diagnosis is made. If this last observation is valid, it is inconsistent with traditional neurobiologic models of mental disorders, such as metabolic encephalopathy, posttraumatic condition, or neurodegenerative disorder, all of which implicate pathology that is either progressive or that occurs close to the onset of the illness. If the brain findings in schizophrenia are clues to its pathogenesis, which seems likely, then it may be useful to consider other models of illness. The following discussion illustrates that this recent evidence fits surprisingly well into a neurodevelopmental model that, while speculative, may at the least explain the three inescapable clinical facts mentioned above. A preliminary discussion of this model has appeared elsewhere.[2]

It will be proposed that schizophrenia is a neurodevelopmental disorder in which a fixed brain lesion from early in life interacts with certain normal maturational events that occur much later. The thesis rests on the clinical maxim that the manifestations of a brain lesion vary with the state of brain maturation and involution.[4] The thesis is only peripherally about etiology. It holds that what is pathophysiologically distinct about schizophrenia is neither the location nor the cause of its "lesion"; it is, instead, the interaction between this "lesion" and the normal course of maturation of the neural system affected by it. This thesis is a variation on a theme that has had many previous incarnations in the neuropsychiatric literature.

First, a brief summary of data implicating brain pathology in schizophrenia will be presented. This section is not intended to be a critical review of the data. Rather, it will take the position that if recent research is correct and pathology of the limbic system and prefrontal cortex exists in schizophrenia, then this pathology is probably congenital

Accepted for publication Sept 9, 1986.

From the Clinical Brain Disorders Branch, Intramural Research Program, National Institute of Mental Health, Washington, DC.

Reprint requests to Clinical Brain Disorders Branch, Intramural Research Program, National Institute of Mental Health, William A. White Building, Saint Elizabeths Hospital, Washington, DC 20032 (Dr Weinberger).

Schizophrenia and Brain Development—Weinberger

18

and static. This section will also argue that the pathology is not sufficient explanation for the illness. The second section presents the argument that the critical factor in the onset of the illness is the normal course of brain maturation. In the third section, aspects of the role of dopaminergic neural systems will be considered. In particular, it will be argued that dopaminergic function is an important element in understanding both of the preceding sections, that its role in normal behavioral responses to stress is compromised by the "lesion" in schizophrenia, and that the course of schizophrenia is related in part to the normal maturation and regression of brain dopamine systems.

BRAIN PATHOLOGY IN SCHIZOPHRENIA

Recent controlled studies of postmortem brain tissue have found nonspecific but objective evidence of anatomical pathology in the periventricular limbic and diencephalic areas and in the prefrontal cortex in schizophrenia.[5-16] Although these studies have not demonstrated a characteristic lesion or even a consistent pathologic picture, in part because of differing approaches to examining the tissue, they have suggested that in a generic sense, pathology of the limbic system is a replicable phenomenon in schizophrenia (for a detailed review, see Kirch and Weinberger[16]). Since most of these studies have been strictly quantitative, ie, comparisons of mean structure size and/or cellularity, it is not possible to conclude from the data that only some cases are involved, while others are not. This point will be discussed further in the section on etiology.

Numerous controlled investigations by computed tomography (CT) of living patients have also found quantitative evidence of brain pathology in the form of enlarged third and lateral ventricles and increased cortical markings suggestive of reduced gyral mass or atrophy, especially in the prefrontal cortex (for a review, see Shelton and Weinberger[17]). While the CT findings are not proof of periventricular limbic and diencephalic pathology, they certainly are consistent with this possibility and with the results of the postmortem studies. In all of these investigations, both CT and postmortem, the magnitude of the differences between patients and controls is not so extreme as to be qualitatively obvious, and considerable overlap between groups invariably exists. In other words, only a slight reduction in tissue mass or change in cellularity has been found. Indeed, this may explain the failure of some investigators during the first half of this century to observe or appreciate brain pathology in schizophrenia.

Because the neuropathologic findings are subtle and nonspecific, it is impossible to determine on the basis of the available data whether the primary pathology involves all of the implicated structures directly or is more selective and affects some areas only as a result of secondary changes. Since the brain regions implicated are richly interconnected,[18,19] even focal pathology might have far-reaching ramifications, both structural and functional, throughout the system. This is especially the case if the pathology occurs early in development. Thus, as one possible example, prefrontal pathology and/or dysfunction may be secondary to primary pathology in the temporal lobe, or vice versa. In the interest of conciseness, the brain pathology in schizophrenia will be referred to herein as a "lesion," though as discussed in the section on etiology, it is probably premature to conclude that a unitary lesion exists.

On the basis of circumstantial evidence, it can be stated that the clinical features of schizophrenia are at least theoretically consistent with dysfunction of the brain areas implicated as the site of the lesion. From depth-electrode studies in humans, it is apparent that psychotic experiences

such as hallucinations, ineffable and strange experiences, perceptual distortions, and irrational fears can result from electrical discharges in either the temporal cortex, amygdala, or hippocampus.[20,21] Neurologic disorders such as tumors, trauma, and infections are associated with schizophreniform symptomatology much more frequently when they involve the limbic system and diencephalon than when they occur in other brain regions.[21,22] These clinical analogies suggest that florid psychotic experiences and symptoms, or so-called positive psychotic features, reflect dysfunction in these subcortical sites.

While hallucinations and delusions are perhaps the most dramatic clinical aspects of schizophrenia and the cornerstones of current diagnostic criteria, they may not be the most disabling features of the illness. This distinction is often attributed to what are called the defect or negative symptoms[24,25] (eg, flat affect, social withdrawal, lack of initiative and motivation, poor insight and judgment) and for the intellectual impairment that probably characterize the majority of individuals with the disorder.[26,27] These subtle and difficult-to-define characteristics are not typical manifestations of the subcortical neurologic lesions that produce positive symptoms[28] but tend to resemble symptoms seen in patients with lesions of the frontal lobe, especially of the dorsolateral prefrontal cortex (DLPFC).[28,29] This is particularly true of the pattern of cognitive impairment, motivational difficulties, and deficits in social functioning and insight.[29-31] In the case of schizophrenia, there is evidence from recent regional cerebral blood flow studies that the degree of characteristic intellectual deficit is caused by a failure of DLPFC physiological activation (vide infra).[32,33]

Unfortunately, while research evidence for brain pathology in schizophrenia may seem convincing and may provide a theoretical framework for understanding many of the clinical features of the illness, the pathogenic implications of this pathology are not obvious. For example, the lesion is far from unique or specific. It is certainly not by itself a sufficient explanation for the illness because other disorders that are associated with pathology in similar brain areas usually do not present as schizophrenia. For example, schizophrenialike psychoses are not typical of several degenerative disorders that involve similar brain areas, most notably Alzheimer's disease. Many cases of trauma and tumor affect areas involved in schizophrenia, yet relatively infrequently do such patients present with schizophrenialike symptoms. It appears, therefore, that even if the proposed lesion in schizophrenia were a necessary condition for the development of the syndrome, it must exist in combination with other factors for it to be clinically manifest as this disorder.

The relationship of the lesion to the pathogenesis of schizophrenia is made even more obscure by the apparent distance between the occurrence of the lesion and the time of onset of the psychosis. The information that bears most directly on this issue and that is central to the pathogenic model presented herein is the evidence that the structural changes represent an old pathologic event that is no longer active. The postmortem studies have not found signs of an ongoing neuropathologic process, such as reactive gliosis, dying neurons, inclusion bodies, or inflammation. Instead, the findings suggest either an old episode of brain damage or, perhaps, a dysplastic condition. In fact, several investigators have interpreted their findings as indicative of a congenital lesion.[5,6,9,15] The data from CT studies also strongly suggest that the lesion is old and inactive. Ventricular enlargement has been reported in first-episode schizophreniform patients,[34-36] a finding that implicates

19

early developmental pathology since ventricular enlargement would be unlikely to develop acutely during adolescence without concomitant neurologic symptoms. The observation that ventricular size correlates with poor premorbid social adjustment[37-39] and reports of a link between ventricular enlargement and a history of perinatal complications[39,40] also suggest that the pathology exists early in life.

The majority of the CT studies have not found a relationship between ventricular enlargement and duration of illness, a correlation that would be expected if the underlying pathologic process were active and progressive.[17] Moreover, in a prospective study of 15 patients who underwent repeated scanning after eight years of continuous illness, we have found no evidence of progression of CT findings (B. Illowsky, D. Juliano, L. Bigelow, D.R.W., unpublished data, 1987).

A simple pathogenic model would predict that if the disease process responsible for schizophrenia leads to structural pathology of the brain, the development of this pathology would be temporally related to the development of the illness. For example, if schizophrenia is caused by a viral infection in early adult life, then whatever pathology this infection produces should not be apparent before the infection occurs. Alternatively, if schizophrenia is analogous to a metabolic encephalopathy or to a neurodegenerative disorder, then the pathology should parallel the disease process and become more extensive over time as the process continues. Therefore, to the extent that the lesion described above relates to the pathogenesis of schizophrenia, a simple model of brain insult followed *pari passu* by symptomatic brain dysfunction does not seem to apply. The neurodevelopmental model considered in the following discussion may be more appropriate.

IMPLICATIONS OF NORMAL BRAIN DEVELOPMENT

One factor that influences the clinical manifestations of any lesion is the age of the brain. In childhood, there are classic examples of how even fixed congenital lesions produce changing clinical symptoms over time. For instance, perinatal hypoxic encephalopathy may cause cerebral palsy with spastic diplegia or hemiparesis in a 2-year-old child. At 4 years of age, athetosis may develop, and seizures may follow in a few years. The lesion itself is static, but its effects on neurologic function change. This is believed to reflect the fact that the pathways mediating a behavior such as athetosis do not mature until after a few years of life. The message is that if a lesion affects a brain structure or region that has yet to mature functionally, the effects of the lesion may remain silent until that structure or system matures.[4] Another example of this phenomenon, one that is closer to the issue of schizophrenia, is the changing pattern of seizures seen with a congenital scar of the temporal lobe. During childhood, the clinical manifestations of epileptic discharges from the temporal lobe usually include only autonomic phenomena and lapses in consciousness. Psychic experiences rarely appear before adolescence.[41] If the analogy to athetosis is valid, it suggests that the regions mediating the psychic experiences of epilepsy do not mature until adolescence.

In adulthood as well, the time of life when a brain lesion presents is important in understanding its clinical impact. The clinical literature suggests that this may be especially true with lesions that cause psychopathology. Although this has not been systematically studied, in a number of neurologic disorders that frequently present with psychiatric symptoms, the character of the psychopathology seems to be determined more by the age of the patient than by the

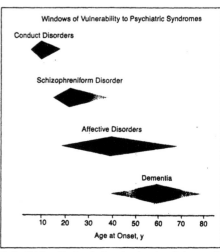

Fig 1.—Relationship of age to character of psychopathology seen in association with various cerebral disorders. See text for discussion.

character of the neuropathology or by the origin of the condition. For example, Huntington's disease has a variable age at onset and often begins with changes in behavior. Although the neuropathologic features do not vary systematically with age of onset, the psychiatric (and motor) features do. Behavioral manifestations are rare in childhood cases; adolescent and early adult onset are more likely to be associated with schizophreniform psychosis than are cases of later onset; onset in the late third and in the fourth decade is more likely to be associated with depression; and later-onset cases typically present with dementia as the psychiatric manifestation.[4,42,43]

A surprisingly similar age-related pattern of behavioral change tends to be seen in other disorders with a variable age of onset. Examples include Wilson's disease,[4,44] metachromatic leukodystrophy,[4,45] ceroid lipofucsinosis,[4] Fahr's syndrome,[46] encephalitis,[47] systemic lupus erythematosus,[48] Creutzfeldt-Jakob disease,[49] head trauma,[50] and brain tumor.[51] In each of these conditions, if psychosis develops, it tends to do so more frequently during the late second and third decades of life than at other times (Fig 1). In some cases the correlation between age and psychosis is well documented and striking. For example, Achte and colleagues,[50] in their landmark study of the prevalence of psychosis in 3552 brain-injured veterans of the Finnish wars, reported that schizophrenialike psychosis was five times more frequent in individuals wounded before 20 years of age than after 35 years of age. Since the neuropathology in each of these neurologic disorders does not vary systematically with age, the predictable behavioral variation appears to represent an interaction between the lesion and age-related aspects of brain physiology. In other words, early adulthood may be a critical period of vulnerability for the expression of psychotic behavior, regardless of the underlying brain disease.

The existence of a critical period of vulnerability for the expression of schizophreniform psychosis suggests that the neural systems mediating this behavior reach a functional

Schizophrenia and Brain Development—Weinberger

20

peak during this period. This may relate to hormonal influences on central nervous system physiology[42] or, more simply, the natural course of the ontological development of psychosis-related systems (*vide infra*). It may also reflect developmental changes in systems that normally inhibit or modulate the psychosis-related systems. In any case, the psychotogenic effects of a lesion affecting the structure and/or function of this neural system, even a static lesion that exists throughout life, might be linked to and perhaps be dependent on this critical phase of brain maturation. It follows from these considerations that a lesion in this neural system conceivably could remain clinically silent or at least not be expressed as a psychosis until early adulthood.

One of the brain areas implicated in schizophrenia that appears to reach functional maturity in early adulthood is the DLPFC. In the monkey, there are specific cell populations in the principal sulcus of the DLPFC that increase their firing rates during the delay period of delayed-response behavioral tasks, a type of task that is a sensitive measure of DLPFC cognitive function. The response of these cells to the delay period becomes most apparent after sexual maturity.[53] In humans, the DLPFC is the last brain area to begin myelination and may be the only area that continues myelination throughout life.[54] The myelogenic cycle for the DLPFC is thought to occur primarily during the second and third decades of life. While the meaning of this in terms of behavior is unclear, it suggests that this area remains relatively "uncommitted" or plastic until adulthood. Recent studies in humans[55] and monkeys[56] have shown that synaptic pruning, ie, the normal developmental regression of excessive interneuronal contacts, does not level off until after puberty. Cognitive behaviors attributable to the DLPFC, such as developing strategies for future behavior based on past experiences,[57] are not characteristic of preadolescent cognition, as illustrated by the work of Piaget.[58] Neuropsychological tests that are thought to be sensitive measures of DLPFC cognitive function in adults (eg, the Wisconsin Card Sorting Test[59]) are difficult for children. In fact, performance on such tests may not reach adult levels before early adolescence.[60] To the extent that ontogeny recapitulates phylogeny, it is not surprising that the most highly evolved—the most human—brain areas should mature the latest.

It might be predicted that since the DLPFC reaches functional maturity relatively late in life, a lesion of the DLPFC would have little impact on behavior during childhood. Experiments in monkeys support this assumption. A DLPFC lesion does not dramatically impair the behavior of infant or prepubescent monkeys, yet it devastates the capacity of the adult monkey to perform delayed-response tasks.[61] Even more striking are reports that some monkeys with infantile DLPFC lesions who do well on delayed-response tasks during childhood lose their ability to perform when they reach early adulthood.[62,63] This is in contrast to monkeys with infantile lesions of the orbital frontal cortex whose performance on delayed-response tasks, while compromised during childhood, becomes normal by adulthood.[63]

These lesion experiments suggest that DLPFC function is not "rate limiting" for many behaviors until adulthood.[63] The data further suggest that a lesion in the DLPFC can be consistently compensated for only before this stage of life. Moreover, these experimental observations provide an animal model of how a fixed congenital lesion could remain relatively unapparent until early adulthood and then have a profound impact on behavior. It is probably an oversimplification to assume that in humans such a lesion would be totally clinically silent before adolescence. It would probably

be associated with subtle behavioral abnormalities, perhaps social awkwardness and shyness, as well as so-called soft neurologic signs. This might explain the tendency for the premorbid history of patients with schizophrenia to be characterized by such traits.[44-46] The clinical observation that at the onset of schizophrenia some patients appear to lose intellectual functions that they used to possess[67] may represent the "coming of age" of a defective DLPFC.

In summary, there are considerable clinical and animal research data to show that the time a brain lesion occurs is not necessarily the time at which it is clinically manifest. Since the symptoms of schizophrenia may be linked to dysfunction of neural systems that normally reach physiological maturity in late adolescence and early adulthood, the clinical onset of the illness may be a function of this normal maturational process. Unfortunately, the clinical and research data that suggest this explanation for the onset of schizophrenia have emphasized the prefrontal cortex, a region not directly implicated in "positive" psychotic symptoms. Furthermore, these considerations do not define the mechanisms by which the symptoms are triggered. How might the physiological and neurochemical changes that occur at this critical time of life interact with the lesion to produce schizophrenic behavior? Would this interaction be affected by stress, as schizophrenic symptoms appear to be? While there are no certain answers to these questions, there is evidence that brain dopaminergic systems play a role in this mystery.

DOPAMINE AND SCHIZOPHRENIA

It is unlikely that dysfunction of any single neurotransmitter system could account for a disorder as complex as schizophrenia or that the brain pathology implicated above would affect only one neurotransmitter system. Nevertheless, there is considerable evidence that dopamine is an important neurochemical variable in the pathophysiology of schizophrenia. For the past quarter century, the dopamine hypothesis has preoccupied researchers with the notion that schizophrenia was related to an excess of dopaminergic activity.[1,66] This hypothesis rested on the clinical observation that dopamimetic drugs can be psychotogenic and on the finding that the potency of neuroleptic drugs in binding to striatal dopamine receptors in vitro directly correlated with their clinical potency in reducing psychotic symptoms.[68]

These clinical aspects of dopamine pharmacology are presumably mediated by mesolimbic dopamine pathways, ie, neurons with cell bodies in the midbrain ventral tegmental area that project to the hypothalamus, amygdala, hippocampus, and nucleus accumbens.[1] While there is no conclusive evidence that mesolimbic dopamine hyperactivity exists in this illness, several recent postmortem neurochemical studies have found increased numbers of limbic dopamine receptors, especially in patients with more florid psychotic symptoms ("positive symptoms").[2,70,71] The usual criticism of these findings, that they represent an effect of prior neuroleptic treatment,[2] has been tempered by a recent positron tomography study that found increased striatal dopamine receptor activity in medication-naive patients.[72]

It is interesting to consider how the anatomic and neurochemical findings might relate to each other. In light of the structural neuropathologic lesion described above, for the mesolimbic dopamine system to be functionally overactive it must be relatively spared by the pathologic process. This is assumed because it is not likely that a neural system would be both structurally compromised and *functionally* enhanced as a result of a direct pathologic insult. While

21

there are examples of structural pathology coexisting with enhanced dopamine receptor activity (eg, Parkinson's disease), the receptor "up-regulation" is a secondary change that does not restore overall dopaminergic function to normal. In other words, if mesolimbic dopaminergic function is relatively *overactive* in schizophrenia, it may well be a secondary phenomenon (eg, because of diminished inhibitory control).

A case can be made that the dopamine system directly affected by the lesion and functionally compromised as a result is the so-called mesocortical system that projects from the midbrain to primarily the prefrontal cortex.[73] Clinical features of schizophrenia that implicate dysfunction of the DLPFC (ie, defect symptoms) could reflect dysfunction of this dopamine system. This possibility is based on the following arguments, which suggest that dopamine afferentation of the prefrontal cortex is an important component of normal prefrontal behavioral function. In the monkey, DLPFC-related cognition (eg, delayed-response test performance) is impaired after dopamine afferents to the cortex are selectively "lesioned."[74] An analogous situation has been reported in humans following ingestion of 1-methyl-4-phenyl-1,2,3,6-tetrahydropuridine (MPTP), a neurotoxin that destroys dopaminergic neurons and produces clinical parkinsonism.[75] Its toxicity is associated with mild cognitive impairment that is suggestive of selective DLPFC dysfunction, possibly because of reduced dopaminergic input to the prefrontal cortex.[76]

In patients with idiopathic Parkinson's disease, cognitive deficits suggestive of DLPFC dysfunction are often present.[77] It has been proposed that this also reflects diminished activity in dopamine terminals of the prefrontal cortex as a result of the degenerative changes that affect dopamine neurons in this illness.[78] Some of the intellectual deficits as well as the flat affect, decreased motivation, and diminished spontaneity of Parkinson's disease are phenomenologically similar to the defect symptoms of schizophrenia. Dopamimetic agents may ameliorate these symptoms not just in Parkinson's disease but also in some cases of schizophrenia.[79,80] Furthermore, dopamine-blocking agents (eg, neuroleptics) do not consistently benefit such symptoms and may even exacerbate them.[81] Unfortunately, since there are no postmortem studies of dopamine metabolism in schizophrenia that selectively assayed the DLPFC, there is no direct evidence of dopaminergic underactivity in this region. There are, however, reports that concentrations of dopamine metabolites in the cerebrospinal fluid, a measure possibly related to DLPFC dopaminergic activity,[82] are inversely correlated with the degree of defect symptoms.[83] Thus, decreased dopamine activity in the prefrontal cortex may be linked to behavioral evidence of prefrontal dysfunction in schizophrenia.

Dopamine activity in the prefrontal cortex also appears to be related to physiological evidence of prefrontal dysfunction. The clearest data that dysfunction of the DLPFC occurs in schizophrenia and accounts for at least part of the behavioral picture comes from recent studies of regional cerebral blood flow during mental activity.[32,33] In these studies, the degree to which blood flow to the DLPFC increased in patients during a test of DLPFC cognitive function over that during a mentally active baseline state correlated directly with performance on the test. This tight coupling of prefrontal physiology and function (ie, cognition) is surprising and suggests a condition of limited prefrontal physiological reserve. Otherwise, it would be improbable for a small change in activation to be associated with a predictable change in cognitive function. In normal individuals[33] and even in patients with Huntington's dis-

ease,[84] this physiological-functional correlation is not foun implying that prefrontal activation is not a primary det minant of performance on this cognitive test in all con tions. In contrast, patients with Parkinson's disease sh the same coupling of DLPFC activation and cognit performance that is seen in schizophrenia.[85] In addition, Parkinson's disease, DLPFC activation also correlates w motor symptoms traditionally linked to dopamine de ciency (eg, rigidity and bradykinesia),[85] suggesting that t mechanism of the DLPFC physiological-functional re tionship common to both illnesses is dopamine deafferen tion.

In more general terms, dopaminergic function appears be one mechanism by which physiological activity DLPFC is enhanced. This is further supported by anim studies that show an increase in prefrontal cortex gluc metabolism following the administration of dopamine a nists.[86] It follows that if an illness is characterized diminished dopamine innervation of the prefrontal corte the capacity to enhance prefrontal metabolism (ie, to ac vate) may be impaired. In such conditions, physiologi activation could become a critical factor in predicting pr frontal behavioral function, consistent with the region cerebral blood flow data in Parkinson's disease and, pos bly, schizophrenia.

The weight of the evidence cited suggests that the lesi in schizophrenia renders mesocortical dopamine functi *underactive*, perhaps because the structural patholo directly involves dopamine projections to the prefront cortex or the synaptic connections of these projections. reconcile this with the evidence that supports the dopami hypothesis of mesolimbic dopamine overactivity and t existence of "positive" psychotic symptoms, one must pc tulate a paradoxical state of inverse levels of cortic subcortical dopaminergic function. It is unknown wheth any lesion or pathologic condition of the human brain cou produce such a peculiar physiological state. In the r however, this state has been produced by a specific lesion the prefrontal cortex. Pycock et al[87] showed that aft selectively destroying dopamine afferents within the pr frontal cortex (a procedure analogous to that of Brozows et al,[74] mentioned above), chronic subcortical dopami hyperactivity develops. The results included both increas dopamine turnover (ie, homovanillic acid concentration) a up-regulation of postsynaptic receptors, findings that a similar to the postmortem neurochemical data in schiz phrenia.[2] This landmark experiment suggests not only th such a peculiar physiological state can exist but also th mesocortical dopamine neurons affect prefrontal cortic neurons that exert feedback control over mesolimbic dop mine activity[88] (Fig 2). If an analogous situation exists humans, then a lesion that affects prefrontal dopami projections and/or their connections could account for bo mesocortical dopaminergic underactivity and mesolimb overactivity and, thereby, the defect and "positive" sym toms of schizophrenia.

At least two physiological roles for dopamine projectio to prefrontal cortex emerge from these considerations. O is to enhance prefrontal metabolism and presumably beha ioral function, and the other is to provide information abo subcortical dopaminergic activity that the prefrontal cort has the capacity to modulate. The exact pathways a neurotransmitter systems involved in the corticolimb feedback that modulates mesolimbic dopaminergic activi are uncertain and probably complex. The prefrontal cort projects directly to dopamine cell bodies in the midbra and to mesocortical terminal fields in the amygdala, nucle accumbens, hypothalamus, and hippocampus, as well

22

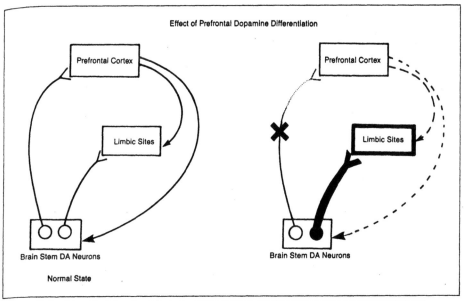

Effect of Prefrontal Dopamine Differentiation

Fig 2.—Schematized interactions between mesolimbic and mesocortical dopamine systems in normal state (left) and after selective lesioning of dopamine input to prefrontal cortex (right), based on the work of Pycock et al.[87] Broken line indicates that specific effect of lesion on corticolimbic feedback (eg, decreased inhibition or increased excitation) is unknown. DA indicates dopamine.

indirectly through numerous other areas that also send projections to the mesocortical dopamine system.

Whatever the precise physiology of this system, it also appears to play an important role in responding to stress. It has long been known that dopamine metabolism in the brain increases when an animal is under physical stress such as pain or shock.[89,90] Only recently, however, have the unique responses of the mesocortical dopamine system to stress been described. If an animal is placed in a cage and administered electric shock, dopamine metabolism increases in both mesolimbic and mesocortical terminal fields.[91] If the animal is returned to the cage but not shocked, dopamine metabolism still increases in the prefrontal cortex but does not change elsewhere.[91] While all dopamine systems respond to visceral stress, the prefrontal afferentation system is uniquely sensitive to experiential stress. A similarly selective response of mesocortical dopamine neurons to a pharmacologic model of anxiety has been reported.[92] It is tempting to infer from these experiments that prefrontal dopamine afferentation is an important physiological mechanism in experiential stress management and that deafferentation would leave an organism at a distinct behavioral disadvantage in managing such stresses.

It is conceivable that mesocortical dopamine projections evolved as a means of increasing prefrontal cortical function when there is a critical need for it, such as at times of stress where judgment and abstract concepts must be called into action. Since responding to experiential and psychological stresses often involves surveying the present in terms of past experience and making choices for the future, it is not farfetched to assume that this process places a heavy demand on dorsolateral prefrontal function. If dopaminergic afferents to the prefrontal cortex are one of the mechanisms involved in meeting this demand, a lesion that disrupts these projections or interferes with their function at the cortical level might render an individual physiologically incapable of making appropriate cognitive responses to stressful situations. Moreover, because the prefrontal cortex may not be receiving appropriate information about the state of mesolimbic dopaminergic activity, it may be incapable of sending appropriate feedback, predisposing to unmodulated mesolimbic dopamine overactivity and psychosis.

These considerations suggest clues as to why stress is associated with clinical decompensation in schizophrenia. If dopaminergic mechanisms involved in the activation of the prefrontal cortex are defective in patients with this illness, then the normal experiential stress response, ie, enhanced mesocortical dopaminergic function and prefrontal activation, will also be compromised. These patients cannot meet the demand for prefrontal function because they are lacking in this highly evolved physiological adaptation mechanism. In other words, stress-related decompensation may represent a failure to respond, not an excessive response.

DOPAMINE AND BRAIN DEVELOPMENT

The final element in this thesis about the pathogenesis of schizophrenia is the similarity in the course of development of the brain's dopamine systems and of the areas affected by the "lesion." If dopamine is an important variable in the

23

pathophysiology of schizophrenia, and normal developmental changes help determine the time of onset of the illness, then one might assume that something special is happening to dopamine systems at this critical time in development. The results of recent research in animals and humans support this assumption and suggest that early adulthood is the time of maximum dopaminergic activity in the brain. In the monkey, the level of dopamine metabolism in the prefrontal cortex peaks at early adulthood.[93] Furthermore, the regional specificity of this activity is most clearly established after sexual maturity.[93] In postmortem studies of the adult human cortex, concentrations of dopamine and its metabolites have been shown to be highest in early adulthood.[94]

A similar age pattern for subcortical dopamine activity has been reported. Studies of postmortem mesolimbic dopamine receptors have suggested that peak activity occurs during early adulthood.[95] The same finding has been observed using radiolabeled methylspiperone and positron emission tomography in studies of subcortical dopamine receptor activity during life.[96]

SYNTHESIS

It thus appears that several developmental factors possibly related to the pathogenesis of schizophrenia converge in early adulthood. It is a time of anatomical and functional maturation for certain highly evolved and complex brain regions that are important for adaptation to the vagaries and challenges of human independent living. It is a time of considerable environmental and psychological adventure, if not stress, for most individuals. It is also a time at which brain dopamine systems reach peak activity. If an individual enters this stage of life with a lesion that compromises these maturing neural systems, especially those of the prefrontal cortex, he or she might be impaired in making necessary physiological and behavioral adaptations. If the lesion does not permit prefrontal dopamine activity to respond appropriately to experiential and psychological stresses and to keep pace developmentally with mesolimbic dopamine activity, a chain reaction could be started that might lead to a schizophrenialike behavioral decompensation.

One scenario for this decompensation might be as follows. Faced with stresses that demand maximum prefrontal cognitive function and a lesion impairing one of the mechanisms that augment this function (ie, dopaminergic afferentation), the individual cannot make the physiological and cognitive adaptations required and instead manifests behavior that seems inappropriate, thinking that is confused, perseverative, and perhaps delusional, and, ultimately, social withdrawal. Faced with mesolimbic dopamine activity that is peaking for normal developmental reasons as well as in response to somatic stresses, and that usually is modulated by corticofugal feedback, the individual cannot control this activity because the lesion is interrupting the mesocortical-corticofugal feedback system, and he or she becomes, as a result, agitated, fearful, and hallucinative. Environmental interventions that limit or arrest this chain reaction may facilitate remission or at least improve function.

In addition, much of the natural course of the defect and psychotic symptoms of schizophrenia, once they are established, may reflect the normal gradual regression of brain dopaminergic function during the adult years. Longitudinal studies of patients with schizophrenia indicate that with time, hallucinations and other "positive" psychotic features tend to become less florid, while defect symptoms become more prominent.[97] To the extent that "positive" features

relate to mesolimbic dopaminergic overactivity, their diminution over time parallels the decline in subcortical dopaminergic activity that has been shown to accompany normal aging.[96,96] Similarly, to the extent that defect symptoms relate to mesocortical dopaminergic underactivity, their increase over time parallels the loss of dopamine from the prefrontal cortex that also accompanies normal aging.[96] Moreover, the time-honored clinical observations that female patients with schizophrenia have a later age at onset and a less malignant course may relate to the findings that dopamine activity peaks later and regresses more slowly in normal women.[96]

THE QUESTION OF ETIOLOGY

The thesis put forth herein does not address etiology. Numerous causes of the "lesion" may exist. Many of the current etiologic hypotheses of schizophrenia could account for the lesion, including a hereditary encephalopathy or predilection to environmental injury, an infection or postinfectious state, damage from an immunologic disorder, perinatal trauma or encephalopathy, toxin exposure early in development, a primary metabolic disease, or other early developmental events. Though they seem highly unlikely, two other possibilities cannot be excluded at the present time. One is that early developmental psychosocial experience could produce a structural brain lesion in plastic neural systems. While basic research has begun to demonstrate that experience can affect neuronal structure,[98,99] it is probably a giant leap to assume that the lesion in schizophrenia could be the result of such factors. The second possibility is that the lesion may not reflect a discrete event or illness process at all, but rather one end of the developmental spectrum that for genetic and/or other reasons 0.5% of the population will fall into. In other words, there may not be a true lesion at all, but simply a relative hypoplasia or dysplasia of the systems implicated, resulting in a quantitative physiological deficit. This possibility could represent the so-called diathesis in diathesis-stress models of schizophrenia,[100] or perhaps the "liability" factor that appears to be inherited.[101]

It has long been appealing to consider that there may be many causes of the lesion and thus of schizophrenia. This could help explain the clinical and biologic heterogeneity that is characteristic of the disorder. It could also explain the apparent variability in the lesion. Researchers have found it productive to view this heterogeneity as an indication that there are subgroups or subtypes of schizophrenia, perhaps based on different causes.[102,103] However, the evidence pointing to a structural lesion has not supported the notion of subgroups. In both the postmortem and the CT anatomical studies, the distributions of the data tend to be normal, not bimodal or polymodal. In other words, there are not segregated clusters of patients with similar findings, as one might expect if discrete pathogenic subgroups existed. Instead, what is almost always reported in these studies is a pathologic continuum. This is analogous to what is found in CT and postmortem anatomical studies of Alzheimer's disease and many other brain disorders. It suggests an alternative approach to clinical heterogeneity, in that the extent of the pathology may determine clinical differences. Patients on one end of the continuum might seem clinically far removed from patients on the other end, despite a common pathogenesis and perhaps even cause. It follows that the more extensive the lesion, the greater will be the prefrontal dysfunction, the more the defect symptoms, and the less the illness will appear to resolve with pharmacologic blockade of subcortical dopamine receptors. Not surprisingly, the larger the lesion, the poorer would be

24

the overall prognosis. These assumptions are supported by studies of the clinical implications of cerebral ventricular size on CT scans, in that patients with more pathology (ie, larger ventricles) tend to have more features associated with poor prognosis.[17]

IMPLICATIONS FOR RESEARCH AND TREATMENT

Many of the experimental findings and much of the speculation presented herein represent fertile ground for future research. With respect to the lesion, it is obvious that the renaissance of anatomical studies in schizophrenia is only beginning. Most of the postmortem findings require extensive replication, necessitating an investment by psychiatry in brain banking and in neuropathologic techniques and expertise. The DLPFC is especially understudied, both anatomically and neurochemically. It is important that future postmortem investigations carefully identify and dissect the DLPFC and not abdicate in favor of a "piece of frontal lobe." It is also imperative that laboratories conducting postmortem histopathologic investigations combine anatomical and neurochemical analyses on the same brains so that the relationship of these variables can be addressed. By utilizing the newer technique of magnetic resonance imaging, it should be possible to test during life whether quantitative limbic and prefrontal pathology exists at the onset of illness and whether prefrontal pathology is limited to the DLPFC.

To test the thesis that onset is determined by maturation of critical brain regions, it might be helpful to identify another biologic covariate of onset. One possibility is sexual maturation. If this variable is a factor in the maturation of the relevant limbic and prefrontal regions, then one could hypothesize that the onset of schizophrenia should be occurring earlier today than it did at the turn of the century. Notwithstanding methodologic problems associated with changes in diagnostic criteria, these data may be retrievable. An alternative approach would be to look at individuals who experience precocious puberty. It would be predicted by the arguments presented herein that if there are patients with schizophrenia among such persons, the onset of the illness would be earlier than in the general population. In testing these hypotheses, however, it must be considered that sexual maturity may be only a coincidental covariate of the maturation of the important brain areas and not a neurobiologic determinant.

The roles of dopamine in DLPFC function and in the normal adaptation to stress are subjects ripe for extensive research. A number of basic animal experiments are needed to define better the mesocortical-corticolimbic dopamine loops, both anatomically and neurochemically. It is likely that other neurotransmitter systems will become implicated as well. Preliminary evidence of the delayed effects of an infantile DLPFC lesion on adult behavior, combined with the experiment of Pycock et al,[87] suggest a primate model of

schizophrenia. If the infantile lesion produces at early adulthood not just specific cognitive deficits but also subcortical dopamine overactivity, we might have a compelling animal model for this illness.

It may be possible to study mesocortical dopamine activity during life with radiolabeled precursors of dopamine, such as levodopa labeled with fluorine 18, or with radiolabeled specific dopamine type 1 receptor agents and positron emission tomography. It would be of interest to study dopamine metabolism during a prefrontal mediated behavior, eg, performance of the Wisconsin Card Sorting Test. This might show whether mesocortical dopamine underactivity was indeed the neurochemical lesion correlated with this behavior in schizophrenia. It might, on the other hand, demonstrate that the lesion in schizophrenia involves an uncoupling of prefrontal dopamine activity and postsynaptic neuronal metabolism. While it is hard to believe that dopamine metabolism has not been studied selectively in postmortem specimens of DLPFC, such is the case, and it should be remedied, despite the possibilities that antemortem medication may obscure any findings and that differences between patients and controls may be related to or obscured by stress.

Finally, there are a number of implications here for the treatment of schizophrenia. If the core neurochemical deficit is mesocortical dopamine deficiency, then replacement therapy should be miraculous! Unfortunately, we lack selective mesocortical dopamimetic agents. Administering regionally nonspecific dopamimetics is usually counterproductive, perhaps because they also increase mesolimbic dopamine activity. It behooves us, therefore, to encourage a basic neuropharmacologic effort to develop regionally selective agents. Preliminary animal data suggest that the pharmacology of dopamine projections to the cortex is sufficiently distinct from that of projections to the limbic system to permit the development of regionally active drugs.[104] In addition, if more can be learned about the neurochemistry of corticolimbic feedback, neuropharmacologic intervention could be directed at this side of the loop, bypassing the afferent deficit.

In the meantime, the role of certain nonpharmacologic interventions can be rationalized by the thesis developed herein. Environmental stress-management techniques are logical and desirable, not just because they are empathic but because they may help reduce the demand on physiologically compromised prefrontal neural systems. By the same token, it is not surprising that social-skill training and occupational therapy lessen the frequency of relapse,[105,106] while insight-oriented psychotherapy may do the opposite.[106] The first two treatments probably reduce the demand for autonomous prefrontal function; the latter treatment probably increases it. A neurobiologic translation of the psychoanalytic notion that patients with schizophrenia require in treatment a "lend-lease ego" may be that they require a surrogate DLPFC!

References

1. Meltzer HY, Stahl SM: The dopamine hypothesis of schizophrenia: A review. *Schizophr Bull* 1976;2:19-76.
2. Weinberger DR, Kleinman JE: Observations on the brain in schizophrenia, in Hales RE, Frances AJ (eds): *Psychiatry Update, American Psychiatric Association Annual Review.* Washington, DC, American Psychiatric Association Press, 1986, vol 5, pp 42-67.
3. Weinberger DR: The pathogenesis of schizophrenia: A neurodevelopmental theory, in Nasrallah HA, Weinberger DR (eds): *The Neurology of Schizophrenia.* Amsterdam, Elsevier Science Publishers, 1986, pp 397-406.
4. Adams RD, Lyons G: *Neurology of Hereditary Metabolic Diseases of Children.* New York, McGraw-Hill International Book Co, 1982, pp 5-6, 376-381.
5. Bogerts B, Meertz E, Schonfeldt-Bausch R: Basal ganglia and limbic system pathology in schizophrenia: A morphometric study. *Arch Gen Psychiatry* 1985;42:784-791.
6. Jakob H, Beckmann H: Prenatal development disturbances in the limbic allocortex in schizophrenics. *J Neural Transm* 1986;65:303-326.
7. Stevens JR: Neuropathology of schizophrenia. *Arch Gen Psychiatry* 1982;39:1131-1139.
8. Brown R, Colter N, Corsellis JAN, Crow TJ, Frith CD, Jagoe R, Johnstone EC, Marsh L: Postmortem evidence of structural brain changes in schizophrenia. *Arch Gen Psychiatry* 1986;43:36-42.
9. Kovelman JA, Scheibel AB: A neurohistological correlate of schizophrenia. *Biol Psychiatry* 1984;19:1601-1621.
10. Lesch A, Bogerts B: The diencephalon in schizophrenia: Evidence for reduced thickness of the periventricular grey matter. *Eur Arch Psychiatry*

25

Neurol Sci 1984;234:212-219.

11. Nieto D, Escobar A: Major psychoses, in Minkler J (ed): *Pathology of the Nervous System.* New York, McGraw-Hill International Book Co, 1972, pp 2654-2665.

12. Averback P: Lesions of the nucleus ansa peduncularis in neuropsychiatric disease. *Arch Neurol* 1981;38:230-235.

13. Bogerts B, Hantsch J, Herzer M: A morphometric study of the dopamine containing cell groups in the mesencephalon of normals, Parkinson patients and schizophrenics. *Biol Psychiatry* 1983;18:951-969.

14. Falkai P, Bogerts B: Cell loss in the hippocampus of schizophrenics. *Eur Arch Psychiatry Neurol Sci,* in press.

15. Benes FM, Davidson J, Bird ED: Quantitative cytoarchitectural studies of the cerebral cortex of schizophrenics. *Arch Gen Psychiatry* 1986;43:31-35.

16. Kirch DG, Weinberger DR: Anatomical neuropathology in schizophrenia: Post-mortem findings, in Nasrallah HA, Weinberger DR (eds): *The Neurology of Schizophrenia.* Amsterdam, Elsevier Science Publishers, 1986, pp 325-348.

17. Shelton RC, Weinberger DR: X-Ray computerized tomography studies of schizophrenia: A review and synthesis, in Nasrallah HA, Weinberger DR (eds): *The Neurology of Schizophrenia.* Amsterdam, Elsevier Science Publishers, 1986, pp 207-250.

18. Fuster J: *The Prefrontal Cortex.* New York, Raven Press, 1980.

19. Isaacson RL. *The Limbic System.* New York, Plenum Publishing Corp, 1982.

20. Gloor P, Olivier A, Quesney LF, Anderman F, Horowitz S: The role of the limbic system in experiential phenomena of temporal lobe epilepsy. *Ann Neurol* 1982;12:129-144.

21. Halgren E, Walter RD, Cherlow DG, Crandall PH: Mental phenomena evoked by electrical stimulation of the human hippocampal formation and amygdala. *Brain* 1978;101:83-117.

22. Davison K, Bagley CR: Schizophrenia-like psychoses associated with organic disorders of the central nervous system. *Br J Psychiatry* 1969;113 (suppl 1):18-69.

23. Davison K: Schizophrenia-like psychoses associated with organic cerebral disorders: A review. *Psychiatr Dev* 1983;1:1-34.

24. Strauss JS, Carpenter WT Jr, Bartko JJ: The diagnosis and understanding of schizophrenia: III. Speculations on the processes that underlie schizophrenic symptoms and signs. *Schizophr Bull* 1974;1:61-69.

25. Andreasen NC: Negative vs positive schizophrenia. *Arch Gen Psychiatry* 1982;39:784-788.

26. Seidman LJ: Schizophrenia and brain dysfunction: An integration of recent neurodiagnostic findings. *Psychol Bull* 1984;94:195-235.

27. Goldberg TE, Weinberger DR: Methodological issues in the neuropsychological approach to schizophrenia, in Nasrallah HA, Weinberger DR (eds): *The Neurology of Schizophrenia.* Amsterdam, Elsevier Science Publishers, 1986, pp 141-156.

28. Stuss DT, Benson DF: Neuropsychological studies of the frontal lobes. *Psychol Bull* 1984;95:3-28.

29. Dimascio A: The frontal lobes, in Heilman KM, Valenstein E (eds): *Clinical Neuropsychology.* New York, Oxford University Press, 1979, pp 360-412.

30. Grafman J, Vance SC, Weingartner H, Salazar AM: Specific effects of orbito-frontal brain wounds upon regulation of mood. *Neuropsychologia,* in press.

31. Hecaen H, Albert ML: Disorders of mental functioning related to the frontal lobes, in Benson DF, Blumer D (eds): *Psychiatric Aspects of Neurological Disease.* New York, Grune & Stratton, 1975, 137-149.

32. Weinberger DR, Berman KF, Zec RF: Physiological dysfunction of dorsolateral prefrontal cortex in schizophrenia: I. Regional cerebral blood flow (rCBF) evidence. *Arch Gen Psychiatry* 1986;43:114-125.

33. Berman KF, Zec RF, Weinberger DR: Physiological dysfunction of dorsolateral prefrontal cortex in schizophrenia: II. Role of medication, attention, and mental effort. *Arch Gen Psychiatry* 1986;43:126-143.

34. Weinberger DR, DeLisi LE, Perman G, Targum S, Wyatt RJ: Computed tomography scans in schizophreniform disorder and other acute psychiatric patients. *Arch Gen Psychiatry* 1982;39:778-783.

35. Nyback H, Berggren BM, Hindmarsh T: Computed tomography of the brain in patients with acute psychosis and in healthy volunteers. *Acta Psychiatr Scand* 1982;65:403-414.

36. Schultz SC, Koller MM, Kishore P: Ventricular enlargement in teenage patients with schizophrenia spectrum disorder. *Am J Psychiatry* 1983;140:1592-1595.

37. Weinberger DR, Cannon-Spoor E, Potkin SG, Wyatt RJ: Poor premorbid adjustment and CT scan abnormalities in chronic schizophrenia. *Am J Psychiatry* 1980;137:1410-1413.

38. DeLisi LE, Schwartz CC, Targum SD, Byrnes SM, Cannon-Spoor E, Weinberger DR, Wyatt RJ: Ventricular brain enlargement and outcome of acute schizophrenic disorder. *J Psychiatr Res* 1983;9:169-171.

39. Williams AO, Reveley MA, Kolakowska T, Andern M, Mandelbrote BM: Schizophrenia with good and poor outcome: II. Cerebral ventricular size and its clinical significance. *Br J Psychiatry* 1985;146:239-246.

40. Turner SW, Toone BK, Brett-Jones JR: Computerized tomographic scan changes in early schizophrenia. *Psychol Med* 1986;16:219-225.

41. Glaser GH: Limbic epilepsy in childhood. *J Nerv Ment Dis* 1967;144:

391-397.

42. Chandler JH, Reed TE, DeJong RN: Huntington's chorea in Michigan: III. Clinical observations. *Neurology* 1960;10:148-153.

43. Garron DC: Huntington's chorea and schizophrenia, in Barbeau A, Chase TN, Paulson O (eds): *Advances in Neurology.* New York, Raven Press, 1973, pp 729-734.

44. Beard AW: The association of hepatolenticular degeneration with schizophrenia. *Acta Neurol Scand* 1959;34:411-428.

45. Manowitz P, Kling A, Kohn H: Clinical course of adult metachromatic leukodystrophy presenting as schizophrenia. *J Nerv Ment Dis* 1978;166: 500-506.

46. Cummings JL, Gosenfeld LF, Houlihan JP, McCaffrey T: Neuropsychiatric disturbances associated with idiopathic calcification of the basal ganglia. *Biol Psychiatry* 1983;18:591-601.

47. Greenbaum JV, Lurie LA: Encephalitis as a causative factor in behavioral disorders of children. *JAMA* 1948;136:923-930.

48. Feinglass EJ, Arnett FC, Dorsch CA, Zizic M, Stevens MD: Neuropsychiatric manifestations of systemic lupus erythematosus: Diagnosis, clinical spectrum and relationship to other features of the disease. *Medicine* 1976;55:323-339.

49. Brown P, Rodgers-Johnson P, Cathala F, Gibbs CJ, Gadjusek DG: Creutzfeldt-Jakob disease of long duration: Clinicopathological characteristics, transmissibility, and differential diagnosis. *Ann Neurol* 1984;16: 295-304.

50. Achte KA, Hillbom E, Salberg V: Psychoses following war brain injuries. *Acta Psychiatr Scand* 1969;45:1-18.

51. Ludwig CL, Smith MT, Godfrey AD, Armbrustmacher V: A clinicopathological study of 323 patients with oligodendrogliomas. *Ann Neurol* 1986;19:15-21.

52. Hruska RE, Silbergeld EK: Increased dopamine receptor sensitivity after estrogen treatment using the rat rotation model. *Science* 1980;208: 1466-1468.

53. Goldman-Rakic PS, Isseroff A, Schwartz ML, Bugbee NM: The neurobiology of cognitive development, in Mussen P (ed): *Handbook of Child Psychology, Biology and Infancy Development.* New York, John Wiley & Sons Inc, 1983, pp 281-344.

54. Yakovlev PI, LeCours A-R: The myelogenetic cycles of regional maturation of the brain, in Minkowski A (ed): *Regional Development of the Brain in Early Life.* Boston, Blackwell Scientific Publications Inc, 1964, pp 3-70.

55. Huttenlocher PR: Synaptic density in human frontal cortex: Developmental changes and effects of aging. *Brain Res* 1979;163:195-205.

56. Rakic P, Bourgeois J-P, Eckenhoff MF, Zecevic N, Goldman-Rakic PS: Concurrent overproduction of synapses in diverse regions of the primate cerebral cortex. *Science* 1986;232:232-235.

57. Ingvar DH: 'Memory of the future': An essay on the temporal organization of conscious awareness. *Hum Neurobiol* 1985;4:127-136.

58. Piaget J: *The Origins of Intelligence in Children.* New York, WW Norton & Co Inc, 1963.

59. Milner B: Effects of different brain lesions on card sorting. *Arch Neurol* 1963;9:100-110.

60. Kirk V, Kelly MS: Children's differential performance in selected dorsolateral prefrontal and posterior cortical functions: A developmental perspective. Presented at the International Neuropsychological Society Annual Meeting, Denver, Jan 17, 1986.

61. Goldman PS, Alexander GE: Maturation of prefrontal cortex in the monkey revealed by local reversible cryogenic depression. *Nature* 1977;267: 613-615.

62. Tucker TJ, Kling A: Differential effects of early and late lesions of frontal granular cortex in the monkey. *Brain Res* 1967;5:377-389.

63. Goldman PS: Functional development of the prefrontal cortex in early life and the problem of neuronal plasticity. *Exp Neurol* 1971;32:366-387.

64. Kraepelin E: *Dementia Praecox and Paraphenia.* Melbourne, Fla, Robert E Krieger Publishing Co Inc, 1971.

65. Bleuler E: *Dementia Praecox or the Group of Schizophrenias.* New York, New York International Press, 1950.

66. Fish B: Neurobiologic antecedents of schizophrenia in children. *Arch Gen Psychiatry* 1977;34:1297-1313.

67. Goldberg T, Weinberger DR: Methodological issues in the neuropsychological approach to schizophrenia, in Nasrallah HA, Weinberger DR (eds): *The Neurology of Schizophrenia.* Amsterdam, Elsevier Science Publishers, 1986, pp 141-156.

68. Carlsson A: Antipsychotic drugs, neurotransmitters and schizophrenia. *Am J Psychiatry* 1978;135:164-173.

69. Creese I, Burt DR, Snyder SH: Dopamine receptor binding predicts clinical and pharmacological potencies of antischizophrenic drugs. *Science* 1976;192:481-483.

70. Crow TJ: Positive and negative schizophrenic symptoms and the role of dopamine. *Br J Psychiatry* 1980;137:383-386.

71. Seeman P, Ulpian C, Bergeron C: Bimodal distribution of dopamine receptor densities in brains of schizophrenics. *Science* 1984;225:728-731.

72. Wong DF, Wagner HN Jr, Tune LE, Dannals RF, Pearlson GD, Links JM, Tamminga CA, Broussolle EP, Ravert HT, Wilson AA, Thomas Toung JK, Malat J, Williams JA, O'Tuama LA, Snyder SH, Kuhar MJ, Gjedde A: Positron emission tomography reveals elevated D₂ dopamine receptors in

26

drug-naive schizophrenics. Science 1986;234:1558-1563.

73. Glowinski J, Tassin JP, Thierry AM: The mesocorticoprefrontal dopaminergic neurons. Trends Neurosci 1984;7:415-418.

74. Brozowski TJ, Brown RM, Rosvold HE, Goldman PS: Cognitive deficit caused by regional depletion of dopamine in prefrontal cortex of rhesus monkey. Science 1979;205:929-932.

75. Langston JW, Ballard P, Tetrud JW, Irwin I: Chronic parkinsonism in humans due to a product of meperidine-analogue synthesis. Science 983;219:979-980.

76. Stern Y, Langston JW: Intellectual changes in patients with MPTP-induced parkinsonism. Neurology 1985;35:1506-1509.

77. Bowen FP, Kamienny RS, Burns MM, Yahr ND: Parkinsonism: Effects of levodopa treatment on concept formation. Neurology 1975;25:701-704.

78. Scatton B, Rouquier L, Javoy-Agid F, Agid Y: Dopamine deficiency in the cerebral cortex in Parkinson disease. Neurology 1982;32:1039-1040.

79. Gerlack J, Luhdorf K: The effect of L-dopa on young patients with simple schizophrenia treated with neuroleptic drugs: A double-blind cross-over trial with madopar and placebo. Psychopharmacology 1975;44:105-110.

80. Ogura C, Kishimoto A, Nakao T: Clinical effects of L-dopa on chizophrenia. Curr Ther Res 1976;20:308-318.

81. Rifkin A, Quitkin F, Klein DF: Akinesia. Arch Gen Psychiatry 975;32:672-674.

82. Elsworth JD, Leahy DJ, Roth RH Jr, Redmond D Jr: Homovanillic acid concentrations in brain, CSF and plasma as indicators of central dopamine function in primates. J Neural Transm 1987;68:51-62.

83. Lindstrom LH: Low HVA and normal 5HIAA CSF levels in drug-free chizophrenic patients compared to healthy volunteers: Correlations to symptomatology and family history. Psychiatry Res 1985;14:265-273.

84. Weinberger DR, Berman KF: Huntington's disease and subcortical dementia: rCBF evidence. Neurology 1985;35(suppl 1):109.

85. Weinberger DR, Berman KF, Chase TN: Prefrontal cortex physiological activation in Parkinson's disease: Effect of L-dopa. Neurology 1986;36 suppl 1):170.

86. McCulloch J, Savaki HE, McCulloch MC: The distribution of altera-ions in energy metabolism in the rat brain produced by apomorphine. rain Res 1982;243:67-80.

87. Pycock CJ, Kerwin RW, Carter CJ: Effect of lesion of cortical opamine terminals on subcortical dopamine in rats. Nature 1980;286:74-77.

88. Thierry A-M, Tassin J-P, Glowinski J: Biochemical and electro-hysical studies of the mesocortical dopamine system, in Descarsies L, Leader TR, Jasper HH (eds): Monoamine Innervation of Cerebral Cortex. New York, Alan R Liss Inc, 1984, pp 233-262.

89. Bliss EL, Ailion J: Relationship of stress and activity to brain opamine and homovanillic acid. Life Sci 1971;10:1161-1169.

90. Thierry AM, Tassin JP, Blanc G, Glowinski J: Selective activation of the mesocortical DA system by stress. Nature 1976;263:242-244.

91. Herman JP, Guilloneau D, Dantzer R: Differential effects of inescapa-ble foot shocks and of stimuli previously paired with inescapable foot shock on dopamine turnover in cortical and limbic areas of the rat. Life Sci 1982;30:2207-2214.

92. Tam S-Y, Roth RH: Selective increase in dopamine metabolism in the prefrontal cortex by the anxiogenic beta-carboline FG 7142. Biochem Pharmacol 1985;34:1595-1598.

93. Goldman-Rakic PS, Brown RM: Postnatal development of monoamine content and synthesis in the cerebral cortex of rhesus monkeys. Dev Brain Res 1982;4:339-349.

94. McGeer PL, McGeer EG: Neurotransmitters in the aging brain, in Darrison AM, Thompson RH (eds): The Molecular Basis of Neuro-pathology. London, Edward Arnold Ltd, 1981, pp 631-648.

95. Bzowej NH, Seeman P: Age and dopamine D2 receptors in human brain. Soc Neurosci Abstr 1985;11:889.

96. Wong DF, Wagner HN Jr, Dannals RF, Links JM, Frost JJ, Ravert HT, Wilson AA, Rosenbaum AE: Effects of age on dopamine and serotonin receptors measured by positron emission tomography in the living human brain. Science 1984;226:1393-1396.

97. Pfohl B, Winokur G: The evolution of symptoms in institutionalized hebephrenic catatonic schizophrenics. Br J Psychiatry 1982;141:567-572.

98. Kandel ER: From metapsychology to molecular biology: Explora-tions into the nature of anxiety. Am J Psychiatry 1983;140:1277-1293.

99. Haracz JL: Neural plasticity in schizophrenia. Schizophr Bull 1985; 11:191-229.

100. Zubin J, Spring B: Vulnerability: A new view of schizophrenia. J Abnorm Psychol 1977;86:103-126.

101. Kendler KS: Genetics of schizophrenia, in Hales RE, Frances AJ (eds): Psychiatry Update, American Psychiatric Association Annual Review. Washington, DC, American Psychiatric Association Press, 1986, pp 42-67.

102. Meltzer HY: Biology of schizophrenia subtypes: A review and proposal for method of study. Schizophr Bull 1979;5:460-479.

103. Crow TJ: Molecular pathology of schizophrenia: More than one disease process. Br Med J 1980;280:66-68.

104. Bannon MJ, Roth RH: Pharmacology of mesocortical dopamine neurons. Pharmacol Rev 1983;35:53-68.

105. Liberman RP, Musser KT, Wallace CT: Social skill training for schizophrenic individuals at risk for relapse. Am J Psychiatry 1986;147: 523-526.

106. Linn MQW, Caffey EM, Klett J, Hogarty GE, Lamb HR: Day treatment and psychotropic drugs in the aftercare of schizophrenic patients. Arch Gen Psychiatry 1979;36:1055-1066.

27

Lifetime Prevalence, Demographic Risk Factors, and Diagnostic Validity of Nonaffective Psychosis as Assessed in a US Community Sample

The National Comorbidity Survey

Kenneth S. Kendler, MD; Timothy J. Gallagher, PhD; Jamie M. Abelson, MSW; Ronald C. Kessler, PhD

Background: We seek to estimate lifetime prevalence and demographic correlates of nonaffective psychosis in the US population assessed by a computer-analyzed structured interview and a senior clinician.

Methods: In the National Comorbidity Survey, a probability subsample of 5877 respondents were administered a screen for psychotic symptoms. Based on the response to this screening, detailed follow-up interviews were conducted by mental health professionals (n=454). The initial screen and clinical reinterview were reviewed by a senior clinician. Results are presented for narrowly (schizophrenia or schizophreniform disorder) and broadly (all nonaffective psychoses) defined psychotic illness.

Results: One or more psychosis screening questions were endorsed by 28.4% of individuals. By computer algorithm, lifetime prevalences of narrowly and broadly defined psychotic illness were 1.3% and 2.2%, respectively. Of those assigned a narrow diagnosis by the computer, the senior clinician assigned narrow and broad diagnoses to 10% and 37%, respectively. By clinician agnosis, lifetime prevalence rates of narrowly and broadly defined psychosis were 0.2% and 0.7%, respectively. clinician diagnosis of nonaffective psychosis was significantly associated with low income; unemployment; a marital status of single, divorced, or separated; and urban residence. Clinician confirmation of a computer diagnosis was predicted by hospitalization, neuroleptic treatment, duration of illness, enduring impairment, and thought disorder.

Conclusions: Lifetime prevalence estimates of psychosis in community samples are strongly influenced by methods of assessment and diagnosis. Although results using computer algorithms were similar in the National Comorbidity Survey and Epidemiologic Catchment Area studies, diagnoses so obtained agreed poorly with clinical diagnoses. Accurate assessment of psychotic illness in epidemiologic samples may require collection of extensive contextual information for clinician review.

Arch Gen Psychiatry. 1996;53:1022-1031

From the Departments of Psychiatry and Human Genetics, Medical College of Virginia/Virginia Commonwealth University, Richmond, Va (Dr Kendler); the Department of Psychiatry, Washington University School of Medicine, St Louis, Mo (Dr Gallagher); and the Institute for Social Research, University of Michigan, Ann Arbor (Ms Abelson and Dr Kessler).

LTHOUGH epidemiologic investigations of psychotic illness have been conducted for many years,[1-5] the interpretation of results continues to be beset by methodological problems.[6] In the general population, psychotic symptoms are rare and their evaluation is problematic, requiring the elimination of respondent misunderstanding, schizotypal traits, drug-induced states, and culturally sanctioned magical or religious beliefs. These epidemiologic studies have relied largely on 2 sources of diagnostic information: psychiatric hospital records and interviews. While hospital records contain information about contemporaneously recorded psychotic symptoms and signs, unless specifically designed for research, they usually vary so widely in detail and

accuracy that applying diagnostic criteria to them is problematic. Depending on the organization of psychiatric care, maintenance of medical records, and consent requirements, such records may be difficult to obtain. Furthermore, hospital records produce estimates of *treated* prevalence. In western countries, 15% to 20% of subjects with schizophrenia in the general population (and probably more with milder psychotic illnesses) have had no prior contact with mental health professionals.[7]

With personal interviews, it is possible to estimate total rather than treated

---

See Subjects and Methods on next page

28

SUBJECTS AND METHODS

SAMPLE

The NCS, a nationwide survey of the US population ages 15 through 54 years, is based on a stratified, multistage area probability sample of the noninstitutionalized civilian population in the 48 coterminous states.[17] The NCS included a nonresponse survey, carried out in a sample of initial nonrespondents who were offered a substantial financial incentive to complete a short form of the diagnostic interview. The survey data were weighted to compensate for this nonresponse. The data were also weighted to adjust for variation in probabilities of selection within households, for differential selection of new households, and for the underrepresentation of difficult-to-reach households. These weighted data, finally, were poststratified by means of an iterative procedure to approximate the national population distributions of the cross-classification of age, sex, race or ethnicity, marital status, education, living arrangements, region, and urbanicity as defined by the 1989 US National Health Interview Survey.[19]

The NCS used a 2-phase sample design, in the first phase of which the part I diagnostic interview was administered to all 8098 respondents. In the second phase, a part II risk factor interview, including a screen for psychotic symptoms, was administered to a probability subsample of 5877 respondents consisting of (a) all part I respondents aged 15 to 24 years, (b) all older part I respondents who were positive on initial questions in 1 or more diagnostic sections of the CIDI (possible cases), and (c) a 1-in-6 random subsample of all remaining part I respondents. All analyses using the part II data were weighted to reflect probability of selection.

INITIAL DIAGNOSTIC ASSESSMENT

The instrument used in the initial assessment, administered by the highly experienced field staff of the Survey Research Center at the University of Michigan, was a modified University of Michigan version of the CIDI[18] (UM-CIDI). Diagnoses were generated by the use of the CIDI diagnostic program.[20] Interviewers completed a 7-day training program for the NCS.

The UM-CIDI contained the 13 probes to screen for psychotic symptoms from the original CIDI plus follow-up questions about treatment, impairment, and possible organic causes. In addition, the UM-CIDI had interviewers rate the presence of 4 "signs" of psychosis contained in the original CIDI: neologisms, thought disorder, flat affect, and "behaves as if hallucinating." While the original CIDI provided only a small space for the interviewer to record examples of psychotic symptoms, the UM-CIDI provided an entire page for each psychotic symptom on which the interviewer was to record verbatim responses to probes about the nature and/or causes of the putative psychotic symptom. The UM-CIDI contains an original CIDI item in which the interviewer assesses whether the putative psychotic symptom was "realistic."

REINTERVIEW

We developed a new instrument ("Section K Telephone Reinterview") to conduct clinical reinterviews with individuals who screened positive for psychosis in the CIDI. While this interview maintained the structure of the original CIDI, it added numerous additional probes for each stem question, inquiring in detail about the putative psychotic symptoms.

To generate a computer diagnosis of psychotic disorders, we applied the CIDI computer algorithm to the reinterview, using only those items derived from the original CIDI. To score a psychotic symptom as present, this algorithm requires that (1) the interviewer rate the symptom as "not realistic"; (2) the symptom be accompanied by either treatment seeking or major impairment ("interfere with life or activities a lot"); and (3) the symptom not be due to illness or injury, medications, drugs or alcohol. In addition to diagnoses of schizophrenia and schizophreniform disorder, we generated computer diagnoses for NAP, which equaled *DSM-III-R*[21] categories of schizophrenia, schizophreniform disorder, schizoaffective disorder, delusional disorder, or psychosis not otherwise specified.

In the NCS 1868 individuals responded yes to at least 1 of the 13 stem questions for psychotic symptoms in the

Continued on next page

prevalence. Pioneered in early Scandinavian studies[8,9] where personal assessments were performed by psychiatrists, this approach was also used in the Epidemiologic Catchment Area (ECA) study,[10] in which lay interviewers administered the Diagnostic Interview Schedule (DIS),[11] which contains sections assessing schizophrenia and schizophreniform disorder.

Personal interviews, however, also have limitations as assessment tools for psychotic illness. They may generate false negatives due to inadequate probing or denial of prior psychotic symptoms.[12-14] Through misinterpretation, lay interviewers may assign false-positive diagnoses of psychosis.[12,14-16]

Herein, we present results on lifetime prevalence (LTP), psychosocial correlates, and patterns of comorbidity of nonaffective psychosis (NAP) from the National Comorbidity Survey (NCS).[17] A unique feature of this study was a 5-tiered approach to assessing psychotic symptoms. First, lay interviewers administered a revised version of the Composite International Diagnostic Interview (CIDI),[18] including a section screening for psychotic symptoms. Second, interviews containing possible psychotic symptoms were sorted into varying categories of the assessed probability of true psychotic illness. Third, a small proportion of subjects from the low-probability and all subjects from the high-probability classes were recontacted by experienced mental health professionals and administered the psychosis section of the CIDI plus extensive additional probes. Fourth, the CIDI computer algorithm was applied to the completed follow-up interviews, generating computer diagnoses of psychotic disorder. Fifth, a senior psychiatric diagnostician (K.S.K.) reviewed all available information and made best estimate clinical diagnoses.

29

lay-administered UM-CIDI. After weighting, 28.4%±1.3% (mean±SE) of the US population was estimated to endorse 1 or more probes for psychosis. We developed a 7-category classification for these interviews in which individuals who responded to more than 1 psychotic probe were assigned the highest score for any item they endorsed. These categories (and the number of individuals so classified) were (1) misunderstood (n=143), (2) realistic (n=418), (3) "light" (n=431, unusual experiences, usually occurring rarely, that raised no suspicion of psychosis), (4) need more information (n=313, insufficient information to form any clear judgment but available information raises little question of true psychosis), (5) possible (n=406, at least a suspicion of psychosis), (6) drug related (n=117, possible or probable psychotic symptoms that occurred only in relation to drug use), and (7) probable or definite (n=40).

Individuals who classified the CIDI interviews and conducted reinterviews had either a Master's or Doctoral degree in a mental health–related field or a Bachelor's degree and at least 4 years of clinical experience. They were trained and supervised by one of us (J.M.A.), a clinical social worker with extensive experience in the evaluation of psychotic patients. Difficulties were discussed with one of us (K.S.K.).

We did not reinterview those classified as "misunderstood" or "realistic," as we were confident that they did not have a psychotic disorder. We reinterviewed 38 individuals with "light" symptoms and 38 "needing more information." As we rated none of these 76 respondents as having true psychotic symptoms, we did not reinterview other individuals in these categories.

We attempted to reinterview all individuals classified as categories 5, 6, or 7, with 1 exception: a subsample of subjects who had been previously recontacted for a validation study of major depression were not recontacted for this study because of concerns about respondent burden. The numbers of individuals whom we tried to reinterview, could not contact, refused, and successfully reinterviewed were for category 5: 368, 83, 9, and 276, respectively; for category 6: 115, 42, 1, and 72, respectively; and for category 7: 38, 7, 1, and 30, respectively.

Reinterviewers were provided, for each respondent, information concerning religion, employment, education,

CIDI diagnoses of major depression, mania or generalized anxiety disorder, and previous responses to the CIDI Psychotic Disorders probes. They were instructed to probe items initially responded to positively plus any additional relevant items. The reinterview lasted an average of 24 minutes (range, 5-120 minutes), and editing time averaged 40 minutes.

The diagnostic arbiter (K.S.K.) in this study has had extensive experience diagnosing psychotic disorders in nonclinical populations with high reliability.[22-26] Blind to prior classification, he reviewed interviews, associated demographic information, reinterviews, and relevant sections of the original CIDI for 172 individuals: 30 randomly selected from the group classified as "easy," all 138 from the group classified as "difficult," and 4 "probable or definite" CIDI cases not successfully reinterviewed. The 30 "easy" and 138 "difficult" cases were also reviewed by the second diagnostician (J.M.A.). For NAP, raw and chance-corrected agreements (κ)[27] between the 2 diagnosticians were 0.93 and 0.82, respectively.

ANALYSIS PROCEDURES

The data analyzed in this report were obtained from a stratified multistage sample and were subsequently weighted to adjust for differential probabilities of selection and nonresponse. Poststratification to the total US population in the target age range was also made. As a result of this complex sample design and weighting, estimates of SEs based on the usual assumptions of equal-probability simple random sampling are biased. More complex analysis methods are needed to obtain appropriate SEs. Estimates of SEs of proportions were obtained using the Taylor series linearization method.[28] The PSRATIO program in OSIRIS[29] was used to make these calculations. Estimates of standard errors of logistic regression coefficients were obtained using the method of balanced repeated replication (BRR).[30,31] This procedure began by generating 44 balanced subsamples of the survey data. The LOGISTIC program in SAS[32] was used to make individual calculations for each of these 44 replicate subsamples. A SAS BRR macro[30-32] was used to compute estimates of the SEs of model coefficients from the distribution of the coefficients in the 44 replicates.

ARCH GEN PSYCHIATRY/VOL 53, NOV 1996
1024

CIDI DIAGNOSIS: SCHIZOPHRENIA OR SCHIZOPHRENIFORM DISORDER

We present LTP and demographic correlates for narrow psychotic illness (schizophrenia or schizophreniform disorder) and broad psychotic illness (all NAP). Applying the CIDI diagnostic program[20] to follow-up interviews, LTP was estimated at 1.3%±0.2% for narrowly defined psychotic illness and 1.1%±0.2% for schizophrenia alone. Descriptive data on the sociodemographic distributions of these computer-based diagnoses are seen in **Table 1**. The associations are presented as odds ratios (ORs) estimated from logistic regression equations in each of which dummy variables defining categories of a single sociodemographic variable were used to predict 1 of the 2 di-

agnostic measures. The ORs are reported in relation to an omitted category of each sociodemographic variable that has an implicit OR of 1.0. Because of the small number of affected individuals, confidence intervals (CIs) are presented at the 90% level. In addition, likelihood-ratio χ^2 tests are provided (with significance noted at 10% level 2-tailed) to evaluate the significance of the overall association. The latter tests are useful in evaluating joint significance in cases where the sociodemographic variable has 3 or more categories.

The overall χ^2 test showed significant associations of CIDI diagnoses with income, employment, religion region, and "area raised." An increased probability of computer-diagnosed narrowly defined psychotic illness was associated with unemployment, non-Catholic religious affiliation, living in the West, and being raised in a nonrural area. The association with income was complex with

Table 1. Demographic Correlates of the CIDI Computer Diagnosis of Narrowly Defined Psychosis and the Clinician Diagnosis of NAP in the National Comorbidity Survey*

| | CIDI Narrow Psychosis† | | | | | | | | Clinician NAP | | | | | | | |
| | | | Cases | | | Noncases | | | | | Cases | | | Noncases | | |
Variable Categories	OR	90% CI	%	SE	n	%	SE	n	OR	90% CI	%	SE	n	%	SE	n
Age, y	χ^2_4= 0.39								χ^2_4= 3.02							
15-24	0.82	0.32-2.13	22.9	8.1	17	25.9	1.0	1504	2.17	1.15-4.10‡	36.2	8.1	15	25.8	1.0	1507
25-34	1.04	0.39-2.73	34.3	7.1	25	30.9	1.0	1793	1.49	0.73-3.01	29.7	7.1	12	30.9	1.0	1806
35-44	0.88	0.38-2.08	25.9	6.7	19	27.4	1.0	1589	1.35	0.63-2.88	23.9	6.7	10	27.4	0.9	1598
45-54	1.00	...	16.9	2.9	12	15.8	0.9	917	1.00	...	10.3	2.9	4	15.9	0.9	926
15-54, linear	1.02	0.99-1.04	...	...	...	...	...	...	0.98	0.95-1.01	...	...	...	...	...	...
Sex	χ^2_1= 0.90								χ^2_1= 0.94							
Male	1.00	...	42.1	8.0	31	47.9	1.4	2781	1.00	...	39.9	8.0	16	47.9	1.4	2796
Female	1.26	0.78-2.05	57.9	8.0	43	52.1	1.4	3023	1.39	0.79-2.44	60.1	8.0	24	52.1	1.4	3041
Race or ethnicity	χ^2_3= 1.55								χ^2_3= 2.75							
White	1.00	...	71.7	8.6	53	76.4	2.4	4433	1.00	...	64.7	8.6	26	76.4	2.4	4459
Black	1.34	0.69-2.61	14.3	5.6	11	11.4	1.1	659	1.92	0.93-3.98	18.5	5.6	7	11.3	1.1	662
Hispanic	1.02	0.34-3.02	8.6	5.2	6	9.0	1.9	522	1.51	0.47-4.85	11.5	5.2	5	8.9	1.9	523
Other	1.77	0.69-4.54	5.5	3.4	4	3.3	0.6	190	1.92	0.36-10.42	5.4	3.4	2	3.3	0.6	192
Education, y	χ^2_3= 5.03								χ^2_3= 3.68							
0-11	2.24	1.02-4.93‡	25.9	5.9	19	23.2	1.4	1346	2.32	1.04-5.20‡	34.6	5.9	14	23.2	1.4	1351
12	2.23	0.99-5.04	40.7	7.5	30	36.7	1.3	2127	1.58	0.63-3.93	37.3	7.5	15	36.7	1.3	2142
13-15	2.24	0.98-5.13	24.2	5.4	18	21.7	1.0	1259	1.16	0.46-2.88	16.2	5.4	7	21.8	1.0	1271
16+	1.00	...	9.2	4.8	7	18.5	1.3	1071	1.00	...	11.8	4.8	5	18.4	1.3	1073
0-16+, linear	0.92	0.83-1.03	...	...	...	...	...	...	0.91	0.78-1.06	...	...	...	...	...	...
Household income, ×$1000/y	χ^2_3= 9.54§								χ^2_3= 4.99§							
0-19	1.47	0.89-2.41	40.6	9.1	30	27.7	1.8	1609	2.18	1.11-4.29‡	44.6	9.1	18	27.8	1.8	1621
20-34	0.47	0.24-0.94‡	11.3	5.7	8	24.0	1.2	1393	1.12	0.60-2.09	19.8	5.7	8	23.9	1.2	1394
35+	1.00	...	48.1	7.1	36	48.3	2.0	2801	1.00	...	35.7	7.1	14	48.4	2.0	2822
0-120+, linear	0.95	0.91-0.99‡	...	...	...	...	...	...	0.92	0.87-0.98‡	...	...	...	...	...	...
Marital status	χ^2_2= 0.63								χ^2_2= 5.78§							
Married	1.00	...	64.2	7.4	47	62.1	1.0	3605	1.00	...	45.3	7.4	18	62.3	1.0	3634
Separated, widowed, or divorced	1.19	0.63-2.24	11.8	4.8	9	9.6	0.6	559	2.72	1.42-5.21‡	18.9	4.8	8	9.6	0.6	560
Never married	0.82	0.42-1.58	23.9	7.3	18	28.2	0.9	1639	1.75	0.98-3.11	35.8	7.3	14	28.1	0.9	1642
Employment	χ^2_3= 20.10§								χ^2_3= 11.13§							
Working	1.00	...	55.8	6.8	41	60.9	1.4	3537	1.00	...	52.9	6.8	21	60.9	1.4	3557
Student	0.62	0.29-1.30	10.3	5.1	8	18.4	1.0	1067	0.81	0.34-1.92	12.9	5.1	5	18.3	1.0	1069
Homemaker	0.79	0.27-2.35	9.1	4.0	7	12.7	1.1	735	0.80	0.34-1.86	8.7	4.0	4	12.6	1.1	738
Other	3.58	2.09-6.14‡	24.8	6.9	18	8.0	0.9	464	3.84	2.06-7.18‡	25.6	6.9	10	8.1	0.9	472
Religion	χ^2_3= 16.50§								χ^2_3= 1.66							
Protestant	2.15	1.09-4.26‡	53.9	6.9	40	52.4	1.8	3041	0.86	0.41-1.79	44.9	6.9	18	52.5	1.8	3063
No preference	3.13	1.31-7.48‡	13.9	5.4	10	9.3	0.7	541	1.54	0.56-4.23	14.3	5.4	6	9.4	0.7	546
Other	5.29	2.30-12.15‡	17.0	4.0	12	6.8	0.6	397	1.38	0.43-4.49	9.4	4.0	4	6.9	0.6	406
Catholic	1.00	...	15.2	7.8	11	31.4	1.9	1824	1.00	...	31.4	7.9	13	31.2	1.9	1822
Household composition	χ^2_3= 2.07								χ^2_3= 5.88							
Lives alone	0.84	0.28-2.54	4.9	3.1	4	5.6	0.5	323	2.37	0.77-7.31	9.6	3.1	4	5.5	0.5	323
Lives with parent	0.72	0.37-1.41	15.7	5.5	12	11.9	0.8	689	1.55	0.69-3.49	22.3	5.5	9	11.9	0.8	692
Lives with other	1.31	0.68-2.53	15.2	6.8	11	21.2	0.9	1229	2.62	1.15-5.94‡	22.8	6.8	9	21.1	0.9	1231
Lives with spouse	1.00	...	64.2	7.4	47	61.4	1.0	3561	1.00	...	45.3	7.4	18	61.5	1.0	3591
Region	χ^2_3= 9.32§								χ^2_3= 4.63							
Northeast	0.51	0.21-1.25	17.6	7.4	13	20.3	2.2	1177	0.60	0.27-1.33	20.4	7.4	8	20.2	2.2	1181
Midwest	0.36	0.12-1.05	15.6	9.1	11	25.4	2.6	1472	0.46	0.12-1.67	19.5	9.1	8	25.3	2.6	1475
South	0.56	0.24-1.29	32.4	7.1	24	34.2	2.1	1983	0.45	0.22-0.93‡	25.9	7.1	10	34.2	2.1	1997
West	1.00	...	34.4	7.9	25	20.2	1.2	1171	1.00	...	34.2	7.9	14	20.3	1.2	1183
Urban/city	χ^2_2 = 2.56								χ^2_2= 12.32§							
Large metropolitan area	1.69	0.83-3.46	53.9	7.7	40	46.8	3.5	2715	5.81	3.17-10.63‡	72.5	7.7	29	46.7	3.5	2725
Small metropolitan area	1.45	0.72-2.95	31.4	7.6	23	31.7	4.2	1839	2.57	1.14-5.77‡	21.8	7.6	9	31.8	4.2	1853
Rural	1.00	...	14.7	2.0	11	21.5	2.9	1250	1.00	...	5.8	2.0	2	21.6	2.9	1258
Area raised	χ^2_4= 8.82§								χ^2_4= 6.65							
City	3.13	1.68-5.83‡	37.8	5.5	28	25.9	1.4	1504	5.03	2.09-12.11‡	40.3	5.5	16	25.9	1.4	1515
Suburb	1.94	0.78-4.85	14.4	4.2	11	15.9	1.1	925	2.13	0.70-6.53	10.5	4.2	4	15.9	1.1	931
Midsize town	1.63	0.63-4.20	8.7	6.3	6	11.4	0.9	662	4.24	1.18-15.22‡	14.8	6.3	6	11.3	0.9	662
Small town	2.39	1.18-4.83‡	28.0	5.8	21	25.1	1.1	1459	3.09	1.19-8.02‡	23.9	5.8	10	25.2	1.1	1470
Rural	1.00	...	11.1	5.2	8	21.6	1.4	1254	1.00	...	10.4	5.2	4	21.6	1.4	1258

*CIDI indicates Composite International Diagnostic Interview; NAP, nonaffective psychosis; OR, odds ratio; CI, confidence interval; and subscript in χ^2, the degrees of freedom.
†Schizophrenia or schizophreniform disorder.
‡Unity is outside 90% CI of OR.
§χ^2 is significant at the .10 level.

the lowest risk found in the middle-income range. However, when coded as a linear variable, income was significantly and inversely related to risk for a computer-diagnosed narrowly defined psychotic illness. Although the overall χ^2 test for education was not significant, a significantly increased risk of computer-diagnosed narrowly defined psychotic illness was associated with having less than a high school education.

CIDI DIAGNOSIS: NAP

The LTP of broadly defined NAP, diagnosed by computer algorithm from the follow-up interview, was 2.2%±0.3%. A CIDI diagnosis of NAP was significantly associated with income, employment, religion, region, and area raised. Demographic correlates of NAP differ from those for the more narrow diagnoses in having a different relationship with income (the significant effect now being an elevated risk associated with the lowest income) and having a lower risk associated with both Catholic and Protestant religious affiliations. In addition, a significantly increased risk is found for broadly defined psychosis in Hispanics.

CLINICIAN DIAGNOSIS

Based on clinician diagnoses, LTP was estimated at 0.16%±0.06% for narrowly defined psychotic illness and 0.15%±0.05% for schizophrenia alone. These disorders were too infrequently diagnosed (a total of 9 cases) to permit meaningful risk factor analyses. In a number of cases, the diagnostician (K.S.K.) was confident about the presence of NAP, but information was lacking to enable a more specific DSM-III-R diagnosis to be given with certainty. In further analyses of clinician-defined psychotic illness, we focused on the broader category of NAP, with an estimated LTP of 0.7%±0.1%.

Crude ORs for the demographic correlates of clinician NAP diagnoses are seen in Table 1. On the basis of an overall χ² test, the risk of illness was significantly associated with income, marital status, employment, and urbanicity. Specifically, an increased risk of a clinician NAP diagnosis was associated with unemployment; residing in a metropolitan area; low income levels; and a marital status of separated, widowed, or divorced. In the absence of an overall significant χ² test, significant associations were also noted with young age, less than a high school education, living with nonrelatives, residing outside the south, or being raised in a city or town.

The wide age range of the NCS respondents complicates the interpretation of the association between marital status and psychopathology. When we examine the clinician diagnosis of NAP only in individuals aged 30 years or older, the OR is somewhat greater among those who are single (OR=3.84; 90% CI, 1.00 to 14.80) than among those separated, widowed, or divorced (OR=3.47; 90% CI, 1.88 to 6.38). This difference is more marked in those aged 35 years or older: OR=10.20 (90% CI, 2.17 to 47.86) for single individuals and OR=5.62 (90% CI, 2.37 to 13.39) for separated, widowed, or divorced.

Since both childhood and current residence are significantly associated with risk for clinician-defined NAP, we attempted to clarify the nature of these relationships by examining a combined model. In this model, current residence in a metropolitan or other urban area was associated with significantly greater risk than residence in rural areas (OR=5.90; 90% CI, 2.95 to 11.77 and OR=2.54; 90% CI, 1.08 to 5.96, respectively). However, compared with being raised in a rural area, neither being raised in a city (OR=1.25; 90% CI, 0.75 to 2.08) nor in a suburb (OR=0.52; 90% CI, 0.21 to 1.25) was significantly asso-

Table 2. Patterns of Lifetime Comorbidity for Clinician Diagnosis of NAP*

	Prevalences of Other Disorders Among Respondents With NAP, %	OR	95% CI
Affective disorders			
Major depression	66.6	9.4	5.2-16.7†
Dysthymia	28.3	5.4	2.8-10.4†
Mania	20.9	15.7	6.6-37.2†
Any	73.4	10.7	5.6-21.8†
Anxiety disorders			
Generalized anxiety disorder	30.9	8.0	3.8-16.8†
Agoraphobia	27.5	5.1	2.4-10.6†
Simple phobia	30.8	3.4	1.8-6.3†
Social phobia	39.5	4.1	1.9-9.0†
Panic disorder	25.5	9.1	4.0-21.1†
Posttraumatic stress disorder	28.9	4.9	2.2-10.7†
Any	71.4	5.9	2.4-14.6†
Substance use disorder			
Alcohol dependence	43.2	4.4	2.4-8.1†
Drug dependence	37.7	7.1	3.6-14.0†
Alcohol abuse or dependence	57.0	4.2	2.2-8.2†
Drug abuse or dependence	44.8	6.2	3.1-12.5†
Any	58.5	3.7	1.8-7.3†

*NAP indicates nonaffective psychosis; OR, odds ratio; and CI, confidence interval.
†Unity is outside 95% CI.

ciated with the risk for psychosis controlling for current urbanicity.

Individuals receiving a clinician diagnosis of NAP were at significantly increased risk for a wide range of CIDI diagnoses assigned *without* diagnostic hierarchies including all anxiety disorders, alcohol and drug abuse and dependence, and affective disorders (**Table 2**). Only 7% of NAP cases did *not* receive at least 1 additional psychiatric diagnosis.

THE RELATIONSHIP BETWEEN CIDI AND CLINICIAN DIAGNOSES

Only 10.5% of weighted cases assigned a CIDI computer diagnosis of narrowly defined psychosis were so diagnosed by K.S.K., an additional 26.1% being diagnosed as another NAP. Of cases diagnosed as NAP by the CIDI computer algorithm, 28.4% were so diagnosed by the senior clinician (K.S.K.). Of the cases diagnosed by the CIDI as being broad but not narrowly defined psychosis, none and 9.8% were judged by K.S.K. to have narrowly and broadly defined psychosis, respectively.

We examined whether information recorded in the CIDI reinterview could predict a clinician diagnosis of NAP among those cases diagnosed by the CIDI computer algorithm as (1) narrowly or (2) broadly defined psychosis. Individual psychotic symptoms recorded on the CIDI did not strongly predict clinician diagnosis of psychosis (**Table 3**); however, they were more predictive in cases with a narrow than with a broad CIDI di-

32

	Predicting a Clinical Diagnosis of NAP Among Subjects With a CIDI Computer Diagnosis of			
	Schizophrenia or Schizophreniform Disorder		NAP	
Predictor Variable	OR	95% CI	OR	95% CI
K1, Spying or following	2.10	0.65-6.80	2.40	0.77-7.45
K2, Experimenting, poisoning	0.68	0.19-2.43	0.89	0.28-2.75
K3, Reading mind	0.90	0.07-12.25	0.79	0.14-4.58
K4, Others hear your thoughts	0.52	0.06-4.41	0.39	0.07-2.01
K5, Hear others' thoughts	0.90	0.15-5.34	0.91	0.20-4.21
K6, Under control of force	1.68	0.40-7.14	1.00	0.27-3.67
K7, Thoughts into mind	4.29	1.07-17.17†	3.07	0.79-11.85
K8, Sent messages	3.24	1.12-9.41†	1.85	0.29-11.71
K9, Hypnotized, lasers, x-rays	2.49	0.26-24.24	3.50	0.35-34.75
K10, Visions	6.26	1.40-27.96†	3.56	0.54-23.37
K11, Voices	3.76	0.91-15.49	2.07	0.56-7.71
K12, Strange smells	1.02	0.11-9.42	0.55	0.09-3.26
K13, Unusual feelings	2.10	0.52-8.47	0.85	0.21-3.54
No. of symptoms				
Low	1.00	...	1.00	...
Medium	6.86	0.88-53.55	2.12	0.14-32.47
High	14.79	1.64-133.64†	4.19	0.29-60.45
Delusions and hallucinations	1.00	...	1.00	...
Delusions only	0.02	0.00-0.13†	0.39	0.00-85.57
Hallucinations only	0.20	0.03-1.24	0.25	0.04-1.48
Thought disorder	...	...	4.86	1.01-23.40†
Flat affect	1.54	0.30-7.84	2.30	0.47-11.39
Impairment during symptoms	1.13	0.74-1.72	1.27	0.83-1.94
Enduring impairment	1.96	1.09-3.52†	2.16	1.13-4.15†
Duration	1.13	1.00-1.28†	1.14	1.03-1.26†
Neuroleptic treatment	2.80	0.89-8.82	4.27	1.26-14.53†
Seeking help	0.89	0.34-2.29	1.02	0.46-2.27
Hospitalization	7.02	1.43-34.35†	8.99	2.20-36.71†
Age at onset	0.93	0.86-1.01	0.96	0.90-1.02

CIDI indicates Composite International Diagnostic Interview; NAP, nonaffective psychosis; OR, odds ratio; and CI, confidence interval.
Unity is outside 95% CI.

nosis. Endorsement of 4 items assessing common perceptory delusions (K2) and various aspects of "thought transfer" (K3-5) predicted a decreased probability of a clinician diagnosis of psychosis. Given a CIDI diagnosis of narrowly defined psychosis, items assessing auditory and visual hallucinations, delusions of thought insertion (K7), and ideas of reference from the television or radio (K8) were significantly associated with an increased probability of a clinician diagnosis of psychosis.

Could the total number or kind of endorsed psychotic symptoms predict clinician diagnosis? In those with narrow computer-CIDI diagnosis, the clinician diagnosis of psychosis was significantly predicted both by to-number of endorsed psychotic symptom items and by the combination of delusions and hallucinations. Subjects who endorsed only items reflecting delusions were particularly unlikely to be confirmed as psychotic by the clinician.

Of the 4 "signs" of psychosis rated by interviewers, neologisms and "behaves as if hallucinating") were too few to analyze. While flat affect did not predict clinician diagnosis, an interviewer rating of "thought disorder" did significantly predict the clinician diagnosis of NAP in those with a CIDI broad diagnosis.

In cases with a CIDI diagnosis of either narrowly or broadly defined psychosis, several other clinical characteristics of the respondents significantly predicted a clinician diagnosis of psychosis, including respondent reports of enduring impairment, duration of their psychotic symptoms, treatment with neuroleptic drugs, or hospitalization.

Among respondents diagnosed by the CIDI-computer algorithm with narrowly defined psychosis, we created a summary variable of the 8 significant predictors of clinician diagnosis seen in Table 3. Using weighted data, individuals with between 0 and 3, 4, or 5 or more of these 8 variables were diagnosed by K.S.K. as psychotic 20.0%, 84.4%, and 79.1% of the time, respectively. However, of the cases that were diagnosed by K.S.K. as psychotic, only 40.5% had 5 or more "predictor" variables.

COMMENT

CIDI DIAGNOSES

In a representative sample of the US population, we found, by applying a computer algorithm for DSM-III-R diagnoses to CIDI questions from our follow-up interview, an LTP of schizophrenia of 1.1%. Despite methodologic differences in the various studies, the diagnostic algorithms for psychotic disorders in the UM-CIDI and DIS are sufficiently similar to warrant comparing our results with those obtained with the DIS in epidemiologic samples. The standardized LTP of schizophrenia in the ECA study was similar, ie, 1.3.[5] Other studies using the DIS in general population samples report a range of LTPs of schizophrenia from 0.3% to 1.6%.[33-38]

Demographic predictors of a computerized diagnosis of schizophrenia were generally similar in the NCS and ECA studies.[5] Both found higher rates of disorder significantly associated with low socioeconomic status, younger age, unemployment, and a marital status of single, divorced, or separated. Both studies found a nonsignificant 30% to 35% higher rate of illness in female individuals. However, the ECA study reported significantly lower rates of disorder in Hispanics, while we found no significant differences across race or ethnicity, but a trend toward *higher* prevalences in nonwhite individuals.

How do the prevalence estimates for schizophrenia found by the CIDI in the NCS compare with those obtained using hospital diagnoses or examinations by psychiatrists? In a review of prevalence studies of schizophrenia, Torrey[3] finds that, although nearly all studies used a diagnostic approach to schizophrenia broader than *DSM-III-R,* only 1 of 17 found an LTP of schizophrenia exceeding 1%. Including studies reporting shorter prevalence periods, 4 of 76 reported prevalences of schizophrenia that were 1% or greater. Only 2 studies of selected small populations with suspected high LTPs[39,40] produced estimates substantially in excess of those estimated from the CIDI interviews in the NCS. The LTP of schizophrenia from the NCS, generated by a computer analysis of the CIDI, is toward the very upper end, if not outside the range, of prevalence estimates found by more traditional methods. If this difference in LTP estimates does not reflect true population differences or cohort effects, then the higher rate of schizophrenia and associated disorders found by the CIDI is likely to result from either false negatives using other methods or false positives from the CIDI. The diagnostic follow-up procedure built into the NCS permits us to directly evaluate this issue.

COMPARISON OF CIDI AND CLINICIAN DIAGNOSES

Built into the NCS study of psychosis was a follow-up interview, conducted by mental health professionals, which contained the psychosis section from the CIDI and extensive additional probes to assess psychotic symptoms. Clinical diagnoses based on this interview suggested that a large proportion of the CIDI diagnoses of psychosis were false positives.

In 2 prior large-scale studies where clinicians reevaluated epidemiologic samples of individuals who received diagnoses of schizophrenia by the DIS, the DIS diagnoses were confirmed only 22%[14] and 16% of the time.[41] In a study examining psychiatric outpatients and community subjects,[16] clinicians confirmed 30.2% of cases diagnosed as schizophrenic by the DIS. A lay-administered psychosis screening questionnaire predicted, in the general population, to produc[e] true-positive rate of 17%.[42]

Our results, consistent with previous findings, [sug]gest that standard structured psychiatric interviews, a[na]lyzed by computer, are a questionable method of c[ase] detection for psychotic illnesses in the general popula[tion] and generate an unacceptably high proportion of f[alse] positives. Given the rarity of psychotic illness in the g[en]eral population, the false-positive rate will be low o[nly] if the method of assessment has a higher specificity t[han] can be achieved with the current methods.

We attempted to understand the high fa[lse] positive rates generated by the CIDI-computer a[lgo]rithm. Among the criteria for a "psychotic" sympto[m is] the interviewer judgment that it is not "p[lau]sible" or "realistic." This is too low a threshold. A n[um]ber of beliefs or hallucinatorylike experiences judge[d by] the clinician as nonpsychotic were assessed by the [in]terviewers as unrealistic. Examples would include s[ub]cultural beliefs (eg, witchcraft), schizotypal sympt[oms] (eg, isolated ideas of reference), or brief hallucinatory [ex]periences (eg, seeing a ghost or a recently deceased r[ela]tive). In addition, interviewers sometimes coded as [un]realistic responses we considered likely to reflect [real] experiences.

PREDICTION OF CLINICAL DIAGNOSIS FROM THE CIDI INTERVIEW

Given the poor agreement between CIDI-computer [and] clinician diagnoses, could other information in the C[IDI] better predict clinical assessment? In general, clinical [cor]relates were stronger predictors than were psychotic sy[mp]toms themselves. A clinician diagnosis of psychosis [was] strongly predicted by a history of psychiatric hospi[tal]ization or neuroleptic drug treatment. A similar patt[ern] was seen in the follow-up of the Baltimore ECA samp[le.] Other clinical correlates, including duration and end[ur]ing impairment, also predicted clinician diagnoses.

There was a wide variability in the relationship [be]tween endorsement of individual psychotic symptoms [and] the final clinician diagnosis. In particular, endorsem[ent] of items assessing common persecutory themes a[nd] "thought transfer"–like experiences were associated w[ith] a lower probability of a clinical diagnosis of psycho[sis.] In general population samples, these items appear to [per]form particularly poorly at assessing true psychotic sy[mp]tomatology, probably because the questions are [fre]quently misunderstood by respondents and answers [are] often misinterpreted by interviewers. Diagnoses base[d on] interviews with individuals who endorsed only de[lu]sions had an especially low rate of validation by the [cli]nician, suggesting that assessment of delusions by str[uc]tured interview is particularly difficult and likely to l[ead] to false-positive diagnoses.

We then tried to develop a scale from the 8 ite[ms] that significantly predicted a clinician diagnosis of p[sy]chosis among those with a CIDI-computer diagnosi[s of] narrowly defined psychotic illness. If rigorous criteria w[ere] used, it was possible to define a group of psychotic s[ub]jects with a relatively low rate of false positives. H[ow]

34

ever, such criteria would end up missing over 50% of cases considered psychotic by the senior clinician. Based on these results, it is difficult to be optimistic about the development of a structured interview assessment for the general population to be used by lay interviewers that has high both sensitivity and specificity for the assessment of psychotic illness.

CLINICAL DIAGNOSIS

We also examined LTP and sociodemographic correlates of NAP, as assessed by the senior clinician's diagnosis. This diagnostic assessment, which is likely, in our judgment, to be more valid than CIDI-computer diagnoses, produced an estimated LTP of NAP of 0.7%±0.1%. This figure is toward the upper end of the range of LTPs reported in Torrey's[3] detailed review. This is to be expected, because the diagnosis of NAP is broader than most definitions of schizophrenia used in previous epidemiologic surveys.

One of the major disappointments in this study was our inability to confidently report LTP for schizophrenia in the NCS using clinician diagnoses. While we were able to assign this diagnosis in a small number of cases, there were a significant number of individuals who were clearly psychotic and may have had schizophrenia, but whom we could not assign diagnoses with confidence with the available information. Therefore, our LTP estimates for schizophrenia by clinician diagnosis should be interpreted only as a plausible lower limit.

Consistent with nearly all prior studies,[4] we found psychotic illness to occur disproportionately among the disadvantaged (as assessed by income, education, or employment) and among those who were single or divorced. Our results, however, do not address the question of the causal relationship between psychotic illness and these measures. Somewhat less anticipated was the strong relationship found between psychotic illness and both current and childhood residence. Limited previous evidence[44,45] has suggested a positive association between rates of psychosis and residence in and, more rarely, having been raised in an urban area. Our results, however, are most consistent with the hypothesis that rates of psychosis are lower among those raised in and/or currently residing in rural areas.

We attempted to gain insight into the possible causal relationship between place of residence and risk of psychosis by jointly examining current and childhood residence. When both sets of variables were examined in a single model, the results indicated that the effect resulted entirely from current residence. These findings would suggest that the association most plausibly results from in-migration of individuals prone to psychosis from rural to more urban areas. We also examined 2 further models that included either current residence (destination) or childhood residence (origination) and a variable that reflected "movement" in either a more or a less urban direction. The "destination-movement" model again suggested that the association with psychosis resulted entirely from the place of current residence. However, the "origination-movement" model produced more complex results, suggesting a significant association with risk

of psychosis for both urban childhood environment and movement into a more urban area.

Because of their greater probable validity, we examined patterns of comorbidity only, using NAP as assessed by the senior diagnostician. Consistent with many prior clinical reports,[46-48] as well as results from the ECA study,[49] we found high rates of comorbidity; when diagnoses were made without hierarchies, individuals with NAP were at substantially increased risk for anxiety disorders, affective disorders, and substance use disorders.

LIMITATIONS

This article should be interpreted in the context of 4 potential methodologic limitations, all of which would tend to produce an *underestimate* of the LTP of psychotic illness in the NCS.

First, our LTP estimates may be underestimated because participants in the NCS were selected from residential units. Using 1990 US Census rates,[50] and estimates of the LTP of psychotic illness in various nonresidential populations,[5,51] we calculated that the bias introduced by excluding nonresidential populations was modest: their inclusion increased the LTP of clinical NAP by no more than 0.1%.

Second, we reinterviewed only 10% of the individuals classified as "light" or "needs more information." Although none of these was found to have true psychosis, the upper 95% CI on this estimate is 3.8%. Although unlikely, such a "worst-case" scenario would substantially increase our LTP estimates for NAP from 0.7 to around 1.2%.

Third, the NCS was unable to interview 18% of the predesignated respondents, usually because they refused.[17] In a follow-up survey of a probability subsample of these nonrespondents, we obtained screening information from slightly less than half of those contacted. By comparing this and other information (eg, small-area Census data, household observations) obtained from initial nonrespondents with the information obtained from NCS respondents, we generated a probability-of-nonresponse score for each respondent in the main survey.[52] An increased rate of NAP was found among respondents with high scores on this measure. Based on these results, a nonresponse weight was developed and applied to the entire NCS sample to adjust for biases in LTP estimates owing to nonresponse. If we markedly underestimated the prevalence of NAP in the initial nonrespondents whom we could not interview, then our LTP estimates of NAP may be considerably too low.

Fourth, we initially conducted follow-up interviews only with individuals who responded positively to 1 or more psychotic symptoms in their initial CIDI interview. What proportion of individuals with psychotic illness would deny all of the 13 specific probes in the CIDI? While we are unaware of any definitive answer to this question, the proportion may not be trivial.[13,43] In an attempt to explore this issue, we reviewed the interviews of all 56 respondents who denied psychotic symptoms but were rated, by the lay interviewer, as having 1 or more of the "signs" of psychosis. Of these individuals, we were confident that 42 did not have NAP. We attempted to con-

35

duct a follow-up interview with the remaining 14 respondents, but we succeeded only in 4. Of these, none had a history of psychosis. While far from ideal, these results do not suggest that we are missing large numbers of psychotic individuals by our CIDI screen.

IMPLICATIONS

A substantial proportion of the general population respond positively to questions assessing a history of psychotic experiences.[42,53-55] Rigorously studying the epidemiology of psychosis requires the accurate identification of the large proportion of such responses that are false positives. The CIDI interview, in our hands, did not succeed at this task. Although further efforts at developing standardized assessments might be successful, including more intensive training courses for lay interviewers, our current recommendation for population-based studies of psychotic illness is either to have experienced clinicians as interviewers or, more realistically, to collect extensive contextual information about putative psychotic symptoms to be reviewed by a senior diagnostician.

Accepted for publication January 3, 1996.

The NCS is a collaborative epidemiologic investigation of the prevalence, causes, and consequences of psychiatric morbidity and comorbidity in the United States. The NCS is supported by the National Institute of Mental Health (grants MH46376 and MH49098), with supplemental support from the National Institute of Drug Abuse (through a supplement to MH46376) and the W. T. Grant Foundation (grant 90135190). Ronald C. Kessler, MD, is the Principal Investigator. Collaborating NCS sites and investigators are: The Addiction Research Foundation, Toronto, Ontario (Robin Room, PhD); Duke University Medical Center, Durham, NC (Dan Blazer, MD, PhD, and Marvin Swartz, MD); The Johns Hopkins University, Baltimore, Md (James Anthony, PhD, William Eaton, PhD, and Philip Leaf, PhD); the Max-Planck Institute of Psychiatry, Munich, Germany (Hans-Ulrich Wittchen, PhD); the Medical College of Virginia, Richmond (Kenneth S. Kendler, MD); the University of Michigan, Ann Arbor (Lloyd Johnston, PhD, and Ronald C. Kessler, PhD); New York University, New York (Patrick Shrout, PhD), State University of New York at Stony Brook (Evelyn Bromet, PhD); The University of Toronto (R. Jay Turner, PhD); and Washington University School of Medicine, St Louis, Mo (Linda Cottler, PhD). Preparation of this report was also supported by Research Scientist Development Awards to Drs Kendler (grant MH01277) and Kessler (grant MH00507).

We thank Kate McGonagle, PhD, Barbara Salem, MSW, and the staff and interviewers for their work on this project.

A complete list of NCS publications can be obtained from the NCS Study Coordinator, Room 1006, Institute for Social Research, the University of Michigan, Box 1248, Ann Arbor, MI 48106-1248. A complete list of NCS publications, study documentation, and interview schedules can be obtained directly from the NCS Homepage by using the URL: http://www.umich.edu/~ncsum/. Appendix materials for the present paper can be found in document P13.WP

within this file. A public use NCS data file can also reached through: gopher.icpsr.umich.edu.

Reprints: Kenneth S. Kendler, Department of Ps chiatry, Medical College of Virginia, Box 980710, Ric mond, VA 23298-0710.

REFERENCES

1. Mishler EG, Scotch NA. Sociocultural factors in the epidemiology of schi phrenia: a review. *Psychiatry.* 1963;26:315.
2. Eaton WW. Epidemiology of schizophrenia. *Epidemiol Rev.* 1985;7:105-12
3. Torrey EF. Prevalence studies in schizophrenia. *Br J Psychiatry.* 1987;1 598-608.
4. Eaton WW, Day R, Kramer M. The use of epidemiology for risk factor resea in schizophrenia: an overview and methodologic critique. In: Tsuang MT, Simps JC, volume eds, and Nasrallah HA, series ed: *Handbook of Schizophrenia, Nosology, Epidemiology and Genetics.* Amsterdam, the Netherlands: Elsev Science Publishers BV; 1988:169-204.
5. Keith SJ, Regier DA, Rae DS. Schizophrenic disorders. In: Robins LN, Reg DA, eds. *Psychiatric Disorders in America: The Epidemiologic Catchment A Study.* New York, NY: The Free Press; 1991:33-52.
6. Bromet E, Davies M, Schulz SC. Basic principles of epidemiologic research schizophrenia. In: Tsuang MT, Simpson JC, volume eds, and Nasrallah HA, ries ed. *Handbook of Schizophrenia, 3: Nosology, Epidemiology and Genetic* Amsterdam, the Netherlands: Elsevier Science Publishers BV; 1988:151-168.
7. Link B, Dohrenwend BP. Formulation of hypotheses about the ratio of t treated to treated cases in the true prevalence studies of functional psychiat disorders in adults in the United States. In: Dohrenwend BP, Dohrenwend E Gould MS, Link B, Neugebauer R, Wunsch-Hitzig R, eds. *Mental Illness in United States: Epidemiological Estimates.* New York, NY: Praeger Publishe 1980:133-149.
8. Sjögren T. Genetic-statistical and psychiatric investigations of a West Swed population. *Acta Psychiatr Neurol Suppl.* 1948;52.
9. Larsson T, Sjögren T. A methodologic, psychiatric and statistical study o large Swedish rural population. *Acta Psychiatr Neurol Scand Suppl.* 1991.
10. Robins LN, Regier DA, eds. *Psychiatric Disorders in America.* New York, N The Free Press; 1991.
11. Robins LN, Helzer JE. *Diagnostic Interview Schedule (DIS): Version III-A.* Louis, Mo: Washington University School of Medicine; 1985.
12. Spengler PA, Wittchen H-U. Procedural validity of standardized symptom que tions for the assessment of psychotic symptoms: a comparison of the D with two clinical methods. *Compr Psychiatry.* 1988;29:309-322.
13. Pulver AE, Carpenter WT, Jr. Lifetime psychotic symptoms assessed with t DIS. *Schizophr Bull.* 1983;9:377-382.
14. Helzer JE, Robins LN, McEvoy LT, Spitznagel E. A comparison of clinical and agnostic interview schedule diagnoses. *Arch Gen Psychiatry.* 1985;42:657-66
15. Wittchen H-U, Semler G, Von Zerssen D. A comparison of two diagnostic met ods: clinical *ICD* diagnoses vs *DSM-III* and Research Diagnostic Criteria usi the Diagnostic Interview Schedule (Version 2). *Arch Gen Psychiatry.* 1985;4 677-684.
16. Canino GJ, Bird HR, Shrout PE, Rubio-Stipec M, Bravo M, Martinez R, Se man M, Guzman A, Guevara LM, Costas H. The Spanish diagnostic intervie schedule: reliability and concordance with clinical diagnoses in Puerto Ric *Arch Gen Psychiatry.* 1987;44:720-726.
17. Kessler RC, McGonagle KA, Zhao S, Nelson CB, Hughes M, Eshleman S, Wittch H-U, Kendler KS. Lifetime and 12-month prevalence of *DSM-III-R* psychiatr disorders in the United States: results from the National Comorbidity Surve *Arch Gen Psychiatry.* 1994;51:8-10.
18. World Health Organization. *Composite International Diagnostic Interview (CI Version 1.0).* Geneva, Switzerland: World Health Organization; 1990.
19. US Department of Health and Human Services. *National Health Interview Su vey, 1989* [computer file]. Hyattsville, Md: National Center for Health Stati tics; 1992.
20. World Health Organization. *Composite International Diagnostic Interview Co puter Programs (Version 1.1).* Geneva, Switzerland: World Health Organiza tion; 1990.
21. American Psychiatric Association. *Diagnostic and Statistical Manual of Men Disorders, Third Edition, Revised.* Washington, DC: American Psychiatric A sociation; 1987.
22. Kendler KS, Gruenberg AM. An independent analysis of the Copenhagen samp of the Danish Adoption Study of Schizophrenia, VI: the relationship betwe psychiatric disorders as defined by *DSM-III* in the relatives and adoptees. *Ar Gen Psychiatry.* 1984;41:555-564.

36

23. Kendler KS, Gruenberg AM, Tsuang MT. Psychiatric illness in first-degree relatives of schizophrenic and surgical control patients: a family study using DSM-III criteria. *Arch Gen Psychiatry.* 1985;42:770-779.

24. Kendler KS, McGuire M, Gruenberg AM, O'Hare A, Spellman M, Walsh D. The Roscommon Family Study, I: methods, diagnosis of probands and risk of schizophrenia in relatives. *Arch Gen Psychiatry.* 1993;50:527-540.

25. Su Y, Burke J, O'Neill FA, Murphy B, Nie L, Kipps B, Bray J, Shinkwin R, Ni Nuallain M, MacLean CJ, Walsh D, Diehl SR, Kendler KS. Exclusion of linkage between schizophrenia and the D_2 dopamine receptor gene region of chromosome 11q in 112 Irish multiplex families. *Arch Gen Psychiatry.* 1993;50:205-211.

26. Kendler KS, Gruenberg AM, Kinney DK. Independent diagnoses of adoptees and relatives as defined by DSM-III in the provincial and national samples of the Danish Adoption Study of Schizophrenia. *Arch Gen Psychiatry.* 1994;51:456-468.

27. Cohen J. A coefficient of agreement for nominal scales. *Educ Psychol Meas.* 1960;20:37-46.

28. Woodruff RS, Causey BD. Computerized method for approximating the variance of a complicated estimate. *J Am Stat Assoc.* 1976;71:315-321.

29. University of Michigan. *OSIRIS VII.* Ann Arbor, Mich: Institute for Social Research, The University of Michigan; 1981.

30. Kish L, Frankel MR. Balanced repeated replications for standard errors. *J Am Stat Assoc.* 1970;65:1071-1094.

31. Woodruff RS. An application of multivariate analysis to complex sample survey data. *J Am Stat Assoc.* 1972;67:780-782.

32. SAS Institute. *SAS/STAT User's Guide, Version 6, Fourth Edition.* Cary, NC: SAS Institute Inc; 1990;1, 2.

33. Hwu H-G, Yeh E-K, Chang L-Y. Prevalence of psychiatric disorders in Taiwan defined by the Chinese Diagnostic Interview Schedule. *Acta Psychiatr Scand.* 1989;79:136-147.

34. Wells JS, Bushnell JA, Hornblow AR, Joyce PR, Oakley-Browne MA. Christchurch psychiatric epidemiology study, I: Methodology and lifetime prevalence for specific psychiatric disorders. *Aust N Z J Psychiatry.* 1989;23:315-326.

35. Wittchen H-U, Essau CA, Von Zerssen D, Krieg J-C, Zaudig M. Lifetime and six-month prevalence of mental disorders in the Munich Follow-up Study. *Eur Arch Psychiatry Clin Neurosci.* 1992;241:247-258.

36. Lee CK, Kwak YS, Yamamoto J, Rhee H, Kim YS, Han JH, Choi JO, Lee YH. Psychiatric epidemiology in Korea, I: gender and age differences in Seoul. *J Nerv Ment Dis.* 1990;178:242-246.

37. Bland RC, Orn H, Newman SC. Lifetime prevalence of psychiatric disorders in Edmonton. *Acta Psychiatr Scand Suppl.* 1988;338:24-32.

38. Canino GJ, Bird HR, Shrout PE, Rubio-Stipec M, Bravo M, Martinez R, Sesman M, Guevara LM. The prevalence of specific psychiatric disorders in Puerto Rico. *Arch Gen Psychiatry.* 1987;44:727-735.

39. Book JA. A genetic and neuropsychiatric investigation of a North-Swedish population with special regard to schizophrenia and mental deficiency. *Acta Genet Stat Med.* 1953;4:1-100.

40. Torrey EF, McGuire M, O'Hare A, Walsh D, Spellman MP. Endemic psychosis in Western Ireland. *Am J Psychiatry.* 1984;141:966-970.

41. Anthony JC, Folstein M, Romanoski AJ, Von Korff MR, Nestadt GR, Chahal R, Merchant A, Brown CH, Shapiro S, Kramer M, Gruenberg EM. Comparison of the lay Diagnostic Interview Schedule and a standardized psychiatric diagnosis: experience in eastern Baltimore. *Arch Gen Psychiatry.* 1985;42:667-675.

42. Bebbington P, Nayani T. The Psychosis Screening Questionnaire. *Int J Meth Psychiatr Res.* 1995;5:11-19.

43. Eaton WW, Romanoski A, Anthony JC, Nestadt G. Screening for psychosis in the general population with a self-report interview. *J Nerv Ment Dis.* 1991;179:689-693.

44. Lewis G, David A, Andreasson S, Allebeck P. Schizophrenia and city life. *Lancet.* 1992;340:137-140.

45. Freeman H. Schizophrenia and city residence. *Br J Psychiatry.* 1994;164 (suppl 23):39-50.

46. Freed EX. Alcoholism and schizophrenia: the search for perspectives. *J Stud Alcohol.* 1975;36:853-881.

47. Johnson DAW. Studies of depressive symptoms in schizophrenia, I: The prevalence of depression and its possible causes. *Br J Psychiatry.* 1981;139:89-101.

48. Tsuang MT, Simpson JC, Kronfol Z. Subtypes of drug abuse with psychosis: demographic characteristics, clinical features, and family history. *Arch Gen Psychiatry.* 1982;39:141-147.

49. Boyd JH, Burke JD, Gruenberg E, Holzer CE,III, Rae DS, George LK, Karno M, Stoltzman R, McEvoy L, Nestadt G. Exclusion criteria of DSM-III: a study of co-occurrence of hierarchy-free syndromes. *Arch Gen Psychiatry.* 1984;41:983-989.

50. US Bureau of the Census. *Statistical Abstract of the United States, 1994.* 114th ed. Washington, DC: US Government Printing Office; 1994.

51. Fischer PJ, Breakey WR. The epidemiology of alcohol, drug, and mental disorders among homeless persons. *Am Psychol.* 1991;46:1115-1128.

52. Kessler RC, Little RJA, Groves RM. Advances in strategies for minimizing and adjusting for survey nonresponse. *Epidemiol Rev.* 1995;17:192-204.

53. Rees WD. The bereaved and their hallucinations. In: Schoenberg B, Gerber I, Wiener A, Kutscher AH, Peretz D, Carr AC, eds: *Bereavement: Its Psychosocial Aspects.* New York, NY: Columbia University Press; 1975.

54. The Roper Organization. *Unusual Personal Experiences: An Analysis of the Data From Three National Surveys.* Las Vegas, Nev: Bigelow Holding Corp; 1992.

55. Ross CA, Joshi S. Schneiderian symptoms and childhood trauma in the general population. *Compr Psychiatry.* 1992;33:269-273.

37

Obstetric Complications and the Risk of Schizophrenia

A Longitudinal Study of a National Birth Cohort

Ý. ®. - ¬² ¿ Ü¿ ³ ¿² ôÓ ÜâÐ» ₥® ß ´» ¾ ¼µôÓ ÜôÐ‚ Üâ Ö± ¿² Ý« ´´¾ ®¹ ôÓ Üâ Ý ‚¿ ®´±⊤ Ù® «² »© ‚¿ ´¼ôÓ ÜôÐ‚ Üâ Ó ¿´ ⊠±⊦®

Background: Numerous epidemiological studies found an increased risk of schizophrenia among persons exposed to various obstetric complications. The underlying mechansims are unknown.

Objective: To study specific risk factors, as well as sets of risk factors, representing 3 different etiologic mechanisms: (1) malnutrition during fetal life; (2) extreme prematurity; and (3) hypoxia or ischemia.

Methods: In this longitudinal cohort study, information in the National Birth Register was linked to the National Inpatient Register. We followed up 507 516 children born between 1973 and 1977 with regard to a diagnosis of schizophrenia between 1987 and 1995 (238 cases). By record linkage, we also had access to data on psychiatric illness in the mother. Occurrence of schizophrenia was measured by the Mantel-Haenszel test and logistic regression.

Results: A number of specific risk factors were associated with an increased risk of schizophrenia. The relative risk (95% confidence interval) for preeclampsia was 2.5 (1.4-4.5); vacuum extraction, 1.7 (1.1-2.6); and malformations, 2.4 (1.2-5.1). In logistic regression models, we found that indicators of all 3 etiologic mechanisms were associated with increased point estimates of schizophrenia, although at lower risk levels. Preeclampsia, an indicator of fetal malnutrition, was the only risk factor with statistically significant increased risk after control for all potentially confounding factors.

Conclusion: This study supports the theory of an association between obstetric complications and schizophrenia. Although preeclampsia was the strongest individual risk factor, there was evidence of increased risk associated with all 3 etiologic mechanisms.

ß ®½ Ù»² Ð·§½½· ¿ ⁴§ôï ççç æ ê â ¦ î î â ì â ð

Two-column body text begins:

HE ORIGIN of schizophrenia is largely unknown. A vulnerability originating from disturbances in the central nervous system (CNS) during the embryonal, fetal, or neonatal period may possibly explain some of the reason for the occurrence of schizophrenia.[1]

Numerous epidemiological studies have been published on the association between obstetric complications and schizophrenia. In a meta-analysis[2] of 18 studies, an overall odds ratio of 2.03 (95% confidence interval [CI], 1.6-2.4) was found for schizophrenia following obstetric complications of any kind. Interestingly, the only 2 historical cohort studies[3,4] in that analysis failed to find a significant association. However, the number of schizophrenic or psychotic patients was small in those studies.

Many studies have used the summary scale of obstetric complications by Lewis et al,[5] which is unspecific and thus gives little clue to the underlying cause. McNeil et al[6] showed that the kind of scale used has consequences for the results obtained, with higher risk estimates if a weighted scale is used.[7]

Several studies found 1 or 2 (rarely 3) significant risk factors that are seldom confirmed in other studies. Suggested risk factors are preeclampsia,[8-10] small head circumference,[11,12] low birth weight,[13-17] Rh incompatibility,[18] fetal distress,[19] body weight heavy for length (weight/length, ≥ 1 SD),[20] and abnormal presentations.[21-23] Most of these studies are relatively small, including fewer than 100 patients, and, thus, the results are not precise regarding risk estimates. In some studies,[13,24] maternal recall has been used instead of case records, which implies an information bias risk.

Other types of evidence for prenatal risk factors for schizophrenia are the increased occurrence of minor physical anomalies (for example, epicanthal fold and syndactylia) in individuals with

Ù®⫫ ¬» í ⫨ ⫪‚ ±° Ý± ² ¹
Ý‚ · ´ ¼¿ ² ¼ß ¼ø ± ¬ · ¿ ² ¼ø ± ¬ · ¿² ¼ø‚ ¬· Ü· ½
Ø» ¿¿ ² ¼ô ¹ ¹ô·¹ · ¹
Ü«± ‚ ·⊠® »¹ › ·® · Ñ⊠ §¸ ½ ¹ ª± ´ ¹ ⊸ Ñ ¦
ª » ¸ ¹ ¼± ⊠ Ø ·¿² ¼ô ¹ ¹± Ò â ¼ ¹ ¹ ¹ ¹¹ ² ¹
Û² · ﹐ ﹐⫫²² ¹
Ñ⊠ « Ù» ¸¹ · ½ ¹ ß ¼ø ± ¬ · ¿² ¼ø ¬ · ¿²

38

MATERIALS AND METHODS

BIRTH RECORDS

By using the National Birth Register,[41,42] we obtained data on obstetric complications in all Swedish children born between 1973 and 1977 (507 516 children). The National Birth Register has been in operation since 1973 and contains information on all children born in Sweden, around 100 000 every year. Data are based on forms completed by midwives and the pediatricians in charge and sent to the National Board of Health and Welfare with information on risk factors in pregnancy, events during delivery, anthropometric data on the child, and conditions present in the neonatal period. Diagnoses were given according to ×ˀ ˧®¹ ¿ó ¬±² ¿ ´Ÿ ¿-- ·²/¿¬±² ±²Ü ¬¬¬»¿-ôÜ ·¹, ¬, Ì »ˡ ¬¬±² ®×ˀÜ ǽ±.[43] The proportion of missing data is around 1%.

Anthropometric data and malformations are classified in the register. Small for gestational age and large for gestational age are classified according to a method used by the National Board of Health and Welfare based on birth weight in relation to gestational age (based on information regarding the last menstruation). Cutoff points for these and other anthropometric measures are defined according to Maršál et al[44] (standard curves ± 2 SDs based on mean measurements of 759 ultrasonic estimates of Scandinavian children). Malformations are classified into types 1 and 2 in the register. Type 1 includes all registered malformations except preauricular appendix, retractile testis, hydrocele testis, hip-joint luxation, and nevus. Type 2 includes malformations that are known to be more accurately and completely recorded than those in type 1. These are the malformations in the CNS, lungs, and intestinal canal, serious malformations of the heart, ears, or eyes, choanal atresia, facial clefts, esophageal atresia, intersexuality, and hypospadias.

PSYCHIATRIC RECORDS

Psychiatric Illness in Offspring

By means of the unique personal identity number, the cohort was followed up in the National Inpatient Register that covers between 97% and 98% of all episodes of inpatient care. They were given clinical diagnoses according to the Nordic version of ×ˀ ˧®² ¿¬±² ¿ ´Ÿ ¿-- ·²/¿¬±² ±²Ü ¬¬¬-¬-ô

schizophrenia[25,26] and findings from the Dutch Famine Study by Susser et al,[27] in which malnutrition was found to be related to neurodevelopmental disturbances including schizophrenia.

Men have an earlier onset of illness, lower premorbid functional level, and poorer outcome than women.[28,29] Thus, an interesting question is whether there is a sex difference in the risk of schizophrenia following obstetric complications; the results of previous studies are inconsistent in this respect.[11,30-33] Another question that has been raised is whether obstetric complications are more common in cases with an early age of onset.[8,22,30]

Central nervous system disturbances can arise through several mechanisms. In this study, we considered the following 3 possible etiologic mechanisms that might ex-

ð ·²¬, Ì »ˡ ¬¬±² ®×ˀÜ ǽ+[45] during 1987 to 1996. We recorded all admissions with a diagnosis of schizophrenia (×ˀ Ü ǽ code 295) between 1987 and 1995, which included 238 persons (99 women and 139 men).

Psychiatric Illness in Mothers

Data on the mother in the birth records enabled us to search for data on psychiatric care in the National Inpatient Register from 1973 onward. We collected data on psychotic illness (codes 295-299 according to ×ˀ Ü ǽ until 1986; codes 295-298 according to ×ˀ Ü ǽ from 1987) in the mothers for the period from 1973 to 1995.

CLASSIFICATION OF ETIOLOGIC MECHANISMS

Variables reflecting the 3 types of etiologic mechanisms described herein were grouped to identify states reflecting the following:

1. Fetal malnutrition: preeclampsia during pregnancy (×ˀ Ü ǽ code 637.03-637.99), small for gestational age, ponderal index less than 0.2, which is a measurement of leanness (weight/length³).

2. Extreme prematurity: delivery before the onset of week 33 (based on information about last menstruation).

3. Hypoxia or ischemia around birth: cesarean section and vacuum extraction in combination with a diagnosis of threatening fetal distress or intrauterine anoxia (×ˀ Ü ǽ codes 776.30-776.40), breech delivery (×ˀ Ü ǽ codes 650.6-662.6), placental abruption (×ˀ Ü ǽ code 651.4), an Apgar score of 0 to 6 at 1 and 5 minutes, respectively, according to a definition of neonatal distress.[46]

DATA ANALYSIS

We calculated relative risk (RR) estimates with the Mantel-Haenszel test and 95% CIs.[47] Logistic regression analysis was used to take into account other obstetric complications as confounders for each other. By logistic regression analyses, we estimated odds ratios (ORs) for particular variables, controlling for the other variables included in each hypothesized etiologic mechanism. We also used logistic regression analysis to study the impact of each mechanism while controlling for the other 2 hypothesized mechanisms. Finally, we constructed a logistic regression model with the most important variables from all 3 mechanisms.

plain the association between obstetric complications and schizophrenia. In particular, we wanted to distinguish these mechanisms since they require different preventive approaches and also correlate, with an overlap, to different types of neuropathologic characteristics.[34]

1. Reduction in the supply of nutrients, such as oxygen, iodine, glucose, and iron, to the fetus may lead to impaired development of the CNS[35] as well as intrauterine growth restriction. In these cases, the lack of metabolites and states of hypoxia are repeated over time and the basal ganglia is at particular risk of being damaged.[34] A more narrow definition of this state would be chronic fetal hypoxia.[4]

2. Prematurity increases the risk for intracranial hemorrhages,[36] periventricular leukomalacia,[34] and also

39

Table 1. Relative Risk (RR) for Schizophrenia in Relation to Selected Risk Factors*

Variable	No. of Exposed Cases	RR (95% Confidence Interval)		
		All	Female	Male
Male	139	1.3 (1.0-1.7)	...	...
Birth hospital category				
Regional (highly specialized)	56	1.1 (0.8-1.6)	1.0 (0.5-1.8)	1.2 (0.8-2.0)
County (main hospital)	122	1.0 (0.7-1.4)	1.3 (0.8-2.0)	0.9 (0.6-1.4)
Others	60	...	...	...
Psychotic illness of mother	19	7.8 (5.2-11.6)	4.8 (2.1-10.9)	9.9 (6.3-15.6)
Mother's marital status				
Unmarried	85	1.3 (1.0-1.8)	1.2 (0.7-1.9)	1.4 (1.0-2.1)
Unknown	19	2.2 (1.2-3.8)	2.8 (1.1-6.8)	1.8 (0.9-3.7)
Mother's age, y				
≤18	14	1.4 (0.8-2.5)	2.1 (1.0-4.5)	1.0 (0.4-2.2)
19-39	220			
≥40	4	2.0 (0.8-5.3)	0 (0)	3.5 (1.4-8.9)

Ellipses indicate not applicable.

for interstitial respiratory distress syndrome and infections,[37] which may also cause brain damage.

3. Hypoxia or ischemia due to complications during delivery could result in brain damage, especially in the regions of the hippocampus and cortex.[34]

Although all these etiologic mechanisms are plausible, there is also an association between a psychotic disorder in the mother and an increased risk of obstetric complications (shown by Sacker et al[38] and also in our data). Therefore, the occurrence of psychotic disorders in mothers should be taken into account.

The possibility of linking the Swedish National Birth Register with the National Inpatient Register[39,40] enabled us to address several of the issues mentioned herein. Data on obstetric complications were available for all Swedish children born between 1973 and 1977 (507 516 children). The children were observed with regard to diagnosis of schizophrenia to a maximum age of 22 years. Furthermore, the birth records could be linked to data on psychiatric illness in the mother, which enabled us to control for maternal psychotic illness in the analyses. We wanted to study specific risk factors as well as sets of risk factors that were indicators of the 3 etiologic mechanisms mentioned herein.

<hr>

RESULTS

The RRs associated with the major risk factors are presented in **Table 1**. These factors are controlled for in the analyses presented below. There was an 8-fold increased risk of schizophrenia among offspring to mothers who had had a psychotic disorder (including schizophrenia) during their adult life. The risk of obstetric complications, defined as any of the complications included as indicators of the 3 mechanisms, was also increased (RR, 1.3 [95% CI, 1.2-1.3]) in this group of mothers. Children born to mothers younger than 19 or older than 39 years had an increased risk of schizophrenia, although this risk was not statistically significant, except for males born to mothers older than 39 years (RR, 3.5 [95% CI, 1.4-8.9]) and females born to young mothers

(RR, 2.3 [95% CI, 1.1-4.7]). The risk was also increased, although it was not statistically significant, if the mother was unmarried or if her marital status was unknown at the time of delivery.

Table 2 shows the RRs of schizophrenia among children born with various obstetric complications. We found that several risk factors during pregnancy, as well as during the time around delivery, significantly increased the risk of schizophrenia: preeclampsia, gestational age younger than 33 weeks, a ponderal index less than 20, respiratory illness, and type 2 malformations. Adjustments for the variables presented in Table 1 did not dramatically alter the results. There was a clear difference between the sexes. Being the fourth child and small for gestational age were associated with a significantly increased risk of schizophrenia in males, while a birth weight of less than 1500 g significantly increased the risk of schizophrenia among females.

In **Table 3**, we analyzed by logistic regression the impact of the variables included in each etiologic group. Among the hypoxia or ischemia variables, low Apgar scores at 5 minutes and vacuum extraction or cesarean section on indication of fetal distress were associated with the highest risks, although these risks were not statistically significant. Among the indicators of malnutrition, preeclampsia and low ponderal index (leanness) were the strongest risk factors. The third group consisted of only 1 factor, extreme prematurity, which was associated with a significantly increased risk. The separate ORs for each mechanism, without adjustments for the 2 other mechanisms, are also shown in Table 3.

In the next set of regression models, we studied the impact of each etiologic mechanism adjusted for the other 2 mechanisms. The results are shown at the bottom line of the specific mechanisms in Table 3. There is an increased risk, although the risk was not statistically significant, among those who had been exposed to indicators of fetal malnutrition (a total of 24 individuals with schizophrenia) and a gestational age younger than 33 weeks (5 individuals). In the hypoxia or ischemia group, the risk estimate was lower.

40

Table 2. Relative Risk (RR) for Schizophrenia Associated With Specific Risk Factors*

Variable	No. of Exposed Cases	RR (95% Confidence Interval)			
		All (Crude Data)	All†	Female‡	Male‡
Born between January and April	95	1.2 (0.9-1.5)	1.2 (0.8-1.4)	1.2 (0.8-1.7)	1.2 (0.8-1.7)
Born in a town with fewer than 250 000 inhabitants	43	1.3 (0.9-1.9)	1.3 (0.9-1.8)	1.4 (0.9-2.4)	1.2 (0.7-1.9)
Pregnancy					
Maternal history of prior stillbirth or death of child during first week of life	9	1.7 (0.9-3.3)	1.6 (0.8-3.2)	2.8 (1.3-6.2)	0.9 (. . .)
Parity					
1	121	1.3 (1.0-1.8)	1.3 (1.0-1.6)	1.1 (0.7-1.7)	1.4 (1.0-2.0)
2-3	100	...	...	...	...
≥4	17	1.7 (1.0-2.8)	1.5 (0.9-2.6)	0.5 (0.1-1.9)	2.2 (1.2-4.1)
Twin birth	5	1.3 (0.5-3.2)	1.3 (0.5-3.1)	0.6 (0.1-4.3)	1.8 (0.7-4.8)
Preeclampsia	11	2.5 (1.3-4.5)	2.5 (1.4-4.5)	1.1 (0.3-4.6)	3.5 (1.8-6.6)
Bleeding during pregnancy	7	1.8 (0.9-3.9)	2.0 (1.0-4.2)	1.4 (0.3-5.7)	2.4 (1.0-5.7)
Threatening premature delivery	6	2.0 (0.9-4.4)	2.3 (1.0-5.0)	2.8 (0.9-8.6)	1.8 (0.6-5.7)
Urinary tract infection	3	0.9 (0.3-2.8)	0.8 (0.3-2.5)	2.2 (0.7-6.6)	0 (0)
Gestational age, wk (based on information on last menstruation)					
23-32	5	3.4 (1.4-8.2)	2.7 (1.0-7.0)	3.3 (0.8-12.7)	2.2 (0.6-8.8)
33-36	11	1.2 (0.6-2.2)	1.1 (0.6-2.0)	0.5 (0.1-2.1)	1.5 (0.7-2.9)
37-42	215	...	...	...	...
≥43	3	0.4 (0.1-1.3)	0.4 (0.1-1.2)	0.3 (0.0-1.9)	0.5 (0.1-1.8)
Delivery					
Other than vertex	21	0.8 (0.5-1.2)	0.8 (0.5-1.2)	0.8 (0.4-1.5)	0.7 (0.4-1.3)
Breech	5	0.8 (0.3-1.9)	0.8 (0.3-1.8)	0.6 (0.2-2.5)	0.9 (0.3-2.7)
Prolonged	20	1.5 (1.0-2.4)	1.6 (1.0-2.5)	1.4 (0.6-3.1)	1.7 (1.0-2.9)
Uterine inertia	17	2.3 (1.4-3.7)	2.4 (1.5-3.9)	1.6 (0.6-4.5)	2.8 (1.6-4.9)
Cesarean section	15	0.8 (0.5-1.4)	0.8 (0.5-1.4)	0.9 (0.4-2.0)	0.8 (0.4-1.6)
Cesarean section for fetal distress	2	2.7 (0.6-10.7)	2.7 (0.7-10.3)	3.9 (0.6-24.3)	2.1 (0.3-14.25)
Vacuum extraction	21	1.7 (1.1-2.7)	1.7 (1.1-2.6)	1.2 (0.5-3.1)	1.9 (1.1-3.2)
Vacuum extraction for fetal distress	2	1.7 (0.4-6.8)	1.5 (0.3-7.2)	0 (0)	2.3 (0.5-10.9)
Use of forceps	0	0 (0)	0 (0)	0 (0)	0 (0)
Placental abruption	1	1.3 (0.2-9.4)	1.1 (0.1-9.1)	0 (0)	1.6 (0.2-13.9)
Offspring					
Apgar score					
At 1 min, 0-6/7-10	12/222	1.2 (0.7-2.2)	1.2 (0.6-2.1)	0.8 (0.3-2.5)	1.4 (0.7-2.7)
At 5 min, 0-6/7-10	6/228	2.2 (1.0-5.0)	1.9 (0.9-4.4)	3.1 (0.9-10.9)	1.4 (0.5-4.2)
Length, cm					
<48	41	1.0 (0.7-1.4)	1.0 (0.7-1.4)	0.8 (0.5-1.4)	1.2 (0.7-1.9)
49-54	186	...	...	...	...
≥55	9	1.3 (0.7-2.6)	1.3 (0.6-2.4)	2.1 (0.7-6.3)	1.0 (0.5-2.4)
Birth weight, g					
≤1499	2	3.0 (0.7-12.0)	2.9 (0.8-11.4)	6.0 (1.7-21.4)	0 (0)
1500-2499	14	1.7 (1.0-3.0)	1.5 (0.9-2.7)	0.8 (0.2-2.5)	2.2 (1.1-4.1)
2500-4499	217	...	...	...	...
≥4500	5	0.8 (0.3-1.9)	0.7 (0.3-1.8)	0.6 (0.1-4.2)	0.8 (0.3-2.2)
Ponderal index <20 (weight/length³)	3	3.4 (1.1-10.5)	3.4 (1.1-10.1)	2.5 (0.4-16.9)	4.1 (1.1-15.5)
Large for gestational age	5	0.8 (0.4-2.1)	0.8 (0.3-2.1)	0.4 (0.1-3.1)	1.1 (0.4-3.0)
Small for gestational age	13	1.3 (0.7-2.2)	1.2 (0.7-2.1)	0.4 (0.1-1.6)	1.9 (1.1-3.6)
Head circumference, cm					
≤31	11	1.6 (0.9-2.9)	1.4 (0.8-2.7)	0.8 (0.3-2.5)	2.1 (1.0-4.6)
32-37	215	...	...	...	...
≥38	8	1.4 (0.7-2.8)	1.3 (0.6-2.7)	0.8 (0.1-6.0)	1.4 (0.6-3.1)
Respiratory illness	21	1.7 (1.1-2.6)	1.5 (1.0-2.4)	1.6 (0.7-3.3)	1.5 (0.8-2.7)
Neonatal hyperbilirubinemia	15	1.1 (0.7-1.8)	1.1 (0.6-1.8)	1.3 (0.6-2.9)	1.0 (0.5-1.9)
Malformation					
Type 1	8	1.7 (0.9-3.5)	1.7 (0.9-3.4)	1.8 (0.6-5.7)	1.7 (0.7-4.0)
Type 2	7	2.5 (1.2-5.2)	2.4 (1.2-5.1)	2.3 (0.6-9.0)	2.5 (1.1-5.9)

*Controlling for confounders listed in Table 1. Ellipses indicate not applicable. See "Materials and Methods" for definition of type 1 and type 2 malformations.
†Adjusted for psychotic illness in mother, mother's age and marital status, the child's year of birth, birth hospital, and sex.
‡Adjusted for psychotic illness in mother, mother's age and marital status, the child's year of birth, and birth hospital.

41

Table 3. Odds Ratios (ORs) for Schizophrenia: The Impact of Indicators Included in Each Etiologic Mechanism and the Mechanisms in Relation to Each Other Using Logistic Regression Models*

Indicator	No. of Exposed Cases	All†	Female‡	Male
Hypoxia/Ischemia				
Placental abruption	1	1.1 (0.2-8.2)	...	1.8 (0.2-13.4)
Cesarean section for fetal distress	2	2.6 (0.6-10.9)	3.8 (0.5-28.9)	1.9 (0.3-14.1)
Vacuum extraction for fetal distress	2	1.6 (0.4-6.6)	...	2.3 (0.6-9.4)
Apgar score				
At 1 min, 0-6	12	1.0 (0.5-1.9)	0.5 (0.1-1.9)	1.3 (0.6-2.8)
At 5 min, 0-6	6	2.0 (0.8-5.2)	3.9 (1.0-14.8)	1.3 (0.4-4.7)
Breech delivery	5	0.8 (0.3-1.9)	0.7 (0.2-2.8)	0.9 (0.3-2.7)
Exposed to any of the indicators listed above	22	1.3 (0.8-2.0)	1.1 (0.5-2.3)	1.4 (0.8-2.5)
Adjusted for the 2 other mechanisms	22 (8 female, 14 male)	1.1 (0.7-1.7)	0.9 (0.4-2.0)	1.2 (0.7-2.1)
Malnutrition				
Preeclampsia	11	2.3 (1.3-4.3)	1.2 (0.3-4.7)	3.0 (1.5-8.6)
Small for gestational age	13	1.1 (0.6-1.9)	0.4 (0.1-1.6)	1.6 (0.9-3.1)
Ponderal index <20 (weight/length³)	3	3.0 (0.9-9.7)	3.7 (0.5-27.8)	2.7 (0.6-11.5)
Exposed to any of the indicators listed above	24	1.6 (1.1-2.5)	0.8 (0.3-1.9)	2.3 (1.4-3.8)
Adjusted for the 2 other mechanisms	24 (5 female, 19 male)	1.5 (1.0-2.3)	0.7 (0.3-1.8)	2.1 (1.3-3.4)
Prematurity				
Gestational age <33 wk	5	3.1 (1.3-7.6)	5.0 (1.6-16.0)	2.0 (0.5-8.0)
Adjusted for the 2 other mechanisms	5 (3 female, 2 male)	2.7 (1.0-7.3)	4.3 (1.0-18.1)	1.9 (0.5-8.0)

*Ellipses indicate not applicable.
†Adjusted for psychotic illness in mother, mother's age and marital status, the child's year of birth, and birth hospital.
‡Adjusted for psychotic illness in mother, mother's age and marital status, the child's year of birth, birth hospital, and sex.

Table 4. Odds Ratios (ORs) for Schizophrenia: Comparison Between the Strongest Risk Factors in a Logistic Regression Model

Factor	All — No. of Exposed Cases	All — OR* (95% Confidence Interval)	Female — No. of Exposed Cases	Female — OR† (95% Confidence Interval)	Male — No. of Exposed Cases	Male — OR† (95% Confidence Interval)
Hypoxia/Ischemia						
Cesarean section or vacuum extraction for fetal distress	4	2.1 (0.8-5.6)	1	1.6 (0.2-11.3)	3	2.3 (0.7-7.4)
Apgar score at 5 min, 0-6	6	1.5 (0.6-3.6)	3	1.6 (0.4-6.6)	3	1.4 (0.4-4.6)
Malnutrition						
Preeclampsia	11	2.1 (1.1-4.1)	2	1.1 (0.3-4.4)	9	2.8 (1.4-5.8)
Ponderal index <20 (weight/length³)	3	2.5 (0.8-8.3)	1	1.8 (0.3-14.8)	2	3.0 (0.7-13.1)
Prematurity						
Gestational age <33 wk	5	2.5 (0.9-7.2)	3	3.6 (0.8-16.1)	2	1.9 (0.5-8.4)

*Adjusted for psychotic illness in mother, mother's age and marital status, the child's year of birth, and birth hospital.
†Adjusted for psychotic illness in mother, mother's age and marital status, the child's year of birth, birth hospital, and sex.

By comparing the unadjusted and the adjusted ORs for each of the 3 mechanisms in Table 3, we were able to study the effects of confounding between the different mechanisms. The risk estimate for prematurity was reduced, which could be interpreted as if some of the risk was explained by factors of malnutrition during pregnancy and hypoxia or ischemia at birth. The ORs of malnutrition and hypoxia or ischemia were less reduced in this procedure. Notably, the risks were still increased, which indicates independent effects.

The risks were unevenly distributed between the sexes (Table 3). Indicators of malnutrition were associated with higher risk in males (OR, 2.1 [95% CI, 1.3-3.4]), while the females had increased risk following pre-

maturity (OR, 4.3 [95% CI, 1.0-18.1]). Proportionally more males were exposed to the obstetric complications (Table 3).

In a final model, the strongest risk factors from each etiologic group in Table 3 were entered in a logistic regression model to assess the separate effects of the most important risk factors of the 3 etiologic mechanisms (**Table 4**). The risk associated with a low Apgar score, low ponderal index, and prematurity was reduced, especially among the females, compared with the findings in Table 3. However, the point estimates were increased for complications of all 3 mechanisms, although only preeclampsia remained significantly associated with an increased risk of schizophrenia.

42

In this population-based cohort study, controlling for psychotic illness in mothers and other known risk factors, we found that several complications during pregnancy and delivery were associated with an increased risk of schizophrenia. A possible explanation of the fact that we found more obstetric risk factors than those found in previous studies is that our study included a relatively large and homogeneous group of patients with an early age at onset of schizophrenia. Two previous studies[8,22] focused on patients with early age at onset and suggested that obstetric complications might be a stronger risk factor in this group. This finding has been supported by other authors.[19,29,31,48]

When reviewing previous findings regarding obstetric risk factors, the patterns of causes are difficult to discern. Attempts have been made to understand the underlying mechanisms. McNeil et al[6] found an increased risk when using a weighted scale[7] compared with other scales.[5,23] In a cohort study,[4] there was no association with specific subcategories of exposure (chronic fetal hypoxia, prematurity, or other complications), but the number of patients with psychoses was small.

To understand more about the underlying mechanisms, we grouped possible risk factors based on previous clinical knowledge and studies of the disease. This resulted in 3 sets of risk factors: malnutrition during fetal life, extreme prematurity, and hypoxia or ischemia around birth. The etiologic mechanisms have some features in common but still seem to be independent of each other. Hypoxia is a factor in common for the mechanism of malnutrition during fetal life as well as hypoxia or ischemia around birth. Nevertheless, we made this classification based on clinical practice and the knowledge that brain damage following chronic hypoxia during fetal life differs from that following an acute episode of hypoxia at birth. Prematurity is associated with a number of different conditions, such as intraventricular hemorrhages, periventricular leukomalacia, interstitial respiratory distress syndrome, infections, as well as hypoxia or ischemia around birth and fetal malnutrition. Despite this, the results of the logistic regression analysis favor our hypothesis that all 3 subcategories represent different possible mechanisms although some features are mutual.

We tried to be strict in our selection of the indicators to avoid unnecessary dilution of the results. Nevertheless, the factors are more or less good indicators of the conditions they are defined as representing. For example, breech delivery does not automatically result in hypoxia or ischemia. The term -³ ¿ ″ º℗ ¹ »- ⊤⁻ ±¿ ´¿¹ » used herein as an indicator of malnutrition is only a description independent of the cause, which could be genetic influence, chromosomal abbreviations, or infections, although it is often caused by malnutrition.

Preeclampsia was found to be the strongest risk factor for schizophrenia, which has been described in previous studies.[8-10] Geddes et al[49] concluded in their meta-analysis that an association is found only when using birth records instead of maternal recall. In our study, data were based on ЖÜ₡ and ЖÜ₡ codes from the birth records. A possible cause for increased risk of schizophrenia might

be that in preeclampsia there is an abnormal fetal blood flow, which is associated with reduced supply of nutrition to the fetus.[41,50] Interestingly, Ley[51] found an increased occurrence of minor neurological dysfunctions and intellectual impairment at 7 years of age following abnormal blood flow during fetal life.

The risk of schizophrenia following obstetric complications was higher in males than in females. This is in accordance with findings by some authors[9,27-32] but not with others.[8,11,22,33] The difference between the sexes is perhaps more pronounced for cases with an early age at onset of schizophrenia.

Because this longitudinal study included a national sample of mothers and their offspring, in other words, it was a population-based study, the risk for selection bias was reduced. The information is based on case records that are consecutively collected in the National Birth Register. Any misclassification should therefore be randomly distributed in the study. The register has been validated regarding errors of recording[41] and proved to be of acceptable quality, except for information about methods of anesthesia during delivery and metabolic testing of the newborn.

Concerning potential confounders, we were able to adjust for mother's psychotic illness during her adult life (1973-1995) by linkage with the National Inpatient Register. To our knowledge, this has not been possible in other studies. The size of the hospital and age of the mother were controlled for, and they were also proxy factors for being a citizen of a large town at birth and parity, respectively, which is why we were able to omit these suspected confounders from the analysis. We did not have specific information on social class, which is a possible confounder in studies on obstetric complications. For example, are low birth weight and young gestational age more common in lower social classes?[52] We collected data on marital status, which, in previous studies of the National Birth Register, proved to be a good indicator of social position.[42]

Our conclusion from the findings of this national cohort study including cases of schizophrenia with an early age at onset supports the theory that some of the occurrence of schizophrenia could be associated with a vulnerability originating from obstetric complications. Although preeclampsia, which is a cause of fetal malnutrition, was the strongest individual risk factor, there was evidence of increased risk associated with the other 2 mechanisms that were studied: extreme prematurity and hypoxia or ischemia at birth. The increased risks associated with the different etiologic mechanisms remained, although at lower risk levels, in the logistic models, which indicates independent effects. Thus, it seems as if these etiologic mechanisms are acting in different ways but may result in the same future vulnerability for schizophrenia. One explanation could be that the different pathways result in the same kind of damage. Schizophrenia could result from many different disturbances that may cause an altered balance in the CNS of a rather unspecific nature. Nevertheless, knowledge of specific risk factors for schizophrenia is a public health interest, since at least some of the obstetric risk factors we confirmed can potentially be prevented.

43

ß 1½½° ¬¼°₤°«¾· ½¬₤ Ü»¼³ ¾®èôîççèò
Ì₂»-¬¬¼₈© ¿·-«°°₤®¬¼¾₈¹®¿²¬₌®₤¬₇»ƒ©»¼-
Ó»¼½¼²Ì₂»¬¿₍®½Ý±²½´¿²¼¬¬₨₄₂¾₄₄⁴₍ôž·¹-µ¿Ú±²ó
¼₂¬₤ôî¬₤¼₂₤³ôî©»¼²ò
        É»¬¿²¿µÔ±¿²Ù»²⁺òóÜôÐ¸Üô°₤°°»¼¿₄½¼¼·½
¿²¼₤₃²¬₤₈Ú¿ª·₄₍ôÎÝÐ₈½½ô¿²₄Ù₈²Ô©·-ôÎÝÐ₈½½ó
°₤°®₍»-₄¼¼-¼₄---₤-¿²¼°₤°¼₤³»²¬²²¹₤¬²-¿®¬½ò
É»¿·¬±¬¿²µÞ»²¹-Ðª¿¬¹»²½ôÐÜô°₤°-₇¬¬¬¬½¼¼·½ò
        Ýₑ®®®·°₤¼₂¹¿·₍»¬₤ª»Ý¿®®¬²¿¿¼Ú¿¹¿²²ôôÜÜô¼¬
¼¿¿₍Ì₤¼¼¿₤³-î¶µ¿ªª¼¼₤©¾¼óÚ»°¿₍®⁰¹»²²¬₤¬ÐÐ₈½½·¿ó
®₄₈óÈ²¹-¬²¹₤₤ÞÞ₈½½±·-Ì»»»₍©¹¼óÐÈ²Ð±ììôîôîô₤¿ôîèè
Ì¬₤¼²₤₤³ôî©»¼²øøî₍·₌⁄½®¬¬²²¿»¾¼½³¿²à-³»¾¾³½»⁻è

REFERENCES

1. Murray RM, Lewis SW, Reveley AM. Towards an aetiological classification of schizophrenia. Lancet. 1985;1:1023-1026.
2. Geddes JR, Lawrie SM. Obstetric complications and schizophrenia: a meta-analysis. Br J Psychiatry. 1995;167:786-793.
3. Done DJ, Johnstone EC, Frith CD, Golding J, Shepherd PM, Crow TJ. Complications of pregnancy and delivery in relation to psychosis in adult life: data from the British Perinatal Mortality Survey sample. BMJ. 1991;302:1576-1580.
4. Buka SL, Tsuang MT, Lipsitt LP. Pregnancy/delivery complications and psychiatric diagnosis. Arch Gen Psychiatry. 1993;50:151-156.
5. Lewis SW, Owen MJ, Murray RM. Obstetric complications and schizophrenia: methodology and mechanisms. In: Schulz SC, Tamminga CA, eds. Schizophrenia: Scientific Progress. New York, NY: Oxford University Press Inc; 1989:56-68.
6. McNeil TF, Cantor-Graae E, Sjöström K. Obstetric complications as antecedents of schizophrenia: empirical effects of using different obstetric complication scales. J Psychiatr Res. 1994;28:519-530.
7. McNeil TF, Sjöström K. The McNeil-Sjöström OC Scale: A Comprehensive Scale for Measuring Obstetric Complications. Malmö, Sweden: Lund University; 1994.
8. Kendell RE, Juszczak E, Cole SK. Obstetric complications and schizophrenia: a case control study based on standardised obstetric records. Br J Psychiatry. 1996; 168:556-561.
9. McNeil TF, Kaij L. Obstetric factors in the development of schizophrenia: complications in the births of preschizophrenics and in reproduction by schizophrenic parents. In: The Nature of Schizophrenia. New York, NY: John Wiley & Sons Inc; 1978:401-429.
10. O'Dwyer JM. Schizophrenia in people with intellectual disability: the role of pregnancy and birth complications. J Intellect Disabil Res. 1997;41:238-251.
11. Kunugi H, Takei N, Murray RM, Saito K, Nanko S. Small head circumference at birth in schizophrenia. Schizophr Res. 1996;20:165-170.
12. McNeil TF, Cantor-Graae E, Nordström LG, Rosenlund T. Head circumference in "preschizophrenic" and control neonates. Br J Psychiatry. 1993;162:517-523.
13. Rifkin L, Lewis S, Jones P, Toone B, Murray R. Low birth weight and schizophrenia. Br J Psychiatry. 1994;165:357-362.
14. Lane E, Albee GW. Comparative birth weights of schizophrenics and their siblings. J Psychol. 1966;64:227-231.
15. Torrey EF. Birth weights, perinatal insults, and HLA types: return to "original sin." Schizophr Bull. 1977;3:347-351.
16. Lewis SW, Chitkara B, Reveley AM, Murray RM. Family history and birthweight in monozygote twins concordant and discordant for psychosis. Acta Genet Med Gemellol (Roma). 1987;36:267-273.
17. Jones PB, Rantakallio P, Hartikainen AL, Isohanni M, Sipila P. Schizophrenia as a long-term outcome of pregnancy, delivery, and perinatal complications: a 28-year follow-up of the 1966 north Finland general population birth cohort. Am J Psychiatry. 1998;155:355-364.
18. Hollister JM, Laing P, Mednick SA. Rhesus incompatibility as a risk factor for schizophrenia in male adults. Arch Gen Psychiatry. 1996;53:19-24.
19. O'Callaghan E, Givson T, Colohan HA, Buckley P, Walshe DG, Larkin C, Waddington JL. Risk of schizophrenia in adults born after obstetric complications and their association with early onset of illness: a controlled study. BMJ. 1992; 305:1256-1259.
20. Hultman CM, Öhman A, Cnattingius S, Wieselgren IM, Lindström LH. Prenatal and neonatal risk factors for schizophrenia. Br J Psychiatry. 1997;170:128-133.
21. Günther-Genta F, Bovet P, Hohlfeld P. Obstetric complications and schizophrenia: a case-control study. Br J Psychiatry. 1994;164:165-170.
22. Verdoux H, Geddes JR, Takei N, Lawrie SM, Bovet P, Eagles JM, Heun R, McCreadie RG, McNeil TF, O'Callaghan E, Stöber G, Willinger MU, Wright D, Murray RM. Obstetric complications and age at onset in schizophrenia: an international collaborative meta-analysis of individual patient data. Am J Psychiatry. 1997;154:1220-1227.
23. Parnas J, Schulsinger F, Teasdale TW, Schulsinger H, Feldman PM, Mednick SA. Perinatal complications and clinical outcome with the schizophrenia spectrum. Br J Psychiatry. 1982;140:416-420.
24. McCreadie RG, Hall DJ, Berry IJ, Robertson LJ, Ewing JI, Geals MF. The Nithsdale schizophrenia surveys, X: obstetric complications, family history, and abnormal movements. Br J Psychiatry. 1992;160:799-805.
25. Guy JD, Majorski LV, Wallace CJ, Guy MP. The incidence of minor physical anomalies in adult male schizophrenics. Schizophr Bull. 1983;9:571-582.
26. Green MF, Satz P, Gaier DJ, Ganzell S, Kharabi F. Minor physical anomalies in schizophrenia. Schizophr Bull. 1989;15:91-99.
27. Susser E, Hoek HW, Brown A. Neurodevelopmental disorders after prenatal famine: the story of the Dutch Famine Study. Am J Epidemiol. 1998;147:213-216.
28. Strömgren E. Changes in the incidence of schizophrenia? Br J Psychiatry. 1987; 150:1-7.
29. Lewis S. Sex and schizophrenia: vive la différence. Br J Psychiatry. 1992;161: 445-450.
30. Kirov G, Jones PB, Harvey I, Lewis SW, Toone BK, Rifkin L, Sham P, Murray RM. Do obstetric complications cause the earlier age at onset in male than female schizophrenics? Schizophr Res. 1996;20:117-124.
31. Lewis SW, Murray RM. Obstetric complications, neurodevelopmental deviance, and risk of schizophrenia. J Psychiatr Res. 1987;21:413-421.
32. Lewis SW, Stewart A. Complications of pregnancy and delivery and psychosis in adult life. BMJ. 1991;303:582.
33. Verdoux H, Bourgeois M. A comparative study of obstetric history in schizophrenics, bipolar patients and normal subjects. Schizophr Res. 1993;9:67-69.
34. Volpe JJ. Neurology of the Newborn. 2nd ed. Philadelphia, Pa: WB Saunders Co; 1987.
35. Dobbing J. Nutrition and brain development. In: Thallummer O, Baumgarten K, Poltak A, eds. Perinatal Medicine. New York, NY: Thieme-Stratton Inc; 1979.
36. Alvarez MD, Villamil M, Keyes G. Predictive factors in the genesis of intraventricular hemorrhage in premature infants. P R Health Sci J. 1994;13:251-254.
37. Bherman RE, Kliegman RM, Arvin AM. Nelson Textbook of Pediatrics. 15th ed. Philadelphia, Pa: WB Saunders Co; 1996.
38. Sacker A, Done DJ, Crow TJ. Obstetric complications in children born to parents with schizophrenia: a meta-analysis of case-control studies. Psychol Med. 1996: 26:279-287.
39. Kristjansson E, Allebeck P, Wistedt B. Validity of the dianosis schizophrenia in a psychiatric inpatient register. Nord J Psychiatry. 1987;41:229-234.
40. Mortensen PB, Allebeck P, Munk-Jorgensen P. Population-based registers in psychiatric inpatient register. Nord J Psychiatry. 1996;50(suppl 36):67-72.
41. Cnattiagius S, Ericson A, Gunnarskog J, Källén B. A quality study of a medical birth registry. Scand J Soc Med. 1990;18:143-148.
42. Ericson A, Eriksson M, Källen B, Zetterström R. Methods for the evaluation of social effects of birth weight: experiences with Swedish population registries. Scand J Soc Med. 1993;21:69-76.
43. World Health Organization. International Classification of Diseases, Eighth Revision (ICD-8). Geneva, Switzerland: World Health Organization; 1977.
44. Maršâl K, Persson P-H, Larsen T, Lilja H, Selbing A, Sultan B. Intrauterine growth curves based on ultrasonically estimated foetal weights. Acta Paediatr. 1996;85: 843-848.
45. World Health Organization. International Classification of Diseases, Ninth Revision (ICD-9). Geneva, Switzerland: World Health Organization; 1977.
46. Thornberg E. Birth asphyxia: incidence, clinical course and outcome in a Swedish population. Acta Paediatr. 1995;84:927-932.
47. Armitage P, Berry G. Statistical Methods in Medical Research. 2nd ed. Cambridge, Mass: Blackwell Publishers; 1986.
48. Pamas J. Schizophrenia: etiological factors in the light of longitudinal high risk research. In: Kringlen E, Larrik NJ, Torgersen S, eds. Etiology of Mental Disorders. Oslo, Norway: Dept of Psychiatry, Vindern; 1990:49-61.
49. Geddes JR, Verdoux H, Takei N, Lawrie SM, Bovet P, Eagles JM, McCreadie RG, McNeil TF, O,Callaghan E, Stöber G, Willinger U, Murray RM. Schizophrenia and complications of pregnancy and labour: an individual patient data meta-analysis. Schizophr Bull. In press.
50. Chamberlain G, ed. Tumbull's Obstetrics. 2nd ed. New York, NY: Churchill Livingstone Inc; 1995.
51. Ley D. Intrauterine Growth Retardation and Abnormal Fetal Blood Flow: Implications for the Newborn Infant and the Growing Child [thesis]. Malmö, Sweden: Lund University; 1997.
52. Jacobsen G, Schei B, Hoffman HJ. Psychosocial factors and small for gestational age infants among parous Scandinavian women. Acta Obstet Gynecol Scand Suppl. 1997:165:14-18.

ARCH GEN PSYCHIATRY/VOL 56, MAR 1999
240

44

EFFECTS OF FAMILY HISTORY AND PLACE AND SEASON OF BIRTH ON THE RISK OF SCHIZOPHRENIA

Preben Bo Mortensen, D.M.Sc., Carsten Bøcker Pedersen, M.Sc., Tine Westergaard, M.D.,
Jan Wohlfahrt, M.Sc., Henrik Ewald, D.M.Sc., Ole Mors, Ph.D., Per Kragh Andersen, D.M.Sc.,
and Mads Melbye, D.M.Sc.

ABSTRACT

Background Although a family history of schizophrenia is the best-established risk factor for schizophrenia, environmental factors such as the place and season of birth may also be important.

Methods Using data from the Civil Registration System in Denmark, we established a population-based cohort of 1.75 million persons whose mothers were Danish women born between 1935 and 1978. We linked this cohort to the Danish Psychiatric Central Register and identified 2669 cases of schizophrenia among cohort members and additional cases among their parents.

Results The respective relative risks of schizophrenia for persons with a mother, father, or sibling who had schizophrenia were 9.31 (95 percent confidence interval, 7.24 to 11.96), 7.20 (95 percent confidence interval, 5.10 to 10.16), and 6.99 (95 percent confidence interval, 5.38 to 9.09), as compared with persons with no affected parents or siblings. The risk of schizophrenia was associated with the degree of urbanization of the place of birth (relative risk for the capital vs. rural areas, 2.40; 95 percent confidence interval, 2.13 to 2.70). The risk was also significantly associated with the season of birth; it was highest for births in February and March and lowest for births in August and September. The population attributable risk was 5.5 percent for a history of schizophrenia in a parent or sibling, 34.6 percent for urban place of birth, and 10.5 percent for the season of birth.

Conclusions Although a history of schizophrenia in a parent or sibling is associated with the highest relative risk of having the disease, the place and season of birth account for many more cases on a population basis. (N Engl J Med 1999;340:603-8.)
©1999, Massachusetts Medical Society.

T WIN and adoption studies strongly suggest that genetic transmission accounts for most of the familial aggregation of schizophrenia.[1,2] However, little is known about the contribution of familial aggregation to the occurrence of schizophrenia in the general population and the mode of inheritance of the disease. Environmental risk factors have also been suggested, including maternal obstetrical complications,[3,4] influenza infection during the mother's pregnancy,[5] season of

birth,[6] urban place of birth or upbringing,[7] and low social class.[8]

Questions about the relative importance of genetic and environmental risk factors for mental disorders, as well as their possible interaction, remain to be answered.[9] Such questions would ideally be addressed by large studies of incident cases of schizophrenia in representative samples of the general population. Population-based studies of family history as a risk factor for schizophrenia[10] have been based on prevalence rather than incidence and have not evaluated or quantified the relative contributions of, or interactions between, genetic and environmental risk factors for schizophrenia.

We used Danish population-based registries to study the effects of family history, nonfamilial risk factors, and their interactions on the risk of schizophrenia.

METHODS

The study was approved by the Danish Scientific Ethics Committees. All live-born children and new residents in Denmark are assigned a unique personal identification number, and information about them is recorded in the Civil Registration System.[11] Individual information is kept under the personal identification number in all national registers, thus ensuring accurate linkage of information between registers without the necessity to reveal a person's identity. We used data from the Danish Civil Registration System to obtain a large and representative set of data on children born to Danish women. As described in detail elsewhere,[12] we identified all women born in Denmark between April 1, 1935, and March 31, 1978, and all their offspring (2,043,492 people) who were alive on April 1, 1968, or who were born between that date and December 31, 1993. The identity of the father was available for 1,996,726 (97.7 percent) of the offspring. The offspring constituted the study population. A person could be included both as an offspring and as a mother or a father.

The study population (mothers, fathers, and offspring) were then linked with the Danish Psychiatric Central Register. The Danish Psychiatric Central Register has been computerized since April 1, 1969.[13] It contains data on all admissions to Danish psychiatric inpatient facilities and at present includes data on approximately 340,000 persons and 1.4 million admissions. There are no private facilities for inpatient psychiatric treatment in Denmark.

From the Department of Psychiatric Demography, Institute for Basic Psychiatric Research, Psychiatric Hospital, Aarhus University Hospital, Risskov (P.B.M., H.E., O.M.), and the Department of Epidemiology Research, Danish Epidemiology Science Center, Statens Serum Institut, Copenhagen (C.B.P., T.W., J.W., P.K.A., M.M.) — both in Denmark. Address reprint requests to Dr. Mortensen at the Department of Psychiatric Demography, Institute for Basic Psychiatric Research, Psychiatric Hospital, Aarhus University Hospital, Skovagervej 2, 8240 Risskov, Denmark, or at ph.ph1.pbm@aaa.dk.

The diagnostic system used during the study period was the *International Classification of Diseases, 8th Revision* (ICD-8),[14] and the diagnosis of interest was schizophrenia (ICD-8 code 295). In ICD-8 schizophrenia is defined by prototypic descriptions of symptoms, such as bizarre delusions, delusions of control, abnormal affect, autism, hallucinations, and disorganized thinking,[15] whereas in the third edition, revised, and fourth edition of the *Diagnostic and Statistical Manual of Mental Disorders* (DSM-III-R and DSM-IV, respectively) and the *International Classification of Diseases, 10th Revision* (ICD-10), most of the same symptoms have been transformed into explicit criteria. However, in a Danish register sample of 53 patients with schizophrenia as defined by ICD-8, 48 patients (91 percent) also met the criteria for schizophrenia as defined by DSM-III-R,[16] suggesting that the vast majority of persons whom we identified as having schizophrenia would meet the DSM-III-R criteria for the disorder.

Overall, 1.75 million offspring were followed from their fifth birthdays or April 1, 1970, whichever came later, until the date of onset of schizophrenia, the date of death, the date of emigration, or December 31, 1993, whichever came first. Offspring were recorded as having schizophrenia if they had been admitted to a psychiatric hospital with a diagnosis of the disorder. The date of onset was defined as the first day of the first admission leading to a diagnosis of schizophrenia. Parents were recorded as having schizophrenia if they had ever been admitted with this diagnosis. The register was assumed to be almost 100 percent complete during the study period.[13]

The relative risk of schizophrenia among the offspring was estimated by log-linear Poisson regression[17] with the SAS GENMOD procedure.[18] All relative risks were adjusted for age, sex, interactions between age and sex, calendar period when schizophrenia was diagnosed (1970 to 1974, 1975 to 1979, 1980 to 1984, 1985 to 1989, or 1990 to 1993), and age of the mother and father at the time of the child's birth. Age, calendar period of diagnosis, and schizophrenia in a sibling were treated as time-dependent variables, whereas schizophrenia in a parent was treated as a variable that was independent of time. The place of birth was classified according to the degree of urbanization: capital, suburb of the capital, provincial city with more than 100,000 inhabitants, provincial town with more than 10,000 inhabitants, or rural area.

The effect of the month of birth was modeled as a sine function with a period of 12 months and with both the amplitude and the time of the peak risk estimated. The variance of the time of the peak risk and that of the amplitude were calculated by the delta method.[19] The adjusted-residual test[20] suggested that the final regression model was not subject to overdispersion. P values were based on two-tailed likelihood-ratio tests, and 95 percent confidence limits were calculated by Wald's test.[21]

The population attributable risk is an estimate of the fraction of the total number of cases of schizophrenia in the population that would not have occurred if the effect of a specific risk factor had been eliminated — that is, if the risk could have been reduced to that of the exposure category with the lowest risk. The estimation was carried out as described by Bruzzi et al.,[22] on the basis of adjusted relative risks and the distribution of exposure in the cases. The population attributable risk for season of birth, a continuous variable, was estimated by using a categorical approach in which the fitted sine function was used to estimate relative risks for the 15th day of each month.

RESULTS

Table 1 shows the distribution of persons in whom schizophrenia developed and the person-years of exposure to risk in the study population, according to risk factors. Schizophrenia was diagnosed in a total of 1857 sons and 812 daughters during the nearly 25 million person-years of follow-up. Among these patients, 79 had a mother with schizophrenia, 33 had a father with schizophrenia, and 4 had two parents

TABLE 1. DISTRIBUTION OF 2669 CASES OF SCHIZOPHRENIA AND 24.9 MILLION PERSON-YEARS AT RISK IN A POPULATION-BASED COHORT OF 1.75 MILLION PEOPLE

VARIABLE	NO. OF CASES	PERSON-YE
Age (yr)		
5–14	35	13,594,8
15–19	635	5,234,2
20–24	1152	3,539,8
25–29	659	1,894,8
30–34	170	602,7
≥35	18	66,5
Sex		
Male	1857	12,831,5
Female	812	12,101,5
Place of birth		
Capital	860	4,256,5
Suburb of capital	233	2,251,5
Provincial city (>100,000 population)	350	3,284,9
Provincial town (>10,000 population)	737	9,047,3
Rural area	400	5,665,5
Greenland	11	47,5
Other countries	74	342,0
Unknown	4	37,6
Family history of schizophrenia		
Parent		
Father affected, mother affected	4	1,0
Father affected, mother not affected	33	44,2
Father not affected, mother affected	64	55,6
Father not affected, mother not affected	2317	24,144,7
Father unknown, mother affected	15	5,4
Father unknown, mother not affected	236	681,8
Sibling		
One or more affected siblings	59	25,5
No affected siblings	2610	24,907,5

with schizophrenia. Fifty-nine patients had at least one sibling with schizophrenia at the time that they received their own diagnosis of the disorder. Overall there were 52 sibships with 2 affected siblings, 2 sibships with 3 affected siblings, and 1 sibship with 4 affected siblings.

The relative risks associated with the risk factors identified in our study are shown in Table 2. Schizophrenia in a parent or sibling, here referred to as family history of schizophrenia, was associated with the highest relative risk of having the disease. There was a slight reduction in the estimated risk associated with any specific category of family history after adjustment for a family history of schizophrenia (Table 2, second adjustment). Further adjustment for place and season of birth (the full model) resulted in only a slight additional reduction in the association between family history and schizophrenia (Table 2). In the following discussion, we will refer only to the results of the full model.

The risk of schizophrenia was increased by a history of schizophrenia in the mother (relative risk, 9.31; 95 percent confidence interval, 7.24 to 11.96) the father (relative risk, 7.20; 95 percent confidence

TABLE 2. ADJUSTED RELATIVE RISK OF SCHIZOPHRENIA ACCORDING TO FAMILY HISTORY, PLACE OF BIRTH, AND SEASON OF BIRTH.

VARIABLE	RELATIVE RISK (95% CI)*		
	FIRST ADJUSTMENT	SECOND ADJUSTMENT	THIRD ADJUSTMENT (FULL MODEL)
Family history			
Parent			
Father affected, mother affected	65.49 (24.55–174.73)	59.74 (22.39–159.45)	46.90 (17.56–125.26)
Father affected, mother not affected	8.34 (5.91–11.76)	7.97 (5.65–11.24)	7.20 (5.10–10.16)
Father not affected, mother affected	11.33 (8.84–14.53)	10.19 (7.93–13.09)	9.31 (7.24–11.96)
Father not affected, mother not affected†	1.00	1.00	1.00
Father unknown, mother affected	20.99 (12.59–35.00)	17.12 (10.24–28.64)	14.18 (8.48–23.70)
Father unknown, mother not affected	2.48 (2.14–2.88)	2.45 (2.11–2.84)	2.00 (1.72–2.32)
Sibling			
One or more affected siblings	9.04 (6.97–11.72)	7.33 (5.63–9.53)	6.99 (5.38–9.09)
No affected siblings†	1.00	1.00	1.00
Other factors			
Place of birth			
Capital	2.49 (2.21–2.80)	2.49 (2.20–2.80)	2.40 (2.13–2.70)
Suburb of capital	1.64 (1.40–1.93)	1.64 (1.40–1.93)	1.62 (1.37–1.90)
Provincial city (>100,000 population)	1.57 (1.36–1.81)	1.57 (1.36–1.81)	1.57 (1.36–1.81)
Provincial town (>10,000 population)	1.24 (1.10–1.41)	1.24 (1.10–1.41)	1.24 (1.10–1.41)
Rural area†	1.00	1.00	1.00
Greenland	3.71 (2.03–6.75)	3.71 (2.04–6.76)	3.71 (2.04–6.76)
Other countries	3.52 (2.74–4.52)	3.52 (2.73–4.52)	3.45 (2.69–4.44)
Unknown	1.28 (0.48–3.42)	1.26 (0.47–3.39)	1.22 (0.46–3.27)
Season of birth (amplitude of sine function)‡	1.12 (1.06–1.18)	1.11 (1.06–1.18)	1.11 (1.06–1.18)

*The relative risk was adjusted initially for age–sex interaction, calendar year of diagnosis, and ages of the father and mother (first adjustment) and then for family history or, alternatively, other factors as well (second adjustment). The third adjustment (full model) was for all the variables listed. CI denotes confidence interval.

†This was the reference category.

‡For all three adjustments, the estimated peak of the sine function was at March 6 (95 percent confidence interval, February 6 to April 5).

interval, 5.10 to 10.16), or a sibling (relative risk, 6.99; 95 percent confidence interval, 5.38 to 9.09). The risk associated with having a sibling with schizophrenia was not affected by the sex of the sibling, and the risk associated with having a parent with schizophrenia was not significantly affected by which parent had the disease. The relative risk was 46.90 (95 percent confidence interval, 17.56 to 125.26) if both the father and the mother had been hospitalized with schizophrenia, and there was no statistical interaction between the father's status and the mother's status with respect to the disorder. The risk of schizophrenia for persons with unknown fathers and no maternal history of schizophrenia was twice the risk for persons with no parental history of the disorder (the reference group).

Among the other risk factors for schizophrenia, the strongest was an urban place of birth. As compared with persons born in rural areas, those born in the capital (Copenhagen) had a relative risk of 2.40 (95 percent confidence interval, 2.13 to 2.70), those born in provincial cities with more than 100,000 inhabitants or in suburbs of the capital had relative risks of approximately 1.6, and those born in towns with more than 10,000 inhabitants had a rel-

ative risk of 1.24 (95 percent confidence interval, 1.10 to 1.41). The risk of schizophrenia was also increased for children born to Danish mothers in countries other than Denmark (relative risk, 3.45; 95 percent confidence interval, 2.69 to 4.44) or in Greenland (relative risk, 3.71; 95 percent confidence interval, 2.04 to 6.76).

Figure 1 shows the effect of the month of birth on the risk of schizophrenia. The amplitude of the sine function was estimated to be 1.11 (Table 2), which means that the maximal and minimal relative risks associated with the month of birth were 1.11 and 1/1.11, respectively. The time of the peak risk was estimated to be March 6, which means that children born in early March had a risk that was 1.1 times (95 percent confidence interval, 1.06 to 1.18) the risk for those born in early June or early December.

There was no interaction between season of birth and the other variables in the model. There was a weak interaction (P=0.03) between the variables for the presence or absence of a family history of schizophrenia and those for place of birth. However, if an urban place of birth is seen as involving exposure to an unknown urban factor, there is no clear trend in the interaction. Thus, it appears that family history

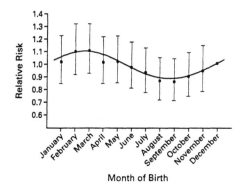

Figure 1. Relative Risk of Schizophrenia According to Month of Birth.

The data points and vertical bars show the relative risks and 95 percent confidence intervals, respectively, with the month of birth analyzed as a categorical variable, and the curve shows the relative risk as a fitted sine function of the month of birth. The reference category is December.

TABLE 3. POPULATION ATTRIBUTABLE RISK ACCORDING TO FAMILY HISTORY, PLACE OF BIRTH, AND SEASON OF BIRTH.

VARIABLE	POPULATION ATTRIBUTABLE RISK (%)
Schizophrenia in one or both parents	3.8
Schizophrenia in one or more siblings	1.9
Schizophrenia in parent or sibling	5.5
Place of birth	34.6
Season of birth	10.5
Place and season of birth	41.4
All variables listed above	46.6

was more important in association with birth in a suburb of the capital or in a provincial town and less so in association with birth in the capital, a provincial city, or a rural area.

There were no interactions between sex or age and the variables shown in Table 2. Exclusion of the youngest age group (5 to 14 years), in which the risk of schizophrenia was very low, resulted in no changes in the risk estimates or only minor changes (data not shown).

The population attributable risks associated with the risk factors in the full model are shown in Table 3. A family history of schizophrenia accounted for 5.5 percent of the cases of schizophrenia, the season of birth accounted for 10.5 percent, and an urban

place of birth accounted for 34.6 percent. The risk factors in Table 3 are not mutually exclusive, and the estimates of attributable risk are not additive.

DISCUSSION

Schizophrenia in a parent or sibling was associated with the highest risk of schizophrenia in this study. The estimate of the risk associated with a family history of schizophrenia could have been artificially increased if clinicians were more likely to diagnose the disorder in a person with one or more family members who had the same disorder than in a person with no affected family members. However, our risk estimates were very similar to those in studies that used standardized diagnostic procedures and case-finding methods that were independent of psychiatric treatment.[1,10] Therefore, we do not believe that this potential bias had any substantial effect on our results.

Some studies have reported higher rates of schizophrenia among the relatives of female patients with schizophrenia than among the relatives of male patients with schizophrenia.[23] However, in line with a population-based study reported in 1995,[24] we found no support for such differences. Our finding of an excess number of men with schizophrenia is consistent with the results of other register-based studies.[25] The effects of the risk factors included in our study were identical for men and women.

We found a twofold increase in the risk of schizophrenia among persons with unknown fathers as compared with persons with known fathers without schizophrenia. This difference might be explained by the lower socioeconomic status of the mothers of these offspring or by difficulties in growing up in a family without a father. If the difference was due to a higher proportion of cases of schizophrenia among unknown fathers, at least 16 percent of the fathers of the 46,766 offspring with unknown fathers must have had schizophrenia. Such a large proportion of unknown fathers with schizophrenia is highly unlikely, since it is of the same order of magnitude as the total number of men hospitalized during the study period for schizophrenia in Denmark. We must conclude that there is no strong empirical evidence to support any of these hypotheses, although the finding itself seems to be robust.

The prevalence of schizophrenia is higher in urban areas than in rural areas.[7,26,27] The difference has been ascribed to selective migration from rural to urban areas before the onset of schizophrenia, but this hypothesis does not explain our finding of a higher risk among people born in urban areas. Other possible explanations include increased exposure to infections during pregnancy and childhood because of more crowded living conditions or more perinatal complications in urban areas. Alternatively, one could hypothesize that persons with an unexpressed genetic predisposition for schizophrenia are more likely to migrate to urban areas, but a family history of schizophrenia does not explain or affect the urban–rural differences we observed. Furthermore, we estimated that if the risk of schizophrenia for persons born in the capital or its suburbs as compared with the risk for those born elsewhere in Denmark (relative risk, 1.74) could be explained by the presence of undiagnosed schizophrenia in parents, 9.5 percent of the 435,124 children who were born in the capital or its suburbs must have had a parent who transmitted a genetic risk equal to that transmitted by a parent with diagnosed schizophrenia. This proportion seems unrealistically high. Finally, differences in the availability of psychiatric services might explain urban–rural differences. This seems unlikely, however, because distances are small in Denmark, services are free, and place of birth, not place of residence, was the variable studied.

An interesting finding was the highly increased risk of schizophrenia in persons born to Danish women outside Denmark. This increase is probably not due to a tendency for mentally ill parents to leave the country temporarily, since the mothers and fathers of these persons did not have an increased likelihood of having schizophrenia. A possible explanation is the theory proposed by Wessely et al.[28] These authors reported an increased risk of schizophrenia in second-generation black Caribbean immigrants living in London and suggested that it could be explained by maternal exposure to infective agents uncommon in their country of origin.

The effect of season of birth on the risk of schizophrenia was of the expected magnitude and had the expected periods of maximal risk (February and March) and minimal risk (August and September).[6] We replicated a previous finding that there was no interaction between season of birth and family history of schizophrenia.[29] However, we did not replicate a previous finding that the association between winter birth and schizophrenia occurred only among persons born in urban areas.[30] Lewis[31] suggested that an association between the season of birth and schizophrenia is a methodologic artifact due to the so-called age–incidence effect — that is, persons born in January are older than those born later in the year within the same age category and thus have spent more time at risk for schizophrenia. This concern was not relevant to our cohort study, however, since all age-specific person-years were calculated exactly for each person.

There is strong evidence that the most important risk factors in families with more than one affected member are genetic.[32,33] However, the absence of consistent interactions between the family-history variables and the variables that are less likely to be genetically determined means that our results do not support the notion that birth in February or March

and an urban place of birth are less important risk factors in cases in which there is a family history of schizophrenia.

Although a family history of schizophrenia was the strongest risk factor in terms of relative risk, by far the most important factors in terms of attributable risk were the place of birth and the season of birth. Obviously, neither of these factors is relevant as a direct basis for intervention, nor are they plausible in terms of biologically meaningful exposure affecting the human brain. Instead, place and season of birth must be seen as proxy variables for factors that contribute more directly to the risk of schizophrenia. Our estimates of attributable risk do not exclude the possibility that genetic factors are necessary causes of schizophrenia in most or all cases. They do, however, suggest that such factors are not sufficient and that environmental factors are major determinants of schizophrenia.

Supported by the Theodore and Vada Stanley Foundation and the Danish National Research Foundation.

We are indebted to Dr. A. Bertelsen for his helpful comments and suggestions.

REFERENCES

1. Gottesman II. Schizophrenia genesis: the origins of madness. New York: W.H. Freeman, 1991.
2. Kendler KS, Diehl SR. The genetics of schizophrenia: a current, genetic-epidemiologic perspective. Schizophr Bull 1993;19:261-85.
3. McNeil TF. Perinatal risk factors and schizophrenia: selective review and methodological concerns. Epidemiol Rev 1995;17:107-12.
4. Geddes JR, Lawrie SM. Obstetric complications and schizophrenia: a meta-analysis. Br J Psychiatry 1995;167:786-93.
5. Barr CE, Mednick SA, Munk-Jorgensen P. Exposure to influenza epidemics during gestation and adult schizophrenia: a 40-year study. Arch Gen Psychiatry 1990;47:869-74.
6. Cotter D, Larkin C, Waddington JL, O'Callaghan E. Season of birth in schizophrenia: clue or cul-de-sac? In: Waddington JL, Buckley PF, eds. The neurodevelopmental basis of schizophrenia. Austin, Tex.: R.G. Landes, 1996:17-30.
7. Lewis G, David A, Andreasson S, Allebeck P. Schizophrenia and city life. Lancet 1992;340:137-40.
8. Eaton WW, Day R, Kramer M. The use of epidemiology for risk factor research in schizophrenia: an overview and methodologic critique. In: Tsuang MT, Simpson JC, eds. Nosology, epidemiology and genetics of schizophrenia. Vol. 3 of Handbook of schizophrenia. Amsterdam: Elsevier, 1988:169-204.
9. Kendler KS. Genetic epidemiology in psychiatry: taking both genes and environment seriously. Arch Gen Psychiatry 1995;52:895-9.
10. Kendler KS, McGuire M, Gruenberg AM, O'Hare A, Spellman M, Walsh D. The Roscommon Family Study. I. Methods, diagnosis of probands, and risk of schizophrenia in relatives. Arch Gen Psychiatry 1993; 50:527-40.
11. Malig C. The civil registration system in Denmark. IIVRS technical papers no. 66. Bethesda, Md.: International Institute for Vital Registration and Statistics, December 1996:1-9.
12. Westergaard T, Andersen PK, Pedersen JB, et al. Birth characteristics, sibling patterns, and acute leukemia risk in childhood: a population-based cohort study. J Natl Cancer Inst 1997;89:939-47.
13. Munk-Jorgensen P, Mortensen PB. The Danish Psychiatric Central Register. Dan Med Bull 1997;44:82-4.
14. Manual of the international statistical classification of diseases, injuries, and causes of death. Vol. 1. Geneva: World Health Organization, 1967.
15. Glossary of mental disorders and guide to their classification. Geneva: World Health Organization, 1974.
16. Munk-Jorgensen P. Faldende forstegangsindlaeggelsesrater for skizofreni i Danmark 1970–1991. (Doctoral dissertation. Århus, Denmark: Århus University, 1995.)

49

17. Breslow NE, Day NE. Statistical methods in cancer research. Vol. 2. The design and analysis of cohort studies. Lyon, France: International Agency for Research on Cancer, 1987. (IARC scientific publications no. 82.)
18. The GENMOD procedure. In: SAS/STAT software: changes and enhancements for release 6.12. Cary, N.C.: SAS Institute, 1996:23-41.
19. Agresti A. Categorical data analysis. New York: John Wiley, 1990.
20. Breslow NE. Generalized linear models: checking assumptions and strengthening conclusions. Stat Applicata 1996;8:23-41.
21. Clayton D, Hills M. Statistical models in epidemiology. Oxford, England: Oxford University Press, 1993.
22. Bruzzi P, Green SB, Byar DP, Brinton LA, Schairer C. Estimating the population attributable risk for multiple risk factors using case-control data. Am J Epidemiol 1985;122:904-14.
23. Goldstein JM, Faraone SV, Chen WJ, Tolomiczencko GS, Tsuang MT. Sex differences in the familial transmission of schizophrenia. Br J Psychiatry 1990;156:819-26.
24. Kendler KS, Walsh D. Gender and schizophrenia: results of an epidemiologically-based family study. Br J Psychiatry 1995;167:184-92.
25. Jablensky A, Eaton WW. Schizophrenia. Baillieres Clin Psychiatry 1995;1:283-306.
26. Takei N, Sham PC, O'Callaghan E, Glover G, Murray RM. Schizo-
phrenia: increased risk associated with winter and city birth — a case-control study in 12 regions within England and Wales. J Epidemiol Community Health 1995;49:106-7.
27. Torrey EF, Bowler A. Geographical distribution of insanity in America: evidence for an urban factor. Schizophr Bull 1990;16:591-604.
28. Wessely S, Castle D, Der G, Murray R. Schizophrenia and Afro-Caribbeans: a case-control study. Br J Psychiatry 1991;159:795-801.
29. Hettema JM, Walsh D, Kendler KS. Testing the effect of season of birth on familial risk for schizophrenia and related disorders. Br J Psychiatry 1996;168:205-9.
30. O'Callaghan E, Gibson T, Colohan HA, et al. Season of birth in schizophrenia: evidence for confinement of an excess of winter births to patients without a family history of mental disorder. Br J Psychiatry 1991;158:764-9.
31. Lewis MS. Age incidence and schizophrenia. I. The season of birth controversy. Schizophr Bull 1989;15:59-73.
32. Gottesman I, Bertelsen A. Confirming unexpressed genotypes for schizophrenia: risks in the offspring of Fischer's Danish identical and fraternal discordant twins. Arch Gen Psychiatry 1989;46:867-72.
33. Kendler K. Familial risk factors and the familial aggregation of psychiatric disorders. Psychol Med 1990;20:311-9.

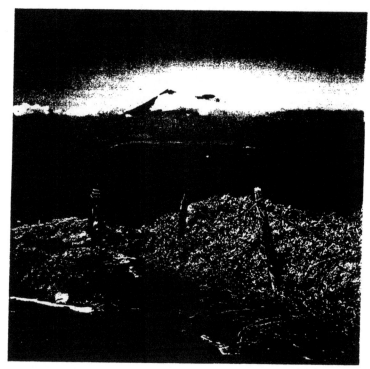

Fuji-San, Japan

DIETER LUFT, M.D.

50

> ## This Month's Special Section
> # Some Aspects of Schizophrenia

Mental Illness in the Biological and Adoptive Families of Adopted Schizophrenics

BY SEYMOUR S. KETY, M.D., DAVID ROSENTHAL, PH.D., PAUL H. WENDER, M.D., AND FINI SCHULSINGER, M.D.

Adoption has been used as a means of separating genetic and environmental factors in the transmission of schizophrenia among family members. In the study reported here, a significantly higher than usual prevalence of schizophrenia-related illness was found among the biological relatives of adopted schizophrenics, but not among their adoptive relatives. The findings support a genetic transmission of vulnerability to schizophrenia, but also imply the requirement of nongenetic, environmental factors for the development of clinical schizophrenic illness.

T HE RELATIVELY HIGH incidence of schizophrenia that is consistently found in the parents, siblings, or children of schizophrenics (1) is compatible with both genetic and environmental transmissability of the disorder since close family members share both types of factors. Monozygotic twins, except for the relatively few who are separated at an early age, also share considerably more environmental components and psychological identification than do the dizygotic

twins of the same sex (2). It was for these reasons that the suggestion was made in 1959 (2) that adopted children, who receive their genetic endowment from one family and their environmental interactions from another, constitute a uniquely useful population for disentangling these two groups of variables in the transmission of schizophrenia.

In 1963 we initiated a collaborative effort to carry out several studies utilizing adoption as a means of disentangling hereditary and environmental influences in schizophrenia (3-5). This paper is based on the report of one of these studies (3), which examined the prevalence and nature of mental illness in the biological and adoptive parents, siblings, and half-siblings of individuals who were adopted at an early age by families not biologically related to them and who eventually became schizophrenic.

Methods

A detailed description of the methods employed was presented in the original report (3). In order to avoid selective bias it was important to begin with a total sample of adopted individuals. Through the cooperation of the State Department of Justice of Denmark, access to the complete file of adoption records was granted with appropriate safeguards regarding their confidentiality. From the total sample of legal adoptions a subsample was obtained that included all adoptions that met the following criteria: 1) adoption granted by the City and County of Copenhagen (the study is now being extended to all of Denmark), 2) adoption granted between 1924 and 1948 inclusive, and 3) adoption by persons not biologically related to the child. This yielded 5,483 adop-

Read at the 123rd annual meeting of the American Psychiatric Association, San Francisco, Calif., May 11-15, 1970.

Dr. Kety is Professor of Psychiatry at Harvard Medical School and Director of the Psychiatric Research Laboratories, Massachusetts General Hospital, Boston, Mass. 02114. Drs. Rosenthal and Wender are with the National Institute of Mental Health, Bethesda, Md., where Dr. Rosenthal is Chief of the Laboratory of Psychology and Dr. Wender is Research Psychiatrist. Dr. Schulsinger is Director of the Psychiatric Service at the Kommunehospitalet, Copenhagen, Denmark.

This work was supported in part by the Intramural Research Program of the National Institute of Mental Health, by Public Health Service grant MH-15602 from NIMH, and by grants from the Schizophrenia Research Program of the Scottish Rite and from the Foundations' Fund for Research in Psychiatry.

[82]

tions and constituted our sample of adoptees.

For the purpose of this study we agreed that we would include as "schizophrenic" those individuals whose psychiatric history was characteristic of "chronic schizophrenia," "acute schizophrenic reaction," or "borderline schizophrenia" as these terms are commonly used in the United States. The characteristics of each group were stipulated (3). It was then necessary to find a group of schizophrenic index cases among the total sample of 5,483 adoptees.

Since 1920 the Psychiatric Register of the Institute of Human Genetics has recorded with little loss the names of those admitted to any psychiatric facility. A search of these records, supplemented by individual searches in specific hospitals, revealed that 507 adoptees had been admitted to a psychiatric facility for any reason. It was from this group that the index cases were selected. Because schizophrenia is more narrowly defined in Denmark and in Europe generally, English abstracts of the psychiatric histories of each of these 507 adoptees were prepared and independently examined by each of us. Where agreement could be reached on a diagnosis of schizophrenia, that adoptee became an index case. In this way, 33 index cases were agreed upon. For each of these a control was selected from the pool of adoptees with no known psychiatric history and who matched the index case in sex, age, socioeconomic class of the adoptive parents, time spent with the biological family, and preadoption history.

These 66 names were then randomly pooled and used in a search through the adoption records and the very complete population register of Denmark in order to identifiy for each individual the biological and adoptive parents, siblings, and half-siblings. In this way 463 such relatives were identified.

The Psychiatric Register, the files of the 14 major psychiatric hospitals, records of the Mothers' Aid Organization, police records, and military records were then searched for the names of any of the 463 identified relatives of the index cases and their controls. This yielded 67 relatives to whom some mental or behavioral aberration could be attributed.

Since the diagnosis of mental illness in the biological and adoptive families of the probands was the crucial determination of the

study, every effort was made to insure that this diagnosis was made independently by each of the four collaborators and in the absence of any knowledge that might bias his evaluation. For each of these relatives, the case records were obtained from the respective institutions and an English summary of each was prepared by a Danish psychiatrist who was not aware of the specific hypotheses being tested and not informed of the relationship of any relative to index or control probands. These summaries were transcribed and the transcriptions were edited to delete all personal names, diagnostic opinions, and any information that might suggest to a sophisticated reviewer that the subject in question was a biological or an adoptive relative of an index case or of a control.

Operating on the hypothesis that schizophrenia need not be transmitted as such but as a broader spectrum of disorders (6), we postulated in advance that this "schizophrenia spectrum" would include clear-cut schizophrenia of the chronic, acute, or borderline type as well as cases where the diagnosis could not be as certain, which would be designated "possible schizophrenia" of one of the three subtypes. Our experience with the selection of index cases caused us to recognize the existence of a group similar in quality to the borderline schizophrenic but of considerably less intensity. This group is best described as "inadequate personality" in the standard nomenclature and it was included as the mildest of the disorders of the schizophrenia spectrum. After independent evaluation by each of the collaborators, a consensus was arrived at in all but four of the cases and these four were excluded from the subsequent analysis.

Results

The adoptive relatives differed from the biological ones in age, in the number of siblings, and especially in the number of half-siblings. In addition, the adoption agency would have employed some type of screening, which might have tended to reduce psychopathology among them, while it would be expected that emotional instability and psychopathology would be higher in the sample of biological parents, who were usually unmarried, than in the population at

TABLE 1

Incidence of Schizophrenia Spectrum Disorders
Among the Biological and Adoptive Relatives
of Schizophrenic Index Cases and Controls

SAMPLE	BIOLOGICAL RELATIVES	ADOPTIVE RELATIVES
Total sample		
Index cases (N = 33)	13 out of 150	2 out of 74
Controls (N = 33)	3 out of 156	3 out of 83
Significance*	p = .0072	n.s.
Subsample: separated within one month of birth		
Index cases (N = 19)	9 out of 93	2 out of 45
Controls (N = 20)	0 out of 92	1 out of 51
Significance*	p = .0018	n.s.

* P is one-sided, from exact distribution.

large. On the other hand, such differences
would not be expected to exist between the
families of index cases and their controls,
whether biological or adoptive. Thus, the
prevalence of particular types of mental illness in each group of relatives of the index
cases can appropriately be compared with
that in the corresponding relatives of the
controls, permitting the separate testing of
hypotheses based on genetic or environmental factors in the transmission of schizophrenia.

Mental illness other than that in the schizophrenia spectrum showed a random distribution among the biological and adoptive
relatives of index cases and controls. On the
other hand (see table 1) there was a highly
significant concentration of disorders in the
schizophrenia spectrum in the biological
relatives of the index cases as compared with
the similar relatives of the controls. When
the examination was confined to those index
cases and controls who spent the shortest
period of time with their biological relatives
(less than one month), the difference became
even more significant, probably by virtue of
eliminating some among the controls where
mental illness in the biological family may
have been a factor in putting the child out for
adoption. Of the 13 biological relatives of
index cases who were found to have disorders
in the schizophrenia spectrum, seven were
paternally related half-siblings with whom
the index cases would have had in common
not even an *in utero* environment but only
some degree of genetic overlap.

The conclusion appears warranted that
genetic factors operate significantly in the
transmission of schizophrenia, and that the
higher than expected prevalence of schizo-

phrenia in the families of naturally reared
schizophrenics is a manifestation of such
transmission.

The prevalence of disorders in the schizophrenia spectrum in the adoptive relatives
of the index cases is low and it is not significantly different from the prevalence that
exists in the adoptive relatives of the controls.
Although this does not support hypotheses
that depend on the acquisition of schizophrenic behavior by learning from or imita-
tion of other members of the family, it should
be pointed out that our findings do not argue
against the importance of environmental
factors in the etiology of these disorders.
Besides the presence in the household of an
individual who exhibits some of the features
of schizophrenia, there are many other aspects of life experience—including subtle
personality characteristics, child rearing
practices, nutritional habits, or even exposure
to toxic or infectious agents—that may serve
to evoke and elaborate one or another type
of disorder in the schizophrenia spectrum
in a genetically vulnerable individual. In an
effort to obtain more information that may
help to define such environmental variables,
systematic interviews are being conducted
with these biological and adoptive relatives.
From the numerous questions relating to
early life experience, education, peer relationships, parental qualities, and history of
physical and emotional illness, it may be
possible to derive some hypotheses regarding
environmental factors that differentiate
from the rest those adoptive families in which
a schizophrenic illness has occurred.

Examination of the types of schizophrenia
spectrum disorder discovered in the biological relatives of the index cases (table 2) indicates a broad distribution over the whole
spectrum with no tendency for the type of
schizophrenia in the index case to be reflected
in the type or intensity of illness in the relatives. This appears to be more compatible
with a polygenic form of inheritance rather
than with any simple monogenic mode. A
parsimonious explanation of the findings,
and the one that we prefer, since it helps to
account for many of the observations of
other workers, is that schizophrenia is not
transmitted genetically as such but as a vulnerability or predisposition that requires
the operation of other factors, probably en-

[84]

Amer. J. Psychiat. 128:3, September 1971

TABLE 2
Distribution of Schizophrenia Spectrum Disorders
in the Biological Relatives of 33 Schizophrenic Index Cases

INDEX CASES	TOTAL NUMBER OF RELATIVES	SCHIZOPHRENIA CHRONIC	SCHIZOPHRENIA ACUTE	SCHIZOPHRENIA BORDERLINE	POSSIBLE SCHIZOPHRENIA CHRONIC	POSSIBLE SCHIZOPHRENIA ACUTE	POSSIBLE SCHIZOPHRENIA BORDERLINE	INADEQUATE PERSONALITY
Chronic schizophrenia (N = 16)	82	1		3			2	1
Acute schizophrenic reaction (N = 7)	30							
Borderline schizophrenia (N = 10)	38			3	1		1	1

vironmental. The presence or absence of schizophrenia, the position on the schizophrenia spectrum, or the extent to which the individual is eccentric or even creative may be determined by an interaction between these genetic and environmental variables.

The data on the distribution of disorders in the schizophrenia spectrum among the biological relatives of the index cases also permits some inferences regarding the nosology of schizophrenia. None of the biological relatives of the index cases diagnosed as "acute schizophrenic reaction" were found to have schizophrenia spectrum disorders, nor did any of the relatives of any index cases receive that diagnosis themselves. This serves to call into question the appropriateness of classifying all such acute psychotic reactions as schizophrenic disorders without further evidence from premorbid personality characteristics or the later course of the illness. On the other hand, it is noteworthy that the biological relatives of the index subjects whom we had diagnosed as having "borderline schizophrenia" showed a pattern of schizophrenia spectrum disorders that was not significantly different from that of the biological relatives of the chronic schizophrenic index cases. We suggest that this constitutes compelling evidence for continuing to regard such borderline states as forms of schizophrenia.

It is interesting that although there is a roughly ten percent prevalence of disorders in the schizophrenia spectrum among the biological relatives of the index cases, there is a much lower prevalence of chronic schizophrenia than one would have been led to expect from the prevalence reported for that disorder in the families of naturally reared schizophrenics (1). Thus, among the 82 identified biological relatives of the chronic schizophrenic index cases only one could be diagnosed as having chronic schizophrenia, a prevalence of a little over one percent. Six others whom we classified in our

deliberately broad schizophrenia spectrum would probably not have fulfilled the traditional criteria for schizophrenia. One possible explanation may be that the presence of a diagnosed schizophrenic in a family that is living together makes more intensive the search for and more likely the discovery of mental disorders or abnormal traits in other members and their diagnosis as schizophrenic. In our sample, on the other hand, the transfer of information regarding the existence of mental illness between the adoptee and the biological family was extremely unlikely by virtue of his early transfer from the biological family, by the fact that most of the schizophrenia spectrum disorders occurred in half-siblings, and because most of the mental illness in the biological family occurred after the separation of the index cases. In our study of adoptees (7), it was found that 87 percent of the schizophrenic biological parents had their first admissions to a psychiatric facility some time after the birth of the child.

If it can be shown that the higher incidence of more severe types of schizophrenia in the families of naturally reared schizophrenics is not an artifact of ascertainment or diagnosis, another explanation could be entertained for the relatively low intensity of schizophrenia in the biological relatives of the index cases. If schizophrenia does in fact depend upon an interaction of environmental and genetic factors, the risk of their combination should be highest in the families of naturally reared schizophrenics, while adoption, by placing a predisposed individual in an environment with only a chance distribution of schizophrenogenic factors, should tend to decrease the risk of occurrence and the severity of schizophrenia. We are now engaged in collecting a sample of nonadopted individuals who can be matched with the 5,483 adoptees in age, sex, and social class as the basis for a comparison group of naturally reared schizophrenics in whose relatives we shall seek to determine the prevalence and type of schizophrenia spectrum disorders using the same diagnostic criteria we have used in the sample of adoptees.

Summary

Adoption has been used as a means of separating genetic and environmental factors in the transmission of schizophrenia among family members. Among the 5,483 adoptions granted in the City and County of Copenhagen from 1924 to 1948 to adoptive parents who were not biologically related to the child, 33 adoptees were found whose psychiatric history warranted a diagnosis of schizophrenia. Of these, 16 were diagnosed as having chronic schizophrenia, seven as having acute schizophrenic reaction, and ten as having borderline schizophrenia. These and an equal number of matched control adoptees with no history of mental hospitalization yielded, by search of the Danish population registers, 306 identified biological parents, siblings, or half-siblings and 157 adoptive relatives in similar relationships. Of these 463 relatives, 67 had at some time been admitted to a psychiatric facility. These records were abstracted and edited to remove prejudicial information; they then served as the basis for our independent and consensus diagnoses.

There was a very significantly greater prevalence of schizophrenia-related disorders in the biological families of the 33 schizophrenic index cases than among those of the controls. The significance of the increased prevalence was even greater for the biological families of the 19 index cases who had been separated from their families within the first month of life. The prevalence of these disorders in the adoptive families was lower and was randomly distributed between index cases and controls.

The pattern of schizophrenia-related disorders in the biological families was the same for the 16 index cases diagnosed as "chronic schizophrenia" as for ten diagnosed as "borderline schizophrenia," which supports the inclusion of this syndrome among the schizophrenias. On the other hand, the seven index cases diagnosed as "acute schizophrenic reaction" showed no schizophrenia-related disorder in the biological relatives, which raises some questions regarding the relationship of that state to schizophrenia.

There was no correlation between the type and intensity of schizophrenia-related disorders in the biological relatives and those in the index cases.

The findings provide support for a theory of genetic transmission of vulnerability to schizophrenia, but they also imply the requirement of nongenetic, environmental factors for the development of clinical schizophrenic illness.

REFERENCES

1. Slater E: A review of earlier evidence on genetic factors in schizophrenia, in The Transmission of Schizophrenia. Edited by Rosenthal D, Kety SS. Oxford, Pergamon Press, 1968, pp 15-26
2. Kety, SS: Biochemical theories of schizophrenia. Science 129:1528-1532; 1590-1596, 1959
3. Kety SS, Rosenthal D, Wender PH, et al: The types and prevalence of mental illness in the biological and adoptive families of adopted schizophrenics, in The Transmission of Schizophrenia. Edited by Rosenthal D, Kety SS. Oxford, Pergamon Press, 1968, pp 345-362
4. Rosenthal D, Wender PH, Kety SS, et al: Schizophrenics' offspring reared in adoptive homes. Ibid, pp 377-392
5. Wender P, Rosenthal D, Kety SS: A psychiatric assessment of the adoptive parents of schizophrenics. Ibid, pp 235-250
6. Rosenthal D: Theoretical overview: a suggested conceptual framework, in The Genain Quadruplets: A Case Study and Theoretical Analysis of Heredity and Environment in Schizophrenia. Edited by Rosenthal D. New York, Basic Books, 1963, pp 505-579
7. Rosenthal D, Wender PH, Kety SS, et al: The adopted-away offspring of schizophrenics. Amer J Psychiat 128:307-311, 1971

[86]   *Amer. J. Psychiat. 128:3, September 1971*

56

An Independent Analysis of the
Danish Adoption Study of Schizophrenia

VI. The Relationship Between Psychiatric Disorders
as Defined by *DSM-III* in the Relatives and Adoptees

Kenneth S. Kendler, MD, Alan M. Gruenberg, MD

● In this report, modified *DSM-III* criteria were applied to all
the available interviews with adoptees from the greater
Copenhagen sample of the Danish Adoption Study of Schizophrenia. In the adoptees, reasonable agreement was found
between our *DSM-III* diagnoses and the original diagnoses
using global *DSM-II*-based criteria by Kety et al for their
categories of chronic and acute, but not borderline, schizophrenia. Comparing *DSM-III*-based diagnoses in adoptees and
relatives, schizophrenia, schizotypal personality disorder, and
paranoid personality disorder were all significantly more
common in the biologic relatives of schizophrenic v screened
control adoptees. These three diagnoses, which together form
a tentative "schizophrenia spectrum," were also significantly
concentrated in the biologic relatives of adoptees with schizoaffective disorder, mainly schizophrenic subtype, and schizotypal personality disorder, but not in biologic relatives of
adoptees with schizophreniform disorder or atypical psychosis.

(Arch Gen Psychiatry 1984;41:555-564)

In 1968, Kety and co-workers published the first report
from an adoption study of schizophrenia carried out in
Denmark.[1] This study began with the identification of 34
adopted persons from the greater Copenhagen area who
suffered what the original investigators called "chronic,"
"borderline," or "acute" schizophrenia. These global diagnostic categories, a detailed description of which is available
in the original publication, were based in part on the *DSM-II*.[2]
To each of these "index" adoptees, the investigators
matched a control adoptee who had no record of psychiatric

hospitalization. The psychiatric registry was then searched
for all identified biologic or adoptive parents, siblings, and
half siblings of the index and control adoptees who had ever
undergone psychiatric hospitalization. Abstracts were
made of these hospital records and then they were blindly
reviewed. A significant excess of chronic, borderline, and
uncertain schizophrenia, as defined by the original investigators, was found in the biologic relatives of the index
adoptees.

The next major results from this study were published in
1975.[3] In the intervening years, an attempt was made to
interview personally all available biologic and adoptive
relatives of the index and control adoptees. In addition, if
available and cooperative, control adoptees were also personally interviewed. No attempt was made to interview
index adoptees. In 1975, the preliminary results of a blind
review of these psychiatric interviews were reported, using
the same diagnostic criteria that had originally been applied
to the hospital records. The results replicated and extended
the results found in the original report. Chronic, borderline, and uncertain schizophrenia, as defined by the
original investigators, again were significantly concentrated in the biologic relatives of the index adoptees.

Since this adoption study was conceptualized in the late
1960s, the approach to psychiatric diagnosis has undergone
considerable change. Particularly, emphasis has shifted
from the global diagnostic descriptions of *DSM-II* to
operationalized diagnostic criteria. These and other
changes in psychiatric diagnosis have prompted three major
reexaminations of the interviews collected by Kety et al.
First, Spitzer et al applied the Research Diagnostic Criteria (RDC)[4] to a subset of the interviews with relatives and
adoptees that contained all the cases diagnosed as chronic,
borderline, acute, or uncertain schizophrenia by Kety et al.[5]
They found a high rate of agreement with the diagnoses of
Kety et al, especially in those cases initially diagnosed as
chronic schizophrenia. Second, Gunderson et al examined
another subset of these interviews with the specific goal of
defining more clearly the characteristics of the "schiz-

Accepted for publication Aug 1, 1983.
From the Departments of Psychiatry and Human Genetics, Medical
College of Virginia, Richmond (Dr Kendler); and the Yale Psychiatric
Institute and Department of Psychiatry, Yale University School of Medi-
cine, New Haven, Conn (Dr Gruenberg).
Reprint requests to Department of Psychiatry, Medical College of
Virginia, PO Box 710, Richmond, VA 23298 (Dr Kendler).

57

Table 1.—Definitions of the Diagnostic Groupings Used in This Report

Term	Definition
"Schizophrenia spectrum"	Cases (adoptees or relatives) meeting *DSM-III* criteria for schizophrenia, schizoaffective disorder (mainly schizophrenic subtype by Research Diagnostic Criteria [RDC]), schizotypal personality disorder, or paranoid personality disorder*
"Psychotic nonspectrum"	Adoptees meeting *DSM-III* criteria for schizoaffective disorder (mainly affective or other subtype by RDC), schizophreniform disorder, paranoid disorder, atypical psychosis, or psychotic affective illness
"Nonpsychotic nonspectrum"	Adoptees meeting *DSM-III* criteria for personality disorders other than schizotypal or paranoid, or meeting criteria for other nonpsychotic mental disorders
"Nonpsychotic spectrum"	Adoptees meeting *DSM-III* criteria for schizotypal or paranoid personality disorder
All controls	All control adoptees initially selected by Kety et al[1]
Screened controls	Those controls for whom personal interviews were available and who did not receive a diagnosis within the "schizophrenia spectrum"

*No cases of schizoaffective disorder were diagnosed in interviewed relatives, and no cases of paranoid personality disorder were diagnosed in adoptees. Therefore, our "schizophrenia spectrum" is not identical as operationalized in adoptees and relatives.

otype."[6] In addition to recording the presence or absence of a wide variety of specific psychiatric symptoms, they made both clinical and *DSM-III*–based[7] diagnoses of borderline and schizotypal personality disorder. They found an identifiable personality syndrome in the biologic relatives of schizophrenic adoptees, which was particularly characterized by social dysfunction, eccentricity, poor interpersonal rapport, and suspiciousness.

The third major reexamination of results from the adoption study of Kety et al began in 1979 as a collaboration between us and John Strauss, MD. Using a select group of *DSM-III* disorders, we reviewed and diagnosed all the available interviews with the relatives collected by Kety and co-workers. Our major focus at that time was to use the adoption method to clarify the nosologic relationships between various psychiatric disorders and schizophrenia. In a series of reports, we examined the distribution of anxiety disorder,[8] schizotypal personality disorder,[9] major depressive disorder,[10] and paranoid personality disorder[11] as defined by *DSM-III*, in the relatives of the index and control adoptees. In addition, we examined the distribution in the relatives of a new disorder, called "delusional disorder" which was related to but not identical with the *DSM-III* category of paranoid disorder.[12] We found that schizotypal and paranoid personality disorders, but not anxiety disorder, major depressive disorder, or delusional disorder, were significantly concentrated in the biologic relatives of the index adoptees.

A methodologic limitation of our earlier reports was that the diagnostic criteria applied to the adoptees and relatives were different. Except for the diagnosis of delusional disorder, the relatives were all diagnosed using *DSM-III* criteria.[7] The adoptees' diagnoses used, however, were the ones originally assigned by Kety and co-workers[1] using global *DSM-II*–based diagnostic criteria. To correct this deficiency, in 1982 we blindly reviewed and applied *DSM-III* criteria to all the available interviews with the index and control adoptees.

In this report, we first compare our diagnoses of the

adoptees with those originally made by Kety and co-workers.[1] Then, we examine the relationship between certain psychiatric disorders as defined by *DSM-III* in th[e] adoptees and their interviewed biologic and adoptive rela[-]tives.

SUBJECTS AND METHODS

The methodologies of the Danish Adoption study[1,3] and ou[r] independent analysis of the interviews with relatives[5] have bee[n] reviewed elsewhere. Briefly, Kety et al[1] identified 34 index adop[-]tees from the greater Copenhagen area who met their criteria fo[r] chronic, borderline, or acute schizophrenia. They made thei[r] psychiatric diagnoses on the basis of a symptom checklist and i[n] case of initial disagreement a one- to two-page synopsis of hospita[l] records. They also identified a group of control adoptees who ha[d] never been hospitalized for psychiatric reasons and who were matched to the index adoptees for sex, age, length of time spen[t] with biologic relatives, institutions or foster families, age a[t] transfer to adoptive parents, and socioeconomic status of adoptiv[e] family. All the biologic and adoptive relatives of the index an[d] control adoptees were then identified and efforts made to inte[r]view them personally. Of the available relatives, 90% were succes[s]fully interviewed. Those who refused were evenly distributed i[n] the four groups of relatives. However, significantly more of th[e] biologic relatives of the index than control adoptees had died and[,] hence, were unavailable for interview.[3]

Interviews were also conducted with all available control adop[-]tees. Based on an extensive review of hospital records, detaile[d] pseudointerviews were constructed for all of the index adoptees[.] These pseudointerviews contained more detailed information o[n] the index adoptees than had been available to Kety and co-worker[s] when they made their initial diagnoses. However, although the[y] contained a detailed account of the psychiatric illness, the hospita[l] records did not contain all the information normally present i[n] sections of the real interviews dealing with such factors as person[al] history or living environment. This difference in informatio[n] content as well as other differences in format made it impossible t[o] be "blind" to whether an adoptee interview was a real intervie[w] with a control adoptee or a pseudointerview with an index adoptee[.]

For this report, we reviewed all available real and pseudointe[r]views with adoptees and applied *DSM-III* criteria to them. Lik[e] the interview with relatives, the real and pseudointerviews wit[h] the adoptees had been edited to remove any mention of adoptive o[r] biologic relatives. Therefore, this diagnostic review was conducte[d] blind to the presence of any psychiatric illness in the relatives of th[e] adoptees. Because this review was conducted three years after ou[r] examination of the interviews with relatives, the reliability of ou[r] diagnoses was reexamined. Each of us blindly rated ten random[ly] chosen index and ten randomly chosen control interviews. Of thes[e] 20 interviews, our *DSM-III* diagnoses agreed in 18 (90% agree[-]ment, K=.86).

Information was not always present in the interviews to rat[e] definitively the presence or absence of all *DSM-III* criteri[a.] Therefore, as in the review of the interview with relatives[,] diagnoses were assigned as definite, probable, or possible. In th[is] report, the diagnoses used in the adoptees and relatives are thos[e] primary diagnoses rated as definite, probable, or possible (ie, th[e] broad definition used previously[8-12]). A number of index adopte[es] had both prominent personality disorders and clearly psychot[ic] episodes. In most of these cases, the primary diagnosis assigne[d] was that of psychosis.

Diagnoses used in this report are as defined in *DSM-III* with tw[o] exceptions. First, as previously reported in our analysis of inte[r]views with relatives, the diagnosis of delusional disorder was giv[en] priority over *DSM-III* diagnosis (usually paranoid disorder [or] atypical psychosis). Only one adoptee met criteria for delusion[al] disorder, and this subject also met *DSM-III* criteria for paranoi[d] disorder. Second, the *DSM-III* criteria for schizoaffective disord[er] contain neither specific inclusion nor exclusion criteria. Furthe[r]more, *DSM-III* provides no criteria for further subtyping th[is] probably heterogeneous diagnostic entity. Therefore, any adopte[e] considered schizoaffective by *DSM-III* was categorized using th[e] RDC[4] as mainly schizophrenic, mainly affective, or other.

Based on earlier results of ours[9,11] and others[4,5] from this Dani[sh]

58

Table 2.—Comparison of Diagnoses Assigned to Index Adoptees by Kety and Co-workers Using Global Criteria Based on *DSM-II* and by Us Using Modified *DSM-III* Criteria

	Diagnoses by Kety and Co-workers		
DSM-III Diagnosis	Chronic Schizophrenia	Borderline Schizophrenia	Acute Schizophrenia
Schizophrenia	11	2	0
Schizoaffective disorder,* mainly schizophrenic	3	0	0
Schizotypal personality disorder	1	1	1
Schizoaffective disorder,* other	0	0	1
Schizophreniform disorder	0	0	5
Delusional disorder†	0	1	0
Atypical psychosis	0	3	0
Bipolar disorder‡	0	1	0
Other personality disorder§	1	2	0
Other nonpsychotic mental disorder	1	0	0
Total	17	10	7

*Subtyped by the Research Diagnostic Criteria.
†Also meets *DSM-III* criteria for paranoid disorder.
‡With psychotic features.
§Two cases—mixed personality disorder, one case (initially diagnosed as borderline schizophrenia)—and borderline personality disorder.

adoption study, as well as other studies[12] and clinical intuition, prior to our examination of the adoptee interviews, we defined a tentative "schizophrenia spectrum" as consisting of four disorders: schizophrenia, schizoaffective disorder meeting RDC criteria for the mainly schizophrenic subtype, schizotypal personality disorder, and paranoid personality disorder. In this report, we will always place quotation marks around this proposed diagnostic grouping to emphasize both the tentative nature of this group and to remind readers that this group differs in some respects from the schizophrenia spectrum concept initially articulated by Kety and co-workers.[1,3] By chance, we found no cases of paranoid personality disorder in the relatives and no cases of schizoaffective disorder in the relatives. Therefore, our "schizophrenia spectrum," as found in the adoptees and relatives, is not the same. In the adoptees, the "schizophrenia spectrum" refers to cases meeting criteria for schizophrenia; schizoaffective disorder, mainly schizophrenic subtype; and schizotypal personality disorder. In the relatives, the "schizophrenia spectrum" refers to cases meeting criteria for schizophrenia and schizotypal and paranoid personality disorders.

As originally done by Kety and co-workers[3] we divided the control adoptees into two groups for analysis: all controls and screened controls. The screened controls were those for whom, in our judgment, sufficient information was available to determine that they had no psychiatric disorder within our "schizophrenia spectrum." All controls consisted of the screened and nonscreened controls. Our intent was to classify as nonscreened any control adoptee who either had a psychiatric disorder within the "schizophrenia spectrum" or for whom insufficient information was available to make a psychiatric diagnosis. However, only the latter criterion was used, as none of the control adoptees for whom sufficient information was available were assigned a diagnosis within the "schizophrenia spectrum." Our division of control adoptees into screened and nonscreened categories was not identical to that made by Kety and co-workers.[3]

Although 34 index adoptees had initially been identified by Kety et al,[1] there were only 33 biologic families because two of the index adoptees were members of a twin pair. Fortunately, we did not have to decide how to analyze their biologic relatives if these two twins were assigned different diagnoses because they had no interviewed biologic relatives.

In the three years since our original analysis of the interviews with relatives, results from the Copenhagen sample of the Danish adoption study have been continually updated. When results from the present adoptee analysis were compared with those previously reported by us,[5,12] a discrepancy of one was revealed. One relative, considered by us to be free of psychiatric illness, was reclassified

from a biologic relative of a control to a biologic relative of an index adoptee.

There are conflicting statistical approaches to the analysis of 2×2 contingency tables with small expected cell frequencies such as found in the results of this report. There is general agreement that when all expected values exceed 5, the χ^2 test is appropriate and accurate.[14] More recent work suggests that the χ^2 test without correction provides a good estimate for type I error rates when the number is greater than 20 with expected values as low as 1.[15,16] Our approach to this uncertain area was as follows. For any contingency table where all expected values exceeded 5, the χ^2 test without correction was used. When expected values fell between 1 and 5, both the uncorrected χ^2 and a modified exact test[17] were applied. However, in every such case, the difference in results between these two methods was trivial, so only the results of the χ^2 analyses are presented. Finally, for any contingency table, when expected values fall below 1 or the total number is less than 20, the results of a modified exact test are reported. For the χ^2 test, two-tailed P values are reported, whereas the exact test is a one-sided test. Unless otherwise noted, reported χ^2 tests have a df of 1. "Not significant" refers to P values greater than .05.

Because we use several new, and potentially confusing, diagnostic groupings in this report, for the sake of clarity, Table 1 provides definitions of these groupings.

RESULTS

DSM-III Diagnoses in Index and Control Adoptees

A comparison of the original diagnoses given to the index adoptees by Kety and co-workers[1] and our *DSM-III* diagnoses is given in Table 2. Of the 17 cases with original diagnoses of chronic schizophrenia by Kety et al, we diagnosed 11 (64.7%) as meeting *DSM-III* criteria for schizophrenia; three (17.6%) as meeting criteria for schizoaffective disorder, mainly schizophrenic subtype; and one each meeting criteria for schizotypal personality disorder, other personality disorder, and other nonpsychotic mental disorder. Of the seven cases with original diagnoses of acute schizophrenia, five (71.4%) met *DSM-III* criteria for schizophreniform disorder and one each for schizoaffective disorder, other subtype, and schizotypal personality disorder. The ten cases with original diagnoses of borderline schizophrenia by Kety and co-workers[1] met criteria for the following *DSM-III* diagnoses: schizophrenia (two), schizotypal personality disorder (one), atypical psychosis (three), psychotic bipolar disorder (one), and other personality disorder (two). In addition, one adoptee originally given a diagnosis of borderline schizophrenia met criteria for delusional disorder (and *DSM-III* criteria for paranoid disorder).

59

Table 3.—Distribution of Various Psychiatric Disorders in All Interviewed Biologic Relatives of Index Adoptees According to Their DSM-III Diagnosis*

DSM-III Adoptee Diagnosis	No.	Relatives With DSM-III Diagnosis				
		Schizophrenia	SPD	PPD	Anxiety Disorder	Major Depressive Disorder
Schizophrenia	35	2	5	2	4	2
Schizoaffective disorder,† mainly schizophrenic	28	1	2	0	3	1
SPD	6	0	2	1	1	0
Schizoaffective disorder, other†	5	0	0	0	0	1
Schizophreniform disorder	13	0	0	1	5	1
Delusional disorder‡	3	0	0	0	1	0
Atypical psychosis	10	0	0	0	3	1
Bipolar disorder	3	0	0	0	1	0
Other personality disorder	1	0	1	0	0	0
Other nonpsychotic mental disorder	2	0	1	0	0	1

*SPD indicates schizotypal personality disorder; PPD, paranoid personality disorder; other, other personality disorders and other nonpsychotic mental disorder.
†Subtyped by Research Diagnostic Criteria.
‡Also meets DSM-III criteria for paranoid disorder.

Table 4.—Frequency of 'Schizophrenia Spectrum' Disorders in All Interviewed Biologic Relatives of Index Adoptees With Schizophrenia, 'Schizophrenia Spectrum,' and 'Psychotic Nonspectrum' Disorders*

Adoptees	No.	Relatives			
		Schizophrenia No. (%)	SPD† No. (%)	PPD No. (%)	"Schizophrenia Spectrum" No. (%)
Schizophrenia	35	2 (5.7)	5 (14.3)	2 (5.7)	9 (25.7)
"Schizophrenia spectrum"	69	3 (4.3)	9 (13.0)	3 (4.3)	15 (21.7)
"Psychotic nonspectrum"	34	0 ...	0 ...	1 (2.9)	1 (2.9)

Comparison Groups of Adoptees	Significance of Difference In Frequency		
	Relatives		
	SPD	"Schizophrenia Spectrum"	"Nonpsychotic Spectrum"
Schizophrenia v "psychotic nonspectrum"	.022	.007	.027
"Schizophrenia spectrum" v "psychotic nonspectrum"	.027	.013	.038

*Statistical analysis by χ^2. No statistically significant difference was found in the frequency of either schizophrenia or paranoid personality disorder (PPD) in the interviewed biologic relatives of either the schizophrenic or "schizophrenic spectrum" adoptees v interviewed biologic relatives of "psychotic nonspectrum" adoptees.
†SPD indicates schizotypal personality disorder.

Sufficient information was present in our opinion to classify 24 of the control adoptees as screened controls. The DSM-III diagnoses assigned to these cases were major depressive disorder (one), anxiety disorder (three), conversion disorder (one), and no psychiatric diagnosis (19).

Psychiatric Disorders in the Interviewed Biologic Relatives

The distribution of various psychiatric disorders in the interviewed biologic relatives of the index adoptees, divided by their DSM-III diagnoses, is given in Table 3. Given the small number of interviewed biologic relatives of the index adoptees and the large number of diagnoses assigned to these adoptees, statistical analy-

sis required that they be divided into a few rational categories. Therefore, we analyzed the index adoptees using the following four overlapping groups: (1) schizophrenia, (2) "schizophrenia spectrum," (3) psychotic disorders outside the spectrum (termed "psychotic nonspectrum"), and (4) nonpsychotic disorders outside the spectrum (termed "nonpsychotic nonspectrum") (see Table 1 for definitions).

The frequency of the "schizophrenia spectrum" disorders in the interviewed biologic relatives of the first three subgroups of the index adoptees is given in Table 4. Schizotypal personality disorder, the "nonpsychotic spectrum" disorders (ie, schizotypal and paranoid personality disorders), and all the "schizophrenia spec-

Schizophrenia—Kendler & Gruenberg

60

Table 5.—Frequency of 'Schizophrenia Spectrum' Disorders In All Interviewed Biologic Relatives of Adoptees With Schizophrenia, 'Schizophrenia Spectrum,' and Screened Control and All Control Adoptees

Adoptees	No.	Relatives			
		Schizophrenia No. (%)	SPD* No. (%)	PPD* No. (%)	"Schizophrenia Spectrum" No. (%)
Schizophrenia	35	2 (5.7)	5 (14.3)	2 (5.7)	9 (25.7)
"Schizophrenia spectrum"	69	3 (4.3)	9 (13.0)	3 (4.3)	15 (21.7)
Screened control	91	0 ...	0 ...	0 ...	0 ...
All control	137	0 ...	2 (1.5)	1 (0.7)	3 (2.2)

Comparison Groups of Adoptees	Significance of Difference In Frequency				
	Relatives				
	Schizophrenia	SPD*	PPD*	"Schizophrenia Spectrum"	"Nonpsychotic Spectrum"
Schizophrenia v screened control	.038†	.0002	.038†	.0000005	.00001
Schizophrenia v all control	.02†	.0006	.057†	.000001	.00006
"Schizophrenia spectrum" v screened control	.04	.0004	.04	.000003	.00004
"Schizophrenia spectrum" v all control	.014	.0005	.08	.000003	.00007

*SPD indicates schizotypal personality disorder; PPD, paranoid personality disorder.
†Statistical analysis by modified exact test; all others by χ^2 analysis.

trum" disorders were significantly more common in the biologic relatives of the schizophrenic adoptees than in the biologic relatives of the "psychotic nonspectrum" adoptees. The results were similar if the biologic relatives of the "schizophrenia spectrum" adoptees were compared with the biologic relatives of the "psychotic nonspectrum" adoptees.

Major depressive disorder was more frequent in the interviewed biologic relatives of the "psychotic nonspectrum" adoptees (3/34 [8.8%]) than in the biologic relatives of either the schizophrenic (2/35 [5.7%]) or "schizophrenia spectrum" (3/69 [4.3%]) adoptees, but these differences were not statistically significant. Anxiety disorder was also more common in the biologic relatives of the "psychotic nonspectrum" adoptees (10/34 [29.4%]) than in the biologic relatives of the schizophrenic (4/35 [11.4%]) or "schizophrenia spectrum" adoptees (8/69 [11.6%]). This difference reached statistical significance comparing the biologic relatives of the "schizophrenia spectrum" v "psychotic nonspectrum" adoptees ($\chi^2 = 5.01$, $P = .025$).

Of the three interviewed biologic relatives of index adoptees with a "nonpsychotic nonspectrum" diagnosis, two received diagnoses of schizotypal personality disorder (Table 3).

Of the 137 interviewed biologic relatives of control adoptees, 91 were relatives of screened controls and 46 of unscreened controls. No significant difference was found in the frequency of either anxiety disorder or major depressive disorder in the two groups of relatives. However, though no case of "schizophrenia spectrum" disorder was found in the biologic relatives of the screened controls, three cases (6.5%) (two cases schizotypal personality disorder, one case paranoid personality disorder) were found in the biologic relatives of the unscreened controls. This difference was significant ($\chi^2 = 6.07$, $P = .01$).

Frequency of Psychiatric Disorders In Interviewed Biologic Relatives of Schizophrenic v Control Adoptees

Schizophrenia and schizotypal personality disorder were significantly more common in the biologic relatives of adoptees with a diagnosis of schizophrenia than in the biologic relatives of either the screened or all the control adoptees (Table 5). Paranoid per-

sonality disorder was significantly more common in the biologic relatives of the schizophrenic v screened control adoptees (Table 4). However, the excess of paranoid personality disorder in the biologic relatives of the schizophrenic v all control adoptees was of only marginal statistical significance (ie, $P < .10$) (Table 5).

"Nonpsychotic spectrum" disorders were significantly more common in the biologic relatives of the schizophrenic v screened control or all control adoptees (Table 5). To a high degree of statistical significance ($P < .000005$), "schizophrenia spectrum" disorders were more common in the biologic relatives of the schizophrenic adoptees than in the biologic relatives of either the screened or all control adoptees (Table 5).

No significant difference was found in the frequency of anxiety disorder or major depressive disorder in the biologic relatives of the schizophrenic adoptees when compared with the biologic relatives of either the screened or all control adoptees (Table 6).

Frequency of Psychiatric Disorders In Interviewed Biologic Relatives of "Schizophrenia Spectrum" v Control Adoptees

In addition to adoptees with a diagnosis of schizophrenia, those with a diagnosis of schizoaffective disorder mainly schizophrenic and schizotypal personality disorder were combined into our tentative "schizophrenia spectrum." In the biologic relatives of adoptees receiving diagnoses of schizoaffective disorder, mainly schizophrenic, "schizophrenia spectrum" disorders were more common (3/28 [10.7%]) than they were in the biologic relatives of either the screened controls (modified exact $P = .008$) or all the controls ($\chi^2 = 4.82$, $P = .03$). "Schizophrenia spectrum" disorders were also significantly more common in the biologic relatives of adoptees with schizotypal personality disorder (3/6 [50.0%]) than in the biologic relatives of either the screened controls (modified exact $P = .00007$) or all the control adoptees (modified exact $P = .0004$).

Because these results support the validity of our tentative "schizophrenia spectrum," we examined the frequency of various psychiatric disorders in the biologic relatives of the "schizophrenia spectrum" adoptees v screened control or all control adoptees

(Table 5). Results were very similar to those found when the biologic relatives of only the schizophrenic adoptees were examined. Schizophrenia, schizotypal personality disorder, "nonpsychotic spectrum" disorders, and the "schizophrenia spectrum" disorders were all significantly more common in the biologic relatives of the "schizophrenia spectrum" adoptees compared with the biologic relatives of either the screened or all the control adoptees. No significant difference was found in the frequency of either anxiety disorder or major depressive disorder in the biologic relatives of the "schizophrenia spectrum" v screened control or all control adoptees (Table 6).

"Schizophrenia Spectrum" Disorders in First- and Second-Degree Biologic Relatives of Schizophrenic and Control Adoptees

The biologic relatives of the index and control adoptees from the Danish Adoption Study consist of both first-degree relatives (parents and full siblings) and second-degree relatives (maternal and paternal half siblings). The proportion of all relatives who are

first-degree relatives does not significantly differ in the biologic relatives of the following four groups of adoptees: schizophrenic (10/35 [28.6%]), "schizophrenia spectrum" (17/69 [24.6%]), screened control (31/91 [34.1%]), and all control (47/137 [34.3%]). The frequency of "schizophrenia spectrum" disorders in these four groups of relatives divided into first-degree and second-degree relatives is given in Tables 7 and 8, respectively. The frequency of "schizophrenia spectrum" disorders was twice as great in the first-degree relatives of the schizophrenic adoptees (4/10 [40.0%]) compared with their second-degree relatives (5/25 [20.0%]), but this difference was not statistically significant. A similar trend was seen in the first- v second-degree relatives of the "schizophrenia spectrum" adoptees (35.3% v 17.3%, respectively).

In both the first-degree and second-degree (Table 8) relatives of the schizophrenic adoptees, there is a significant excess of "schizophrenia spectrum" disorders compared with either the biologic relatives of the screened or all control adoptees. Similar results are found when the first- and second-degree relatives of the "schizophrenia spectrum" adoptees are examined (Table 6).

Matching Control With Schizophrenic Adoptees

Each index adoptee selected by Kety and co-workers[1] was matched on a variety of variables to a control adoptee. In the aforementioned analyses, we compared the biologic relatives of the schizophrenic and "schizophrenia spectrum" adoptees with the biologic relatives of either all the control or just the screened control adoptees. These analyses did not use pairs of matched control and index adoptees. To determine whether such an analysis would produce different results, we repeated these analyses using the original control adoptees that had been matched to the schizophrenic and "schizophrenia spectrum" adoptees. There were only nine pairs of matched control and schizophrenic adoptees where at least one biologic relative of both adoptees had been interviewed. (Of the 13 potential pairs, in three the schizophrenic adoptee and in one the control adoptee had no interviewed biologic relatives.) The frequency of "schizophrenia spectrum" disorders was significantly greater in the biologic relatives of the schizophrenic v matched control adoptees (9/34 v 0/40, $\chi^2 = 12.05$, $P = .0005$). There were 15 pairs of matched control and "schizophrenia spectrum" adoptees where at least one biologic relative of both adop-

Table 6.—Frequency of Anxiety Disorder and Major Depressive Disorder in Interviewed Biologic Relatives of Schizophrenic and Control Adoptees*

Adoptees	Relatives, No.	Anxiety Disorder, No. (%)	Major Depressive Disorder, No. (%)
Schizophrenia	35	4 (11.4)	2 (5.7)
"Schizophrenia spectrum"	69	8 (11.6)	3 (4.3)
Screened control	91	15 (16.5)	10 (10.9)
All control	137	21 (15.3)	12 (8.8)

*By χ^2 analysis, no significant difference was found in the frequency of anxiety disorder or major depression disorder in the interviewed biologic relatives of the following comparison groups of adoptees: schizophrenia v screened control, schizophrenia v all control, "schizophrenia spectrum" v screened control, and "schizophrenia spectrum" v all control.

Table 7.—Frequency of 'Schizophrenia Spectrum' Disorders in Interviewed First-Degree Biologic Relatives of Adoptees With Schizophrenia, 'Schizophrenia Spectrum,' and Screened Control and All Control Adoptees

		Relatives			
		Schizophrenia	SPD*	PPD*	"Schizophrenia Spectrum"
Adoptees	No.	No. (%)	No. (%)	No. (%)	No. (%)
Schizophrenia	10	1 (10.0)	2 (20.0)	1 (10.0)	4 (40.0)
"Schizophrenia spectrum"	17	1 (5.9)	3 (17.6)	2 (11.2)	6 (35.3)
Screened control	31	0 ...	0 ...	0 ...	0 ...
All control	47	0 ...	1 (2.1)	0 ...	1 (2.1)

	Significance of Difference in Frequency	
	Relatives	
Comparison Groups of Adoptees	"Schizophrenia Spectrum"	"Nonpsychotic Spectrum"
Schizophrenia v screened control	.001†	.006†
Schizophrenia v all control	.001†	.008†
"Schizophrenia spectrum" v screened control	.0004	.001
"Schizophrenia spectrum" v all control	.0002	.0009

*SPD indicates schizotypal personality disorder; PPD, paranoid personality disorder.
†Statistical analysis by modified exact test; all others by χ^2 analysis.

62

Table 8.—Frequency of 'Schizophrenia Spectrum' Disorders in Interviewed Second-Degree Biologic Relatives of Adoptees With Schizophrenia, 'Schizophrenia Spectrum,' and Screened Control and All Control Adoptees

		Relatives			
		Schizophrenia	SPD*	PPD*	"Schizophrenia Spectrum"
Adoptees	No.	No. (%)	No. (%)	No. (%)	No. (%)
Schizophrenia	25	1 (4.0)	3 (12.0)	1 (4.0)	5 (20.0)
"Schizophrenia spectrum"	52	2 (3.8)	6 (11.5)	1 (1.9)	9 (17.3)
Screened control	60	0 ...	0 ...	0 ...	0 ...
All control	90	0 ...	1 (1.1)	1 (1.1)	2 (2.2)

	Significance of Difference in Frequency†	
	Relatives	
Comparison Groups of Adoptees	"Schizophrenia Spectrum"	"Nonpsychotic Spectrum"
Schizophrenia v screened control	.0004	.002
Schizophrenia v all control	.001	.006
"Schizophrenia spectrum" v screened control	.0008	.003
"Schizophrenia spectrum" v all control	.001	.008

*SPD indicates schizotypal personality disorder; PPD, paranoid personality disorder.
†Statistical analysis by χ^2.

tees had been interviewed. "Schizophrenia spectrum" disorders were significantly more common in the biologic relatives of the "schizophrenia spectrum" adoptees (15/68 [22.1%]) than in the biologic relatives of their matched control adoptees (2/73 [2.7%]) ($\chi^2 = 12.40$, $P = .0004$).

Morbid Risk for Schizophrenia

Schizophrenia is a disorder with a variable age of onset. Therefore, the frequency of the disorder in a population is often not as useful a figure as is the morbid risk (MR), which corrects for the fact that the disorder may yet develop in certain unaffected individuals later in life. To permit a comparison of this and other reports, we calculated the MR for schizophrenia in the biologic relatives of the schizophrenic adoptees using the abridged Weinberg method with the age of risk of 15 to 39 years. The MR ($\pm$ SE) for schizophrenia in all their relatives is 8.2% $\pm$ 5.5%. In their first-and second-degree relatives, the MR is, respectively, 10.5% $\pm$ 9.9% and 6.7% $\pm$ 6.5%. Because of the small number of affected and total relatives, the standard errors of these estimates are very large.

Table 9.—Schizophrenia and 'Schizophrenia Spectrum' Disorders and Delusional Disorder in Interviewed Relatives*

		Relatives		
Adoptee Group	No.	Delusional Disorder	"Schizophrenia Spectrum"	Other
"Schizophrenia spectrum"	69	0	15	54
All other	260	5	8	247

*The difference in prevalence is significant by a 2×3 χ^2 analysis ($\chi^2 = 30.16$, $df = 2$, $P = .0000003$). Difference between delusional disorder and "schizophrenia spectrum" is significant by nonindependent 2×2 χ^2 analysis ($\chi^2 = 7.02$, $P = .008$) or by modified exact test ($P = .007$) (alpha level was corrected from .05 to .0125).

Delusional Disorder

Only five cases of delusional disorder were diagnosed in the 329 interviewed relatives in this sample. Although none of these relatives was biologically related to an index adoptee, the five cases were distributed in each of the other three groups of relatives (ie, biologic relatives of control and adoptive relatives of index and control adoptees). Because of the small number of affected relatives, it is necessary for analysis to divide the relatives into only two groups: those genetically related v not genetically related to a "schizophrenia spectrum" adoptee. When divided in these two groups, the distribution of delusional disorder is significantly different from that of "schizophrenia spectrum" disorders (Table 9). The single adoptee receiving the diagnosis of delusional disorder had no biologic relative with the diagnosis of a "schizophrenia spectrum" disorder (Table 3). This finding is consistent with the genetic independence of delusional disorder and the "schizophrenia spectrum" disorders.

Distribution of "Schizophrenia Spectrum" Disorders in Biologic Families of Adoptees

In addition to the distribution of psychiatric illness in individual relatives, it is also of interest to examine the distribution of these disorders in families. Considering biologic families with at least one interviewed member, "schizophrenia spectrum" disorders were significantly more common in the biologic families of schizophrenic adoptees (5/10 [50%]) than in either the biologic families of the screened control adoptees (0/21 [0%]) ($\chi^2 = 12.52$, $P = .0004$) or all the control adoptees (2/31 [6.5%]) ($\chi^2 = 10.13$, $P = .002$). Similar results were obtained when the frequency of "schizophrenia spectrum" disorders was examined in the biologic families of the "schizophrenia spectrum" (9/17 [52.9%]) v either the biologic families of the screened control adoptees ($\chi^2 = 14.57$, $P = .0001$) or all the control adoptees ($\chi^2 = 13.42$, $P = .0002$). These analyses were repeated using only the matched pairs of index and control adoptees. "Schizophrenia spectrum" disorders were significantly more common in the biologic families of the schizophrenic adoptees (5/9 [55.6%]) than in the biologic families of their matched control adoptees (0/9) (modified exact $P = .007$). "Schizophrenia spectrum" disorders were also significantly more

63

DSM-III Adoptee Diagnosis	No.	Relatives With DSM-III Diagnosis				
		Schizophrenia	SPD	PPD	Anxiety Disorder	Major Depressive Disorder
Schizophrenia	12	0	0	0	3	0
"Schizophrenia spectrum"	21	0	0	1	6	0
"Psychotic nonspectrum"	12	0	0	0	1	3
"Nonpsychotic nonspectrum"	5	0	0	0	0	0
Screened control	34	0	0	0	9	2
All control	48	0	0	1	0	10	4

*SPD indicates schizotypal personality disorder; PPD, paranoid personality disorder. Of 12 adoptive relatives of adoptees with diagnosis of schizophrenia, were adoptive parents and two adoptive siblings. No statistically significant differences were found in frequency of any of diagnostic categories in adop relatives of schizophrenia, schizophrenia plus "schizophrenia spectrum," psychotic nonspectrum, or other adoptees v either screened control or all con adoptees. However, there was significantly greater frequency of major depressive disorder in adoptive relatives of psychotic nonspectrum adoptees (25%) t in adoptive relatives of the schizophrenia plus "schizophrenic spectrum" adoptees (0%) ($\chi^2 = 5.78$, $P = .016$, modified exact $P = .02$).

common in the biologic families of the "schizophrenia spectrum" adoptees (9/16 [56.3%]) than in the biologic families of their matched control adoptees (1/16 [6.3%]) ($\chi^2 = 9.31$, $P = .002$).

Psychiatric Illness in Interviewed Adoptive Relatives

The distribution of the diagnosed psychiatric disorders in the interviewed adoptive relatives of the various groups of adoptees is given in Table 10. Major depressive disorder was significantly more common in the adoptive relatives of the "psychotic nonspectrum" v the "schizophrenia spectrum" adoptees. Otherwise, no significant differences in the frequency of psychiatric disorders were found among the different groups of adoptive relatives. No "schizophrenia spectrum" disorders were found in the 12 interviewed adoptive relatives (ten parents and two siblings) of schizophrenic adoptees.

COMMENT
Original v DSM-III Diagnoses in Index Adoptees

We blindly applied modified DSM-III criteria to all available interviews with the adoptees from the greater Copenhagen sample of the Danish Adoption Study of Schizophrenia. Agreement was reasonable between our DSM-III–based diagnoses and the original DSM-II–based global diagnoses of Kety et al for their categories of chronic and acute but not borderline schizophrenia. We found that 64.7% of their chronic schizophrenic adoptees met DSM-III criteria for schizophrenia and an additional 17.6% met criteria for schizoaffective disorder, mainly schizophrenic subtype (by RDC criteria[4]). Of the adoptees originally called acute schizophrenics, 71.4% met DSM-III criteria for schizophreniform disorder. However, of the adoptees originally receiving diagnoses of borderline schizophrenia, only 10% were assigned what might be considered the DSM-III equivalent of this diagnosis: schizotypal personality disorder.

In the case of adoptees with diagnoses of chronic schizophrenia by Kety et al,[1] these results confirm the previous good rate of agreement found between the original diagnosis and the diagnosis of chronic schizophrenia as defined by the RDC and applied by Spitzer and Endicott (see Kety et al[4]). Though differences in the diagnoses that we assigned to the adoptees using DSM-III criteria and those given by Kety and co-workers[1] using global DSM-II–based diagnoses may result from differences in diagnostic criteria, these diagnoses may also be discrepant because they were made from different information sources. Kety et al[1] made

their adoptee diagnoses based on symptom checklists and certain cases relatively brief hospital abstracts, where our diagnoses were made on the basis of the more extens information later summarized in the pseudointerviews.

Pattern of DSM-III Disorders in Adoptees and Biologic Relatives

The presence of DSM-III diagnoses in both adoptees a relatives permits an examination of the relationship b tween certain psychiatric disorders in these two grouj Results of this examination confirmed our previously i ported findings that had relied on the initial global dia noses of the adoptees.[8,12] Schizotypal personality disorde and paranoid personality disorder were both significant more frequent in the biologic relatives of the schizophrei adoptees than in the biologic relatives of the screen controls. These results confirm the previous findings[3,5,6] that, in this sample, certain nonpsychotic schizophreniali syndromes are genetically linked to schizophrenia. The frequency of neither anxiety disorder nor major depressi disorder was significantly different in the biologic relativ of the schizophrenic and control adoptees, thereby suppo ing our previous hypotheses that these two disorders ha no genetic link to schizophrenia.[8,10] The distribution delusional disorder and "schizophrenia spectrum" disc ders was significantly different in the biologic relatives the "schizophrenia spectrum" adoptees v all other relative which supports our previous finding that in this samp delusional disorder is not part of the "schizophrenia spe trum."[12]

Several conclusions are evident from this report tl were not contained in our previous analyses. First, schiz phrenia itself was significantly more common in the biolog relatives of the schizophrenic v control adoptees. The results provide direct support for a role of genetic factors the etiology of schizophrenia as defined by DSM-III. Se ond, the significantly increased frequency of "schizophrer spectrum" disorders and the low frequency of major depre sive disorder in the biologic relatives of the three adopte with diagnoses of schizoaffective disorder, mainly schiz phrenic subtype, suggest that this type of schizoaffecti disorder is genetically part of the "schizophrenia spectrur and not genetically related to affective illness. Because the small number of adoptees, these results should l

64

regarded as quite tentative, but they are consistent with those recently found using a family study method.[13]

Third, the low concentration of "schizophrenia spectrum" disorders in the biologic relatives of the "psychotic non-spectrum" adoptees suggests that these disorders have little genetic relationship to schizophrenia. Although again limited by the small sample size, these results support the distinction in *DSM-III* between schizophrenia and particularly schizophreniform and atypical psychosis. It is important to note that adoptees with diagnoses of schizophreniform disorder in this study had all been observed to recover from psychotic episodes within a six-month period. This may define a different patient population than would be found if subjects were included who had not recovered from their schizophrenialike illness but had not yet been ill six months.

Fourth, anxiety disorder was concentrated in the biologic relatives of the "psychotic nonspectrum" adoptees. These results are consistent with a previous report of Welner and Stromgren where a high concentration of "neurosis" but a low concentration of schizophrenia was found in the relatives of patients with "benign schizophreniform psychosis."[18] These results raise the possibility that anxiety disorder may be genetically related to acute, remitting psychotic disorders. Further research will be needed to test this hypothesis more definitively.

Fifth, although the numbers are quite small, the high frequency of schizotypal personality disorder in the biologic relatives of adoptees with the same diagnosis suggests that the genetic liability to this disorder can be directly transmitted. Previous reports have only shown that schizotypal personality disorder may be genetically related to schizophrenia.

Sixth, an unexpected result was the high concentration of schizotypical personality disorder in the few biologic relatives of the "nonpsychotic nonspectrum" adoptees. The disorders of these adoptees were difficult to diagnose and often had some schizophrenialike clinical features. However, in our judgment they did not meet criteria for either schizotypal or paranoid personality disorder. These results suggest the existence of other "schizophrenia spectrum" syndromes not covered by the current *DSM-III* criteria for either schizotypal or paranoid personality disorder.

Seventh, the results of the initial review of the interviews with the relatives by Kety and co-workers[3] have been criticized because of the finding of a greater concentration of their schizophrenia spectrum disorders in the second-degree v first-degree relatives of the index adoptees.[19] Furthermore, no significant difference is found in the frequency of the schizophrenia spectrum as defined by Kety et al in the first-degree relatives of index and control adoptees. In this regard, our results using *DSM-III* diagnoses differ from those of Kety and co-workers. Our "schizophrenia spectrum" disorders were more common in the first- v second-degree relatives of the schizophrenic adoptees. Furthermore, a significant excess of "schizophrenia spectrum" disorders was found in only the first- or only the second-degree relatives of the schizophrenic v control adoptees.

Comparison With the Report of Gunderson et al

Gunderson et al have analyzed a subset of the interviews from this adoption study.[5] Their specific aim was to clarify the symptoms and signs that characterize the "schizotype." It is useful to compare and contrast their findings with those reported herein. Like us, they found that the adoptees given diagnoses by Kety et al of borderline schizophrenia differed from the relatives with such diagnoses. Of the 16 biologic relatives of index adoptees given diagnoses by Kety et al of borderline or uncertain borderline schizophrenia for whom we also gave a psychiatric diagnosis, we assigned nine (56.3%) a diagnosis of schizotypal or paranoid personality disorder. However, of the ten index adoptees considered by Kety and co-workers to be borderline schizophrenic, we gave only one (10%) a diagnosis of schizotypal or paranoid personality disorder. Like them, we also noted that a number of the adoptees considered to be borderline schizophrenic by Kety et al[1] had prominent personality disorder, many with borderline features. In fact, we gave a primary and one a secondary *DSM-III* diagnosis of borderline personality disorder. However, when we were forced to assign a best primary *DSM-III* diagnosis to the index borderline schizophrenic adoptees, we assigned five (50%) of them a nonschizophrenic psychotic diagnosis (three, atypical psychosis; one, paranoid or delusional disorder; one, psychotic affective disorder).

Gunderson et al noted that nine of the ten borderline schizophrenic adoptees met *DSM-III* criteria for borderline schizophrenia. The probable source of this discrepancy is differing diagnostic orientations of the two groups of investigators. Presented with a case with a mixture of psychotic symptoms and prominent features of a personality disorder, our tendency was to diagnose a primary psychotic disorder. Gunderson and colleagues, however, when confronted with such a clinical picture, tended to view the psychotic symptoms as consistent with a primary personality disorder (J. Gunderson, MD, written communication, June 1983).

Potential Limitations

Several potential limitations of the current investigation are worth considering while interpreting the results presented. First, by the nature of the interviews, we could not be blind to whether an adoptee was classified by Kety et al[1] as index or control. However, we assigned a wide variety of diagnoses to the index adoptees. Furthermore, a large difference was found in the pattern of psychiatric illness in the biologic relatives of the different subgroups of the index adoptees (Table 4). Therefore, it seems unlikely that our lack of blindness to the overall group to which the adoptee belonged was responsible for the findings reported herein.

Second, the criteria for schizotypal personality disorder were developed using a subset of the interviews with relatives from this study.[5,20] It cannot therefore be claimed that our demonstration of the concentration of cases of schizotypal personality disorder in the biologic relatives of schizophrenic adoptees is an entirely independent verification of the genetic link between these two disorders. Furthermore, our putative "schizophrenia spectrum" is in part a post hoc diagnostic formulation. Only after our initial series of reports did we find, by a reexamination of the interviews, that paranoid personality disorder concentrated in the biologic relatives of the index adoptees.[11] However, independent verification of the validity of this "schizophrenia spectrum" is now available from two new study populations, one examined by the family history method[22] and the other by the family study method.[21]

Third, the interviewed relatives from the greater Copenhagen sample of the Danish Adoption Study of Schizophrenia were not a random sample of all the relatives. Nearly three times as many of the biologic relatives of the index v control adoptees had died prior to the time the interviews were conducted. The precise impact of this bias on the results observed is not certain. Schizophrenia is associated with an increased mortality,[23,24] and it is probable, but unverified, that this would also apply to the other "schizophrenia spectrum" disorders. Therefore, persons with "schizophrenia spectrum" disorders were probably overrepresented in the biologic relatives of the index adoptees who died prematurely. If anything, this biased ascertainment of relatives for interview would result in an underestimation of the concentration of "schizophrenia spectrum" disorders in the biologic relatives of the index v control adoptees.

CONCLUSIONS

Given these potential limitations, what can be concluded from this study regarding the possible role of genetic and nongenetic familial factors in the cause of schizophrenia as defined by DSM-III? First, genetic factors appear to play an etiologic role in schizophrenia. The likelihood that a person adopted at an early age and reared by nonrelatives will suffer schizophrenia is substantially increased if at least one of his biologic relatives has a "schizophrenia spectrum" disorder. This study does not provide information to conclude that genetic factors are sufficient to cause schizophrenia. The results of this study are compatible with the hypothesis that schizophrenia occurs through an interaction of genetic susceptibility and environmental "stress." Second, these results suggest that the genetic factors underlying the liability to schizophrenia also increase the risk for several schizophrenialike syndromes that in this study appear to include schizoaffective disorder, mainly schizophrenic subtype, and schizotypal and paranoid personality disorder. Third, these results confirm the "specificity" of the genetic factors involved in schizophrenia as they do not appear to increase the liability to other psychiatric disorders, specifically anxiety disorder, major depressive disorder, or delusional disorder. Furthermore, this study suggests that there is little or no genetic relationship between schizophrenia and the other nonaffective psychotic disorders in DSM-III. Although the genetic predisposition to schizophrenia may manifest itself as either a chronic psychotic disorder or a chronic schizophrenialike personality disorder, it does not, in this sample, appear to increase the liability to acute, remitting psychotic illness.

This study also permits some tentative conclusions regarding the etiologic role of nongenetic familial factors in schizophrenia. No case of "schizophrenia spectrum" disorder was found in the ten interviewed adoptive parents of the schizophrenic adoptees. Being raised by a person with a "schizophrenia spectrum" disorder is not necessary for the development of schizophrenia.

This research was supported in part by research associate award from the Veterans Administration (Dr Kendler).

John Strauss, MD, assisted in the earlier phases of this project. Hal Morgenstern, PhD, provided statistical consultation. Seymour Kety, MD, David Rosenthal, PhD, Paul Wender, MD, Fini Schulsinger, MD, and Bjørn Jacobsen, MD, allowed us to review their data from the Danish Adoption Study of Schizophrenia. Sandy Cole, MA, provided technical assistance.

References

1. Kety SS, Rosenthal D, Wender PH, Schulsinger F: The types and prevalence of mental illness in the biological and adoptive families of adopted schizophrenics. J Psychiatr Res 1968;6:345-362.
2. American Psychiatric Association Committee on Nomenclature and Statistics: Diagnostic and Statistical Manual of Mental Disorders, ed 2. Washington, DC, American Psychiatric Association, 1968.
3. Kety SS, Rosenthal D, Wender PH, Schulsinger F, Jacobsen B: Mental illness in the biological and adoptive families of adopted individuals who have become schizophrenic: A preliminary report based on psychiatric interviews, in Fieve R, Rosenthal D, Brill H (eds): Genetic Research in Psychiatry. Baltimore, Johns Hopkins Press, 1975, pp 147-165.
4. Spitzer RL, Endicott J, Robins E: Research Diagnostic Criteria for a Selected Group of Functional Disorders, ed 2. New York, New York Psychiatric Institute, 1975.
5. Kety SS, Rosenthal D, Wender PH: Genetic relationships within the schizophrenia spectrum: Evidence from adoption studies, in Spitzer RL, Klein DF (eds): Critical Issues in Psychiatric Diagnosis. New York, Raven Press, 1978, pp 213-223.
6. Gunderson JG, Siever LJ, Spaulding E: The search for a schizotype: Crossing the border again. Arch Gen Psychiatry 1983;40:15-22.
7. American Psychiatric Association Committee on Nomenclature and Statistics: Diagnostic and Statistical Manual of Mental Disorders, ed 3. Washington, DC, American Psychiatric Association, 1980.
8. Kendler KS, Gruenberg AM, Strauss JS: An independent analysis of the Copenhagen sample of the Danish Adoption Study of Schizophrenia: I. The relationship between anxiety disorder and schizophrenia. Arch Gen Psychiatry 1981;38:973-977.
9. Kendler KS, Gruenberg AM, Strauss JS: An independent analysis of the Copenhagen sample of the Danish adoption study of schizophrenia: II. The relationship between schizotypal personality disorder and schizophrenia. Arch Gen Psychiatry 1981;38:982-984.
10. Kendler KS, Gruenberg AM, Strauss JS: An independent analysis of the Copenhagen sample of the Danish Adoption Study of Schizophrenia: IV. The relationship between major depressive disorder and schizophrenia. Arch Gen Psychiatry 1982;39:639-642.
11. Kendler KS, Gruenberg AM: Genetic relationship between paranoid personality disorder and the 'schizophrenia spectrum' disorders. Am J Psychiatry 1982;139:1185-1186.

12. Kendler KS, Gruenberg AM, Strauss JS: An independent analysis of the Copenhagen sample of the Danish Adoption Study of Schizophrenia: III. The relationship between paranoid psychosis (delusional disorder) and schizophrenia. Arch Gen Psychiatry 1981;38:985-987.
13. Baron M, Gruen R, Asnis L, Kane J: Schizoaffective illness, schizophrenia and affective disorders: Morbidity risk and genetic transmission. Acta Psychiatr Scand 1982;65:253-262.
14. Siegel S: Nonparametric Statistics for the Behavioral Sciences. New York, McGraw-Hill Book Co, 1956, p 110.
15. Camilli G, Hopkins KD: Applicability of chi-square to 2×2 contingency tables with small expected cell frequencies. Psychol Bull 1978;85:163-167.
16. Bradley DR, Bradley TD, McGrath SG, Cutcomb SD: Type I error rate of the chi-square test of independence in R×C tables that have small expected frequencies. Psychol Bull 1979;86:1290-1297.
17. Miettinen OS: Comment. J Am Stat Assoc 1974;69:380-382.
18. Welner J, Strømgren E: Clinical and genetic studies on benign schizophreniform psychoses based on follow-up. Acta Psychiatr Scand 1958;33:377-399.
19. Lidz T, Blatt S: Critique of the Danish-American studies of the biological and adoptive relatives of adoptees who became schizophrenic. Am J Psychiatry 1983;140:426-434.
20. Spitzer RL, Endicott J, Gibbon M: Crossing the border into borderline personality and borderline schizophrenia: The development of criteria. Arch Gen Psychiatry 1979;36:17-24.
21. Kendler KS, Masterson CC, Ungaro R, Davis KL: A family history study of schizophrenia related personality disorders. Am J Psychiatry 1984; 141:424-427.
22. Baron M: Schizotypal personality disorders: Family studies. Read before the annual meeting of the American Psychiatric Association, New York, May 4, 1983.
23. Weiner BP, Marvit RC: Schizophrenia in Hawaii: Analysis of cohort mortality risk in a multi-ethnic population. Br J Psychiatry 1977;131:497-503.
24. Tsuang MT, Woolson RF: Excess mortality in schizophrenia and affective disorders: Do suicides and accidental deaths solely account for this excess? Arch Gen Psychiatry 1978;35:1181-1185.

66

Am. J. Hum. Genet. 68:299–312, 2001

REVIEW ARTICLE
Genetics of Schizophrenia and the New Millennium: Progress and Pitfalls

Miron Baron

Department of Psychiatry, Columbia University, and Department of Medical Genetics, New York State Psychiatric Institute, New York

Introduction

Schizophrenia (MIM 181500) is a severe and common psychiatric disorder afflicting 1% of the world population. The disease is characterized by psychotic symptoms and by cognitive, affective, and psychosocial impairment. As a leading cause of psychiatric admissions, schizophrenia accounts for a considerable portion of health-care expenditures and is viewed as a major public health concern.

Despite extensive research, our knowledge of the structural or functional pathology of schizophrenia is limited. The only etiological factor with a reasonably firm foundation is inheritance, as evidenced by family, twin, and adoption studies that point to substantial heritability (Gottesman and Shields 1982; Gottesman 1991; Kendler and Diehl 1993).

In the premolecular era, attempts to discern the underlying genetic mechanism consisted of (1) segregation analysis, testing the fit of observed familial patterns to specific genetic formulations (e.g., single–major-locus, oligogenic, and multifactorial-polygenic models); (2) searching for genetic susceptibility traits, also known as "biological markers," that segregate with the disorder in families (e.g., neurotransmitter enzymes, receptor proteins, or metabolites; attentional and electroencephalographic measures; and indices based on brain imaging); and (3) linkage studies that used classical gene markers (e.g., leukocyte antigens, blood groups, or serum proteins). However, in spite of numerous studies, the genetic underpinnings of schizophrenia remain elusive. The disorder, which is confounded by a host of factors (e.g., phenotypic diversity, etiologic heterogeneity, incomplete penetrance, unknown mode of inheritance, uncertainty about the number of loci involved and about their interactions, and the existence of nongenetic cases or phenocopies), was consigned to a complex multifactorial etiology, with no firmly established

Received December 4, 2000; accepted for publication December 6, 2000; electronically published January 17, 2001.

Address for correspondence and reprints: Dr. Miron Baron, Department of Psychiatry, Columbia University, 1051 Riverside Drive, Unit 6, New York, NY 10032. E-mail: mb17@columbia.edu

© 2001 by The American Society of Human Genetics. All rights reserved.
0002-9297/2001/6802-0002$02.00

biological correlates (Baron 1986a and 1986b; Risch 1990b; Kendler and Diehl 1993). A single major locus is unlikely as a common mode of inheritance. Oligogenic or polygenic models are plausible alternatives.

The advent of molecular genetics was a turning point in schizophrenia research, enabling the systematic application of both reverse genetics (studying random, anonymous DNA markers spanning the genome) and forward-genetics (testing candidate-gene polymorphisms with presumed functional relevance for the disease) (Martin 1987; Baron and Rainer 1988; Owen and Craddock 1996). In this article I review molecular genetic findings about schizophrenia, with an eye toward methodological issues and future research.

Findings

The search for schizophrenia genes appeared to be off to an auspicious start when Sherrington et al. (1988) reported strong statistical evidence of linkage to DNA markers on chromosome 5q11-13, in British and Icelandic pedigrees (a LOD score of 6.49, under a dominant model of inheritance and a broad disease definition). However, failure to replicate this finding in independent samples, coupled with heightened awareness of phenotypic and genetic complexities, dimmed the initial optimism, and the disease was dubbed a "graveyard for molecular geneticists" (Owen 1992). The initial finding was eventually retracted after a more extensive analysis of the original sample and consideration of additional data (Kalsi et al. 1999).

Conflicting results may arise because of complex inheritance that leads to reduced power and to difficulties in distinguishing a true-positive result from a false-positive one (type 1 error) and in distinguishing a true-negative result from a false-negative one (type 2 error). But a host of other factors must be considered, including diagnostic uncertainties, variability among studies in methods of data collection and interpretation, selection bias, incomplete genotypic information, and statistical artifacts. Several methodological advances have occurred to counter these problems (Baron 1990, 1995; Baron et al. 1990; Risch 1990a; Pauls 1993; Spence et al. 1993; Cloninger 1994; Lander and Kruglyak 1995; Owen and Craddock 1996). These include operation-

Am. J. Hum. Genet. 68:299–312, 2001

alized diagnostic constructs and practices, which enhance diagnostic reliability and consensus among researchers; focus on conservative definitions of the phenotype, to diminish phenotypic ambiguities; maintainenance of scrupulous "blindness" between those conducting diagnostic procedures and those performing genotyping, to avert systematic errors; systematic ascertainment of subjects and pedigrees, to counter selection bias; power simulations, to assess the suitability of clinical samples; a range of analytical models for gene detection; dense genetic maps that allow genomewide searches; and statistical guidelines for the prudent interpretation of results (e.g., adjusting for multiple testing and performing simulations to determine power and levels of significance).

Coupled with advances in other complex disorders (e.g., Alzheimer disease, diabetes, and certain types of cancer), the improved methodology has rekindled interest in the genetics of schizophrenia. A new harvest of findings has been reported, including results of genome searches using linkage mapping and results of studies of candidate genes and chromosomal aberrations. Findings are compiled in the World Congress on Psychiatric Genetics chromosome workshops (Crow and DeLisi 1998; DeLisi and Crow 1998; DeLisi et al. 1999). To narrow the scope of this review, I focus on findings that seem promising by virtue of statistical significance or some consistency across studies. It must be stressed, however, that criteria for significance in the genetic analysis of complex disease are not well established and that positive results are often followed by attempts at replication that yield negative or equivocal findings.

Linkage Studies

Linkage studies are the mainstay of gene-finding strategies in psychiatric genetics. Significant or suggestive evidence of linkage (Lander and Kruglyak 1995) (see the "Linkage Methods" subsection, below) has been reported in several chromosomal regions: 1q21-22, 1q32-41, 4q31, 5p13-14, 5q22-31, 6p22-24, 6q21-22, 8p21-22, 9q21-22, 10p11-15, 13q14-32, 15q15, 22q11-13, and Xp11. There are preliminary results from other genome scans or candidate regions, but evaluation must await the full published reports.

Chromosome 1q21-22. — Brzustowicz et al. (2000) reported a genomewide scan in 22 Canadian pedigrees, which showed pronounced linkage to 1q21-22. A maximum heterogeneity LOD score of 6.50 was found between markers D1S1653 and D1S1679, under a recessive model and a narrow disease definition, and ~75% of the families were linked to this locus. The strength of the evidence is unusual for a complex disorder such as

schizophrenia, especially given an outbred population and a relatively small sample. The authors attributed their apparent success to the dense pedigrees selected for study and to a fortuitous sample variation. Marginal support for linkage to 1q22-23 was noted in an earlier study (Shaw et al. 1998). A potassium-channel gene (hKCa3/KCNN3) mapped to 1q21 was reportedly associated with schizophrenia in one study (Dror et al. 1999), although linkage analysis in an independent sample found no evidence for the involvement of hKCa3/KCNN3 in the disease (Austin et al. 1999).

Chromosome 1q32-41. — Hovatta et al. (1999) reported a three-stage genomewide scan in 69 families from a Finnish population isolate. They observed a maximum LOD score of 3.82 at marker D1S2891, under a dominant model and a narrow disease definition, with no evidence of locus heterogeneity. A putative haplotype, which might narrow the chromosomal region implicated, was observed in some core families.

Chromosome 4q31. — Hovatta et al. (1999) also observed a maximum LOD score of 2.74 at marker D4S1586, under a dominant model and a narrow diagnostic model. Positive LOD scores occurred on a fairly large region, and the evidence was supported by affected sib-pair analysis with the same marker (LOD score of 2.09; P = .00097).

Chromosome 5p13-14. — Silverman et al. (1996) reported a maximum LOD score of 4.37 at locus D5S111, under dominant inheritance and a broad disease definition (including putative schizophrenia-related phenotypes), in one large Puerto Rican pedigree. However, the LOD score was not robust to sensitivity analysis (testing the impact of diagnostic misclassifications on the evidence for linkage), and 23 other families examined concurrently showed no evidence of linkage to this region, suggesting that the putative disease gene is rare.

Chromosome 5q22-31. — After a genome scan of 265 Irish pedigrees, Straub et al. (1997) reported a maximum heterogeneity LOD score of 3.35 (P = .0002) at marker D5S804, under a recessive genetic model and a narrow diagnostic model, and ~10%–25% of the families linked to this locus. D5S804 is mapped to 5q22, but positive LOD scores were in evidence across the entire 5q22-31 region. Schwab et al. (1997) reported additional support, albeit at a lower level of significance, for linkage to this region (marker D5S399 at 5q31), in German and Israeli families.

Chromosome 6p22-24. — Straub et al. (1995), following up on a report on a subset of the data in the same German and Israeli families (Wang et al. 1995), studied 265 Irish families for linkage to 6p22-24. They reported a maximum LOD score of 3.51 (P = .0002) at marker D6S296, under an additive genetic model and a broad definition of schizophrenia (including putative schizophrenia-related disorders). An estimated 15%–30% of the families were presumed linked to this region. The evidence of linkage declined substantially when the narrow disease definition was used. Additional, support for linkage to this region was reported by Schwab et al. (1995 and 2000) in German and Israeli families, by Moises et al. (1995) in 65 European, Canadian, U.S., and Taiwanese families, and by Antonarakis et al. (1995) in 57 U.S. families.

Chromosome 6q21-22.—Cao et al. (1997) reported possible linkage to 6q21-22 in two independent U.S. samples: $P = .00018$ at locus D6S474 using sib-pair analysis in 63 independent sib pairs, and $P = .00095$ at D6S424 (~14 cM proximal to D6S474) in a second sample of 87 independent sib pairs. The same group of researchers reported modest support for linkage to D6S424 in a third sample consisting of 54 U.S. and Australian sib pairs; when these researchers combined samples (141 independent sib pairs), they observed a nonparametric LOD score of 3.82 ($P = .000014$) (Martinez et al. 1999).

Chromosome 8p21-22.—Using a narrow disease definition in a genome scan of 54 U.S. pedigrees, Blouin et al. (1998) observed a nonparametric LOD score of 3.64 ($P = .0001$) at D8S1771. They obtained additional support from a dominant-model analysis (dominant heterogeneity LOD score of 4.54, assuming 70% of the families are linked) and from a follow-up sample of 51 pedigrees. When a broad disease definition was used in this sample, support for linkage increased, yielding a nonparametric LOD score of 6.17 ($P = .0000008$) (Pulver et al. 2000). Previously, Pulver et al. (1995) published preliminary evidence of linkage to this region. Some additional support came from Kendler et al. (1996), who found a maximum LOD score of 2.34, using a dominant genetic model and a broad disease definition, in 265 Irish pedigrees. Further support for linkage to 8p21 was reported by Brzustowicz et al. (1999), with a maximum LOD score of 3.49 at marker D8S136, under a dominant model and narrow disease phenotype, in 21 Canadian families.

Chromosome 9q21-22.—In their Finnish study (see the "Chromosome 1q32-41" subsection, above), Hovatta et al. (1999) also observed a maximum LOD score of 1.95 at marker D9S922, under a dominant model. Other investigators (Moises et al. 1995; Levinson et al. 1998) reported some support for linkage to this region, although at marginal statistical significance.

Chromosome 10p11-15.—Faraone et al. (1998) reported a genome scan of 43 U.S. nuclear families, with suggestive linkage in 50 independent sib pairs using a narrow disease definition. The nonparametric LOD scores at markers D10S1423 and D10S582 were 3.4 ($P = .0004$) and 3.2 ($P = .0006$), respectively. Supportive evidence was provided by Schwab et al. (1998a), with a nonparametric LOD score of 3.2 ($P = .0007$) at

marker D10S1714, in 72 German and Israeli families. Straub et al. (1998) observed a multipoint heterogeneity LOD score of 1.91 ($P = .006$) at with markers D10S1426 and D10S674 in 265 Irish pedigrees.

Chromosome 13q14-32.—Blouin et al. (1998) reported a nonparametric LOD score of 4.18 ($P = .00002$), near D13S174 on 13q32, using a narrow disease phenotype in a genome scan of 54 U.S. pedigrees. The maximum heterogeneity LOD score for this region, under a dominant genetic model, was 4.5. This finding was supported in a follow-up sample of 51 families, with a nonparametric LOD score of 2.36 ($P = .007$) at D13S779, ~7 cM distal to the peak obtained in the first sample. Further support for this finding was furnished by Brzustowicz et al. (1999), with a maximum heterogeneity LOD score of 4.42 at D13S793 (~10 cM distal to D13S779), under a recessive model and a broad disease definition, in 21 Canadian pedigrees. Other work (Lin et al. 1997; Shaw et al. 1998) also supported this finding, although at lower significance levels.

Chromosome 15q13-15.—Stober et al. (2000) reported linkage to 15q15 in a genome scan of 12 German pedigrees, segregating the periodic catatonia subtype of schizophrenia. They found a nonparametric LOD score of 3.57 ($P = .000026$) and a maximum LOD score of 2.75 at marker D15S1012, under a dominant model. Marginal support for linkage to15q13-15 in U.S. schizophrenia pedigrees was suggested by Coon et al. (1994b) and Leonard et al. (1998). The 15q-candidate region overlaps with a putative schizophrenia locus defined by a neurophysiological impairment in the P50 auditory sensory gating (Freedman et al. 1997). It also contains the $\alpha7$ nicotinic acetylcholine receptor gene (CHRNA7), a potential candidate gene.

Chromosome 22q11-13.—Pulver et al. (1994a) observed a maximum LOD score of 2.82 at marker locus IL2RB, in 39 U.S. pedigrees. Affected sib-pair analysis in an expanded sample of 57 U.S. pedigrees was consistent with linkage to the same general region ($P = .009$) (Lasseter et al. 1995). Other investigators (Polymeropoulos et al. 1994; Coon et al. 1994a; Stober et al. 2000) also reported modest support for linkage. The implicated region is near the velocardiofacial syndrome (VCFS) deletion, which is reportedly associated with psychotic features (see the "Chromosomal aberrations" subsection, below). It also harbors a putative candidate gene, which may influence two neurophysiological functions, P50 auditory sensory gating and antisaccade ocular motor performance (Myles-Worsley et al. 1999).

Chromosome Xp11.—This region is of interest, because it harbors the monoamine oxidase B (MAOB) gene, a potential candidate gene for neuropsychiatric disease. The Finnish isolate study (Hovatta et al. 1999; see the "Chromosome 1q32-41" subsection, above) reported a maximum LOD score of 2.01 at the MAOB

Am. J. Hum. Genet. 68:299–312, 200

locus, using a recessive model and a narrow disease definition. Earlier reports found positive LOD scores in the close vicinity of MAOB, at marker DXS7 (DeLisi et al. 1994a; Dann et al. 1997).

Candidate Genes and Chromosomal Aberrations

In contrast to most linkage studies (which typically involve genomewide searches), studies of candidate genes and chromosomal aberrations target specific genomic sites.

Candidate genes. — Candidate genes for schizophrenia (genes that encode products with neurobiological function such as neurotransmitter receptors or enzymes) are commonly studied by way of association studies. Whereas linkage analysis tests for cosegregation of a gene marker and disease phenotype in families, association studies examine the co-occurrence of a marker and disease at the population level, using a case-control design (unrelated cases and population-based controls). Family-based controls can also be studied using a trio consisting of an affected child (case) and two parents (controls).

Most association studies have focused on genes involved in dopaminergic or serotonergic neurotransmission. Disturbances in dopaminergic or serotonergic systems have long been implicated in the pathogenesis of schizophrenia, primarily because of their role as sites for antipsychotic drug action. Numerous association studies have been reported, with conflicting results. Because association studies are largely concerned with genes of minor effect, studies of large, statistically powerful samples may produce more compelling results than the more typical small-scale studies have done. Two such studies, which aimed to pursue previously reported suggestive results, warrant attention and are described below.

Spurlock et al. (1998) examined polymorphisms in the dopamine DRD2 and DRD3 receptor genes in a large European multicenter sample. They studied two polymorphisms: Ser311Cys (in exon 7 of DRD2) and Ser9gly (in exon 1 of DRD3) in samples of 373 and 413, and 311 and 306 patients and controls, respectively. They found no evidence of allelic association with the DRD2 polymorphism and no homozygotes for this variant. However, an excess of homozygotes for both alleles of the DRD3 polymorphism was noted in the patient group ($P = .003$), as well as a significant excess of the 1:1 (Ser9Ser) genotype ($P = .004$), with no allelic association. They concluded that an association exists between increased homozygosity of the DRD3 variant and the disease.

Williams et al. (1996) studied the serotonin polymorphism T102C of the gene for 5-hydroxytryptamine type 2a (5-H2Ta) receptor, in a large European multicenter sample of 571 patients and 631 matched controls.

They observed significant association between the disease and allele 2 ($P = .003$), as well as a significant excess of the ½:½ genotype in patients ($P = .008$). The concluded that the 5-HT2a receptor gene—or a locus i linkage disequilibrium with it—confers susceptibility t schizophrenia.

Association studies with specific genes that may be involved in genetic anticipation (progressively earlier ag at onset or increased severity in successive generations have also been of interest (1) because these genes, which are characterized by trinucleotide repeat expansions, ar common in human brain, and (2) because anticipatio has been reported in schizophrenia. However, the searc for such genes has yielded conflicting results, with n evidence for a clear-cut relationship between the tr nucleotide-repeat size and age at onset of the diseas (Sasaki et al. 1996; Morris et al. 1995; O'Donovan e al. 1995). Also, the evidence for anticipation in schizc phrenia may be fraught with ascertainment bias (Ash erson et al. 1994).

Chromosomal aberrations. — Chromosomal aberra tions have been instrumental in identifying disease gene There are numerous accounts of associations betwee schizophrenia and chromosomal aberrations, includin the partial trisomy of 5q11-13 (Bassett et al. 198& which led to the claimed linkage to DNA markers i this region (see the "Linkage Studies" subsectior above). In a separate publication, Bassett (1992) re viewed earlier reports. Later accounts include trans locations such as t(2;18)(p11.2;p11.2) (Maziade et a 1993) and t(1;7)(p22;q22) (Gordon et al. 1994), inver sions such as 9p11-9q13 (Nanko et al. 1993) an 4p15.2-q21.3 (Palmour et al. 1994), trisomies of 5p14. (Malaspina et al. 1992) and 8 (Ong and Robertso 1995), fragile sites at 8q24 and 10q24 (Garofalo et a 1993), deletions at 22q11.1 (Karayiorgou et al. 1995 and 5q21-23.1 (Bennett et al. 1997), and sex aneuplo idies (reviewed in DeLisi et al. 1994b).

Because of the high prevalence of schizophrenia, an the fact that most of the reported chromosomal aber rations are confined to isolated cases, it is likely that th great majority of these associations are spurious. Con fidence in the potential relevance of a particular findin can be enhanced by (1) increasing the rate of the chr mosomal anomaly in the patient population, (2) increas ing the rate of the disease among patients with the chr mosomal anomaly, or (3) finding independent evidenc of linkage between the disease and the specific genomi region. One of the reported aberrations—the deletion a 22q11, which overlaps the region involved in VCF (Karayiorgou et al. 1995; also see the "Linkage Studies subsection, above)—appears to meet these criteria an warrants further study.

Methodological Issues

Although some of the aforementioned results show promise, the failure of attempts to replicate results and the limited power to detect and replicate gene effects, as well as limited power to distinguish true-positive results from false-positive ones, continue to mar the search for susceptibility genes in schizophrenia. Methodological refinements that may expedite this search involve new perspectives on phenotype definition and new analytical approaches.

The Phenotype

The lack of external validating criteria and the considerable variability in clinical manifestations present a challenge to genetic studies. Strategies that attempt to redress this problem include (1) dissecting the phenotype to clinical subtypes that cluster in families and that may have distinct underlying genetic bases and (2) supplanting discrete phenotypes by quantitative measures, such as symptom-based algorithms and biological endophenotypes, that may be more closely related to the underlying genetic vulnerability. The use of quantitative measures may also provide a greater power to detect linkage than the power provided by use of discrete phenotypes. Another strategy to overcome the challenges of genetic studies is to blur the diagnostic boundaries between schizophrenia and other major psychiatric disorders, such as bipolar disorder, to examine genetic commonality. Several investigators have recently applied these strategies, with varying degrees of success.

Clinical Subtypes

As mentioned (see the "Linkage Studies" subsection, above), Stober et al. (2000) found evidence for a major locus for the periodic catatonia subtype of schizophrenia on chromosome15q15. Elsewhere they reported high familial aggregation of this syndrome, with an estimated prevalence of 0.1% in the general population (Stober et al. 1995). Their finding suggests that periodic catatonia is a genetically homogeneous subtype of schizophrenia that is linked to a major locus on 15q15.

It should be noted, however, that catatonic schizophrenia is uncommon and that other recent attempts to determine whether schizophrenia subtypes cluster in families produced negative results (Leboyer et al. 1992; Kendler et al. 1994). This suggests that the finding reported by Stober et al. (2000), although potentially relevant for a subset of schizophrenia, may not have general applicability.

Symptom-Based Analysis

Brzustowicz et al. (1997) studied quantitative clinical traits, using positive-symptom (psychotic), negative-

symptom (deficit), and general-psychopathology-symptom scales for schizophrenia. Using categorical phenotypes, they found evidence of linkage between the positive-symptom trait and marker D6S1960 ($P = .0000054$) on chromosome 6p11-21, slightly proximal to the 6p21-24 region previously implicated in schizophrenia (see the "Linkage Studies" subsection, above). The somewhat different localization may result from differences in phenotypic classification and marker coverage or from the presence of two distinct susceptibility loci. Interestingly, there was no evidence of linkage when categorical diagnoses were used. This supports the notions that (1) the use of a quantitative trait may, indeed, have increased the power to detect linkage and (2) positive symptoms show more pronounced correlation with genetic vulnerability at the 6p putative locus.

A different symptom-based approach was taken by Kendler et al. (2000), who tested for linkage of symptom and outcome variables to chromosomes 5q21-31, 6p22-24, 8p21-22, and 10p11-15, all of which are regions implicated in previous linkage studies using discrete diagnoses (see the "Linkage Studies" subsection, above). There was no evidence of linkage to 5q, 6p, or 10p, but affected individuals from families with prior evidence of linkage to 8p21-22 had more affective deterioration, more thought disorder, fewer depressive symptoms, and poorer outcome than did affected individuals from other families. These clinical features are characteristic of the core, poor-outcome form of schizophrenia. Notwithstanding methodological limitations (Kendler et al. 2000), the study suggests that a locus on 8p21-22 confers susceptibility to this syndrome.

Biological Endophenotypes

Much attention has focused on two neurobiological dysfunctions associated with familial schizophrenia: impaired gating of the auditory evoked response (Judd et al. 1992; Freedman et al. 1997) and ocular motor dysfunctions (Holzman et al. 1988; Levy et al. 1993). Impaired sensory gating, commonly measured by recording the P50 wave of the auditory evoked response, reflects a dysfunction in the brain's processing of sensory stimuli. Ocular motor dysfunctions include impaired smooth-pursuit eye movement and deficient antisaccade ocular motor performance. The P50 auditory sensory gating and antisaccade ocular performance are specific measures of inhibitory neurophysiological functioning. Physiological deficits in these measures occur in most schizophrenics and in many of their unaffected relatives, an observation consistent with the hypothesis that vulnerability to the disease is inherited.

Both putative endophenotypes were tested for linkage to schizophrenia (see the "Linkage Studies" subsection, above). Freedman et al. (1997) reported linkage of the

Am. J. Hum. Genet. 68:299–312, 2001

P50 sensory gating deficit to chromosome 15q13-14, the site of the α7-nicotinic receptor locus, in nine U.S. schizophrenia pedigrees (LOD score of 5.3, using a dominant model). Their neurobiological studies suggest that decreased function of the α7-nicotinic receptor could underlie the P50 sensory gating defect, a finding that suggests this gene may have a role in the pathophysiology of schizophrenia. In a follow-up study of eight of these families, Myles-Worsley et al. (1999) reported linkage between a composite biological phenotype— combining the P50 sensory gating and antisaccade ocular motor performance—and marker D22S315 on chromosome 22q11-12 (LOD of 3.55, using a dominant model). This composite endophenotype appeared to identify nearly 80% of nonschizophrenic relatives as abnormal in at least one inhibitory processing domain.

It must be emphasized, however, that the evidence of linkage between the clinical phenotype and the two chromosomal regions, in this sample and in samples reported by others (see the "Linkage Studies" subsection, above), is less pronounced than the linkage reported for the endophenotypes. Also, the endophenotypes appeared to be governed by dominant major genes, a genetic model unlikely for schizophrenia generally.

Diagnostic Boundaries

Ordinarily, the disease phenotype can range from schizophrenia proper (a narrow definition) to broader phenotype definitions that include what are known as "spectrum" disorders (disease states that aggregate in families of schizophrenic patients but do not meet the criteria for schizophrenia). However, recent data suggest a broader perspective on this matter. Specifically, although schizophrenia and bipolar affective disorder do not show significant coaggregation in families and are generally considered distinct nosological entities, there is evidence for some overlap (Baron et al. 1982; Gershon et al. 1988; Maier et al. 1993). In particular, families both of schizophrenic and of bipolar patients are at increased risk for schizoaffective disorder (a syndrome combining schizophrenic and affective features) and unipolar depression. Also, relatives of schizoaffective patients show increased rates of schizophrenia, bipolar illness, and unipolar depression. There is, additionally, some resemblance in epidemiological and clinical features: the two disorders have similar prevalence and age at onset, show no gender preference, are lifelong conditions, and have some common psychotic features.

The apparent partial overlap of schizophrenia and bipolar disorder has drawn attention to the notion of shared susceptibility loci. Indeed, examination of recent linkage studies shows several chromosomal regions that are implicated in both disorders. In particular, 1q32, 10p11-15, 13q32, and 22q11-13, which were linked to schizophrenia in some studies (see the "Linkage Studies" subsection, above), have also been implicated in bipolar disorder. For example, Detera-Wadleigh et al. (1999) observed evidence of linkage at 1q32 (LOD score of 2.67; $P = .00022$), 13q32 (LOD score of 3.5; $P = .000028$), and 22q11-13 (LOD score of 2.1; $P = .00094$) in 22 U.S. pedigrees with bipolar illness. Foroud et al. (2000) reported a LOD score of 2.5 ($P = .001$) at 10p14, in 97 U.S. pedigrees with bipolar illness. Another region of potential interest is 18p11, where Schwab et al. (1998b) reported modest evidence of linkage to schizophrenia (LOD score of 1.76 at marker D18S53) in 59 German and Israeli families. The LOD score increased to 3.1 when the phenotype definition was broadened to include bipolar disorder and unipolar depression. Possible linkage of bipolar disorder to 18p11 was reported in an independent sample of 22 U.S. pedigrees (Berrettini et al. 1994), although the status of this linkage is unclear (Baron and Knowles 2000). Evidence of shared genetic susceptibility between schizophrenia and affective disorders may provide cross-validation of genetic findings and a rationale for some latitude in phenotype definition.

Analytical Approaches

There is an ongoing debate as to the optimal study design and analytical methods for complex traits such as schizophrenia. Issues that warrant attention include linkage and association methods, meta-analyses, and novel analytical models.

Linkage Methods

Linkage analysis examines familial cosegregation of a gene marker and a disease phenotype, to determine whether the marker and the disease are physically linked. Controversial issues include sample configuration (sib pairs in nuclear families vs. extended high-density pedigrees), type of analysis (model-free [nonparametric] methods, e.g., sib-pair analysis, vs. model-based [parametric] methods, e.g., LOD scores in pedigrees), and definition of significant findings.

The advantages and disadvantages of various sample configurations and types of analysis have been discussed elsewhere (Vieland et al. 1992; Greenberg et al. 1997 and 1998; Goldgar and Easton 1997; Kruglyak 1997; Terwilliger 1998; Ott and Hoh 2000) and can be summarized as follows:

Sample configuration.—Proponents of the sib-pair approach argue that extended pedigrees may be error-prone for two main reasons: (1) reduced power for linkage detection may result from intrafamilial heterogeneity caused by "extraneous" genes entering the pedigree through marrying-in spouses and (2) selection bias in favor of a particular form of familial disease with a dominantlike, single-gene effect may accompany a failure to consider more representative mechanisms for complex traits, such as oligogenic inheritance and multiple genes of modest effect. It may be argued, however, that (1) extended pedigrees can be divided into component nuclear families to account for intrafamilial heterogeneity; (2) sib pairs in small families are also susceptible to intrafamilial heterogeneity (phenocopies may be more common because of low illness density); (3) extended pedigrees contain more genetic information than small families do, and this results in increased statistical power, especially when heterogeneity is accounted for; and (4) although the dominantlike appearance of some extended pedigrees may favor the detection of rarer, large-effect genes, such genes can be more easily traceable, and their biological impact may be greater than that of genes of minor effect.

Type of analysis. — Advocates of model-free methods argue that these methods are more suitable for complex disorders whose mode of inheritance is uncertain, because such methods make no assumptions about the underlying genetic transmission. It may be argued, however, that (1) model-based LOD score analysis has greater power and is largely robust to model misspecification, if more than one model is tested; (2) with model-based methods, several different models can be used, covering a range of genetic hypotheses with adequate power and with little risk of missing a true linkage; (3) there is no systematic evidence that model-free methods have a greater sensitivity for linkage detection than do model-based methods.

Clearly, there is no one correct method for linkage detection. The studies reviewed in this article (see the "Linkage Studies" subsection, above) used a variety of methods, including nuclear families with sib pairs, extended pedigrees, and model-free and model-based analysis. Given the acknowledged complexities, the use of complementary methods might be advisable, provided the advantages and disadvantages of the various approaches are recognized.

Statistical significance. — As mentioned, simulation studies suggest guidelines for genomewide significance of linkage results in studies of complex traits (Lander and Kruglyak 1995). In parametric analysis, the categories of significant and suggestive linkage correspond to LOD scores of 3.3 and 1.9, respectively; the corresponding pointwise P values in sib-pair analysis are .000022 (LOD score of 3.6) and .00074 (LOD score of 2.2). Once significant linkage is observed, a P value in an independent study is required for replication. However, although these guidelines are widely used (see the "Linkage Studies" subsection, above), debate continues about what constitutes appropriate thresholds for significance. What appears to be significant linkage can be a false-positive result, even in the presence of presumed replication. Conversely, linkage findings that fall

short may be worth pursuing, especially if contiguous markers in the candidate region show positive results.

Linkage versus association. — As mentioned, there are numerous association studies of candidate genes. Although linkage studies continue to play a pivotal role, association mapping is becoming a competing strategy. The advantages and disadvantages of linkage and association mapping have been widely debated (Crowe 1993; Kidd 1993; Risch and Merikangas 1996; Owen et al. 1997; Terwilliger and Weiss 1998; Risch 2000; Weiss and Terwilliger 2000; Ott and Hoh 2000; Baron 1997 and in press). The advantages of association studies can be summarized as follows: (1) Most of the genetic variance in complex disease is due to genes of modest effect. Such genes are probably detectable by association analysis but may not be amenable to the linkage approach, which is best suited for genes of larger effect. (2) The sample-size requirements for linkage detection are much higher (possibly beyond reach) than those for association mapping. (3) The slow progress in linkage mapping of complex disease attests to the constraints of this approach. (4) The emergent maps of high-density single-nucleotide polymorphisms (SNPs) should enable genomewide association studies with tens of thousands of candidate-SNPs. This may allow systematic assessment of all candidate genes for complex traits such as psychiatric disease.

There are, however, caveats. First, although linkage analysis is, indeed, geared toward genes of moderate-to-large effect, a few examples of common disease alleles of modest effect have been detected by linkage analysis. Two examples are apolipoprotein E (ApoE), which predisposes to both a common form of Alzheimer dementia and to cardiovascular disease, and HLA, which predisposes to type I diabetes. Some simulations show that modest-effect genes (genotypic relative risk = 2) are detectable by linkage analysis with realistic sample sizes (~400 sib pairs) (Hauser et al. 1996). Second, enrichment of the sample for disease-allele carriers, by using clinical subtypes or biological endophenotypes, can augment the power to detect linkage. Examples of the success of this approach include early-onset familial breast and prostate cancer and, possibly, the aforementioned linkages to catatonic schizophrenia (15q13-15) and to the putative schizophrenia endophenotypes P50 (15q13-15) and the P50-antisaccade composite (22q11-13). Third, as mentioned (see the "Candidate genes" subsection, above), the pattern of conflicting results in association studies is at least as pronounced as that in linkage studies. Also, seemingly significant disease-marker associations are more likely than not to be spurious, because of the infinitesimally small odds of selecting a likely candidate gene from among the multitude of genes expressed in human brain. To curtail false-positive results, the requirements for statistical significance

Am. J. Hum. Genet. 68:299–312, 2001

would have to be much more stringent, even in samples substantially larger than those that are deemed feasible. A further complication arises from spurious results caused by sample stratification (in case-control designs), although this can be rectified by using family-based controls. Second, although systematic genome searches with SNPs can circumvent limitations in current designs that focus on a few favored candidate genes, there are potential drawbacks. For example, given the vast number of test results, there are questions concerning the statistical thresholds required to curb false-positive results. Also, in the presence of substantial allelic heterogeneity, there may never be enough power for the confident detection of modest gene effects, even with huge population samples. There are also questions about the efficiency of SNP mapping. For example, the number of required markers may have to be severalfold larger (hundreds of thousands, including noncoding SNPs), compounding the effects of multiple testing and augmenting an already substantial and costly genotyping effort. Also, a linkage disequilibrium map is needed for the entire genome, given the high variability across the genome. Further statistical, computational, and technological advances are needed to render this approach fully applicable.

Joint linkage and association. — It may be argued that a two-stage procedure would be more feasible and cost-effective than the aforementioned genomewide association strategy, namely, initial genome scan using linkage analysis followed by high-density association (linkage disequilibrium) mapping with candidate SNPs, only in target regions identified by the preceding linkage analysis (Baron in press). For example, pursuant to the initial accounts of linkage between schizophrenia and chromosome 6p21 (see the "Linkage Studies" subsection, above), Wei and Hemmings (2000) conducted a linkage disequilibrium test with densely spaced DNA markers (including SNPs) in the major histocompatibility complex region, which is mapped to 6p21. They showed that two haplotypes for the gene NOTCH4, which may be involved in neurogenesis, are strongly associated with schizophrenia ($P = .0000078$ and $P = .000011$, respectively). Of course, a potential drawback is that genes of minor effect may elude detection in the initial linkage stage.

The presence of allelic association can, in turn, augment the power of linkage analysis to uncover gene effects that might otherwise remain ambiguous. For example, a joint linkage and association test has revealed evidence for two complex disease genes: a major locus for psoriasis, on chromosome 6p21 (Trembath et al. 1997), and the type 1 angiotensin II receptor gene related to essential hypertension (Kainulainen et al. 1999).

Meta-analyses. — Sample-size requirements for linkage detection in complex traits depend on the underlying gene effects. For example, a locus with a genotypic relative risk of 2 may require 400 sib pairs for adequate power (Hauser et al. 1996), whereas a smaller relative risk may necessitate much larger samples (Risch and Merikangas 1996). The samples required for replication may be larger yet (Suarez et al. 1994). Large samples may augment weak linkage signals found in small data sets (if linkage is present) and are less susceptible to random statistical fluctuations that may lead to false-positive results in smaller samples. Because samples of this magnitude are generally not available in single studies, meta-analyses of multiple independent data sets have been proposed as an alternative. Several analyses have been reported that focus on chromosomal regions with prior evidence of possible linkage.

Gill et al. (1996), following up on a previous, smaller meta-analysis of chromosome 22q11-13 (Pulver et al. 1994*b*), analyzed a combined sample of 620 sib pairs in 574 pedigrees collected by 11 independent research groups. They focused on marker D22S278 because it showed the strongest evidence for linkage in three previous studies. When a narrow disease definition was used, the combined sib-pair analysis showed modest support for excess allele sharing at D22S278 ($P = .001$ or $P = .006$, depending on the availability of parental genotypes).

Subsequently, 14 research groups studied 14 markers on chromosomes 3p, 6p, and 8p in 567 pedigrees, including 687 independent sib pairs (Schizophrenia Linkage Collaborative Group for Chromosomes 3p, 6p, and 8p 1996). There was no evidence for linkage to chromosome 3p. When a narrow diagnostic model was used, suggestive support for linkage was observed for chromosomes 6p22-24 (sib-pair analysis, $P = .0004$ for the combined sample, $P = .001$ after removing the sample in which the first linkage finding was reported) and 8p21-22 (heterogeneity LOD score of 3.06, $P = .00018$ for the combined sample, LOD score of 2.22, $P = .0014$ with the original sample removed).

Recently, Levinson et al. (2000) analyzed candidate regions on chromosomes 5q, 6q, 10p, and 13q in 734 pedigrees, including 824 independent sib pairs, collected by eight research groups. They found modest support for linkage to chromosome 6q21-22 (a LOD score of 3.10, $P = .0036$, sib-pair analysis; nonparametric LOD score of 2.47, $P = .0046$; recessive LOD score of 2.47), with or without the sample in which linkage evidence was first reported. Weak support for linkage was observed on chromosome 10p11-15, with no evidence for linkage to chromosomes 5q or 13q.

At face value, these multicenter studies support previously reported linkage to some chromosomal regions (6p, 6q, 8p, and 22q), although the evidence is far from conclusive in spite of the sizable sample. The evidence in other implicated regions (10p and 13q) is substantially weaker than that in the original reports. However, there are drawbacks that limit the interpretation of results (Rice et al. 1997). These include differences among samples—in ascertainment, diagnostic and laboratory methods, marker density and informativeness, or other factors—and possible selection bias resulting from (1) the inclusion of the original positive data sets or (2) the proclivity of researchers to study more intensively chromosomal regions in which they already have evidence of linkage or to select these regions prior to others, to the exclusion of a more systematic study of the genome. A potential bias of this type may have occurred in the 22q-multicenter study (Gill et al. 1996), which included the original samples with linkage evidence at marker D22S278.

Meta-analyses may be useful in guiding the search for disease genes. However, in most cases, a single sizable study involving a systematic genomewide search (or a set of studies with a common design) is preferable to a post hoc meta-analysis of multiple data sets collected under various conditions. Several such studies are under way.

Novel analytical models.—Most current models do not allow the simultaneous consideration of susceptibility loci from various chromosomal regions. Instead, they treat separate disease loci as if they were independent of each other. As a result, these models may not have sufficient power to detect the various genes involved in complex disease, in particular genes of small effect. Recently, new statistical methods have been developed to address this issue. For example, Cox et al. (1999) described an approach to assessing statistical interactions between different chromosomal regions whereby the evidence for linkage at one region is taken into account in assessing the evidence for linkage elsewhere in the genome. Using this approach, they showed an interaction between loci on chromosomes 2 and 15 that increases susceptibility to non–insulin-dependent diabetes (NIDD1). Interestingly, conventional linkage analysis failed to detect linkage to chromosome 15 in the initial genome scan. Because the genetic complexity of schizophrenia appears comparable to that of diabetes, this example is of potential interest. The use of other novel techniques that involve neural networks is proposed to examine the inheritance of all markers jointly over the entire genome (Lucek et al. 1998; Hoh and Ott 2000). This approach may uncover interactions among the multiple genes that underlie complex disorders such as schizophrenia. Power to detect genes of small effect can also be increased by methods that analyze multiple tightly linked markers, an approach that can extract more information on genetic linkage than is provided by existing statistical models (Zhao et al. 2000). It may also be possible to enhance the abilities of linkage and association analysis to detect genes of small effect by the combined use of path analysis, segregation analysis, and linkage/association analysis (Rao and Province 2000). This method may allow systematic examination of multiple risk factors, both genetic and nongenetic. Finally, the recent emergence of technologies based on microarrays (DNA chips) may enable an extensive evaluation of interactions among thousands of genes in the entire genome, a task that exceeds the capacity of current linkage and association mapping (Ott and Hoh 2000).

Summary and Outlook

Methodological issues notwisthanding, the available evidence supports multiple candidate regions as possible sites for schizophrenia-susceptibility genes—in particular, chromosomes 1q, 4q, 5p, 5q, 6p, 6q, 8p, 9q, 10p, 13q, 15q, 22q, and Xp. However, as with other complex diseases, not all studies agree. Most of the positive results are at the suggestive level; and the chromosomal regions implicated are large, thereby complicating the search for disease genes. It remains to be seen which, if any, of these hypothesis-generating findings will result in gene discovery. The definitive studies have yet to be done. In particular, (1) the collection of large-scale, well-characterized data sets (including detailed phenotypic information and cell lines from extended pedigrees, sib pairs, simplex families, and population-based case-control samples) using common, standardized research protocols; (2) marker-intensive genomewide searches for linkage and association, using the ever-improving genomic maps and gene catalogue; (3) application of novel technologies such as DNA pooling, DNA-chip methods, and high-speed SNP testing, as well as advanced statistical and biocomputing tools. These approaches are better suited than hitherto published efforts to the identification of genes for schizophrenia and to the improvement of cost-effectiveness. All the same, existing studies with promising results need not await the completion of the more definitive large-scale efforts such as phenotypic refinement, application of new statistical tools, and intensive molecular studies of candidate regions may bear fruit in some cases. It may well be that genes of moderate-to-large effect will be the first to be identified, if such genes exist. The search for multiple genes of minor effects will be more painstaking.

Electronic-Database Information

Accession number and URL for data in this article are as follows:

Online Mendelian Inheritance in Man (OMIM), http://www .ncbi.nlm.nih.gov/Omim/ (for schizophrenia [MIM 181500])

References

Antonarakis SE, Blouin JL, Pulver AE, Wolyniec P, Lasseter VK, Nestadt G, Kasch L, Babb R, Kazazian HH, Dombroski B, Kimberland M, Ott J, Housman D, Karayiorgou M, MacLean CJ (1995) Schizophrenia susceptibility and chromosome 6p24-22. Nature Genet 11:235–236

Asherson P, Walsh C, Williams J, Sargeant M, Taylor C, Clements A, Gill M, Owen MJ, McGuffin P (1994) Imprinting and anticipation: are they relevant to genetic studies of schizophrenia? Br J Psychiatry 164:619–624

Austin CP, Holder DJ, Ma L, Mixson LA, Caskey CT (1999) Mapping of hKCa3 to chromosome1q21 and investigation of linkage of CAG repeat polymorphism to schizophrenia. Mol Psychiatry 4:261–266

Baron M (1986a) Genetics of schizophrenia. I. Familial patterns and mode of inheritance. Biol Psychiatry 21:1051–1066

Baron M (1986b) Genetics of schizophrenia. II. Vulnerability traits and gene markers. Biol Psychiatry 21:1189–1211

Baron M (1990) Genetic linkage in mental illness. Nature 346: 618

Baron M (1995) Genes and psychosis: old wine in new bottles? Acta Psychiatr Scand 92:81–86

Baron M (1997) Association studies in psychiatry: a season of discontent. Mol Psychiatry 2:278–281

Baron M (2001) The search for complex disease genes: fault by linkage or fault by association? Mol Psychiatry 6: 143–149

Baron M, Rainer JD (1988) Molecular genetics and human disease: implications for modern psychiatric research and practice. Br J Psychiatry 152:741–753

Baron M, Knowles JA (2000) Bipolar disorder and chromosome 18p11: uncertainties redux. Psychiatr Genet 10:55–58

Baron M, Gruen R, Asnis L, Kane J (1982) Schizoaffective illness, schizophrenia and affective disorders: morbidity risk and genetic transmission. Acta Psychiatr Scand 65:253–262

Baron M, Endicott J, Ott J (1990) Genetic linkage in mental illness: limitations and prospects. Br J Psychiatry 157: 645–655

Bassett AS (1992) Chromosomal aberrations and schizophrenia: autosomes. Br J Psychiatry 161:323–334

Bassett AS, McGillivray BC, Jones BD, Pantzar JT (1988) Partial trisomy chromosome 5 cosegregating with schizophrenia. Lancet 1:799–801

Bennett RL, Karayiorgou M, Sobin CA, Norwood TH, Kay M (1997) Identification of an interstitial deletion in an adult female with schizophrenia, mental retardation, and dysmorphic features: further support for a putative schizophrenia susceptibility locus At 5q21-23.1. Am J Hum Genet 61:1450–1454

Berrettini WH, Ferraro TN, Goldin LR, Weeks DE, Detera-Wadleigh S, Nurnberger JI, Gershon ES (1994) Chromosome 18 DNA markers and manic-depressive illness: evidence for a susceptibility gene. Proc Natl Acad Sci USA 91: 5918–5921

Blouin J-L, Dombroski BA, Nath SK, Lasseter VK, Wolyniec PS, Nestadt G, Thornquist M, Ullrich G, McGrath J, Kasch L, Lamacz M, Thomas MG, Gehrig C, Radhakrishna U, Snyder SE, Balk KG, Neufeld K, Swartz KL, Demarchi N,

Papadimitriou GN, Dikeos DG, Stefanis CN, Chakravar A, Childs B, Pulver AE, et al. (1998) Schizophrenia susceptibility loci on chromosomes 13q32 and 8p21. Nature Genet 20:70–73

Brzustowicz LM, Hodgkinson KA, Chow EWC, Honer WC Bassett AS (2000) Location of a major susceptibility locus for familial schizophrenia on chromosome 1q21-22. Science 288:678–682

Brzustowicz LM, Honer WG, Chow EWC, Hogan J, Hodgkinson K, Bassett AS (1997) Use familial schizophrenia t chromosome 6p: 1,396 familial schizophrenia to chromosome 6p. Am J Hum Genet 61:1388–1396

Brzustowicz LM, Honer WG, Chow EWC, Little D, Hogan Hodgkinson K, Bassett AS (1999) Linkage of familial schizophrenia to chromosome 13q32. Am J Hum Genet 6. 1096–1103

Cao Q, Martinez M, Zhang J, Sanders AR, Badner JA, Craw chik A, Markey CJ, Beshah E, Guroff JJ, Maxwell ME Kazuba DM, Whiten R, Goldin LR, Gershon ES, Gejma PV (1997) Suggestive evidence for a schizophrenia susceptibility locus on chromosome 6q and a confirmation in a independent series of pedigrees. Genomics 43:1–8

Cloninger RC (1994) Turning point in the design of linkag studies of schizophrenia. Am J Med Genet 54:83–92

Coon HS, Holik J, Hoff M, Reimherr F, Wender P, Myles Worsley M, Waldo M, Freedman R, Lepper M, Byerley V (1994a) Analysis of chromosome 22 markers in nine schizo phrenia pedigrees. Am J Med Genet 54:72–79

Coon HS, Jensen M, Holik J, Hoff M, Myles-Worsley M Reimherr F, Wender P, Waldo M, Freedman R, Leppert M Byerley W (1994b) Genome scan for genes predisposing t schizophrenia. Am J Med Genet 54:59–71

Cox NJ, Frigge M, Nicolae DL, Concannon P, Hanis CL, Be GI, Kong A (1999) Loci on chromosomes 2 (NIDD1) an 15 interact to increase susceptibility to diabetes in Mexica Americans. Nature Genet 21:213–215

Crow TJ, DeLisi LE (1998) The chromosome workshops a the 5th International Congress of Psychiatric Genetics: th weight of the evidence from genome scans [Workshop re ports, pp 63-129]. Psychiat Genet 8:59–62

Crowe RR (1993) Candidate genes in psychiatry: an epide miological perspective. Am J Med Genet 48: 74–77

Dann J, DeLisi LE, Devoto M, Laval S, Nancarrow DJ, Shield G, Smith A, et al (1997) A linkage study of schizophreni to markers within Xp11 near the MAOB gene. Psychiatr Res 70:131–143

DeLisi LE, Crow TJ (1998) Chromosome Workshops 1998 Current state of psychiatric linkage [Workshop reports, p 219-286]. Am J Med Genet 88:215–218

DeLisi LE, Devoto M, Lofthouse R, Poulter M, Smith A Shields G, Bass N, Chen G, Vita A, Morganti C, Ott J, Crov TJ (1994a) Search for linkage to schizophrenia on the and Y chromosomes. Am J Med Genet 54:113–121

DeLisi LE, Friedrich U, Wahlstrom J, Boccio-Smith A, Forsma A, Eklund K, Crow TJ (1994b) Schizophrenia and sex chro mosome anomalies. Schizophr Bull 20:495–505

DeLisi LE, Craddock N, Detera-Wadleigh S, Foroud T, Gejma P, Kennedy JL, Lendon C, Macciurdi F, Mckeon P, Mynet Johnson L, Nurnberger JI Jr, Paterson A, Schwab S, Va Broeckhoven C, Wildenauer D, Crow TJ (2000) Update o chromosomal locations for psychiatric disorders: report of the interim meeting of chromosome workshop chairpersons from the VII World Congress of Psychiatric Genetics, Monterey, California, October 14-18, 1999. Am J Med Genet 96:434–449

Detera-Wadleigh SD, Badner JA, Berrettini WH, Yoshikawa T, Goldin LR, Turner G, Rollins DY, Moses T, Sanders AR, Karkera JD, Esterling LE, Zeng J, Ferraro TN, Guroff JJ, Kazuba D, Maxwell ME, Nurnberger Jr, JI, Gershon ES (1999) A high-density genome scan detects evidence for a bipolar disorder susceptibility locus on 13q32 and other potential loci on 1q32 and 18p11.2. Proc Natl Acad Sci USA 96:5604–5609

Dror V, Shamir E, Ghanshani S, Kimhi R, Swartz M, Barak Y, Weizman R, Avivi L, Litmanovitch T, Fantino E, Kalman K, Jones EG, Chandy KG, Gargus JJ, Gutman GA, Navon R (1999) hKCa3/KCNN3 potassium channel gene: association of longer CAG repeats with schizophrenia in Israeli Ashkenazi Jews, expression in human tissues and localization to chromosome 1q21. Mol Psychiatry 4:254–260

Faraone SV, Matise T, Svrakic D, Pepple J, Malaspina D, Suarez B, Hampe C, Zambuto CT, Schmitt K, Meyer J, Markel P, Lee H, Harkavy-Friedman J, Kaufmann C, Cloninger CR, Tsuang MT (1998) Genome scan of European- American scizophrenia pedigrees: results of the NIMH genetics initiative and millennium consortium. Am J Med Genet 81: 290–295

Foroud T, Castelluccio PF, Koller DL, Edenberg HJ, Miller M, Bowman E, Rau NL, et al. (2000) Suggestive evidence of a locus on chromosome 10p using the NIMH genetics initiative bipolar affective disorder pedigrees. Am J Med Genet 96:18–23

Freedman R, Coon H, Myles-Worsley M, Orr-Urtreger A, Olincy A, Davis A, Polymeropoulos M, Holik J, Hopkins J, Hoff M, Rosenthal J, Waldo MC, Reimherr F, Wender P, Yaw J, Young DA, Breese CR, Adams C, Patterson D, Adler LE, Kruglyak L, Leonard S, Byerley W (1997) Linkage of a neurophysiological deficit in schizophrenia to a chromosome 15 locus. Proc Natl Acad Sci USA 94:587–592

Garofalo G, Ragusa RM, Argiolas A, Scavuzzo C, Spina E, Barletta C (1993) Evidence of chromosomal fragile sites in schizophrenic patients. Annales de Genetique 36: 132–135

Gershon ES, DeLisi LE, Hamovit J, Nurnberger JI Jr, Maxwell ME, Schreiber J, Dauphinais D, Dingman CW, Guroff JJ (1988) A controlled family study of chronic psychoses: schizophrenia and schizoaffective disorder. Arch Gen Psychiatry 45:328–336

Gill M, Vallada H, Collier D, Sham P, Holmans P, Murray R, McGuffin P, et al (1996)A combined analysis of D22S278 marker alleles in affected sib-pairs: support for a susceptibility locus for schizophrenia at chromosome 22q12. Schizophrenia Collaborative Linkage Group (Chromosome 22). Am J Med Genet 67:40–45

Goldgar DE, Easton DF (1997) Optimal strategies for mapping complex diseases in the presence of multiple loci. Am J Hum Genet 60:1222–1232

Gottesman II (1991) Schizophrenia genesis: the origins of madness. W.H. Freeman, New York

Gottesman II, Shields J (1982) Schizophrenia: The Epigenetic Puzzle. Cambridge University Press, New York

Gordon CT, Krasnewich D, White B, Lenane M, Rapoport JL (1994) Translocation involving chromosomes 1 and 7 in a boy with childhood-onset schizophrenia. J Autism Dev Disord 24:537–545

Greenberg DA, Hodge SE, Vieland VJ, Spence MA (1997) Reply to Farrall. Am J Hum Genet 61:254–255

——— (1998) Reply to Kruglyak. Am J Hum Genet 62: 202–204

Hauser ER, Bohnke M, Guo S-W, Risch N (1996) Affected sib pair interval mapping and exclusion for complex genetic traits. Genet Epidemiol 13:117–137

Hoh JJ, Ott J (2000) Complex inheritance and localizing disease genes. Hum Hered 50: 85–89

Holzman PS, Kringlen E, Matthysse S, Flanagan SD, Lipton RB, Cramer G, Levin S, Lange K, Levy DL (1988) A single dominant gene can account for eye tracking dysfunctions and schizophrenia in offspring of discordant twins. Arch Gen Psychiatry 45:641–647

Hovatta I, Varilo T, Suvisaari J, Terwilliger JD, Ollikainen V, Arajarvi R, Juvonen H, Kokko-Sahin ML, Vaisanen L, Mannila H, Lonnqvist J, Peltonen L (1999) A genomewide screen for schizophrenia genes in an isolated Finnish subpopulation, suggesting multiple susceptibility loci. Am J Hum Genet 65:1114–1124

Judd LL, McAdams L, Budnick B, Braff D (1992) Sensory gating differences in schizophrenia: new results. Am J Psychiatry 149:488–493

Kainulainen K, Perola M, Terwilliger J, Kaprio J, Koskenvuo M, Syvanen AC, Vartiainen E, Peltonen L, Kontula K (1999) Evidence for involvement of the type 1 angiotensin II receptor locus in essential hypertension. Hypertension 33: 844–849

Kalsi G, Mankoo B, Curtis D, Sherrington R, Melmer G, Brynjolfsson J, Sigmundsson T, Read T, Murphy P, Petursson H, Gurling H (1999) New DNA markers with increased informativeness show diminished support for a chromosome 5q11-13 schizophrenia susceptibility locus and exclude linkage in two new cohorts of British and Icelandic families. Ann Hum Genet 63:235–247

Karayiorgou M, Morris MA, Morrow B, Shprintzen RJ, Goldberg R, Borrow J, Gos A, Nestadt G, Wolyniec PS, Lasseter VK, Eisen H, Childs B, Kazazian HH, Kucherlapati R, Antonarakis SE, Pulver AE, Housman DE (1995) Schizophrenia susceptibility associated with interstitial deletions of chromosome 22q11. Proc Natl Acad Sci USA 92:7612–7616

Kendler KS, Diehl SR (1993) The genetics of schizophrenia: a current, genetic-epidemiological perspective. Schizophr Bull 19:261–285

Kendler KS, McGuire M, Gruenberg AM,Walsh D (1994) Outcome and family study of the subtypes of schizophrenia in the west of Ireland. Am J Psychiatry 151:849–856

Kendler KS, MacLean CJ, O'Neill FA, Burke J, Murphy B, Duke F, Shinkwin R, Easter SM, Webb BT, Zhang J, Walsh D, Straub RE (1996) Evidence for a schizophrenia vulnerability locus on chromosome 8p in the Irish study of high-density schizophrenia families. Am J Psychiatry 153:1534–1540

Kendler KS, Myers JM, O'Neill FA, Martin R, Murphy B, MacLean CJ, Walsh D, Straub RE (2000) Clinical features of schizophrenia and linkage to chromosomes 5q, 6p, 8p,, ana 10p in the Irish study of high-density schizophrenia families. Am J Psychiatry 157:402–408

Kidd KK (1993) Association of disease with genetic markers: déjà vu all over again. Am J Med Genet 48:71–72

Kruglyak L (1997) Nonparametric linkage tests are model free. Am J Hum Genet 61: 254–255

Lander E, Kruglyak L (1995) Genetic dissection of complex traits: guidelines for interpreting and reporting linkage results. Nature Genet 11:241–247

Lasseter VK, Pulver AE, Wolyniec PS, Nestadt G, Meyers D, Karayiorgou M, Housman D, Antonarakis S, Kazazian H, Kasch L, Babb R, Kimberland M, Childs B (1995) Follow-up report of potential linkage to schizophrenia on chromosome 22q: part 3. Am J Med Genet 60:172–173

Leboyer M, Filteau MJ, Jay M, Campion D, d'Amato T, Guilloud-Bataille M, Hillaire D, Feingold J, des Lauriers A, Widlocher D (1992) Clinical subtypes and age at onset in schizophrenic siblings. Psychiatry Res 41:107–114

Leonard S, Gault J, Moore T, Hopkins J, Robinson M, Oliney A, Adler LE, Cloninger CR, Kaufman CA, Tsuang MT, Faraone SV, Malaspina D, Svrakic DM, Freedman R (1998) Further investigation of a chromosome 15 locus in schizophrenia: analysis of affected sib pairs from the NIMH genetics initiative. Am J Med Genet 81:308–312

Levinson DF, Holmans P, Straub RE, Owen MJ, Wildenauer DB, Gejman PV, Pulver AE, Laurent C, Kendler KS, Walsh D, Norton N, Williams NM, Schwab SG, Lerer B, Mowry BJ, Sanders AR, Antonarakis SE, Blouin J-L, DeLeuze J-F, Mallet J (2000) Multicenter linkage study of schizophrenia candidate regions on chromosomes 5q, 6q, 10p, and 13q: Schizophrenia Linkage Collaborative Group III. Am J Hum Genet 67:652–663

Levinson DF, Mahtani MM, Nancarrow DJ, Brown DM, Kruglyak L, Kirby A, Hayward NK, Crowe RR, Andreasen NC, Black DW, Silverman JM, Edicott J, Sharpe L, Mohs RC, Siever LJ, Walters MK, Lennon DP, Jones HL, Nertney DA, Daly MJ, Gladis M, Mowry BJ (1998) Genome scan of schizophrenia. Am J Psychiatry 155:741-750

Levy D, Holzman PS, Matthysse S, Mandell N (1993) Eye tracking dysfunction and schizophrenia: a critical perspective. Schizophr Bull 19:461–536

Lin MW, Sham P, Hwu HG, Collier D, Murray R, Powell JF (1997) Suggestive linkage of schizophrenia to markers on chromosome 13 in Caucasian but not Oriental populations. Hum Genet 99:417–420

Lucek P, Hanke J, Reich J, Solla S, Ott J (1998) Multi-locus nonparametric linkage analysis of complex trait loci with neural networks. Hum Hered 48:275–284

Maier W, Lichtermann D, Minges J, Hallmayer J, Heun R, Benkert O, Levinson DF (1993) Continuity and discontinuity of affective disorders and schizophrenia: results of a controlled family study. Arch Gen Psychiatry 50:871–883

Malaspina D, Warburton D, Amador X, Harris M, Kaufmann CA (1992) Association of schizophrenia and partial trisomy of chromosome 5p: a case report. Schizophr Res 7:191–196

Martin JB (1987) Molecular genetics: applications to the clinical neurosciences. Science 238:765–772

Martinez M, Goldin LR, Cao Q, Zhang J, Sanders AR, Nancarrow DJ, Taylor JM, Levinson DF, Kirby A, Crowe RR,

Andreasen NC, Black DW, Silverman JM, Lennon DP, Nertney DA, Brown DM, Mowry BJ, Gershon ES, Gejman PV (1999) Follow-up study on a susceptibility locus for schizophrenia on chromosome 6q. Am J Med Genet 88:337–343

Maziade M, Debraekeleer M, Genest P, Cliché D, Fournier JP, Garneau Y, Shriqui C, Roy MA, Nicole L, Raymond V (1993) A balanced 2:18 translocation and familial schizophrenia: falling short of an association. Arch Gen Psychiatry 50:73–75

Moises HW, Yang L, Kristbjarnarson H, Wiese C, Byerley W, Macciardi F, Arolt V, et al (1995) An international two-stage genome-wide search for schizophrenia susceptibility genes. Nature Genet 11: 321–324

Morris AG, Gaitonde E, McKenna PJ, Molton JD, Hunt DM (1995) CAG repeat expansions and schizophrenia: association with disease in females and with early age-at-onset. Hum Mol Genet 4:1957–1961

Myles-Worsley M, Coon H, McDowell J, Brenner C, Hoff M, Lind B, Bennett P, Freedman R, Clementz B, Byerely W (1999) Linkage of a composite inhibitory phenotype to a chromosome 22q locus in eight Utah families. Am J Med Genet 88:544–550

Nanko S, Kunugi H, Sasaki T, Fukuda R, Kawate T, Kazamatsuri H (1993) Pericentric region of chromosome 9 is a possible candidate region for linkage study of schizophrenia. Biol Psychiatry 33:655–658

O'Donovan MC, Guy C, Craddock N, Murphy KC, Cardno AG, Jones LA, Owen MJ, McGuffin P(1995) Expanded CAG repeats in schizophrenia and bipolar disorder. Nature Genet 10:380–381

Ong SH, Robertson JR (1995) Schizophrenia with karyotype mosaic 47,XXY/48, XXY + 8. Psychiatr Genet 5:67–69

Ott J, Hoh J (2000) Statistical approaches to gene mapping. Am J Hum Genet 67:289–294

Owen MJ (1992) Will schizophrenia become a graveyard for molecular geneticists? Psychol Med 22:289–293

Owen MJ, Craddock N (1996) Modern molecular genetic approaches to complex traits: implications for psychiatric disorders. Mol Psychiatry 1:21–26

Owen MJ, Holmans P, McGuffin P (1997) Association studies in psychiatric genetics. Mol Psychiatry 2:270–273

Palmour RM, Miller S, Fielding A, Vekemans M, Ervin ER (1994) A contribution to the differential diagnosis of the "group of schizophrenias": structural abnormality of chromosome 4. J Psychiatry Neurosci 19:270–277

Pauls DL (1993) Behavioral disorders: lessons in linkage. Nature Genet 3:4–5

Polymeropoulos MH, Coon H, Byerley W, Gershon ES, Goldin L, Crow TJ, Rubenstein J, Hoff M, Holik J, Smith AM, Shields G, Bass NJ, Poulter M, Lofthouse R, Vita A, Morganti C, Merril CR, DeLisi LE (1994) Search for a schizophrenia susceptibility locus on human chromosome 22. Am J Med Genet 54:93–99

Pulver AE, Karayiorgou M, Wolyniec PS, Lasseter VK, Kasch L, Nestadt G, Antonarakis S, et al. (1994a) Sequential strategy to identify a susceptibility gene for schizophrenia: report of potential linkage on chromosome 22q12-q13.1. I. Am J Med Genet 54:36–43

Pulver AE, Karayiorgou M, Lasseter VK, Wolyniec P, Kasch

L, Antonarakis S, Housman D, et al. (1994b) Follow-up of a report of a potential linkage for schizophrenia on chromosome 22q12-q13.1. II. Am J Med Genet 54:44–50

Pulver AE, Lasseter VK, Kasch L, Wolyniec P, Nestadt G, Blouin J-L, Kimberland M, Rabb R, Vourlis S, Chen H, Lalioti M, Morris MA, Karayiorgou M, Ott J, Meyers D, Antonarakis SE, Housman D, Kazazian HH (1995) A genome scan targets chromosomes 3p and 8p as potential sites of susceptibility genes. Am J Med Genet 60:252–260

Pulver AE, Mulle J, Nestadt G, Swartz KL, Blouin J-L, Dombroski B, Liang K-Y, Housman DE, Kazazian HH, Antonarakis SE, Lasseter VK, Wolyniec PS, Thornquist MH, McGrath JA (2000) Genetic heterogeneity in schizophrenia: stratification of genome scan data using co-segregating related phenotypes. Mol Psychiatry 5:650–653

Rao DC, Province MA (2000) The future of path analysis, segregation analysis, and combined models for genetic dissection of complex traits. Hum Hered 50:34–42

Rice JP (1997) The role of meta-analysis in linkage studies of complex traits. Am J Med Genet 74:112–114

Risch N (1990a) Genetic linkage and complex diseases, with special reference to psychiatric disorders. Genet Epidemiol 7:3–16

Risch N (1990b) Linkage strategies for genetically complex traits. I. Multilocus models. Am J Hum Genet 46:222–228

Risch N (2000) Searching for genetic determinants in the new millennium. Nature 405:847–856

Risch N, Merikangas K (1996) The future of genetic studies of complex human diseases. Science 273:1516–1517

Sasaki T, Billett E, Petronis A, Ying D, Parsons T, Macciardi FM, Meltzer HY, Lieberman JL, Joffe RT, Ross CA, McInnis MG, Li SH, Kennedy JL (1996) Psychosis and genes with trinucleotide repeat polymorphism. Hum Genet 97:244–246

Schizophrenia Linkage Collaborative Group for Chromosomes 3, 6, and 8 (1996) Additional support for schizophrenia linkage on chromosomes 6 and 8: a multicenter study. Am J Med Genet 67:580–594

Schwab SG, Albus M, Hallmayer J, Honig S, Borrmann M, Lichtermann D, Ebstein RP, Ackenheil M, Lerer B, Risch N, Maier W, Wildenauer DB (1995) Evaluation of a susceptibility gene for schizophrenia on chromosome 6p by multipoint affected sib-pair linkage analysis. Nature Genet 11:325–327

Schwab SG, Eckstein GN, Hallmayer J, Lerer B, Albus M, Borrmann M, Lichtermann D, Ertl MA, Maier W, Wildenauer DB (1997) Evidence suggestive of a locus on chromosome 5q31 contributing to the susceptibility to schizophrenia in German and Israeli families by multipoint affected sib-pair linkage analysis. Mol Psychiatry 2:156–160

Schwab SG, Hallmayer J, Albus M, Lerer B, Hanses C, Kanyas K, Segman R, Borrmann M, Dreikorn B, Lichtermann D, Rietschel M, Trixler M, Maier W, Wildenauer DB (1998a) Further evidence for a susceptibility locus on chromosome 10p14-11 in 72 families with schizophrenia by nonparametric linkage analysis. Am J Med Genet 81:302–307

Schwab SG, Hallmayer J, Lerer B, Albus M, Borrmann M, Honig S, Straub M, Segman R, Lichtermann D, Knapp M, Trixler M, Maier W, Wildenauer DB (1998b) Support for a

chromosome 18p locus conferring susceptibility to functional psychoses in families with schizophrenia, by association and linkage analysis. Am J Hum Genet 63:1139–1152

Schwab SG, Hallmayer J, Albus M, Lerer B, Eckstein GN, Borrmann M, Segman RH, Hanses C, Freymann J, Yakir A, Trixler M, Falkai P, Rietschel M, Maier W, Wildenauer DB (2000) A genome-wide autosomal scan for schizophrenia susceptibility loci in 71 families with affected siblings: support for loci on chromosome 10p and 6. Mol Psychiatry 5:638–649

Shaw SH, Kelly M, Smith AB, Shields G, Hopkins PJ, Loftus J, Laval SH, Vita A, De Hert M, Cardon LR, Crow TJ, Sherrington R, DeLisi LE (1998) A genomewide search for schizophrenia susceptibility genes. Am J Med Genet 81:364–376

Sherrington R, Brynjolfsson J, Petursson H, Potter M, Dudleston K, Barraclough B, Wasmuth J, Dobbs M, Gurling H (1988) Localization of a susceptibility locus for schizophrenia on chromosome 5. Nature 336:164–167

Silverman JM, Greenberg DA, Altstiel LD, Siever LJ, Mohs RC, Smith CJ, Zhou G, Hollander TE, Yang X-P, Kedache M, Li G, Zaccario ML, Davis KL (1996) Evidence for a locus for schizophrenia and related disorders on the short arm of chromosome 5 in a large pedigree. Am J Med Genet 67:162–171

Spence MA, Bishop DT, Boehnke M, Elston RC, Falk C, Hodge SE, Ott J, Rice J, Merikangas K, Kupfer D (1993) Methodological issues in linkage analyses for psychiatric disorders: secular trends, assortative mating, bilineal pedigrees. Hum Hered 43:166–172

Spurlock G, Williams J, McGuffin P, Aschauer HN, Lenzinger E, Fuchs K, Sieghart WC, Meszaros K, Fathi N, Laurent C, Mallet J, Macciardi F, Pedrini S, Gill M, Hawi Z, Gibson S, Jazin EE, Yang H-T, Adolfsson R, Pato CN, Dourado AM, Owen MJ (1998) European Multicentre Association Study of Schizophrenia: a study of the DRD2 Ser311Cys and DRD3 Ser9Gly polymorphisms. Am J Med Genet 81:24–28

Stober G, Franzek E, Lesch KP, Beckmann H (1995) Periodic catatonia: a schizophrenic subtype with major gene effect and anticipation. Eur Arch Psychiatry Clin Neurosci 245:135–141

Stober G, Saar K, Ruschendorf F, Meyer J, Nurnberg G, Jatzke S, Franzek E, Reis A, Lesch K-P, Wienker TF, Beckmann H (2000) Splitting schizophrenia: periodic catatonia-susceptibility locus on chromosome 15q15. Am J Hum Genet 67:1201–1207

Straub RE, MacLean CJ, Martin RB, Ma Y, Myakishev MV, Harris-Kerr C, Webb BT, O'Neill FA, Walsh D, Kendler KS (1998) A schizophrenia locus may be located in region 10p15-p11. Am J Med Genet 81:296–301

Straub RE, MacLean CJ, O'Neill FA, Burke J, Murphy B, Duke F, Shinkwin R, Webb BT, Zhang J, Walsh D, Kendler KS (1995) A potential vulnerability locus for schizophrenia on chromosome 6p24-22: evidence for schizophrenia heterogeneity. Nature Genet 11:287–293

Straub RE, MacLean CJ, O'Neill FA, Walsh D, Kendler KS (1997) Support for a possible schizophrenia vulnerability locus in region 5q22-31 in Irish families. Mol Psychiatry 2:148–155

Am. J. Hum. Genet. 68:299–312, 2001

Suarez BK, Hampe CL, Van Eerdewegh P (1994) Problems of replicating linkage claims in psychiatry. In: Gershon ES, Cloninger CR (eds) Genetic approaches to mental disorders. American Psychiatric Press, Washington, DC, pp 23–46

Terwilliger JD (1998) Linkage analysis is model-based. In: Armitage P, Colton T (eds) Encyclopedia of Biostatitics. Vol 3. Wiley, London, pp 2279–2291

Terwilliger JD, Weiss KM (1998) Linkage disequilibrium mapping of complex disease: fantasy or reality? Curr Opin Biotechnol 9:578–594

Trembath RC, Clough RL, Rosbotham JL, Jones AB, Camp RDR, Frodsham A, Browne J, Barber R, Terwilliger J, Lathrop GM, Barker JN (1997) Identification of a major susceptibility locus on chromosome 6p and evidence for further disease loci revealed by a two-stage genomewide search in psoriasis. Hum Mol Genet 6:813–820

Vieland VJ, Hodge SE, Greenberg DA (1992) Adequacy of single-locus approximations for linkage analyses of oligogenic traits. Genet Epidemiol 9:45–59

Wang S, Sun CE, Walczak CA, Ziegle JS, Kipps BR, Goldin LR, Diehl SR (1995) Evidence for a susceptibility locus for schizophrenia on chromosome 6pter-p22. Nature Genet 10: 41–46

Wei J, Hemmings GP (2000) The NOTCH4 locus is associated with susceptibility to schizophrenia. Nature Genet 25: 376–377

Weiss KM, Terwilliger JD (2000) How many diseases does it take to map a gene with SNPs? Nature Genet 26:151–157

Williams J, Spurlock G, McGuffin P, Mallet J, Nothen MM, Gill M, Aschauer H, Nylander PO, Macciardi F, Owen MJ (1996) Association between schizophrenia and T102C polymorphism of the 5-hydroxytryptamine type 2a-receptor gene. European Multicentre Association Study of Schizophrenia (EMASS) Group. Lancet 347:1294–1296

Zhao H, Zhang S, Merikangas KR, Trixler M, Wildenauer DB, Sun F, Kidd KK (2000) Transmission/disequilibrium tests using multiple tightly linked markers. Am J Hum Genet 67:936–946

Effect of COMT Val[108/158] Met genotype on frontal lobe function and risk for schizophrenia

Michael F. Egan*[†], Terry E. Goldberg*, Bhaskar S. Kolachana*, Joseph H. Callicott*, Chiara M. Mazzanti[‡], Richard E. Straub[§], David Goldman[‡], and Daniel R. Weinberger*

*Clinical Brain Disorders Branch, Building 10, Center Drive, National Institute of Mental Health, Bethesda, MD 20892; [‡]Laboratory of Neurogenetics, 12501 Washington Avenue, Park 5, 451 National Institute of Alcohol Abuse and Alcoholism, Rockville, MD 20852; and [§]Department of Psychiatry, Virginia Commonwealth University, Richmond, VA 23298

Communicated by P. S. Goldman-Rakic, Yale University School of Medicine, New Haven, CT, March 20, 2001 (received for review August 7, 2000)

Abnormalities of prefrontal cortical function are prominent features of schizophrenia and have been associated with genetic risk, suggesting that susceptibility genes for schizophrenia may impact on the molecular mechanisms of prefrontal function. A potential susceptibility mechanism involves regulation of prefrontal dopamine, which modulates the response of prefrontal neurons during working memory. We examined the relationship of a common functional polymorphism (Val[108/158] Met) in the catechol-O-methyltransferase (COMT) gene, which accounts for a 4-fold variation in enzyme activity and dopamine catabolism, with both prefrontally mediated cognition and prefrontal cortical physiology. In 175 patients with schizophrenia, 219 unaffected siblings, and 55 controls, COMT genotype was related in allele dosage fashion to performance on the Wisconsin Card Sorting Test of executive cognition and explained 4% of variance (P = 0.001) in frequency of perseverative errors. Consistent with other evidence that dopamine enhances prefrontal neuronal function, the load of the low-activity Met allele predicted enhanced cognitive performance. We then examined the effect of COMT genotype on prefrontal physiology during a working memory task in three separate subgroups (n = 11–16) assayed with functional MRI. Met allele load consistently predicted a more efficient physiological response in prefrontal cortex. Finally, in a family-based association analysis of 104 trios, we found a significant increase in transmission of the Val allele to the schizophrenic offspring. These data suggest that the COMT Val allele, because it increases prefrontal dopamine catabolism, impairs prefrontal cognition and physiology, and by this mechanism slightly increases risk for schizophrenia.

Schizophrenia is a complex genetic disorder characterized by chronic psychosis, cognitive impairment, and functional disability. Linkage studies have implicated several possible susceptibility loci, including regions on chromosomes 1q, 6p, 8p, 13q, and 22q (1–3). Attempts to replicate these findings have met with limited success, perhaps due to the weak effects of susceptibility loci and limited power of linkage (4, 5). Of genes mapped to 22q11, one common functional polymorphism of catechol-O-methyltransferase (COMT), a methylation enzyme that metabolizes released dopamine (6), has been a popular candidate because of the long hypothesized role of dopamine in schizophrenia (7). Although two family-based association studies using the transmission disequilibrium test (TDT) have provided evidence for a role of COMT in schizophrenia (8–10), several small case-control association studies of COMT alleles have been negative, and it has been unclear how either protein variation would increase risk for schizophrenia (11, 12).

One approach that may improve power to find genes for complex disorders is to target biological traits found in ill subjects and their unaffected relatives, so-called intermediate phenotypes, rather than clinical diagnosis (13, 14). Such traits may be more directly related to the biological effects of susceptibility genes. Abnormal function of the prefrontal cortex, a cardinal aspect of schizophrenia, also may represent an intermediate phenotype related to genetic risk for schizophrenia (15,

16). Stable deficits in cognitive functions referable to the dorsolateral prefrontal cortex and cortical physiological abnormalities during performance of such tasks have been consistently reported in studies of schizophrenia (17–22). Recent evidence indicates that healthy siblings of patients, including monozygotic cotwins, show similar cognitive and physiological abnormalities (14–16, 22, 24).[¶]

Prefrontal deficits also are appealing phenotypes for genetic studies because the molecular mechanisms underlying such deficits have been sufficiently clarified to permit an hypothesis-driven test of candidate functional polymorphisms (25, 26). Electrophysiological studies in primates (27, 28) and rodents (29), and neuroimaging studies in humans (30, 31), have shown that dopamine plays an important role in modulating the activity of prefrontal circuitry during performance of working memory tasks. Although there are many proteins involved in the biological actions of dopamine, COMT, because it metabolizes released dopamine, may be an important factor during such prefrontally mediated tasks. Despite COMT's widespread distribution in nondopaminergic neurons and glia, pharmacological studies have shown that catabolic flux of synaptic dopamine through the COMT pathway is characteristic of the prefrontal cortex in contrast to the striatum (32). Studies of COMT knockout mice, similarly, have demonstrated that dopamine levels are increased only in prefrontal cortex (33) and, remarkably, that memory performance is enhanced.[∥] This regionally selective effect of COMT may be because, in contrast to striatum, in prefrontal cortex dopamine transporters are expressed in low abundance and not within synapses (34, 35). As a consequence, released synaptic dopamine appears to be inactivated by diffusion, receptor internalization, and COMT degradation. These findings strongly support the notion that variation in COMT activity may have neurobiological effects specific to the prefrontal cortex.

The COMT gene contains an evolutionarily recent G to A missense mutation that translates into a substitution of Met for Val at codon 108/158 (Val[108/158] Met) (GenBank accession no. Z26491). The enzyme containing Met is unstable at 37°C and has 1/4 of the activity of the enzyme containing Val (36). The alleles are codominant, as heterozygous individuals have enzyme activity that is midway between homozygote individuals (6). Thus, genetically determined variations in COMT activity might affect prefrontal cortical activity, especially during executive and work-

---

Abbreviations: COMT, catechol-O-methyltransferase; fMRI, functional MRI; WCST, Wisconsin Card Sorting Test; TDT, transmission disequilibrium test; WRAT, Wide Range Achievement Test.

[†]To whom reprint requests should be addressed. E-mail: eganm@intra.nimh.nih.gov.

[¶]Callicott, J., Egan, M., Mattay, V., Bertolino, A., Jones, K., Goldberg, T. & Weinberger, D. (1998) Neuroimage 7, S895 (abstr.).

[∥]Kneavel, M., Gogos, J., Karayiorgou, K. & Luine, V., Society for Neuroscience 30th Annual Meeting, November 5–10, 2000, New Orleans, 571.20 (abstr.).

The publication costs of this article were defrayed in part by page charge payment. This article must therefore be hereby marked "advertisement" in accordance with 18 U.S.C. §1734 solely to indicate this fact.

81

ing memory tasks. We hypothesized that the high-activity Val allele, because it leads to increased dopamine catabolism, would be associated with relatively compromised prefrontal function, and, by virtue of this effect, would increase risk for schizophrenia.

To test these hypotheses, we studied prefrontal executive cognition and physiology in control subjects, patients with schizophrenia, and their unaffected siblings. To measure executive cognition and working memory, we used the Wisconsin Card Sorting Test (WCST). Deficits in WCST performance are enduring and core features of schizophrenia and predict long term-disability, independent of other cognitive deficits (17, 21); healthy siblings of patients with schizophrenia also perform abnormally on it (24, 37). Functional neuroimaging studies have found that the WCST activates the dorsolateral prefrontal cortex (17, 38) and that dopamimetic drugs improve performance on this task in patients with schizophrenia and enhance the signal to noise of the prefrontal physiological response (30, 31). We hypothesized, therefore, that COMT genotype would affect WCST performance and that Val/Val individuals would have the poorest performance.

To assay prefrontal physiology, we used functional MRI (fMRI) while subjects performed the N-back task. This task has been shown to activate dorsolateral prefrontal cortex as well as a distributed cortical working memory network (20, 39). In studies of patients with schizophrenia who perform relatively well on the N-back and similar tasks, fMRI activation of dorsolateral prefrontal cortex is "inefficient," i.e., there is excessive activity for a given level of performance (19, 20). Similar fMRI results have been described in their unaffected siblings,[¶] suggesting that inefficient prefrontal information processing is related to genetic risk for schizophrenia. Using the N-back fMRI paradigm, Mattay et al. recently reported analogous inefficiency in hypodopaminergic patients with Parkinson's disease.[**] In contrast, the efficiency of the N-back fMRI response in dorsolateral prefrontal cortex is enhanced by the dopamimetic drug, amphetamine, in healthy individuals whose performance remains stable (40). Thus, deviations of prefrontal physiology can be appreciated with this *in vivo* fMRI assay even if there is compensation at the level of performance accuracy, and changes in cortical dopaminergic function impact on physiological efficiency during this task. We hypothesized, therefore, that COMT genotype would affect the efficiency of the prefrontal fMRI response during this task and predicted an allele dosage relationship with activation, with Val/Val individuals being least efficient.

Methods

Subjects and Cognitive Testing. Subjects were recruited from local and national sources as volunteers for the Clinical Brain Disorders Branch/National Institute of Mental Health sibling study, as described (41). Briefly, all participants gave written informed consent of an Institutional Review Board-approved protocol. Most families had two eligible full siblings (at least one of whom met DSM-IV criteria for schizophrenia or schizoaffective disorder, depressed subtype). All subjects had to be from 18 to 60 years of age, above 70 in premorbid IQ, and able to give informed consent. Applicants with significant medical problems, history of head trauma, alcohol or drug abuse within the last 6 months were excluded. All subjects were medically screened and interviewed by a research psychiatrist using the Structured Clinical Interview (42).

To reduce the possibility of artifactual association due to ethnic stratification, the final sample included only individuals of

European ancestry born and educated in the U.S. This sample included 175 patients with schizophrenia, 219 healthy siblings, and 55 control subjects.

Subjects performed the WCST. Perseverative errors was used as a dependent measure because it is thought to best reflect prefrontal function. Scores were transformed to *t* scores and normalized for age and education based on population means, a routine convention (43). Thus, better performance is reflected in a higher *t* score. IQ (from the Wechsler Adult Intelligence Scale, revised edition, or WAIS-R) and reading comprehension (using the Wide Range Achievement Test, WRAT, a measure of premorbid IQ) also were collected (44).

Neuroimaging. Two cohorts of siblings (all nonsmokers) and one cohort of probands were randomly selected, based on scanner availability. Blood oxygen level-dependent fMRI was performed while subjects took the two-back and zero-back versions of the N-back task (20). In contrast to the WCST, the N-back is a relatively simple working memory task more suitable for fMRI.

The N-back task was presented via a fiber-optic goggle system and responses were recorded via a pneumatic button box. Stimuli were displayed randomly at a rate of 1.8 per sec. All subjects were first trained to maximal performance. The first group of unaffected siblings (*n* = 16) and the group of patients with schizophrenia (*n* = 11) were studied with an echo planar imaging blood oxygen level-dependent fMRI sequence at 1.5 Tesla (20). The second sibling group (*n* = 11) was studied by using a more rapid scanning pulse sequence, fast spiral imaging also at 1.5 Tesla (45).

Whole brain echo planar imaging data were collected in a modified block design with pseudorandomized intermixing of zero-back and two-back working memory tasks. Fast spiral imaging data were collected by using a simple block design alternating between zero-back and two-back (16 sec/task epoch) occurring during one 256-sec run. All fMRI data were reconstructed, registered, linear detrended, globally normalized, and then smoothed (10 mm Gaussian kernel) before analysis within statistical parametric mapping (SPM) (46). All data were rigorously screened for artifacts as described (20). Individual data from 18 task epochs were collapsed into adjusted means and then entered into a general linear model within SPM96 (for cohort 1) or SPM 99 (for cohort 2) (Wellcome Department of Cognitive Neurology, London). We first estimated parameters that reflected activation as a contrast between the two-back task and the zero-back task. These parameter estimates were then entered into a second analysis to test inferences about differential activations among the three genotype groups. This analysis is formally identical to a random effects analysis where the subject effect is a random effect. Because we had an anatomically specified hypothesis about prefrontal activation, we used an uncorrected threshold of *P* = 0.005 (voxelwise) to identify these regionally specific differences. The resultant statistical maps then were rendered onto a three-dimensional standard brain.

Genetic Analysis. Blood was collected from all subjects as well as all available parents of patients with schizophrenia. DNA was extracted by using standard methods. DNA from 104 pairs of parents were available for the final analysis. COMT Val[108/158] Met genotype was determined as a restriction fragment length polymorphism after PCR amplification and digestion with *Nla*III, similar to a previously described method (47) (details available on request).

To address at a genomic level the issue of potential population admixture, 19 unlinked, short tandem repeat markers, all with heterozygosities >65%, were genotyped by using PCR and gel analysis as described (48) in selected subjects (details available on request). The markers were: D1S1612, D1S1678, D2S1356, D4S1280, D5S1471, D6S1006, D7S2847, D17S1308, D18S843, D18S535, D19S714, D20S604, D20S477, D20S481, D21S1437,

**Mattay, V. S., Tessitore, A., Callicott, J. H., Bertolino, A., Duyn, J., Frank, J. A., Goldberg, T., Chase, T., Hyde, T. & Weinberger, D. R., Society for Neuroscience 30th Annual Meeting, November 5–10, 2000, New Orleans, 746 (abstr.).

82

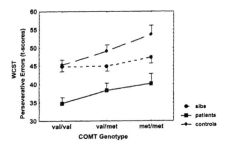

Fig. 1. WCST perseverative error t scores (± SE) by genotype for each group (population mean = 50, SD = 10, lower scores indicate worse performance). Main effect of genotype: F = 4.93, df = 2,224, P = 0.008.

Table 1. Demographics

Variable	Patients (n = 175)	Siblings (n = 219)	Controls (n = 55)
Age	36.1 (8.5)	35.6 (8.8)	33.9 (9.2)
Gender (M/F)	138/37*†	97/122	23/32
Education years	13.7*† (2.1)	15.5 (2.5)	15.7 (2.5)
WRAT	102.0*† (12.1)	106.3 (11.2)	107.3 (11.4)
IQ	92.8*† (13.1)	107.4 (10.6)	109.1 (11.5)
WCST perseverative errors	37.6*† (12.6)	45.2 (9.5)*	49.4 (9.0)

Means ± SD.
*Significantly different compared to controls (P < 0.05).
†Significantly different compared to siblings (P < 0.05).

D21S1446, D22S445, SLC6A3 3′ untranslated region VNTR (GenBank accession no. 162767), and the (TAA) repeat in locus HSMHC3A5 (GenBank accession no. U89335).

Statistical Analyses. Between groups comparisons of demographic data were performed by using paired or unpaired t tests or χ^2, as appropriate. To avoid lack of independence among family members, we used one randomly selected sib per family for comparisons with the control group. The effects of COMT genotype were analyzed several ways. First, groups were compared by using standard parametric techniques (case/control comparisons). Second, to avoid spurious results due to admixture, we used TDT (49, 50), which are family-based methods that substantially sacrifice power.

The effect of COMT genotype on WCST performance was assessed by using two case-control analyses: (i) ANOVA and (ii) multiple regression. With ANOVA, we first included all subjects. Because this assumes independence of individuals, we also report ANOVA results including only patients and controls. Second, using multiple regression we tested the hypothesis that the number of Met alleles was parametrically related to enhanced performance (patients and controls only); diagnostic group was included as the only additional independent variable. Next, we performed a family-based test to examine the effect of COMT genotype on WCST performance (quantitative sib TDT; ref. 50). Subsequently, we examined whether admixture was present in Val/Val and Met/Met groups for patients and controls (Fig. 1) by comparing allele frequencies of 19 unlinked polymorphic genetic markers using an overall χ^2_s as described by Pritchard and Rosenberg (51).

The effect of COMT genotype on risk for schizophrenia was analyzed by using both case-control and family-based methods. The case-control analysis was a comparison of allele frequencies. The family-based analysis used the TDT (49). A critical issue in

assessing the significance of association with phenotypic measures is the likelihood of type I errors. Many genes and phenotypes can be evaluated for schizophrenia and ultimately may be examined in this dataset, but Bonferroni correction for all possible combinations that ultimately may be performed seems overly stringent. The approach here was to selectively analyze a single candidate functional polymorphism, chosen for its biological effect, against a target phenotype likely impacted by this biological effect. Given the role of COMT in prefrontal dopamine metabolism, and the role of dopamine in prefrontal function and working memory, the prior probability of this gene modifying prefrontal function may be high relative to other polymorphisms and phenotypes.

Results

Demographic data are presented in Table 1. Briefly, siblings and controls were well matched on age, gender, education, IQ, and WRAT. There was no difference between patients receiving typical and atypical neuroleptic treatment on any cognitive variable. History of alcohol abuse and dependence did not affect any cognitive measure in this study, most likely because subjects with recent or prolonged abuse or dependence were excluded (41). Patients and siblings scored significantly worse on the WCST compared with the control group (Table 1), as reported (24, 37) ($F = 29.6$, df = 2,440, $P < 0.00001$). An ANOVA for all groups revealed a significant effect of COMT genotype on WCST performance ($F = 6.00$, df = 2,440, $P = 0.003$) with no group by genotype interaction ($F = 1.40$, df = 4,440, $P = 0.23$, Fig. 1). A second ANOVA including only patients and controls also detected a significant effect of genotype ($F = 4.93$, df = 2,224, $P = 0.008$). Post hoc analysis showed that subjects with the Val/Val genotype performed worse than those with the Val/Met and Met/Met genotypes ($P < 0.002$). In contrast, no genotype effect was seen on tasks of general academic ability, e.g., WRAT reading scores or IQ, and no differences were seen between genotype groups in other demographic measures (Table 2).

Using multiple regression, the number of Met alleles was parametrically related to perseverative errors t scores [$r^2 = 0.041$, $t(228) = 3.29, P = 0.001$]. COMT genotype accounted for 4.1% of the variance in performance. Because prior reports have

Table 2. Demographics by genotype for patients and controls

	Patients			Controls		
	Val/Val	Val/Met	Met/Met	Val/Val	Val/Met	Met/Met
Age	37.1 (8.3)	35.7 (8.1)	35.1 (8.3)	34.5 (10.5)	33.7 (10.0)	34.2 (9.5)
Gender (M/F)	49/13	68/17	21/7	6/9	10/20	7/3
Education years	13.9 (2.0)	13.6 (2.0)	13.5 (2.6)	16.3 (2.5)	15.8 (2.3)	15.8 (2.6)
WRAT	102.1 (10.7)	102.4 (11.4)	100.9 (13.4)	108.0 (9.1)	106.8 (10.6)	107.4 (6.0)
IQ	89.9 (13.7)	94.3 (12.0)	94.5 (12.6)	111.5 (8.7)	107.3 (9.2)	110.4 (8.8)

Means ± SD. Within each group (patients or controls), there is no significant difference between genotype for any variable.

Egan et al.

PNAS | June 5, 2001 | vol. 98 | no. 12 | 6919

83

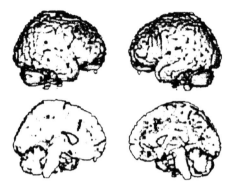

Fig. 2. Effect of COMT genotype on fMRI activation during the two-back working memory task. Regions showing a significant effect of genotype on fMRI activation (voxelwise $P < 0.005$) are in red (shown clockwise from upper left in right lateral, left lateral, right medial, and left medial views, respectively). In dorsolateral prefrontal cortex (e.g., Brodmann area 46; $x = 58$, $y = 32$, $z = 12$; cluster size = 47; $Z = 2.55$) and anterior cingulate (e.g., Brodmann 32; $x = 6$, $y = 60$, $z = 8$; cluster size = 77; $Z = 2.36$), Val/Val individuals showed a greater fMRI response (and by inference, greater inefficiency, as performance is similar) than Val/Met individuals who have greater activation than Met/Met individuals. Post hoc analysis of genotype group contrasts confirmed these significant relationships in dorsolateral prefrontal and cingulate cortices across all groups.

found an effect of gender on COMT expression in animal models (33), we added gender into both the ANOVA and multiple regression analyses. There was no effect of gender or gender by genotype interaction. To exclude other possible spurious effects, we added diagnosis, age, gender, and education to a stepwise multiple regression analysis. This resulted in a small decrease in the r^2 for the COMT effect but its significance at entry remained high (increment in adjusted $r^2 = 0.024$, $P = 0.003$). Using the family-based quantitative sib TDT, a trend was seen for a COMT genotype effect on WCST performance ($F = 2.36$, df = 2,159, $P < 0.10$). Using 19 polymorphic genetic markers, no evidence for population stratification was found between Val/Val and Met/Met groups in patients or controls (omnibus $\chi^2 = 113.5$, df = 112 $P = 0.44$).

Figs. 2 and 3 show the effect of COMT allele load on the fMRI response during the two-back version of the N-back task in the two groups of siblings. The first group (Fig. 2) consisted of five Met/Met individuals, six Val/Met individuals, and five Val/Val individuals. The genotype subgroups used did not differ in mean age, gender, education, handedness, or performance accuracy. The second group (Fig. 3) consisted of three Met/Met, five Met/Val, and three Val/Val individuals; these genotype subgroups did not differ significantly in age, education, gender, handedness, or performance accuracy. In both groups, locales in dorsolateral prefrontal and cingulate cortices show the predicted genotype effects, with Val/Val individuals having the greatest response (i.e., being least efficient), followed by Val/Met and then Met/Met individuals. Similar results were seen in the patient group as well (data not shown).

We next addressed the possibility that in the 104 family trios, the COMT Val allele is a risk factor for schizophrenia, per se. A total of 126 transmissions were counted from heterozygous parents to probands. The Val allele was transmitted 75 times, compared with 51 transmissions of the Met allele. These proportions are different from that predicted by random assortment

($\chi^2 = 4.57$; $P = 0.03$) and indicate that the COMT Val allele is weakly associated with schizophrenia. The odds ratio for the Val/Val genotype is 1.5. Unaffected siblings ($n = 117$) had 77 Val transmissions and 87 Met transmissions, indicating that meiotic segregation distortion is not present. Monte Carlo simulation of 10,000 TDT replicates confirmed that our result would occur at the $P < 0.04$ level of significance. In the case-control analysis, no significant differences in allele ($\chi^2 = 0.92$; df = 1; $P = 0.34$) or genotype ($\chi^2 = 1.25$; df = 2, $P = 0.54$) frequencies were seen comparing patients and controls (Table 3), similar to most (11, 52–54), but not all (55, 56) earlier case-control studies.

Discussion

We report several convergent findings that implicate an effect of COMT genotype on prefrontal cortical function and, as a result, on increased risk for schizophrenia. First, COMT genotype is specifically associated with level of performance on a neuropsychological test of executive cognition that is related to function of prefrontal cortex, but not with general intelligence. This effect of COMT is independent of psychiatric diagnosis and explains 4.1% of the variance on the WCST. The high-activity Val allele is associated with a reduction in performance compared with the Met allele. Second, Val allele load is related to reduced "efficiency" of the physiologic response in the dorsolateral prefrontal cortex during performance of a simple working memory task in three cohorts studied with fMRI. Neural net modeling of the effects of dopamine on working memory circuits predicted that reductions in synaptic dopamine would reduce signal-to-noise ratios, thus reducing efficiency (57). This prediction recently was confirmed in an fMRI study of patients with Parkinson's disease.** It is also consistent with the effect of the Val allele observed in our fMRI data. These convergent findings suggest that the COMT Val allele, presumably by compromising the postsynaptic impact of the evoked dopamine response, may reduce signal to noise in prefrontal neurons and thereby alter working memory function. Third, the Val allele is transmitted slightly more often ($P < 0.04$) to probands with schizophrenia. The association of the Val allele with schizophrenia suggests that this allele, by virtue of its physiological effect on prefrontal information processing, increases susceptibility to schizophrenia.

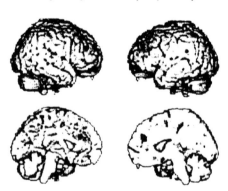

Fig. 3. Effect of COMT genotype on fMRI activation during the two-back working memory task in a second group of subjects. Again, Val/Val individuals showed greater activation (and by inference greater inefficiency) than Val/Met individuals who showed less efficiency than Met/Met individuals in the dorsal prefrontal cortex and several other locales.

84

Table 3. Distribution of genotypes and alleles

Genotype	Patients (n = 175)	Sibs (n = 219)	Controls (n = 55)
Val/Val	62 (35%)	69 (31%)	15 (27%)
Val/Met	85 (49%)	114 (51%)	30 (55%)
Met/Met	28 (16%)	39 (18%)	10 (18%)
Frequency Val	0.60 ± 0.03	0.57 ± 0.02	0.54 ± 0.03
Frequency Met	0.40 ± 0.03	0.43 ± 0.02	0.46 ± 0.03

Frequency is ± SE.

This proposed genetic/neurophysiological mechanism is consistent with prior studies of the neurobiology of schizophrenia. As described above, deficits in prefrontal function are core manifestations of schizophrenia and are related to genetic risk for schizophrenia (15, 16, 24). Neuroimaging and postmortem studies have found evidence of reduced dopaminergic innervation of dorsolateral prefrontal cortex in patients with schizophrenia (17, 58, 59). Thus, the COMT Val allele, by imposing an additional adverse load specifically on prefrontal function, might add to or interact with other causes of prefrontal malfunction in those at risk for schizophrenia and thereby increase their susceptibility. However, the effect of COMT genotype on prefrontal function is small; indeed, it was not significant in the cohort of siblings. This latter negative finding could be due to siblings being a mixed group, in terms of other genetic risk and protective factors. Val/Val siblings who have no psychiatric disorder, for example, could have protective factors positively affecting prefrontal cortical function, otherwise they might themselves have schizophrenia.

With an odds ratio of 1.5, the effect of the Val/Val genotype acting alone on diagnosis is weak. Indeed, a 4.1% variation in prefrontal function by itself may not pose much of a risk for behavioral decompensation. This risk, however, represents an average effect across many individuals. The effect of COMT genotype within any particular individual could be large or small, depending on a variety of background factors. Thus, a gene such as COMT could have an important clinical effect in combination with other genes and environmental factors and could be of value in identifying such factors, especially if their effects are nonadditive. Nevertheless, it seems possible or even likely that most susceptibility genes for schizophrenia will either have a relatively low genotypic relative risk or will be very uncommon in the general patient population and affect only a small portion of patients (5, 60).

Although our results offer a mechanism for how the Val allele might increase susceptibility for schizophrenia, the results of genetic studies, including this one, showing linkage or association between COMT and schizophrenia are, at best, weak. Linkage studies generally have found logarithm of odds scores of 2 or less for markers near 22q11, the chromosomal region containing the COMT gene (3, 61, 62) (see ref. 60 for review). Of previously published TDT-based association studies, one found a significant relationship between schizophrenia and Val transmissions (9); a second also reported an excess (22 vs. 13, $\chi^2 = 2.31$, $P = 0.13$) of Val transmissions (8). In an expanded sample of 198 trios, Li et al. (10) performed a haplotype analysis and again showed a significant association with the Val allele and schizophrenia. Although TDT analyses have been uniformly positive, the results of case control association studies (including our own), which have generally used small sample sizes (relative to those needed to detect a weak genetic effect), have been negative in most (11, 52–54), but not all (55) cases. These negative results are not unexpected, given the lack of power in these studies to detect alleles of minor effect.

Population stratification artifacts are an important consideration in genetic case control analyses and might be an occult factor in our genetic effect on prefrontal function. COMT Val/Met allele frequencies differ across some ethnic groups, although this is probably not the case for the western European populations represented in our study (12). Given that the predicted COMT effect on WCST performance was seen in two unrelated samples (patients and controls) and the predicted effect on cortical physiology was found in three samples, similar stratification would have to be common to all these cohorts and both phenotypes. Furthermore, the genetically distinct subpopulations would have to differ only on prefrontal measures and not on general intelligence, because genotype groups did not differ on other cognitive tests. Nevertheless, we also used two methods to test whether admixture might account for our genetic effect on cognition, a family-based analysis (50), and genomic controls (51). The quantitative sibling TDT used with the WCST data was not significant, although with a trend P value of <0.10, but this is a random effects model with limited degrees of freedom. Using 19 unlinked polymorphic genetic markers, we found no genetic evidence for stratification. The family-based TDT, which found a weakly significant association with schizophrenia, also controls for stratification (49).

A second possible artifact to consider is that the COMT Val/Met polymorphism is not the causative locus but is in linkage disequilibrium with another mutation. We suggest that, given (i) the strong impact of the COMT Val/Met polymorphism on COMT enzyme activity, (ii) the known effects of COMT on prefrontal dopamine metabolism, and (iii) the effect of dopamine on prefrontal neuronal function and working memory, the COMT Val/Met allele is the causative genetic locus for the association with prefrontal function. Using a COMT knockout mouse model, others have shown that prefrontal dopamine levels are increased (33) and that performance on a memory task is actually improved relative to the wild-type animal.[∥] This remarkable improvement in memory performance supports our model that the Met allele, with its reduced activity, accounts for improved prefrontal function, and not another nearby gene.

Finally, is it plausible that a common allele with such weak effects could increase risk for schizophrenia? In some respects, our results with COMT and schizophrenia are similar to the calpain-10 association with diabetes (63), and the association of the APO e4 allele with Alzheimer's disease, although the APO e4 effect is much greater (64). The calpain-10 allele is found in 75% of the general population and in 80% of diabetics, a weak association that is not easily replicated across populations, and the biologic effect of the polymorphism is unknown. It is assumed that such polygenes interact with other genes and environmental factors to incrementally increase risk. The COMT Val allele is certainly not a necessary or sufficient causative factor for schizophrenia, nor is it likely to increase risk only for schizophrenia. However, its biological effect on prefrontal function and the relevance of prefrontal function for schizophrenia susceptibility is a mechanism by which it could increase liability for this disorder. The data presented here provide convergent evidence that the Val allele compromises prefrontal function and thereby impacts directly on the biology of schizophrenia. Despite the apparent disadvantage of the Val allele, the Met allele may increase susceptibility to other disorders, such as estrogenic cancer (23), suggesting that a heterozygote advantage could maintain the high Met and Val allele frequencies observed in a variety of human populations. Finally, it should be noted that the COMT polymorphism affects performance and prefrontal cortical function in both ill and healthy subjects. Thus, the recent Met mutation, which has not been reported in nonhuman primates (12), enhances an important component of normal human cognition, suggesting a possible role in the evolution of human brain function.

We thank the following for their assistance: Lew Bigelow, Mary Weirick, Venkatta Mattay, Tonya Gscheidle, Ashley Bone, Tom Weickert, Andreas Myer-Lindenberg, Alan Barnett, and the patients and their families whose participation made this project possible. This project was supported by funding from the National Institute of Mental Health and the Stanley Foundation (to D.R.W.).

1. Brzustowicz, L. M., Hodgkinson, K. A., Chow, E. W., Honer, W. G. & Bassett, A. S. (2000) *Science* **288**, 678–682.
2. Straub, R. E., MacLean, C. J., O'Neill, F. A., Burke, J., Murphy, B., Duke, F., Shinkwin, R., Webb, B. T., Zhang, J., Walsh, D., *et al.* (1995) *Nat. Genet.* **11**, 287–293.
3. Pulver, A. E., Karayiorgou, M., Wolyniec, P. S., Lasseter, V. K., Kasch, L., Nestadt, G., Antonarakis, S., Housman, D., Kazazian, H. H., Meyers, D., *et al.* (1994) *Am. J. Med. Genet.* **54**, 36–43.
4. Risch, N. & Merikangas, K. (1996) *Science* **273**, 1516–1517.
5. Risch, N. (1990) *Am. J. Hum. Genet.* **46**, 222–228.
6. Weinshilboum, R. M., Otterness, D. M. & Szumlanski, C. L. (1999) *Annu. Rev. Pharmacol. Toxicol.* **39**, 19–52.
7. Carlsson, A., Waters, N., Waters, S. & Carlsson, M. L. (2000) *Brain Res. Brain Res. Rev.* **31**, 342–349.
8. Kunugi, H., Vallada, H. P., Sham, P. C., Hoda, F., Arranz, M. J., Li, T., Nanko, S., Murray, R. M., McGuffin, P., Owen, M., *et al.* (1997) *Psychiatr. Genet.* **7**, 97–101.
9. Li, T., Sham, P. C., Vallada, H., Xie, T., Tang, X., Murray, R. M., Liu, X. & Collier, D. A. (1996) *Psychiatr. Genet.* **6**, 131–133.
10. Li, T., Ball, D., Zhao, J., Murray, R. M., Liu, X., Sham, P. C. & Collier, D. A. (2000) *Mol. Psychiatry* **5**, 77–84.
11. Karayiorgou, M., Gogos, J. A., Galke, B. L., Wolyniec, P. S., Nestadt, G., Antonarakis, S. E., Kazazian, H. H., Housman, D. E. & Pulver, A. E. (1998) *Biol. Psychiatry* **43**, 425–431.
12. Palmatier, M. A., Kang, A. M. & Kidd, K. K. (1999) *Biol. Psychiatry* **46**, 557–567.
13. Freedman, R., Coon, H., Myles-Worsley, M., Orr-Urtreger, A., Olincy, A., Davis, A., Polymeropoulos, M., Holik, J., Hopkins, J., Hoff, M., *et al.* (1997) *Proc. Natl. Acad. Sci. USA* **94**, 587–592.
14. Kremen, W. S., Seidman, L. J., Pepple, J. R., Lyons, M. J., Tsuang, M. T. & Faraone, S. V. (1994) *Schizophr. Bull.* **20**, 103–119.
15. Cannon, T. D., Huttunen, M. O., Lonnqvist, J., Tuulio-Henriksson, A., Pirkola, T., Glahn, D., Finkelstein, J., Hietanen, M., Kaprio, J. & Koskenvuo, M. (2000) *Am. J. Hum. Genet.* **67**, 369–382.
16. Goldberg, T. E., Ragland, J. D., Torrey, E. F., Gold, J. M., Bigelow, L. B. & Weinberger, D. R. (1990) *Arch. Gen. Psychiatry* **47**, 1066–1072.
17. Weinberger, D. R., Berman, K. F. & Zec, R. F. (1986) *Arch. Gen. Psychiatry* **43**, 114–124.
18. Carter, C. S., Perlstein, W., Ganguli, R., Brar, J., Mintun, M. & Cohen, J. D. (1998) *Am. J. Psychiatry* **155**, 1285–1287.
19. Manoach, D. S., Press, D. Z., Thangaraj, V., Searl, M. M., Goff, D. C., Halpern, E., Saper, C. B. & Warach, S. (1999) *Biol. Psychiatry* **45**, 1128–1137.
20. Callicott, J. H., Bertolino, A., Mattay, V. S., Langheim, F. J. P., Duyn, J., Coppola, R., Goldberg, T. E. & Weinberger, D. R. (2000) *Cereb. Cortex* **10**, 1078–1092.
21. Goldberg, T. E. & Weinberger, D. R. (1988) *Schizophr. Bull.* **14**, 179–183.
22. Park, S., Holzman, P. S. & Goldman-Rakic, P. S. (1995) *Arch. Gen. Psychiatry* **52**, 821–828.
23. Lavigne, J. A., Helzlsouer, K. J., Huang, H. Y., Strickland, P. T., Bell, D. A., Selmin, O., Watson, M. A., Hoffman, S., Comstock, G. W. & Yager, J. D. (1997) *Cancer Res.* **57**, 5493–5497.
24. Egan, M., Goldberg, T., Gscheidle, T., Bigelow, L., Hyde, T. & Weinberger, D. R. (2001) *Biol. Psychiatry*, in press.
25. Lidow, M. S., Williams, G. V. & Goldman-Rakic, P. S. (1998) *Trends Pharmacol. Sci.* **19**, 136–140.
26. Gao, W. J., Krimer, L. S. & Goldman-Rakic, P. S. (2001) *Proc. Natl. Acad. Sci. USA* **98**, 295–300. (First Published December 26, 2000, 10.1073/pnas.011524298)
27. Sawaguchi, T. & Goldman-Rakic, P. S. (1991) *Science* **251**, 947–950.
28. Williams, G. V. & Goldman-Rakic, P. S. (1995) *Nature (London)* **376**, 572–575.
29. Seamans, J. K., Floresco, S. B. & Phillips, A. G. (1998) *J. Neurosci.* **18**, 1613–1621.
30. Daniel, D. G., Weinberger, D. R., Jones, D. W., Zigun, J. R., Coppola, R., Handel, S., Bigelow, L. B., Goldberg, T. E., Berman, K. F. & Kleinman, J. E. (1991) *J. Neurosci.* **11**, 1907–1917.
31. Mattay, V. S., Berman, K. F., Ostrem, J. L., Esposito, G., Van Horn, J. D., Bigelow, L. B. & Weinberger, D. R. (1996) *J. Neurosci.* **16**, 4816–4822.
32. Karoum, F., Chrapusta, S. J. & Egan, M. F. (1994) *J. Neurochem.* **63**, 972–979.
33. Gogos, J. A., Morgan, M., Luine, V., Santha, M., Ogawa, S., Pfaff, D. & Karayiorgou, M. (1998) *Proc. Natl. Acad. Sci. USA* **95**, 9991–9996.
34. Lewis, D. A., Sesack, S. R., Levey, A. I. & Rosenberg, D. R. (1998) *Adv. Pharmacol.* **42**, 703–706.
35. Sesack, S. R., Hawrylak, V. A., Matus, C., Guido, M. A. & Levey, A. I. (1998) *J. Neurosci.* **18**, 2697–2708.
36. Lotta, T., Vidgren, J., Tilgmann, C., Ulmanen, I., Melen, K., Julkunen, I. & Taskinen, J. (1995) *Biochemistry* **34**, 4202–4210.
37. Faraone, S. V., Seidman, L. J., Kremen, W. S., Pepple, J. R., Lyons, M. J. & Tsuang, M. T. (1995) *J. Abnorm. Psychol.* **104**, 286–304.
38. Berman, K. F., Ostrem, J. L., Randolph, C., Gold, J., Goldberg, T. E., Coppola, R., Carson, R. E., Herscovitch, P. & Weinberger, D. R. (1995) *Neuropsychologia* **33**, 1027–1046.
39. Cohen, J. D., Perlstein, W. M., Braver, T. S., Nystrom, L. E., Noll, D. C., Jonides, J. & Smith, E. E. (1997) *Nature (London)* **386**, 604–608.
40. Mattay, V. S., Callicott, J. H., Bertolino, A., Heaton, I., Frank, J. A., Coppola, R., Berman, K. F., Goldberg, T. E. & Weinberger, D. R. (2000) *Neuroimage* **12**, 268–275.
41. Egan, M., Goldberg, T. E., Gscheidle, T., Weirick, M., Bigelow, L. & Weinberger, D. R. (2000) *Am. J. Psychiatry* **157**, 1309–1316.
42. First, M. B., Gibbon, M., Spitzer, R. L. & Williams, J. B. W. (1996) *User's Guide for the SCID-I for DSM-IV Axis I Disorders-Research Version* (Biometrics Research, New York).
43. Heaton, R. K., Chelune, G. J., Talley, J. L., Kay, G. G. & Curtiss, G. (1993) *Wisconsin Card Sorting Test Manual* (Psychological Assessment Resources, Odessa, FL).
44. Jastak, S. & Wilkinson, G. S. (1984) *Wide Range Achievement Test* (Jastak Associates, Wilmington, DE).
45. Yang, Y., Glover, G. H., van Gelderen, P., Mattay, V. S., Santha, A. K., Sexton, R. H., Ramsey, N. F., Moonen, C. T., Weinberger, D. R., Frank, J. A. & Duyn, J. H. (1996) *Magn. Reson. Med.* **36**, 620–626.
46. Friston, J. K., Holmes, A. P., Worsley, J., Poline, J. B., Frith, C. D. & Frackowiak, R. S. J. (1995) *Hum. Brain Mapp.* **2**, 189–210.
47. Lachman, H. M., Papolos, D. F., Saito, T., Yu, Y. M., Szumlanski, C. L. & Weinshilboum, R. M. (1996) *Pharmacogenetics* **6**, 243–250.
48. Straub, R. E., Speer, M. C., Luo, Y., Rojas, K., Overhauser, J., Ott, J. & Gilliam, T. C. (1993) *Genomics* **15**, 48–56.
49. Spielman, R. S., McGinnis, R. E. & Ewens, W. J. (1993) *Am. J. Hum. Genet.* **52**, 506–516.
50. Allison, D. B., Heo, M., Kaplan, N. & Martin, E. R. (1999) *Am. J. Hum. Genet.* **64**, 1754–1763.
51. Pritchard, J. K. & Rosenberg, N. A. (1999) *Am. J. Hum. Genet.* **65**, 220–228.
52. Daniels, J. K., Williams, N. M., Williams, J., Jones, L. A., Cardno, A. G., Murphy, K. C., Spurlock, G., Riley, B., Scambler, P., Asherson, P., *et al.* (1996) *Am. J. Psychiatry* **153**, 268–270.
53. Chen, C. H., Lee, Y. R., Wei, F. C., Koong, F. J., Hwu, H. G. & Hsiao, K. J. (1997) *Biol. Psychiatry* **41**, 985–987.
54. Strous, R. D., Bark, N., Woerner, M. & Lachman, H. M. (1997) *Biol. Psychiatry* **41**, 493–495.
55. de Chaldee, M., Laurent, C., Thibaut, F., Martinez, M., Samolyk, D., Petit, M., Campion, D. & Mallet, J. (1999) *Am. J. Med. Genet.* **88**, 452–457.
56. Ohmori, O., Shinkai, T., Kojima, H., Terao, T., Suzuki, T., Mita, T. & Abe, K. (1998) *Neurosci. Lett.* **243**, 109–112.
57. Servan-Schreiber, D., Printz, H. & Cohen, J. D. (1990) *Science* **249**, 892–895.
58. Weinberger, D. R., Berman, K. F. & Illowsky, B. P. (1988) *Arch. Gen. Psychiatry* **45**, 609–615.
59. Akil, M., Pierri, J. N., Whitehead, R. E., Edgar, C. L., Mohila, C., Sampson, A. R. & Lewis, D. A. (1999) *Am. J. Psychiatry* **156**, 1580–1589.
60. Riley, B. P. & McGuffin, P. (2000) *Am. J. Med. Genet.* **97**, 23–44.
61. Pulver, A. E., Karayiorgou, M., Lasseter, V. K., Wolyniec, P., Kasch, L., Antonarakis, S., Housman, D., Kazazian, H. H., Meyers, D., Nestadt, G., *et al.* (1994) *Am. J. Med. Genet.* **54**, 44–50.
62. Gill, M., Vallada, H., Collier, D., Sham, P., Holmans, P., Murray, R., McGuffin, P., Nanko, S., Owen, M., Antonarakis, S., *et al.* (1996) *Am. J. Med. Genet.* **67**, 40–45.
63. Horikawa, Y., Oda, N., Cox, N. J., Li, X., Orho-Melander, M., Hara, M., Hinokio, Y., Lindner, T. H., Mashima, H., Schwarz, P. E., *et al.* (2000) *Nat. Genet.* **26**, 163–175.
64. Roses, A. D. (1998) *Ann. N.Y. Acad. Sci.* **855**, 738–743.

86

Epidemiology and Natural History of Schizophrenia

Evelyn J. Bromet and Shmuel Fennig

The present review explores the descriptive epidemiology of schizophrenia. Risk factors and correlates are divided into three groups based on whether the available evidence is consistent and strong, consistent and potentially strong, or inconsistent. The paper then considers epidemiologic studies of the course of illness, including a description of findings from the Suffolk County Mental Health Project. Given renewed attention to the need for preventive interventions for individuals at high risk for developing a psychotic illness, epidemiologic values have become more and more central to the conduct of clinical research. Biol Psychiatry 1999;46:871–881 © 1999 Society of Biological Psychiatry

Key Words: Schizophrenia, epidemiology, risk factors, Illness course

Introduction

Psychotic disorders are often chronic, debilitating conditions. They are associated with an increase in mortality (Allebeck and Wistedt 1986) and are costly and uniquely distressing for patients and their families (Brown and Birtwistle 1998). Although there is some indication, albeit controversial, that the incidence of schizophrenia has declined during this century (e.g., Eagles and Whalley 1985), the number of people with psychosis may continue to grow as life expectancy increases.

Epidemiology is the study of the frequency and determinants of illness in the population. Thus, epidemiologic studies of schizophrenia focus on the incidence rate and risk factors associated with disease onset, and on the prevalence rate and factors associated with the occurrence and course of illness. Studies designed as epidemiologic inquiries have fundamental features, including the use of representative samples, systematically derived diagnoses, reliable measures, and a comprehensive array of risk factors. Hence, research based on nonrepresentative or convenience samples, clinical or nonreproducible diagnoses, or nonsystematic methods of data collection do not

fall under the rubric of epidemiology. Nevertheless, such research can suggest important hypotheses, and the convergence of evidence across nonepidemiologic studies can serve as a test for these hypotheses in the absence of epidemiologic data. Indeed, the majority of descriptive and follow-up studies of psychosis do not fall within the rubric of epidemiology, but consistent patterns of findings have nonetheless emerged.

The most basic requirement of an epidemiologic study is an accurate diagnosis. In schizophrenia, this requires both a thorough clinical history of the onset and progression of symptoms and evidence that the psychosis is not due to organic causes. Relevant information must be integrated from records, reports of significant others, and patient assessment. Clinical diagnoses of patients treated in academic settings may be relatively more reliable than those given in other types of treatment facilities. Overall, however, even with recent advances in specifying operational criteria for diagnosis, the level of agreement between clinical and research diagnoses remains modest (Fennig et al 1994a).

Another fundamental requirement of epidemiologic studies is specifying the date of onset, or disease acquisition. This is crucial for calculating the incidence rate and identifying risk factors, as opposed to correlates that may be either noncausal in nature or consequences of the illness. Thus, a risk factor is a determinant of disease development and antedates the onset of the illness (Greenberg et al 1996). The best study design for identifying true risk factors is the prospective study, in which the putative risk factors are first ascertained in healthy populations who are then monitored longitudinally for initial signs of psychopathology. This design is expensive and time-consuming to implement. Hence, most risk factor research is based on retrospective information. With newer interview methodologies designed to sharpen memory, such as the Retrospective Assessment of the Onset of Schizophrenia (IRAOS; Häfner et al 1992), the reliability of retrospective data has improved over time. For disorders with insidious onsets, however, the determination of whether a variable is a true risk factor is often difficult, and in these cases, the variables are often conceptualized as "correlates."

The third hallmark of epidemiology is the use of representative samples. If the function of an epidemiologic study is to determine the frequency of occurrence of an

From the Department of Psychiatry and Behavioral Science, State University of New York at Stony Brook, Stony Brook, NY (EJB); and the Shelvata Hospital, Tel Aviv, Israel (SF).

Address reprint requests to Evelyn Bromet, Department of Psychiatry and Behavioral Science, Putnam Hall-South Campus, Stony Brook, NY 11794-8790.

Received October 2, 1998; revised June 8, 1999; accepted June 14, 1999.

1999 Society of Biological Psychiatry

0006-3223/99/$20.00
PII S0006-3223(99)00153-5

87

illness (e.g., the incidence or prevalence rate), only the use of representative samples allows the establishment of accurate rates. Three methods have been employed for this purpose. One is the general population survey in which random samples of the population are administered a structured diagnostic interview (e.g., Kessler et al 1994). The second is the two-stage community survey, in which a large representative sample is screened, and a selected sample participates in a second, more extensive, assessment. For low frequency disorders, the two-stage study has the advantage of efficiently identifying potential cases for additional, and usually much more elaborate and expensive, investigation. The third approach is to identify representative samples through treatment settings. For rare disorders in which the majority of cases are known to treatment, such as schizophrenia (Link and Dohrenwend 1980; van Korf et al 1985), this strategy is often the most feasible. Psychiatric case registries have been used for this purpose. It should be noted, however, that treatment samples of prevalence cases over represent chronically ill patients or high utilizers of services, and under represent patients who, for whatever reason, do not stay in or return to treatment (Cohen and Cohen 1984).

This review covers both descriptive studies and longitudinal studies of illness course and uses findings from the Suffolk County Mental Health Project for illustration (Bromet et al 1996).

Descriptive Studies

Since the late 1970s following the introduction of modern nosological systems, several programs of research have attempted to estimate the prevalence and incidence of schizophrenia. The two most recent estimates, based on studies of representative community samples assessed by structured diagnostic interview in the United States and in Israel, put the lifetime and 6-month prevalence rates at 0.7% (Kendler et al 1996 and Levav et al 1993, respectively). In both studies, the diagnoses were based on clinician reinterview. In a recent case registry study, a similar prevalence rate was reported (lifetime prevalence of 5.23/1000 in Northern Italy; DeSalvia et al 1993). The fact that the recently reported rates are lower than the ~1% lifetime prevalence rate reported in many pre-DSM-III studies reflects both a narrowing of the criteria for diagnosing schizophrenia (with concomitant shifts in the frequencies of other affective and nonaffective psychosis diagnoses [Stoll et al 1993]) and differing ascertainment and assessment methods. Turning to incidence, the best data on schizophrenia come from the World Health Organization (WHO) Determinants of Outcome Study. The median annual incidence rate across the eight participating WHO sites was 0.22/1000 (Bromet et al 1995). After reviewing service contact data from several European countries, Jablensky (1986) placed the incidence of schizophrenia similarly at about 0.2/1000.

Schizophrenia is not randomly distributed in the population, and the search for correlates and risk factors has been ongoing since the classic analysis of Faris and Dunham (1939) on the social ecology of schizophrenia. Three groups of variables have been investigated: demographic characteristics (especially social class, age, gender, and marital status), innate predisposing or protective factors (season of birth, pregnancy and birth complications, rheumatoid arthritis, substance abuse, and family background), and environmental factors. These variables have been explored individually and in combination. number of thoughtful reviews of this body of work have appeared (cf. Eaton et al 1988). In this review, the variables are grouped into those for which the findings are regarded as confirmed and strong, those that have been confirmed and are potentially strong, and those for which the evidence is abundant but inconclusive.

Confirmed and Strong Factors

To date, two variables—family history of schizophrenia and social class—have been found in numerous studies be strongly associated with the onset of schizophrenia.

Family History

Schizophrenia aggregates strongly in families (Jones and Cannon 1998). Over the past two decades, there have been numerous reviews of the genetics of schizophrenia (Murray et al 1986). In their review of genetic studies Gottesman and Shields (1982) calculated the morbid risk in first-degree relatives was 5.6% in the parents of schizophrenics, 12.8% in the children of one schizophrenic parent, and 46.3% in the children of two schizophrenic parents. In dizygotic twins and siblings, the rate about 15%, and in monozygotic twins the rate is over 50% whether they were reared together or apart (Jones and Cannon 1998; Murray et al 1986). The overall heritability estimate for the liability to schizophrenia is 60% to 70 (Jones and Cannon 1998; Kendler 1988). Kendler (198 concluded that in family studies using blind diagnose control groups, personal interviews, and operationalize diagnostic criteria, the risk for schizophrenia in clo relatives of schizophrenics is 5 to 15 times greater than the general population. In the Roscommon Family Stud the risk for schizophrenia in relatives of patients who we directly interviewed was 6.5% (Kendler et al 1993). C special interest is the finding that the risk of schizophren in relatives of patients with other psychotic diagnoses w similar—6.7% for relatives of probands with schizoaffe tive disorder, 6.9% for schizotypal personality disorder, a 5.1% for other nonaffective psychoses. The exception w psychotic affective disorder, where the risk for schizophrenia first-degree relatives was considerably lower, 2.8%. The rate of schizophrenia in the relatives of patients with all diagnoses was significantly higher than the rate in control subjects.

The findings from genetic studies demonstrate the unequivocal importance of heritability. Although they have also been used to imply that 20% to 30% of the variance in the liability to schizophrenia is attributable to environmental or other nongenetic factors, the precise contribution of such variables cannot be ascertained from genetic studies.

Social Class

One of the most consistent epidemiologic findings is an inverse relationship between social class and schizophrenia (Dohrenwend and Dohrenwend 1969; Dohrenwend et al 1992). Eaton et al (1988) calculated that the difference in rates between the lowest and highest class is approximately 3 to 1. Two hypotheses have been suggested to explain this relationship. The first is that adverse environmental conditions precipitate the onset of schizophrenia (social causation). The second is that social selection or social drift explains the relationship. That is, individuals in premorbid, prodromal, or early illness stages fail to achieve their potential and suffer a decline in occupational performance relative to expectation. The second hypothesis has the greatest empirical support and is one of the cardinal features of schizophrenia—the failure ever to achieve one's potential or, once diagnosed, to return to one's best premorbid level of functioning. We have suggested that if schizophrenia is a heterogeneous disease (Bellack and Blanchard 1993), then both hypotheses may have merit in different subgroups of schizophrenic patients (Bromet et al 1995).

Confirmed, Potentially Strong Factors

Several risk factors have been extensively examined in relation to schizophrenia but to date they may be considered to be "potentially" strong either because the evidence is largely circumstantial, or their relative contribution in explaining the distribution of schizophrenia is small, or their etiologic significance is obscure.

Age and Gender

Recent findings indicate a male excess in first-episode schizophrenia (e.g., Murray and Van Os 1998), especially in populations with onset under age 35 years (Iacono and Beiser 1992; Jablensky 1986; Jones et al 1998). In the Suffolk County Mental Health cohort composed of first-admissions with psychosis from all of the inpatient facilities in the County hospitalized from 1989 to 1995, 65.2% (148/227) of people with a research diagnosis of DSM-IV schizophrenia or schizoaffective disorder were male, whereas the proportion of males among those with affective psychosis

was smaller, 49.6% (68/137) of those with bipolar disorder with psychotic features; and 40.7% (35/81) of those with major depressive disorder with psychotic features. It has been consistently reported that compared to women, males have a younger age of onset (Murray and Van Os 1998) and are younger at the time of their first hospital admission. This pattern may not be unique to schizophrenia. In the Suffolk County sample, the males in all three diagnostic groups were younger at the time of admission than the females (25, 23, and 27 years for males with schizophrenia/schizoaffective disorder, psychotic bipolar disorder, and psychotic depression, respectively; and 28, 29, and 33 years for the women in the three groups). Larsen et al (1996) also found, in a sample of 43 first-episode patients in Norway, that the duration of untreated psychosis was significantly longer in males than in females, with 61% of males having a duration longer than 1 year and 80% of females having a duration shorter than 1 year. In the Suffolk sample with schizophrenia, the opposite was true. That is, the length of time between the occurrence of the first psychotic symptom and first hospitalization was longer for women (median of 346 days) than men (median 189 days). Methodological and cross-cultural differences undoubtedly all play a role in explaining the different age and gender patterns across studies conducted in various settings.

Further examination of age and gender effects is important because differences in the timing of onset by age and/or gender might point to potential biologic clues about etiology. One variable, for example, that could contribute to the differences in age and gender patterns, at least in part, is a differential distribution of familial schizophrenia among the samples that have been studied. That is, some studies have shown that the gender difference in age of onset is not observed in familial schizophrenia but is more often found in "sporadic" cases (e.g., DeLisi et al 1994). Another hypothesis was tested by the Mannheim research program suggesting that an "elevated vulnerability threshold for women until menopause" could be due to "the sensitivity-reducing effect of estrogen on D_2 receptors in the central nervous system" (Häfner et al 1998).

While the excess of males and young people among treated cases is significant, the proportion of males versus females who develop schizophrenia is almost the same. For example, the 1-month prevalence rate of schizophrenia in the epidemiologic catchment area (ECA) was 0.6% for males and females, and 0.7% for 18 to 24 year olds of both sexes. The 1-year prevalence rate of nonaffective psychosis in the National Comorbidity Survey was 0.5% for males and 0.6% for females.

Rheumatoid Arthritis

Rheumatoid arthritis rarely occurs in patients with schizophrenia (Eaton et al 1992; Jablensky 1986). Eaton et al reviewed the 14 published studies on this topic. The median prevalence of rheumatoid arthritis was 0.047% in schizophrenia compared to 0.16% in people with other psychiatric diagnoses. In spite of the consistency of this association across the 14 studies, the methodologies were found to be wanting. Nevertheless, the authors emphasized that the potential association with autoimmune disease could open important avenues of research on immunopathology that "hold the key to understanding at least some part of the etiology of schizophrenia" (Eaton et al 1992, p. 189).

Season of Birth

The proportion of people with schizophrenia born during the winter months is about 5% to 15% higher than at other times of the year (Torrey et al 1993). Comparable seasonality has not been found for other psychiatric diagnoses, although it has been reported for Down's syndrome and certain cardiovascular diseases (Jablensky 1986). This differential has been found to be greater in females with schizophrenia (Pulver et al 1981) and in patients without a family history of schizophrenia (O'Callaghan et al 1991). Angst (1991), however, has argued that, statistical significance aside, the contribution of this variable to explaining the occurrence of schizophrenia is very weak. Moreover, season of birth may be a proxy for several underlying factors, such as viral infections, diet, or other variables affecting fetal development.

Obstetric, Birth, and Early Childhood Complications

Several complications of pregnancy have been studied as risk factors for schizophrenia, including preeclampsia, low maternal weight, rhesus incompatibility, small head circumference, and fetal distress. A meta-analysis of 18 studies reported an odds ratio of 2.0 (95% confidence interval 1.6 to 2.4) for schizophrenia following obstetric complications of all kinds, although the authors cautioned that both selection and publication bias could have inflated the association (Geddes and Lawrie 1995). Nevertheless, this odds ratio is impressive since these events are relatively common in the general population and may themselves be associated with risk factors such as low social class.

The three specific classes of variables with the most provocative findings to date are exposure to prenatal nutritional deprivation, prenatal brain injury, and prenatal influenza. The evidence regarding nutritional deprivation comes from case-control and cohort studies. For example, Kendell et al (1996) compared the obstetric records of 115 persons born in Scotland in 1971 through 1974 who were later hospitalized with schizophrenia, to control subjects matched on place and date of birth, gender, maternal age, maternal parity, parental social class, and twin status.

Significant differences were found for pregnancy complications in general, and for preeclampsia in particular. Susser and colleagues conducted an extremely compelling cohort study of nutritional deprivation occurring during the Dutch Hunger Winter of 1944 to 1945 (Susser and Lin 1992; Susser et al 1996). A twofold increase in the risk for schizophrenia was found in both male and female offspring of nutritionally deprived mothers compared to unexposed controls. Recent findings from more than 500,000 children in the Swedish National Birth Register born between 1973 and 1977 also support the increased risk for schizophrenia, particularly early onset schizophrenia, associated with malnutrition (Dalman et al 1999). The latter finding is consistent with the possibility that pre- or perinatal complications confer a somewhat younger age of onset (Verdoux et al 1997).

Children exposed in utero to a viral infection (Jones and Cannon 1998) have also been found to be at increased risk for developing schizophrenia. Most of the evidence on viral infection is circumstantial (inferences drawn from populations who were in utero during a flu epidemic compared to control subjects) rather than direct (fetal exposure to influenza confirmed by blood samples). Current research is underway to confirm and extend these findings in birth cohorts for which extensive tests were obtained in utero and during the early years of life.

Early childhood data also suggest that some individuals who go on to develop schizophrenia had evidence of prenatal brain damage or were impaired as children (Jones et al 1998; Kremen et al 1998). The most persuasive findings are from the 1946 British birth cohort showing that the 30 (out of 4746) children who went on to develop schizophrenia were more likely to have had delayed motor development, more speech problems, lower educational test scores in childhood, and a preference for solitary play (Jones and Cannon 1998).

While the predictive power of prenatal and birth complications is modest, and the findings across the literature have not been entirely consistent, the results have been generally viewed as providing support for the neurodevelopmental model of schizophrenia. Furthermore, from a public health standpoint, the significance of this general area of research rests not only with discovering clues about etiology but also for providing avenues for early identification that can lead to better prevention and intervention efforts (Jones et al 1998; McNeil 1995).

Possible Risk Factors

Several other variables have been studied as risk factors, but to date, the findings have been inconclusive. The most widely investigated factors include substance abuse, stress, and geographic location.

Substance Abuse

While substance use or abuse can provoke a psychotic episode in vulnerable individuals, the question of whether it can serve as a risk factor for schizophrenia or hasten its onset is unresolved. A risk factor does not have to "cause" an illness, but merely must elevate the risk of onset. The most compelling evidence that substances may play such a role comes from the 15-year follow-up of 45,570 Swedish army recruits (Andreasson et al 1987). This study showed that those consuming cannabis on more than 15 occasions were 6 times more likely to develop schizophrenia than less frequent users and nonusers. On the other hand, the opposite interpretation of the data is equally plausible— namely, that preschizophrenic individuals were likely to abuse cannabis. As Jones and Cannon (1998) argue, given the increase in consumption of cannabis over the past three decades, one would expect to see an increase in schizophrenia if cannabis played a causal role in the etiology of schizophrenia, and this has simply not occurred.

Stress

Earlier, we noted that environmental stress was seen as one possible explanation for the relationship between social class and schizophrenia. Two lines of research have addressed the role of stress as an etiologic factor in schizophrenia: maternal stress during pregnancy, and life events and familial strains, particularly excessive emotional response to patients. The most intriguing evidence on maternal stress comes from a recent study of mothers exposed to the bombing in the Netherlands during World War II, showing an increase in schizophrenia among children who were in utero during the first trimester (Van Os and Selten 1998). Similarly, Meijer (1985) suggested that the offspring of mothers exposed during pregnancy to the threat and occurrence of the 6-day Arab-Israeli war displayed developmental delays and behavioral deviance. The interpretation of this relationship is complicated, however, because stress is associated with both biologic changes (e.g., elevations in epinephrine and norepinephrine), changes in health behavior (increased smoking, alcohol, or other substance abuse, dietary changes), and/or preterm delivery.

The role of exogenous environmental events in increasing the risk of onset of various psychoses is rather limited and weak. One study found that stressors increased the risk for first-episode schizophreniform disorder but not schizophrenia (Chung et al 1986). We note that Dohrenwend et al (1992) concluded, from their classic study of the social determinants of mental illness in Israel, that social selection was more important than social causation (e.g., stress) in producing the social class effect in schizophrenia. Since the classic papers by Brown et al (1972) and Vaughn and Leff (1976), many studies have confirmed that people with schizophrenia who live in family settings characterized by high levels of "expressed emotion" (critical and over-protective behavior and verbalizations toward the family member with schizophrenia) have higher rates of relapse after discharge from the hospital (e.g., Falloon 1986). However, it should be emphasized that there is no evidence that this form of stress is associated with the onset of schizophrenia. Moreover, as Vaughn and Leff (1976) originally showed, this behavior pattern is also a predictor of relapse in other psychiatric disorders. A recent meta-analysis of the literature on expressed emotion confirmed the importance of expressed emotion as a predictor of outcome in schizophrenia and its association with outcome in mood and eating disorders (Butzlaff and Hooley 1998).

Geographic Location

The World Health Organization studies of schizophrenia found that the incidence of narrowly defined schizophrenia was similar in diverse populations around the world (Jablensky 1997). In contrast, research conducted in other locations suggested that certain geographic areas have unusually high rates. One line of research compared rates in urban versus rural locations. Although Dohrenwend and Dohrenwend (1974) cast doubt on the importance of this distinction, several studies conducted since their masterful review suggest that being raised in an urban environment is a risk factor for schizophrenia (David et al 1992; Takei et al 1992). Using data from a cohort of close to 50,000 Swedish conscripts, Lewis et al (1992) found that those raised in an urban area had a 1.65 times greater risk of schizophrenia than those raised in rural areas. Other studies focused on specific locations, such as areas of Ireland or Yugoslavia, where the rates of schizophrenia are higher than expected. Even if confirmed, these macro variables combine a host of differences in morbidity, comorbidity, service availability, selective migration, and social and physical environmental parameters, which limit their usefulness for generating hypotheses about the etiology of schizophrenia or other psychoses.

Studies of Illness Course

In addition to understanding the distribution of schizophrenia, another major function of epidemiologic research is to shed light on the natural history of the disorder. A large number of follow-up studies of patients with schizophrenia, other nonaffective psychoses, and affective psychoses have been conducted. Most of these studies are not designed as epidemiologic studies, and contain one or more of the following methodological features that detract from their epidemiologic value: consecutive admission rather than first-admission patients; samples drawn from single sites, usually academic facilities; volunteer samples; exclusion of patients with serious substance abuse histories; unclear method for formulating either a clinical or a research diagnosis; cross-sectional research diagnosis; low response rate; high attrition during follow-up; unsystematic timing of follow-up assessments; and reliance on inexpensive and less reliable follow-up procedures, such as telephone interviewing, to obtain even subtle measures like affective flattening. Thus, it is not surprising that the findings from longitudinal studies regarding the proportion who do well over time and the predictors of good adjustment have been inconsistent.

The most powerful design for studies aimed at understanding illness course is a longitudinal cohort study. The word cohort comes from the Latin *cohors*, or warriors, and this is perhaps an apt description of individuals who agree to become part of a longitudinal study. By definition, a cohort is a homogeneous group who share a common attribute, such as being born in a particular year or residing in a particular area, who are followed over time (Greenberg et al 1996). The most informative clinical cohorts are patients identified at the onset of their illness. In psychiatry, first-admission patients provide the most practical such sample, although first-episode patients represent the ideal for understanding remission and relapse over time. Of course, the optimal strategy is to identify groups before or during the prodromal stage, but this is not practical except for studies of high risk samples. However, high risk samples are not necessarily representative of all patients with a given disorder.

In 1992, we reviewed the follow-up literature focused on first-admission samples with schizophrenia (Ram et al 1992). We divided the studies into three groups: statistical reports from state hospitals, long-term follow-up studies (also referred to as follow-back studies), and prospective studies. The latter are distinguished from the statistical reports and follow-back studies by the use of research diagnoses formulated using structured diagnostic procedures. We concluded from the 13 prospective studies that over a 2-year period, about one-third of patients with schizophrenia had a benign course, while two-thirds either relapsed, failed to recover, or were readmitted to the hospital. In the Vancouver first-episode study, 40/72 psychotic patients were incapacitated at 18-month follow-up (Beiser et al 1988). Since 1992, several longer-term studies of first-admission or first-episode cohorts extended the follow-up to as long as 15 years. One study of 82 first-contact cases in the Netherlands found that only 12% had a single episode followed by complete remission and another 14.6% had two or more episodes also followed by complete remission. However, in the 13-year follow-up of a small cohort in Nottingham, 60.9% had an episodic (as opposed to a progressive downward) course

(Mason et al 1996). Thus, the results are not consistent with regard to the long-term outcome of schizophrenia.

The World Health Organization conducted one of the few epidemiologically based longitudinal studies of psychotic patients. One of the most widely cited findings was that patients in developing countries had a more benign course than patients in developed countries (Leff et al 1992). A recent reanalysis by Craig et al (1997) confirmed the original finding but also suggested that two developed centers (Prague and Nottingham) had outcome results at 2-year follow-up that were similar to developing countries.

Several of the variables associated with the occurrence of schizophrenia have also been studied as predictors of illness course, including age, gender, substance abuse, and family history of schizophrenia and of affective disorder. Many studies found evidence that younger patients, males, and those with a family history of schizophrenia do more poorly. In an especially compelling analysis of four case registers, Eaton et al (1992) showed that while age of onset was a significant predictor of rehospitalization, gender was not a consistent predictor when age of onset was included in the model. The evidence on substance abuse has been particularly inconsistent, with some studies finding that substance abuse predicts better outcome, others reporting that it predicts poorer outcome, and still others finding no association (Rabinowitz et al 1998).

Other prognostic variables that have been studied include premorbid intelligence, premorbid social competence, duration between onset of psychosis and receiving "adequate" neuroleptic treatment, severity of positive symptoms, severity of negative symptoms, and noncompliance with medication treatment (Westermeyer and Harrow 1988). Wyatt et al (1998) concluded that there was compelling evidence to indicate that delayed intervention leads to poorer long-term outcome. Nevertheless, among these variables, the strongest predictor of relapse in schizophrenia is noncompliance with medication after treatment has begun (Ayuso-Gutiérrez and Vega 1997).

At the time of the Ram et al (1992) review, there were few first-admission studies of patients with affective psychosis. There continues to be a remarkable dearth of follow-up studies of first-admission patients with psychotic affective disorder, and those that exist are primarily samples of people hospitalized in academic centers. Coryell et al (1990a, 1990b) published two parallel studies on psychotic depression and psychotic bipolar disorder, finding similar predictors of poorer outcome as was seen in schizophrenia, namely, poorer adolescent social functioning and longer duration of index episode. For bipolar disorder, both Coryell et al (1990b) and Tohen et al (1992) reported that the presence of mood-incongruent delusions predicted poorer outcome. More recently, Strakowski et al (1998) assessed the 12-month course of first-admission patients with affective psychosis and found that the sample had great difficulty recovering from their illness, and that delayed recovery was significantly predicted by low socioeconomic status, poor premorbid functioning, treatment noncompliance, and substance abuse.

The patterns of illness course in schizophrenia and other psychoses have rarely been compared directly (Vetter and Köller 1996). However, the available evidence indicates that people with schizophrenia have poorer short- and long-term outcomes than individuals with other psychosis diagnoses (Bromet et al 1996; Harrow et al 1997; Vetter and Köller 1996). On the other hand, while people with schizophrenia function more poorly over time than non-schizophrenic patients, the existing data do not support the notion of an inevitable progressive deterioration in schizophrenia or a generally positive outcome in affective disorder (Huber 1997).

Our NIMH-funded study of the course of illness in patients entering a treatment facility in Suffolk County, Long Island, provides data on illness course in a more representative sample than has been possible before in North America. Because of the unique epidemiologic nature of the study design, and the inclusion of people with other functional psychotic disorders, data on patterns of illness course from this study are presented to illustrate the differences in 2-year outcomes and its predictors for people with schizophrenia compared to people with other psychotic disorders.

The Suffolk County Mental Health Project

Overview and Design

The Suffolk County study was designed using epidemiologic methods to examine the natural history of psychotic illness. The objectives were to examine the stability of diagnosis and to identify the diagnosis-specific predictors of better and worse outcome in psychosis, particularly premorbid competence, illness severity, substance use, and suicidal behaviors. A cohort of 696 first-admission patients was recruited from all 12 inpatient facilities in Suffolk County, Long Island (population 1.3 million) using the following inclusion criteria: age 15 to 60 years, resident of Suffolk County, clinical evidence of psychosis, or a facility diagnosis indicating psychosis. Patients were excluded if their first lifetime psychiatric hospitalization occurred more than 6 months before the index admission, and if they were deemed noninterviewable because of significant mental retardation or failure to speak English. The recruitment took place between September 1989 and December 1995. The initial response rate was 72%, and more than 85% of the respondents were successfully followed over a 2-year period.

The interviewers were experienced master's level men-

tal health professionals, consistent with the use of a semi-structured diagnostic instrument that required clinical judgment to administer.

The study design was longitudinal, and respondents were reinterviewed every 3 months by telephone, and face-to-face at 6, 24, and 48 month follow-up, with a standard battery of diagnostic and psychosocial interview schedules and rating scales (Bromet et al 1992). Information was also routinely obtained from informants and medical records. Longitudinal consensus diagnoses, integrating information across time from all available sources, were formulated by project psychiatrists after the 6- and 24-month follow-ups using both DSM-III-R and DSM-IV criteria (Fennig et al 1994b). All together, 24-month longitudinal diagnoses were formulated for 614 of the original cohort. The three largest diagnostic groups, using the 24-month research diagnosis, were schizophrenia/schizoaffective disorder (37.0%; $n = 227$), bipolar disorder with psychotic features (22.3%; $n = 137$), and major depressive disorder with psychotic features (12.4%; $n = 86$).

Sociodemographic and Baseline Clinical Characteristics

As noted previously, there were significantly more males with schizophrenia (65.2%) compared to bipolar (49.6%) and major depressive disorder (40.7%; $p < .001$). The average age of respondents with schizophrenia and bipolar disorder was similar, but the major depression group was significantly older (54.7% aged 30+ compared to 37.9% and 36.5% in the schizophrenia and bipolar groups, respectively). The percent never married was highest for schizophrenia (77.8% vs. 60.8% of bipolars and 46.8% of the depressed). While the social class of origin of the three groups was not significantly different, relatively fewer people with bipolar disorder came from unskilled households (14.1% vs. 29.7% for schizophrenia and 22.0% for depression). Using the WHO system for classifying mode of onset, 78.3% of people with schizophrenia had an insidious onset, compared to 11.2% and 41.3% of those with bipolar and major depressive disorder, respectively ($p < .001$). Finally, the median number of days between the appearance of the first psychotic symptom and first lifetime hospitalization was 247.5 for respondents with schizophrenia (189 for males, 346 for females) compared to 10 for those with bipolar disorder (11 for males, 8 for females) and 46 for those with major depression (49 for males, 34 for females).

Other clinical differences were also apparent at the time of first hospitalization. The schizophrenia group evidenced more negative and positive psychotic symptoms on the Scale for the Assessment of Negative Symptoms and the

Table 1. Distribution of Consensus Ratings of 24-Month Course Using the WHO Schema in Respondents with Schizophrenia/Schizoaffective Disorder, Bipolar Disorder with Psychotic Features, and Major Depression with Psychotic Features: Suffolk County Mental Health Project

	Schizophrenia ($n = 209$) (%)	Bipolar psychosis ($n = 132$) (%)	Psychotic depressed ($n = 81$) (%)
Single episode/complete remission	3.8	33.3	32.1
Single episode/incomplete remission	12.4	2.3	8.6
Single episode + nonpsychotic episode/ complete remission	1.4	18.2	7.4
Single episode + nonpsychotic episode/ incomplete remission	1.0	5.3	7.4
2+ episodes/complete remission	8.1	28.8	21.0
2+ episodes/incomplete remission	33.0	8.3	11.1
Continually psychotic	40.2	0.8	3.7
Continually nonpsychotic	0	3.0	11.1

Scale for the Assessment of Positive Symptoms (Andreasen 1983, 1984), poorer premorbid adjustment (Cannon-Spoor et al 1982), and lower GAF scores for the best month of the year before the baseline interview. The depressed group had the highest scores on the anxiety/ depression factor of the Brief Psychiatric Rating Scale (BPRS; Woerner et al 1988) and the highest rate reporting a prior suicide attempt (45.3% vs. 24.3% of the schizophrenia and 15.3% of the bipolar groups). The bipolar group had the highest scores on the BPRS activation factor. The one area where the groups were not significantly different was meeting lifetime criteria for drug or alcohol abuse/dependence (47.3% overall).

Diagnostic Differences in Course and Outcome

We previously presented differences by diagnosis in the 6-month outcomes of a subset of the cohort, showing that people with schizophrenia were. functioning more poorly than the two affective disorder groups (Bromet et al 1996). This overall pattern was sustained at 24-month follow-up. Table 1 presents the 24-month course patterns for the groups using the WHO schema. The schizophrenia group had a very difficult time during the initial 24-month period, with 40.2% being continuously ill (categories 7 and 8) and a total of 46.4% achieving only partial remission (categories 2, 4, and 6). Indeed, only 13.3% achieved a period of complete remission during the 24-month follow-up (category 1). In contrast, one-third of the bipolar subjects had a single episode followed by full remission, and another 47.0% had 2+ psychotic or nonpsychotic episodes followed by complete remission (categories 3 and 5). While the depressed group was better off than those with schizophrenia, their functioning was fraught with more difficulties than was true for the bipolar group. We note that the evidence from the 4-year follow-ups completed to date indicates that while the bipolars

achieved remission more quickly, the depressed eventually caught up.

The Quality of Life Scale (Heinrichs et al 1984) was administered to assess psychosocial adjustment at the 6 and 24-month points, and five factors were derived evaluating social functioning, purpose/motivation, daily living activities, role functioning, and family/relative intimacy. At both 6- and 24-month follow-up, people with schizophrenia had the poorest and people with bipolar disorder had the best functioning across the five scales ($p < .00$ for each of the five at both times). The difference remained statistically significant at 24-month follow-up in analyses after adjusting for level of premorbid functioning between ages 12 to 15 years, the baseline GAF for the best month of the year before hospitalization, and the 6-month score on the same outcome variable. Comparisons between quality of life ratings at 6 and 24 months indicated no significant change in people with schizophrenia, and statistically significant improvements across time in the two affective disorder groups.

Finally, the GAF score for the worst week in the month before the 24-month interview was significantly worse ($p < .001$) for people with schizophrenia (mean standard deviation $= 39.1 \pm 11.9$) than for people with bipolar disorder (58.7 ± 14.8) or psychotic depression (54.9 ± 15.4).

Predictors of Post-Hospital Adjustment

Within each of the diagnostic groups, we used regression analysis to identify the significant baseline predictors of 24-month functioning. Logistic regression was used to identify significant predictors of ever achieving complete remission during the follow-up. Linear regression was used to predict the QLS Social and Role Functioning scores. These variables were chosen to represent aspects of both clinical and psychosocial status. The predictors were the WHO rating of mode of onset, premorbid adjustment at age 12 to 15 years, history of suicide attempt, history of substance use disorder, initial clinical presentation (baseline SANS, SAPS, BPRS anxiety/depression factor, gender, age at admission). Each analysis was done within diagnostic group, and each analysis included two steps. Step 1 included the baseline predictors. Step 2 added the number of months in treatment during the 24-month period.

For respondents with schizophrenia, the predictors accounted for 24.4% and 13.7% of the variance in the QLS Social and Role Functioning scales, respectively. The significant predictors of social functioning were an insidious mode of onset ($p = .003$), greater severity on the SAPS ($p = .003$), and receiving more months of treatment ($p < .05$). Insidious mode of onset and SAPS scores were the only significant predictors ($p < .05$) of role functioning. None of the variables was a significant predictor of whether complete remission was ever achieved, but this may have occurred because only 13% of people with schizophrenia had this outcome.

For respondents with bipolar disorder, the predictors accounted for 33.0% and 12.0% of the variance in the QLS Social and Role Functioning scales, respectively. The only significant predictor of social functioning was premorbid adjustment between ages 12 to 15 years ($p < .001$), and this variable was strongly related to the Social Functioning scale. None of the variables was significant in the equation for role functioning. History of suicide attempt was the only significant predictor of whether or not complete remission was achieved (odds ratio = 6.6; confidence interval 1.6 to 26.6; $p = .008$).

For respondents with psychotic depression, the predictors accounted for a similar percentage of the variance in social and role functioning, 36.3% and 39.2%, respectively. The significant predictors of social functioning were mode of onset ($p = .02$) and premorbid adjustment ($p = .015$), while the BPRS anxiety/depression factor was the sole significant predictor of role functioning ($p = .02$). Three predictors were significantly related to remission status, mode of onset ($p = .02$), premorbid functioning ($p = .02$), and lifetime substance use disorder ($p = .04$).

Thus, the baseline predictors of clinical and psychosocial status at 24-month follow-up varied by diagnosis. For people with schizophrenia, severity of psychosis was most important, while, not surprisingly, for people with an episode of psychotic depression at hospitalization, the BPRS anxiety/depression factor was important. Further analysis of the bipolar group focusing on other aspects of premorbid functioning, including substance use and antisocial behaviors, are being undertaken to explain the outcome patterns for this group.

Conclusion

There continues to be much interest in the epidemiology of psychotic illness in general and schizophrenia in particular. The ultimate goal of such research is to suggest strategies for primary and secondary prevention. This goal assumes that the risk factors associated with onset and the prognostic factors associated with illness course are modifiable. A number of prevention projects are described in a recent issue of the *British Journal of Psychiatry* (1998 supplement 33) involving preventive intervention strategies that identify and aggressively treat people at risk for developing psychosis. Thus, the search for modifiable risk factors is ongoing. Epidemiologic approaches encompassing descriptive and analytic research goals, and social and biologic variables, will continue to extend the value of these enterprises by suggesting ways to minimize sampling bias, maximize diagnostic reliability, and test a comprehensive array of risk factors. While in the past epidemiologic research has favored an empirical rather than a model-testing approach, more recent work is testing specific vulnerability models, thereby pushing the frontiers of epidemiology forward.

Supported in part by NIMH Grant No. 44801.

This work was presented at the conference, Schizophrenia: From Molecule to Public Policy, held in Santa Fe, New Mexico in October 1998. The conference was sponsored by the Society of Biological Psychiatry through an unrestricted educational grant provided by Eli Lilly and Company.

References

Allebeck P, Wistedt B (1986): Mortality in schizophrenia: A ten-year follow-up based on the Stockholm County Inpatient Register. *Arch Gen Psychiatry* 43:650–653.

Andreasen NC (1983): *The Scale for the Assessment of Negative Symptoms (SANS).* Iowa City: University of Iowa.

Andreasen NC (1984): *The Scale for the Assessment of Positive Symptoms (SAPS).* Iowa City: University of Iowa.

Andreasson S, Allebeck P, Engstrom A, Ryberg U (1987): Cannabis and schizophrenia: A longitudinal study of Swedish conscripts. *Lancet* 2:1483–1486.

Angst J (1991): Epidemiology of schizophrenia: Discussion. In: Häfner H, Gattaz WF, editors. *Search for the Causes of Schizophrenia.* Berlin: Springer-Verlag, pp 48–53.

Ayuso-Gutiérrez JL, Vega JMR (1997): Factors influencing relapse in the long-term course of schizophrenia. *Schizophr Res* 28:199–206.

Beiser M, Erickson D, Fleming J, Iacono W (1993): Establishing the onset of psychotic illness. *Am J Psychiatry* 150:1349–1354.

Beiser M, Jonathan AE, Fleming MB, Iacono WG, Lin T (1988): Refining the diagnosis of schizophreniform disorder. *Am J Psychiatry* 145:695–700.

Bellack A, Blanchard JJ (1993): Schizophrenia: Psychopathology. In: Bellack A, Hersen M, editors. *Psychopathology in Adulthood*. Boston: Allyn and Bacon, pp 216–333.

Bromet EJ, Dew MA, Eaton W (1995): Epidemiology of psychosis with special reference to schizophrenia. In: Tsuang M, Tohen M, Zahner G, editors. *Textbook in Psychiatric Epidemiology*. New York: Wiley-Liss, Inc, pp 283–300.

Bromet EJ, Jandorf L, Fennig S, et al (1996): The Suffolk County Mental health project: Demographic, pre-morbid and clinical correlates of 6 month outcome. *Psychol Med* 26:953–962.

Bromet E, Schwartz J, Fennig S, et al (1992): The epidemiology of psychosis: The Suffolk County Mental Health Project. *Schizophr Bull* 18:243–255.

Brown GW, Birley JLT, Wing JK (1972): Influence of family life on the course of schizophrenic disorders: A replication. *Br J Psychiatry* 121:241–258.

Brown S, Birtwistle J (1998): People with schizophrenia and their families. *Br J Psychiatry* 173:139–144.

Butzlaff RL, Hooley JM (1998): Expressed emotion and psychiatric relapse: A meta-analysis. *Arch Gen Psychiatry* 55:547–552.

Cannon-Spoor HE, Potkin SG, Wyatt RG (1982): Measurement of premorbid adjustment in chronic schizophrenia. *Schizophr Bull* 8:470–484.

Chung RK, Langeluddecke P, Tennant C (1986): Threatening life events in the onset of schizophrenia, schizophreniform psychosis and hypomania. *Br J Psychiatry* 148:680–685.

Cohen P, Cohen J (1984): The clinician's illusion. *Arch Gen Psychiatry* 41:1178–1182.

Coryell W, Keller M, Lavori P, Endicott J (1990a): Affective syndromes, psychotic features, and prognosis, I: Depression. *Arch Gen Psychiatry* 47:651–657.

Coryell W, Keller M, Lavori P, Endicott J (1990b): Affective syndromes, psychotic features, and prognosis, I: Mania. *Arch Gen Psychiatry* 47:658–662.

Craig TJ, Siegel C, Hopper K, Lin S, Sartorius N (1997): Outcome in schizophrenia and related disorders compared between developing and developed countries. *Br J Psychiatry* 176:229–233.

Dalman C, Allebeck P, Cullberg J, Grunewald C, Köster M. (1999): Obstetric complications and the risk of schizophrenia. *Arch Gen Psychiatry* 56:234–240.

David AS, Lewis GH, Allebeck P, Andreasson S (1992): Urban-rural differences in place of upbringing and later schizophrenia. *Schizophr Res* 6:101–107.

DeLisi LE, Bass N, Boccio A, Shields G, Morganti C, Vita A (1994): Age of onset in familial schizophrenia. *Arch Gen Psychiatry* 51:334–335.

DeSalvia D, Barbato A, Salvo P, Zadro F (1993): Prevalence and incidence of schizophrenic disorders in Portogruaro: An Italian case register study. *J Nerv Ment Dis* 181:275–282.

Dohrenwend BP, Dohrenwend BS (1969): *Social Status and Psychological Disorder: A Causal Inquiry*. New York: John Wiley & Sons.

Dohrenwend BP, Dohrenwend BS (1974): Psychiatric disorders in urban settings. In: Caplan G, editor. *American Handbook of Psychiatry*, 2nd edition, vol 2. New York: Basic Books, pp 424–447.

Dohrenwend BP, Levav I, Shrout PE, et al (1992): Socioeconomic status and psychiatric disorders: The causation-selection issue. *Science* 255:946–952.

Eagles JM, Whalley LJ (1985): Decline in the diagnosis of schizophrenia among first admissions to Scottish mental hospitals from 1969–1978. *Br J Psychiatry* 146:151–154.

Eaton WW, Day R, Kramer M (1988): The use of epidemiology for risk factor research in schizophrenia: An overview and methodologic critique. In: Tsuang MT, Simpson JC, editors. *Handbook of Schizophrenia, vol 3: Nosology, Epidemiology, and Genetics of Schizophrenia*. New York: Elsevier, pp 169–204.

Eaton WW, Hayward C, Ram R (1992): Schizophrenia and rheumatoid arthritis: A review. *Schizophr Res* 6:181–192.

Eaton WW, Mortensen PB, Herrman H, et al (1992): Long-term course of hospitalization for schizophrenia: Part 1. Risk for rehospitalization. *Schizophr Bull* 18:217–241.

Faris R, Dunham H (1939): *Mental Disorders in Urban Areas: An Ecological Study of Schizophrenia and Other Psychoses*. New York: Hafner.

Falloon IRH (1986): Family stress and schizophrenia. *Psychiatr Clin North Am* 9:165–182.

Fennig S, Craig TJ, Tanenberg-Karant M, Bromet EJ (1994a): Comparison of facility and research diagnoses in first-admission psychotic patients. *Am J Psychiatry* 151:1423–1429.

Fennig S, Kovasznay B, Rich C, et al (1994b): Six-month stability of psychiatric diagnosis in first admission patients with psychosis. *Am J Psychiatry* 151:1200–1208.

Geddes JR, Lawrie SM (1995): Obstetric complications and schizophrenia: A meta-analysis. *Br J Psychiatry* 167:786–793.

Gottesman I, Shields J (1982): *Schizophrenia: The Epigenetic Puzzle*. Cambridge: Cambridge University Press.

Greenberg RS, Daniels SR, Flanders WD, Eley JW, Boring JR (1996): *Medical Epidemiology*, 2nd ed. Norwalk, CT: Appleton & Lange.

Häfner H, an der Heiden W, Behrens S, et al (1998): Causes and consequences of the gender difference in age at onset of schizophrenia. *Schizophr Bull* 24:99–113.

Häfner H, Riecher-Rössler A, Hambrecht M, et al (1992): IRAOS: An instrument for the assessment of onset and early course of schizophrenia. *Schizophr Res* 6:209–233.

Harrow M, Sands JR, Silverstein ML, Goldberg JF (1997): Course and outcome for schizophrenia versus other psychotic patients: A longitudinal study. *Schizophr Bull* 23:287–303.

Heinrichs DW, Hanlon TE, Carpenter WT Jr (1984): The Quality of Life Scale: An instrument for rating the schizophrenic deficit syndrome. *Schizophr Bull* 10:388–398.

Huber G (1997): The heterogeneous course of schizophrenia. *Schizophr Res* 28:177–185.

Iacono W, Beiser M (1992): Where are the women in first-episode studies of schizophrenia? *Schizophr Bull* 18:471–480.

Jablensky A (1986): Epidemiology of schizophrenia: A European perspective. *Schizophr Bull* 12:52–73.

Jablensky A (1997): The 100-year epidemiology of schizophrenia. *Schizophr Res* 28:111–125.

Jones P, Cannon M (1998): The new epidemiology of schizophrenia. *Psychiatr Clin North Am* 21:1–25.

Jones PB, Rantakallio P, Hartikainen A-L, Isohanni M, Sipila P (1998): Schizophrenia as a long-term outcome of pregnancy, delivery, and perinatal complications: A 28-year follow-up of the 1966 North Finland general population birth cohort. *Am J Psychiatry* 155:355–364.

Kendler KS (1988): The genetics of schizophrenia. In: Tsuang MT, Simpson JC, editors. *Handbook of Schizophrenia, vol 3, Nosology, Epidemiology and Genetics.* Amsterdam: Elsevier Science Publishers BV, pp 437–462.

Kendell RE, Juszczak E, Cole SK (1996): Obstetric complications and schizophrenia: A case control study based on standardised obstetric records. *Br J Psychiatry* 168:556–561.

Kendler KS, Gallagher TJ, Abelson JM, Kessler RC (1996): Lifetime prevalence, demographic risk factors, and diagnostic validity of nonaffective psychosis as assessed in a U.S. community sample. *Arch Gen Psychiatry* 53:1022–1031.

Kendler KS, McGuire M, Gruenberg AM, O'Hare A, Spellman M, Walsh D (1993): The Roscommon Family Study: I. Methods, diagnosis of probands, and risk of schizophrenia in relatives. *Arch Gen Psychiatry* 50:527–539.

Kessler R, McGonagle K, Zhao S, et al (1994): Lifetime and 12-month prevalence of DSM-III-R psychiatric disorders in the United States. Results from the National Comorbidity survey. *Arch Gen Psychiatry* 51:8–19.

Kremen WS, Buka SL, Seidman LJ, Goldstein JM, Koren D, Tsuang MT (1998): IQ decline during childhood and adult psychotic symptoms in a community sample: A 19-year longitudinal study. *Am J Psychiatry* 155:672–677.

Larsen TK, McGlashan TH, Moe LC (1996): First-episode schizophrenia: I. Early course parameters. *Schizophr Bull* 22:241–256.

Leff J, Sartorius N, Jablensky A, Korten A, Ernberg G (1992): The International Pilot Study of Schizophrenia: Five-year follow-up findings. *Psychol Med* 22:131–145.

Levav L, Kohn R, Dohrenwend BP, et al (1993): An epidemiological study of mental disorders in a 10-year cohort of young adults in Israel. *Psychol Med* 23:691–707.

Lewis G, David A, Andreasson S, Allebeck P (1992): Schizophrenia and city life. *Lancet* 340:137–140.

Link B, Dohrenwend BP (1980): Formulation of hypotheses about the ratio of untreated to treated cases in the true prevalence studies of functional psychiatric disorders in adults in the United States. In: Dohrenwend BP, Dohrenwend BS, Gould MS, et al, editors. *Mental Illness in the United States: Epidemiological Estimates.* New York: Praeger, pp 133–149.

Mason P, Harrison G, Glazebrook C, Medley I, Croudace T (1996): The course of schizophrenia over 13 years. *Br J Psychiatry* 169:580–586.

McNeil TF (1995): Perinatal risk factors and schizophrenia: Selective review and methodological concerns. *Epidemiol Rev* 17:107–112.

Meijer A (1985): Child psychiatric sequelae of maternal war stress. *Acta Psychiatr Scand* 72:505–511.

Murray RM, Reveley A, McGuffin P (1986): Genetic vulnerability to schizophrenia. *T Psychiatr Clin North Am* 9:3–16.

Murray RM, Van Os J (1998): Predictors of outcome in schizophrenia. *J Clin Psychopharmacol* 18:2S–4S.

O'Callaghan E, Gibson T, Colohan H, et al (1991): Season of birth in schizophrenia: Evidence for confinement of an excess of winter births to patients without a family history of mental disorder. *Br J Psychiatry* 158:764–769.

Pulver A, Sawyer JW, Childs B (1981): The association between season of birth and the risk of schizophrenia. *Am J Epidemiol* 114:735–749.

Rabinowitz J, Bromet EJ, Lavelle J, Carlson G, Kovasznay B, Schwartz JE (1998): Prevalence and severity of substance use disorders and onset of psychosis. *Psychol Med* 28:1411–1419.

Ram R, Bromet E, Eaton W, Pato C, Schwartz J (1992): The natural course of schizophrenia: A review of first-admission studies. *Schizophr Bull* 18:185–207.

Stoll AL, Tohen M, Baldessarini RJ, et al (1993): Shifts in diagnostic frequencies of schizophrenia and major affective disorders at six North American psychiatric hospitals, 1972–1988. *Am J Psychiatry* 150:1668–1673.

Strakowski SM, Keck PE, McElroy SL, et al (1998): Twelve-month outcome after a first hospitalization for affective psychosis. *Arch Gen Psychiatry* 55:49–55.

Susser E, Lin S (1992): Schizophrenia after prenatal exposure to the Dutch hunger winter of 1944–1945. *Arch Gen Psychiatry* 49:983–988.

Susser E, Neugebauer R, Hoek HW, et al (1996): Schizophrenia after prenatal famine: Further evidence. *Arch Gen Psychiatry* 53:25–31.

Takei N, O'Callaghan E, Sham P, Glover G, Murray RM (1992): Winter birth excess in schizophrenia: Its relationship to place of birth. *Schizophr Res* 6:102–108.

Tohen M, Tsuang M, Goodwin D (1992): Prediction of outcome in mania by mood-congruent or mood-incongruent psychotic features. *Am J Psychiatry* 149:1580–1584.

Torrey EF, Bowler AE, Rawlings R, Terrazas A (1993): Seasonability of schizophrenia and stillbirths. *Schizophr Bull* 19: 557–562.

Van Korf M, Nestadt G, Romanoski A, et al (1985): Prevalence of treated and untreated DSM-III community survey. *J Nerv Ment Dis* 173:577–580.

Van Os J, Selten J-P (1998): Prenatal exposure to maternal stress and subsequent schizophrenia. *Br J Psychiatry* 172:324–326.

Vaughn CE, Leff JP (1976): The influence of family and social factors on the course of psychiatric illness: A comparison of schizophrenic and depressed neurotic patients. *Br J Psychiatry* 129:125–137.

Verdoux H, Geddes JR, Takei N, et al (1997): Obstetric complications and age of onset in schizophrenia: An international collaborative meta-analysis of individual patient data. *Am J Psychiatry* 154:1220–1227.

Vetter P, Köller O (1996): Clinical and psychosocial variables in different diagnostic groups: Their interrelationships and value as predictors of course and outcome during a 14-year follow-up. *Psychopathology* 29:159–168.

Westermeyer JF, Harrow M (1988): Course and outcome in schizophrenia. In: Tsuang MT, Simpson JC, editors. *Handbook of Schizophrenia, vol 3, Nosology, Epidemiology and Genetics.* Amsterdam: Elsevier Science Publishers BV, pp 205–244.

Woerner M, Manuzza S, Kane J (1988): Anchoring the BPRS: an aid to improved reliability. *Psychopharmacol Bull* 24:112–124.

Wyatt RJ, Damiani M, Henter I (1998): First-episode schizophrenia: Early intervention and medication discontinuation in the context of course and treatment. *Br J Psychiatry* 72 (suppl 33):77–83.

Stability and Course of Neuropsychological Deficits in Schizophrenia

Robert K. Heaton, PhD; Julie Akiko Gladsjo, PhD; Barton W. Palmer, PhD; Julia Kuck, PhD;
Thomas D. Marcotte, PhD; Dilip V. Jeste, MD

Background: Neuropsychological deficits in schizophrenia appear to predate clinical symptoms of the disease and become more pronounced at illness onset, but controversy exists about whether and when further neuropsychological progression may occur.

Objective: To identify and characterize any subset of patients who evidenced progressive neuropsychological impairment, we compared the longitudinal stability of neuropsychological functioning in schizophrenic outpatients and normal comparison subjects.

Methods: One hundred forty-two schizophrenic outpatients and 206 normal comparison subjects were given annually scheduled comprehensive neuropsychological evaluations during an average of 3 years (range, 6 months to 10 years). Clinically and demographically defined subgroups were compared, and test-retest norms were used to identify individual patients who showed unusual worsening over time.

Results: The schizophrenic group was neuropsychologically more impaired than the normal comparison subjects but showed comparable test-retest reliability and comparable neuropsychological stability over both short (mean, 1.6 years) and long (mean, 5 years) follow-up periods. No significant differences in neuropsychological change were found between schizophrenic subgroups defined by current age, age at onset of illness, baseline level of neuropsychological impairment, and worsening of clinical symptoms, and occurrence of incident tardive dyskinesia. Norms for change also failed to show neuropsychological progression in individuals with schizophrenia.

Conclusions: Neuropsychological impairment in ambulatory persons with schizophrenia appears to remain stable, regardless of baseline characteristics and changes in clinical state. Our results may not be generalizable to the minority of institutionalized poor-outcome patients.

Arch Gen Psychiatry. 2001;58:24-32

T HERE IS a high prevalence of neuropsychological impairment in persons with schizophrenia, ranging from mild deficits to frank dementia.[1-5] Consistent with a neurodevelopmental view, some such deficits appear to predate clinical symptoms and exacerbate with typical illness onset during late adolescence or early adulthood.[6-8]

There remains considerable controversy about whether there is further progression of neuropsychological deficits after the onset of the illness.[9] With a few notable exceptions,[10-12] cross-sectional studies generally have not found evidence of increased neuropsychological deficits in association with duration of illness or (relative to age-matched controls) in older than in younger patients with schizophrenia.[2,13-17] Definitive answers to questions regarding possible progression of neuropsychological deficits in schizophrenia must come from longitudinal studies. The available studies, however, provide conflicting results and have a variety of methodologic limitations (eg, small or nonrepresentative samples, controls, brief follow-ups, and/or limited neuropsychological testing).[2,18-36]

Both neurodevelopmental and neurodegenerative views of neuropsychological deficits in schizophrenia seemingly remain viable.[10] While progression of deficit after illness onset clearly is not universal, or even typical of the disorder, a subset of persons with schizophrenia may evidence cognitive deterioration over time. The size and nature of that subgroup are unclear, but the existing studies suggest that potentially relevant issues include subject age, duration of illness, level of initial neuropsychological impairment, improvement or deteriora-

From the Department of Psychiatry, University of California, San Diego (Drs Heaton, Gladsjo, Palmer, Kuck, Marcotte, and Jeste, and the Veterans Affairs San Diego Healthcare System, San Diego, Calif (Dr Jeste).

98

SUBJECTS AND METHODS

SUBJECTS

Subjects included 142 outpatients with schizophrenia and 206 NCs, who had completed at least 2 comprehensive neuropsychological evaluations. Each patient and NC was a participant in 1 of 3 university-based clinical research centers, and most have contributed baseline neuropsychological data to previously published reports.[37-40] Diagnostic procedures for subjects in both groups included the Structured Clinical Interview for the DSM-III-R or DSM-IV.[41,42] Subjects were also screened by a physician using a physical examination and a structured medical history questionnaire; those with current or past medical conditions likely to affect central nervous system functioning (such as significant head injuries, seizure disorder, or acute medical conditions), as well as those meeting DSM-III-R[43] or DSM-IV[44] criteria for current alcohol or substance abuse or dependence, were excluded. All subjects provided written informed consent before participation in the research.

NEUROPSYCHOLOGICAL EXAMINATIONS

The patients and NCs were assessed with an annually scheduled comprehensive neuropsychological test battery (in actuality, the mean test-retest interval between the first 2 of these evaluations was 16.6 months [SD, 8.6 months; range, 6-81 months]). Eighty-nine schizophrenic patients and 119 NCs completed at least 1 additional neuropsychological follow-up evaluation. The total number of evaluations ranged from 2 to 10 (mean, 3.38; SD, 1.57; median, 3.00). The interval between the first and last neuropsychological evaluations ranged from 6 to 125 months and was not significantly different for the schizophrenic patients vs NCs (mean and SD, 37.0 and 22.3 months vs 37.1 and 25.7 months, respectively; $t_{346}=0.05$, $P=.96$).

Except where otherwise indicated, each of the neuropsychological measures was part of the expanded Halstead-Reitan battery, and details of administration and scoring were as described by Reitan and Wolfson[45] and Heaton and colleagues.[46,47] The individual measures were grouped into 7 ability areas based on the neuropsychological constructs that they are putatively designed to measure. The verbal ability area included the Aphasia Screening Test, Boston Naming Test, and the Controlled Oral Word Association Test.[48,49] Scores on the latter test were unavailable for a few subjects, so the Thurstone (written) Word Fluency task was substituted for 2 subjects at the baseline evaluation and

5 subjects at the first follow-up. The psychomotor ability area included the block design, object assembly, and digit symbol subtests from the Wechsler Adult Intelligence Scale–Revised (WAIS-R)[50] and the Trail Making Test Part A (total time), Tactual Performance Test (total time), and Digit Vigilance Test (time). The abstraction and cognitive flexibility ability area included the Category Test (errors), Trail Making Test Part B (total time), and Wisconsin Card Sorting Test[51] (perseverative responses). The attention ability area included the digit span and arithmetic subtests from the WAIS-R,[50] the Rhythm Test, Speech Sounds Perception Test, and Digit Vigilance (errors). The learning and delayed recall ability areas included those scores from the Figure and Story Memory Tests, and the California Verbal Learning Test.[52] The motor skills ability area included the right- and left-hand scores on Finger Tapping, Grooved Pegboard, and Hand Dynamometer.

We also had data from baseline and at least 1 retest evaluation with an even more comprehensive neuropsychological evaluation on a subsample of patients and NCs, permitting calculation of the WAIS-R Verbal, Performance, and Full-Scale IQs[50] for 81 patients and 86 NCs, and the Halstead-Reitan battery Average Impairment Rating[53] for 74 patients and 82 NCs.

Neuropsychological test raw scores were converted to standardized scaled scores (mean and SD, 10 and 3, respectively, in normal subjects) and age-, education-, and sex-corrected T-scores (mean and SD, 50 and 10, respectively, in normal subjects), by means of previously published normative data.[46-48,51,54] We then calculated the mean scaled scores and T-scores within each ability area, and a composite global scaled score and T-score.

PSYCHIATRIC AND MOTOR SYMPTOM RATINGS

Longitudinal ratings of psychiatric symptoms were also obtained for a subset (n=116) of the schizophrenic patients, as well as a smaller subset of NCs (n=86 to 88). Psychiatric symptom rating scales included the Brief Psychiatric Rating Scale[55] and the Scales for the Assessment of Positive and Negative Symptoms (SAPS and SANS, respectively).[56] Tardive dyskinesia was assessed with the Abnormal Involuntary Movement Scale.[57]

STATISTICAL METHODS AND ANALYSES

The test-retest reliability of neuropsychological measures and symptom rating scales was assessed in terms of

Continued on next page

---

tion in clinical status, and emergence of neuroleptic-induced dyskinesia.[2,29-31]

The current study addressed these issues by longitudinally observing sizable samples of ambulatory schizophrenic patients and normal comparison subjects (NCs) with a comprehensive battery of neuropsychological tests. These groups were compared with respect to test-retest correlations and neuropsychological stability over shorter vs longer follow-up periods. Also compared were schizophrenic subgroups defined on the basis of demographic and clinical variables, as well as initial level of neuropsychological functioning. Finally, data from NCs were

used to define normal test-retest variability; these definitions were then applied to the results of the schizophrenic subjects, in an attempt to identify and characterize any subgroup of individuals who demonstrated unusual decreases in neuropsychological functioning over time.

RESULTS

BASELINE CHARACTERISTICS

As shown in **Table 1**, there were small but statistically significant group differences in age, education, and test-

McGraw and Wong's[58] intraclass correlation coefficients for degree of consistency between measurements at the baseline and 1-year follow-up evaluations. The magnitudes of the intraclass correlation coefficients for the neuropsychological and symptom rating scale scores of patients and NCs were compared by means of Fisher r-to-z transformations for intraclass correlation coefficients.[58] The neuropsychological scaled scores, rather than T-scores, were used for these analyses, since the latter would underestimate the stability of neuropsychological performance by removing variance related to the stable traits of education and sex.

To examine the effects of length of follow-up on neuropsychological stability, patients and NCs were divided into diagnosis–by–length of follow-up groups, wherein "short" follow-up was defined as less than 36 months and "long" follow-up was defined as 36 months or longer. This yielded 121 NCs and 75 schizophrenic patients with short follow-up (mean, 19.5 months; SD, 6.8 months) and 85 NCs and 67 schizophrenic patients with long follow-up (mean, 59.7 months; SD, 19.6 months).

In addition to the primary subject groupings described above, we were interested in examining the possible influence of substantial differences in current age, age at onset of illness, duration of illness, and symptom changes on the stability of neuropsychological performance among the schizophrenic patients. Hence, we conducted a series of analyses in which we dichotomized the schizophrenic patients in terms of these characteristics. The definition of the symptom change groups and the resulting samples are described later. The other groupings included 22 elderly patients (age at study entry, ≥65 years; mean, 69.2 years; SD, 3.3 years) vs 120 younger patients (age at study entry, <65 years; mean, 43.7 years; SD, 13.7 years); 24 patients with late-onset schizophrenia (aged ≥45 years at onset of prodromal symptoms; mean, 55.0 years; SD, 5.6 years) vs 118 with earlier onset (onset at age <45 years; mean, 22.7 years; SD, 7.3 years); and 30 patients with a duration of illness less than 5 years (mean, 2.0 years; SD, 1.4 years) vs 105 subjects with a duration of illness of 5 years or more (mean, 23.6 years; SD, 12.5 years). We also dichotomized patients in terms of sex and initial level of neuropsychological functioning (low [global neuropsychological T-score, ≤39] vs high [global neuropsychological T-score, >45]) and anticholinergic use (receiving vs not receiving anticholinergic medication).

Repeated-measures analysis of variance (ANOVA) was used to examine effects of diagnosis (schizophrenic patients vs NCs) and length of follow-up (as noted above,

short vs long) on changes in neuropsychological performance. These analyses were conducted on T-scores (to correct for changes attributable to the effects of normal aging during long-term follow-up) for the entire neuropsychological battery (global neuropsychological T-score) as well as for each of the specific neuropsychological ability areas. We also used repeated-measures ANOVA to examine the various pairs of schizophrenic subgroups on changes in global neuropsychological performance and the 7 ability domains.

To assess the relationship between clinical change and neuropsychological functioning, patients were categorized into 3 groups based on change in clinical symptom scores from baseline to follow-up. Patients whose clinical symptom score (either SAPS or SANS total score) fell in the lower 25% of the distribution were considered to have a "low" level of symptoms, those in the middle 50% were labeled "middle," and those in the upper 25% of the distribution were categorized as "high." To meet criteria for a clinically significant change in symptoms, a subject had to move at least 1 category from baseline to follow-up, and by at least 3 points. Separate analyses were conducted for the SAPS- and SANS-defined change groups.

We also examined significant decreases in global neuropsychological T-scores of individual subjects, by means of the reliable change index method with adjustments for practice effect.[59,60] This approach involves constructing prediction intervals around each subject's expected follow-up score. The predicted follow-up score is the subject's baseline score, adjusted for practice effects among cognitively stable individuals (as determined from the mean change observed among the NCs). The boundary values of the prediction interval around the predicted follow-up score are determined by the normal variability of baseline to follow-up changes (SE of the difference) determined from the NC group. Specifically, 90% prediction intervals were built around these predicted follow-up scores by multiplying the SD of the difference among NCs by 1.64. Subjects whose observed follow-up scores were below the lower limits of the 90% prediction interval (ie, the bottom 5% of normal controls) were considered to have shown significant declines in neuropsychological functioning. These procedures were conducted twice: once to evaluate changes from baseline to first retest among all patients and NCs, and then again in terms of changes from the first to last neuropsychological assessment among subjects with long follow-ups.

Two-tailed tests were used for all analyses. To help avoid type I errors associated with multiple comparisons, significance was defined as $P<.01$.

retest interval. There were no significant differences in sex or ethnicity. As expected, the patients had substantially greater global neuropsychological impairment and more severe clinical symptoms than the NCs.

There were some differences between subjects with and without WAIS-R IQ scores and Average Impairment Rating scores, which primarily reflected different demographic recruiting emphases and slight differences in neuropsychological protocols among the 3 research centers from which the present sample was drawn. Schizophrenic patients who had WAIS-R IQ scores were different from those without only in age

(mean, 41.4 years [SD, 16.6 years] vs 55.9 years [SD, 9.5 years], respectively; $t_{131.65}=6.55$; $P<.001$). Relative to NCs without WAIS-R IQ scores, those with WAIS-R IQ scores were younger (mean age, 45.4 years [SD, 16.8 years] vs 56.2 years [SD, 21.1 years], respectively; $t_{201.65}=4.09$; $P<.001$); completed slightly more education (mean education, 14.8 years [SD, 2.4 years] vs 13.7 years [SD, 2.9 years], respectively; $t_{200.73}=3.12$; $P=.002$); had higher baseline neuropsychological performance (mean global neuropsychological T-score, 50.8 [SD, 4.0] vs 48.6 [SD, 4.9], respectively; $t_{204}=3.46$, $P=.001$); and were more likely to be male

Table 1. Baseline Characteristics of Normal Comparison Subjects and Patients With Schizophrenia*

	Normal Comparison Subjects (n = 206)	Patients With Schizophrenia (n = 142)	t or χ^2	df	P
Age, y	51.7 (20.1)	47.6 (15.7)	2.12	340.63	.04
Education, y	14.2 (2.8)	12.8 (2.3)	4.85	332.70	<.001
Sex, % M	64.1	69.7	1.20	1	.23
Ethnicity, % white	81.6	79.6	0.21	1	.65
Retest interval, mo	15.6 (5.3)	18.1 (11.7)	2.35	181.10	.02
Total No. of neuropsychological evaluations	3.4 (1.7)	3.3 (1.4)	1.04	338.09	.30
Global neuropsychological T-score	49.5 (4.7)	41.9 (6.5)	12.00	239.57	<.001
BPRS	22.2 (3.7)	33.8 (10.2)	12.13	180.75	<.001
SAPS	1.0 (1.4)	5.8 (3.8)	13.45	181.56	<.001
SANS	1.3 (1.7)	8.6 (5.1)	15.37	171.78	<.001
Age at onset of schizophrenia, y	NA	28.2 (14.0)	NA	NA	NA
Duration of illness	NA	18.8 (14.3)	NA	NA	NA
Paranoid subtype, %	NA	45.8	NA	NA	NA
Median CPZE, mg	NA	313 (n = 101)	NA	NA	NA
Median BZE, mg	NA	4 (n = 49)	NA	NA	NA

*Values represent means (with SD) or proportions for all variables other than medication dosages; these are presented as medians for the subgroups taking the respective types of medication. Significance of differences was assessed with independent t tests for variables involving means and with Pearson χ^2 for those involving proportions. The mean daily dose of antipsychotic medication was 993.1 (SD, 1742.3; range, 29.0-12 250.0) mg CPZE. The mean daily anticholinergic dose was 9.4 (SD, 28.1; range, 0.5-200.0) mg BZE. Twenty-five patients were taking an atypical antipsychotic medication at some point in their participation in this longitudinal study (11 risperidone, 9 clozapine, 2 olanzapine, and 3 ramoxipride). Repeated-measures analysis of variance showed no significant differences in the stability of neuropsychological performance between these patients and the other patients. BPRS indicates Brief Psychiatric Rating Scale; SAPS and SANS, Scales for the Assessment of Positive and Negative Symptoms, respectively; CPZE, daily chlorpromazine equivalent[61]; BZE, daily benztropine equivalent[62]; and NA, not applicable.

(76.7% vs 55.0%; $\chi^2_{1,N=206}$= 10.29; P=.002) and white (94.2% vs 72.5%; $\chi^2_{1,N=206}$= 15.66; P<.001). There were no significant differences between the 2 subgroups of NCs in the interval between the baseline to first-retest neuropsychological evaluation. More important, the same patterns of neuropsychological test-retest change were present for schizophrenic patients and NCs with vs without the Halstead-Reitan battery Average Impairment Rating score.

One concern about participant attrition in a longitudinal study is that nonrandom factors may influence who remains in the study, resulting in nonrepresentative (biased) samples. We used Mann-Whitney tests to compare the baseline characteristics of subjects who completed at least 1 follow-up evaluation with patients who dropped out after completing the baseline assessment. Demographic characteristics (except for age), baseline clinical symptoms and cognitive performance (including IQ), and global neuropsychological functioning did not differ between the groups. Patients who dropped out were, however, older than those with follow-up visits (mean ages, 57 and 48 years, respectively; Mann-Whitney P<.001).

TEST-RETEST RELIABILITY

The test-retest reliability coefficients (intraclass correlation coefficients) of neuropsychological and psychiatric rating scale scores for NCs and patients were highly significant within each group (**Table 2**). With the exception of Performance IQ (where the test-retest reliability was higher in the schizophrenic group), the magnitudes of the test-retest correlations for the patients were not significantly different from those observed among the NCs.

MAGNITUDE OF PRACTICE EFFECTS: BASELINE TO FIRST AND LAST REPEATED ASSESSMENT

There were no significant differences between schizophrenic patients and NCs with respect to practice effects (T-score at first follow-up visit minus T-score at baseline visit) for the WAIS-R IQs, neuropsychological summary scores, or neuropsychological ability area scores (**Table 3**).

The **Figure** depicts the changes in global neuropsychological T-scores from baseline to last follow-up, for subgroups with short vs long follow-up periods. Regardless of length of follow-up, the test-retest changes for schizophrenic patients and NCs were essentially parallel lines. Repeated-measures ANOVAs confirmed this finding, not only for the global neuropsychological score but also for all neuropsychological ability areas. There were highly significant group effects (P<.001), and sometimes significant time effects (reflecting modest improvement because of practice), but no significant diagnostic group×time interactions.

ADDITIONAL SCHIZOPHRENIC SUBGROUP COMPARISONS

To further examine the change in cognitive functioning over time, we compared longitudinal global neuropsychological performance changes in subgroups of schizophrenic subjects defined on the bases of demographic and clinical variables (as listed and defined above). These ANOVAs disclosed no significant group effects. As shown in **Table 4**, with 1 exception there also were no significant group × time interactions, indicating that the characteristics defining the various groups were not related

101

Table 2. Test-Retest Reliability of Neuropsychological and Psychiatric Symptom Rating Scale Scores for Normal Comparison Subjects vs Patients With Schizophrenia*

	Normal Comparison Subjects, ICC (C,1)	Patients With Schizophrenia, ICC (C,1)	z	P
Summary scores				
Global neuropsychological scaled score	0.94 (n = 206)	0.93 (n = 141)	0.52	.61
Average impairment rating raw score	0.88 (n = 82)	0.86 (n = 74)	0.42	.67
WAIS-R				
Verbal IQ	0.86 (n = 86)	0.91 (n = 81)	1.31	.19
Performance IQ	0.72 (n = 86)	0.88 (n = 81)	2.97	.003
Full-Scale IQ	0.85 (n = 86)	0.92 (n = 81)	2.19	.03
Specific neuropsychological ability area scaled scores				
Verbal	0.82 (n = 183)	0.86 (n = 139)	1.33	.18
Psychomotor	0.92 (n = 167)	0.88 (n = 139)	2.14	.03
Abstraction/cognitive-flexibility	0.86 (n = 201)	0.81 (n = 135)	1.22	.22
Attention	0.80 (n = 184)	0.81 (n = 133)	0.41	.68
Learning	0.83 (n = 204)	0.81 (n = 140)	0.64	.52
Delayed recall	0.63 (n = 206)	0.72 (n = 140)	1.45	.15
Motor	0.80 (n = 199)	0.85 (n = 133)	1.57	.12
Psychiatric symptom scales				
BPRS	0.48 (n = 88)	0.45 (n = 116)	0.27	.79
SAPS	0.42 (n = 86)	0.57 (n = 116)	1.37	.17
SANS	0.52 (n = 87)	0.56 (n = 116)	0.41	.68

*Test-retest reliability values are intraclass correlation coefficients for degree of consistency between measurements (ICC [C,1]).[58] The z and P values reflect the comparison of ICC magnitude among normal comparison subjects vs patients with schizophrenia. WAIS-R indicates Wechsler Adult Intelligence Scale-Revised; BPRS, Brief Psychiatric Rating Scale; and SAPS and SANS, Scales for the Assessment of Positive and Negative Symptoms, respectively.

Table 3. Change in Neuropsychological T-Scores (First Retest Minus Baseline T-Score) for Normal Comparison Subjects vs Patients With Schizophrenia*

	Normal Comparison Subjects	Patients With Schizophrenia	t	df	P
Summary score changes					
Global neuropsychological T-score	1.3 (2.4) (n = 206)	1.6 (3.2) (n = 142)	1.30	251.84	.20
Average impairment rating T-score	1.6 (9.2) (n = 82)	3.9 (7.9) (n = 74)	0.94	154.00	.35
WAIS-R					
Verbal IQ T-score	0.9 (4.8) (n = 86)	1.3 (5.6) (n = 81)	0.44	165.00	.66
Performance IQ T-score	3.3 (6.9) (n = 86)	1.9 (5.7) (n = 81)	1.46	165.00	.15
Full-Scale IQ T-score	2.2 (5.1) (n = 86)	1.6 (4.8) (n = 81)	0.73	165.00	.47
Neuropsychological ability area T-score changes					
Verbal	1.5 (5.6) (n = 183)	0.9 (5.4) (n = 140)	0.99	321.00	.32
Psychomotor	1.2 (4.3) (n = 167)	1.6 (4.7) (n = 140)	0.87	305.00	.38
Abstraction/cognitive-flexibility	3.0 (7.3) (n = 201)	4.5 (7.3) (n = 136)	1.87	335.00	.06
Attention	0.7 (4.6) (n = 184)	1.1 (5.0) (n = 134)	0.69	316.00	.49
Learning	1.4 (5.9) (n = 205)	2.8 (6.9) (n = 141)	1.94	269.47	.05
Delayed recall	1.5 (6.7) (n = 206)	1.7 (7.4) (n = 140)	0.23	344.00	.82
Motor	1.0 (5.0) (n = 199)	0.6 (5.7) (n = 135)	0.78	332.00	.44

*Values reflect the mean (and SD) of the difference scores between each subject's score at the first follow-up assessment, and that at baseline. Therefore, positive values reflect improved test performance. WAIS-R indicates Wechsler Adult Intelligence Scale-Revised.

to changes in neuropsychological performance over time. The 1 significant interaction reflected the fact that the schizophrenic subgroup with short duration of illness (mean, 2 years at baseline) had a slightly larger neuropsychological improvement than the subgroup with long duration (mean, 24 years at baseline). The smaller "improvement" (practice effect) shown by the long-duration group was the same as that of the NCs (both means, 1.3 T-score points).

Using the SAPS to categorize clinical change status resulted in 11 patients being classified as worse, 27 as better, and 78 as stable. With the use of repeated-measures ANOVAs, no significant group × time interactions were found for the neuropsychological global score or for scores on any of the 7 ability areas (Table 4). Categorization of schizophrenic patients on the basis of SANS scores yielded 19 subjects identified as significantly worse, 80 subjects as stable, and 17 subjects as better. The results of repeated-measures ANOVAs for the neuropsychological global score were similar to those with the SAPS change groups, ie, no significant group × time interactions.

We also compared patients with initial high vs low global neuropsychological performance (global neuropsychological T-score ≥45 vs ≤39, respectively), and those with vs without tardive dyskinesia as defined by the Schooler and Kane criteria[63] and those used by Wad-

102

dington.[64] Again, the groups did not differ significantly with respect to the change in the global neuropsychological score or the 7 neuropsychological ability domain scores (Table 4).

SUBJECTS WITH UNUSUAL DECREASES IN GLOBAL NEUROPSYCHOLOGICAL T-SCORES

The modified Reliable Change Index method, described above, was used to identify and compare the percentages of individual NCs and schizophrenic patients who evidenced unusual neuropsychological worsening from baseline to first retest. With the use of the 90% prediction interval, 10 NCs were so identified (about 5% of the total sample); the latter proportion did not differ significantly from the 5.6% of patients with schizophrenia who evidenced unusual worsening ($\chi^2_{1,N=348}=0.10$; $P=.75$).

The above procedures were also used to evaluate baseline to final follow-up scores of the 85 individual NCs and 67 patients with schizophrenia with follow-up intervals of 36 months or longer (mean, 59.7 months; SD, 68 months). Again, the proportion of patients below the 90% prediction interval was not significantly different from that of the NCs (7.5% vs 4.7%, respectively; $\chi^2_{1,N=152}=0.51$; $P=.48$).

COMMENT

To our knowledge, this is the first longitudinal study to compare comprehensive neuropsychological test results of large samples of NCs and patients with schizophrenia during a multiyear follow-up period. After comparing the two groups with respect to test-retest reliabilities, we attempted to determine whether the schizophrenic patients, or even a subset of that group, evidenced progressive neuropsychological decline.

Consistent with previous reports,[22,65] presence of psychosis did not appear to affect the reliability of neuropsychological test performance. Across the entire neuropsychological battery, reliability estimates were quite high, and were at least as high for the schizophrenic group as for the NCs. This was true even though clinical symptoms were relatively variable over time (Table 2), and even though the test-retest intervals were longer than those in most previous reliability studies with NCs.[50,66] These stability results support the view that neuropsychological deficits in schizophrenia are stable traitlike dimensions of the disorder, rather than reflecting state-related features.

Acceptable test-retest reliability does not rule out the possibility that neuropsychological deficits may be progressive in at least some patients with schizophrenia. Our results, however, provided no evidence of a deteriorating neuropsychological course in the total schizophrenic group, or in subgroups defined on the basis of age, sex, early vs late or recent vs remote onset of illness, baseline level of neuropsychological impairment, or length of follow-up. In each analysis, the schizophrenic groups showed slight improvements that were comparable with those evidenced by the NCs, and these likely represented practice effects. Even rather extreme

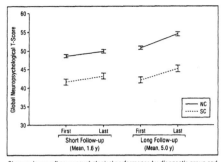

Changes in overall neuropsychological performance by diagnostic group and duration of follow-up. Short follow-up indicates less than 36 months; long follow-up, 36 months or longer; NC, normal comparison group; and SC, schizophrenic patient group. In the short–follow-up groups, sample sizes were 121 for NC and 75 for SC; in the long–follow-up groups, they were 85 for NC and 67 for SC. Vertical lines depict SEMs.

clinical changes did not appear to influence the subjects' neuropsychological performance.

Longitudinal research in institutional settings has shown evidence of neuropsychological decline in some low-functioning, chronically hospitalized patients with schizophrenia.[29-31] Even in those studies, however, such worsening was observed only in small subsets of the groups being followed up. In the absence of longitudinal data from a neurologically stable comparison group, it is unclear whether these observed neuropsychological changes represent true neuropsychological decline, as in a neurodegenerative disorder, or whether they represent the tail of the distribution of test-retest fluctuations in neurologically stable (albeit very low-functioning) persons. It might be argued that the types of change observed in these patients (eg, change in the rated level of dementia) are too gross to be considered "normal fluctuation" and are pathognomonic of a progressive disorder. During approximately a 4-year follow-up interval, however, Ivnik and colleagues[67] found remarkable test-retest differences in neuropsychological performances of some elderly subjects who did not have any neuromedical disorder likely to affect cognition, eg, on neuropsychological factor scores with IQ-type scaling, test-retest differences of 20 or more points were not unusual. Therefore, the outer range of possible fluctuation in performance of neurologically stable persons cannot be assumed and should be established by means of an appropriate comparison group.

The mean global neuropsychological score for our patient group was 1.62 SDs below that of NCs (Table 1), consistent with the range of effect sizes in a recent meta-analytic review of studies comparing controls and schizophrenic patients.[5] Although severely demented patients were not represented in our sample, our "low-functioning" subgroup (n=45; Table 4) was very significantly impaired (ie, more than 3 SDs below NCs on the global neuropsychological T-score).

Limitations of this study include absence of chronically institutionalized patients, and therefore its results may not be generalizable to that minority of patients (but

---

Table 4. Repeated-Measures Analyses of Variance of Schizophrenia Subgroups on Global Neuropsychological Functioning

| | Mean (SD) | | | |
| | Baseline Global Neuropsychological T-Score | Follow-up Global Neuropsychological T-Score | | |
Groups			df	Group × Time F
Age, y				
<65 (n = 120)	41.9 (6.6)	43.8 (7.1) ⎤	1,140	3.28
≥65 (n = 22)	41.5 (5.9)	42.1 (5.5) ⎦		
Sex				
Male (n = 99)	42.2 (6.4)	43.6 (6.5) ⎤	1,140	2.17
Female (n = 43)	41.1 (6.7)	43.4 (7.7) ⎦		
Age at onset of schizophrenia, y				
<45 (n = 118)	41.5 (6.5)	43.3 (6.9) ⎤	1,140	1.30
≥45 (n = 24)	43.4 (6.3)	44.4 (7.0) ⎦		
Duration of illness, y				
<5 (n = 30)	43.6 (6.5)	46.6 (7.0) ⎤	1,133	6.75*
≥5 (n = 105)	41.4 (6.5)	42.7 (6.7) ⎦		
Initial global neuropsychological T-score†				
Low (≤39) (n = 45)	34.2 (3.4)	36.7 (5.2) ⎤	1,94	3.88
High (>45) (n = 51)	48.5 (2.7)	49.9 (3.6) ⎦		
Change in positive symptoms				
Better (n = 27)	42.7 (6.8)	44.0 (7.5) ⎤	1,36	0.03
Worse (n = 11)	45.1 (5.2)	46.6 (6.6) ⎦		
Change in negative symptoms				
Better (n = 17)	41.7 (6.9)	43.3 (7.3) ⎤	1,34	0.29
Worse (n = 19)	42.1 (5.3)	44.2 (5.8) ⎦		
Schooler and Kane tardive dyskinesia criteria				
No tardive dyskinesia (n = 41)	42.0 (6.7)	42.5 (6.9) ⎤	1,52	1.03
Incident tardive dyskinesia (n = 13)	40.8 (8.3)	42.4 (8.4) ⎦		
Waddington orofacial tardive dyskinesia criteria				
No tardive dyskinesia (n = 20)	43.0 (6.9)	43.4 (6.7) ⎤	1,31	0.53
Incident tardive dyskinesia (n = 13)	39.8 (6.0)	39.1 (6.6) ⎦		

*P = .01.
†Because the single score distributions did not meet the repeated-measures analysis of variance requirements for normality and equal variances, the dependent variable in this analysis was the global score Δ.

most contemporary schizophrenic patients are not institutionalized).[68-70] Also, there was limited representation of elderly subjects, and subjects who evidenced substantial clinical change or incident tardive dyskinesias during follow-up (Table 4). Although relatively few of our patients were tested initially very early in the course of their illness, 2 recent studies of first-break schizophrenia showed no significant cognitive decline during the first several years of illness.[35,36] Morover, despite the limited power associated with some of the subgroup analyses in the current study, the data summarized in Table 4 show that these various subject characteristics were associated with clinically trivial effect sizes for changes in cognitive performance.

Considered together, the results of available longitudinal studies strongly suggest that the large majority of people with schizophrenia do not experience progressive neuropsychological decline after the initial onset of their illness. We found no evidence of such decline, even in our ambulatory patients with long follow-up, who were observed for an average of 5 years. It remains possible that a subset of patients with very poor outcome (not represented in our study) do experience progressive neuropsychological decline. Future research with this population should attempt to document such decline by ruling out nonsignificant fluctuations in performance as evidence of progressive impairment. This might be done by

using neuropsychological norms for change developed with a similarly impaired but neurologically stable comparison group, and determining whether any unusual neuropsychological worsening in the schizophrenic patients remains stable or progresses further during a subsequent follow-up period. If future research should conclusively establish progressive neuropsychological decline in a subset of schizophrenic patients, questions arise as to why only a minority are so affected. Is this another example of the heterogeneous manifestations of a common disease,[71-74] or are other factors involved, such as treatment history[75] or comorbid neuromedical conditions (eg, age-related neurodegenerative changes, possibly in combination with schizophrenia-related low "cognitive reserve")?[76] There is a need for larger, collaborative studies using the same methods with patients in different treatment settings.

Accepted for publication July 20, 2000.

This study was supported in part by grants MH43695, MH45131, MH49671, MH19934, MH01452, and MH45294 from the National Institute of Mental Health, Bethesda, Md; State of California (Sacramento) Department of Mental Health grant DMH 89-7000; and the Department of Veterans Affairs, Washington, DC.

Preliminary versions of this work were presented in part at the Mt Sinai Conference on the Role of Cognitive Dysfunc-

104

tion in Schizophrenia, New York, NY, April 6, 1996; the annual meeting of the International Neuropsychological Society, Chicago, Ill, February 16, 1996; and the annual meeting of the American Association of Geriatric Psychiatry, San Diego, Calif, March 10, 1998.

We thank Lou Ann McAdams, PhD, for her comments on an earlier draft of this article.

Reprints: Robert K. Heaton, PhD, Department of Psychiatry, University of California, San Diego, 140 Arbor Dr, San Diego, CA 92103 (e-mail: rheaton@ucsd.edu).

REFERENCES

1. Heaton RK, Crowley TJ. Effects of psychiatric disorders and their somatic treatments on neuropsychological test results. In: Filskov SB, Ball TJ, eds. Handbook of Clinical Neuropsychology. New York, NY: Wiley-Interscience; 1981:481-525.
2. Heaton RK, Drexler M. Clinical neuropsychological findings in schizophrenia and aging. In: Miller NE, Cohen GD, eds. Schizophrenia & Aging. New York, NY: Guilford Press; 1987:145-161.
3. Seidman L. Schizophrenia and brain dysfunction: an integration of recent neurodiagnostic findings. Psychol Bull. 1983;94:195-238.
4. Levin S, Yurgelun-Todd D, Craft S. Contributions of clinical neuropsychology to the study of schizophrenia. J Abnorm Psychol. 1989;98:341-356.
5. Heinrichs RW, Zakzanis KK. Neurocognitive deficit in schizophrenia: a quantitative review of the evidence. Neuropsychology. 1998;12:426-445.
6. Green MF. Schizophrenia From a Neurocognitive Perspective: Probing the Impenetrable Darkness. Boston, Mass: Allyn & Bacon; 1998.
7. Feinberg I. Schizophrenia: caused by a fault in programmed synaptic elimination during adolescence? J Psychiatr Res. 1983;17:319-334.
8. Murray RM. Neurodevelopmental schizophrenia: the rediscovery of dementia praecox. Br J Psychiatry. 1994;25:6-12.
9. Jeste DV. Is schizophrenia a neurodegenerative disorder? a clinical and neurobiological perspective. Biol Psychiatry. 1999;46:729-739.
10. Davidson M, Haroutunian V. Cognitive impairment in geriatric schizophrenic patients. In: Bloom FE, Kupfer DJ, eds. Psychopharmacology: The Fourth Generation of Progress. New York, NY: Raven Press Ltd; 1995:1447-1549.
11. Bilder RM, Turkel E, Lipschutz-Broch L, Lieberman JA. Antipsychotic medication effects on neuropsychological functions. Psychopharmacol Bull. 1992;28:353-366.
12. O'Donnell BF, Faux SF, McCarley RW, Kimble MO, Salisbury DF, Nestor PG, Kikinis R, Jolesz FA, Shenton ME. Increased rate of P300 latency prolongation with age in schizophrenia. Arch Gen Psychiatry. 1995;52:544-549.
13. Hyde TM, Nawroz S, Goldberg TE, Bigelow LB, Strong D, Weinberger DR, Kleinman JE. Is there cognitive decline in schizophrenia? a cross-sectional study. Br J Psychiatry. 1994;164:494-500.
14. Goldberg TE, Greenberg RD, Griffin SJ, Gold JM, Kleinman JE, Pickar D, Schulz SC, Weinberger DR. The effect of clozapine on cognition and psychiatric symptoms in patients with schizophrenia. Br J Psychiatry. 1993;162:43-48.
15. Goldberg TE, Torrey EF, Berman KF, Weinberger DR. Relations between neuropsychological performance and brain morphological and physiological measures in monozygotic twins discordant for schizophrenia. Psychiatry Res Neuroimaging. 1994;55:51-61.
16. Goldstein G, Zubin J. Neuropsychological differences between young and old schizophrenics with and without associated neurological dysfunction. Schizophr Res. 1990;3:117-126.
17. Eyler-Zorrilla LT, Heaton RK, McAdams LA, Zisook S, Jeste DV. Cross-sectional study of older outpatients with schizophrenia and healthy comparison subjects: no differences in age-related cognitive decline. Am J Psychiatry. 2000;157:1324-1326.
18. Moran LJ, Gorham DR, Holtzman WH. Vocabulary knowledge and usage of schizophrenic subjects: a six-year follow-up. J Abnorm Soc Psychol. 1962;61:246-254.
19. Ginnette LE, Moran LJ. Stability of vocabulary performance by schizophrenics. J Consult Psychol. 1964;28:178-179.
20. Smith A. Mental deterioration in chronic schizophrenics. J Nerv Ment Dis. 1964; 139:479-487.
21. Hamlin RM. The stability of intellectual function in chronic schizophrenia. J Nerv Ment Dis. 1969;149:497-503.
22. Klonoff H, Fibiger CH, Hutton GH. Neuropsychological patterns in chronic schizophrenia. J Nerv Ment Dis. 1970;150:291-300.
23. Martin PJ, Friedmeyer MH, Sterne AL, Brittain HM. IQ deficit in schizophrenia: a test of competing theories. J Clin Psychol. 1977;33:667-672.

24. Hamilton V. IQ changes in chronic schizophrenia. Br J Psychiatry. 1963;109: 642-648.
25. Foulds GA, Dixon P, McClelland M, McClelland WJ. The nature of intellectual deficit in schizophrenia, part II: a cross-sectional study of paranoid, catatonic, hebephrenic and simple schizophrenics. Br J Soc Clin Psychol. 1962;1:141-149.
26. Schwartzman AE, Douglas VI. Intellectual loss in schizophrenia, part II. Can J Psychol. 1962;16:161-168.
27. Haywood HC, Moelis I. Effects of symptoms change on intellectual function in schizophrenia. J Abnorm Soc Psychol. 1963;67:76-78.
28. Abrams S, Nathanson IA. Intellectual deficit in schizophrenia: stable or progressive? Dis Nerv Syst. 1966;27:115-117.
29. Harvey PD, Silverman JM, Mohs RC, Parrella M, White L, Powchik P, Davidson M, Davis KL. Cognitive decline in late-life schizophrenia: a longitudinal study of geriatric chronically hospitalized patients. Biol Psychiatry. 1999;45:32-40.
30. Waddington J, Youssef HA. Cognitive dysfunction in chronic schizophrenia followed prospectively over 10 years and its longitudinal relationship to the emergence of tardive dyskinesia. Psychol Med. 1996;26:681-688.
31. Waddington JL, Youssef HA, Kinsella A. Cognitive dysfunction in schizophrenia followed-up over 5 years, and its longitudinal relationship to the emergence of tardive dyskinesia. Psychol Med. 1990;20:835-842.
32. Harvey PD, Lombardi J, Kincaid MM, Parrella M, White L, Powchik P, Davidson M. Cognitive functioning in chronically hospitalized schizophrenic patients: age-related changes and age disorientation as a predictor of impairment. Schizophr Res. 1995;17:15-24.
33. Nopoulos P, Flashman L, Flaum M, Arndt S, Andreasen N. Stability of cognitive functioning early in the course of schizophrenia. Schizophr Res. 1994;14:29-37.
34. De Lisi LE, Tew W, Xiew S, Hoff AL, Sakuma M, Kushner M, Lee G, Shedlack K, Smith AM, Grimson R. A prospective follow-up study of brain morphology and cognition in first-episode schizophrenic patients: preliminary findings. Biol Psychiatry. 1995;38:349-360.
35. Hoff AL, Sakuma M, Wieneke M, Horon R, Kushner M, DeLisi LE. Longitudinal neuropsychological follow-up study of patients with first-episode schizophrenia. Am J Psychiatry. 1999;156:1336-1341.
36. Gold S, Arndt S, Nopoulos P, O'Leary DS, Andreasen NC. Longitudical study of cognitive function in first-episode and recent-onset schizophrenia. Am J Psychiatry. 1999;156:1342-1348.
37. Braff DL, Heaton R, Kuck J, Cullum M, Moranville J, Grant I, Zisook S. The generalized pattern of neuropsychological deficits in outpatients with chronic schizophrenia with heterogeneous Wisconsin Card Sorting Test Results. Arch Gen Psychiatry. 1991;48:891-898.
38. Heaton R, Paulsen J, McAdams LA, Kuck J, Zisook S, Braff D, Harris MJ, Jeste DV. Neuropsychological deficits in schizophrenia: relationship to age, chronicity, and dementia. Arch Gen Psychiatry. 1994;51:469-476.
39. Heaton RK, Grant I, Butters N, White DA, Kirson D, Atkinson JH, McCutchan JA, Taylor MJ, Kelly MD, Ellis RJ, Wolfson T, Velin R, Marcotte TD, Hesselink JR, Jernigan TL, Chandler J, Wallace M, Abramson I, and the HNRC Group. The HNRC 500: neuropsychology of HIV infection at different disease stages. J Int Neuropsychol Soc. 1995;1:231-251.
40. Jeste DV, Harris MJ, Krull A, Kuck J, McAdams LA, Heaton R. Clinical and neuropsychological characteristics of patients with late-onset schizophrenia. Am J Psychiatry. 1995;152:722-730.
41. Spitzer RL, Williams JBW. Structured Clinical Interview for DSM-III-R: Patient Version. New York: Biometric Research Dept, New York State Psychiatric Institute; 1986.
42. First MB, Spitzer RL, Gibbon M, Williams JBW. Structured Clinical Interview for DSM-IV Axis I Disorder: Patient Edition. New York: Biometrics Research Dept, New York State Psychiatric Institute; 1995.
43. American Psychiatric Association. Diagnostic and Statistical Manual of Mental Disorders, Revised Third Edition. Washington, DC: American Psychiatric Association; 1987.
44. American Psychiatric Association. Diagnostic and Statistical Manual of Mental Disorders, Fourth Edition. Washington, DC: American Psychiatric Association; 1994.
45. Reitan RM, Wolfson D. The Halstead-Reitan Neuropsychological Test Battery: Theory and Clinical Interpretation. 2nd ed. Tucson, Ariz: Neuropsychology Press; 1993.
46. Heaton RK. Comprehensive Norms for an Expanded Halstead-Reitan Battery: A Supplement for the Wechsler Adult Intelligence Scale-Revised. Odessa, Fla: Psychological Assessment Resources Inc; 1992.
47. Heaton RK, Grant I, Matthews CG. Comprehensive Norms for Expanded Halstead-Reitan Battery: Demographic Corrections, Research Findings, and Clinical Applications. Odessa, Fla: Psychological Assessment Resources Inc; 1991.
48. Gladsjo AJ, Schuman C, Evans J, Peavy G, Miller S, Heaton RK. Norms for letter and category fluency: demographic corrections for age, education, and ethnicity. Assessment. 1999;6:147-178.
49. Spreen O, Strauss E. A Compendium of Neuropsychological Tests: Administra-

tion, Norms and Commentary. 2nd ed. New York, NY: Oxford University Press; 1998.

50. Wechsler D. *WAIS-R Manual: Wechsler Adult Intelligence Scale–Revised.* New York, NY: Psychological Corp; 1981.

51. Heaton RK, Chelune GJ, Talley JL, Kay GG, Curtiss G. *Wisconsin Card Sorting Test Manual: Revised and Expanded.* Odessa, Fla: Psychological Assessment Resources Inc; 1993.

52. Delis DC, Kramer JH, Kaplan E, Ober BA. *California Verbal Learning Test (CVLT) Manual.* San Antonio, Tex: Psychological Corp; 1987.

53. Russell EW, Neuringer C, Goldstein G. *Assessment of Brain Damage.* New York, NY: John Wiley & Sons Inc; 1970.

54. Norman M, Evans J, Miller S, Heaton R. Demographically corrected norms for the California Verbal Learning Test. *J Clin Exp Neuropsychol.* 2000;22:80-94.

55. Overall JE, Gorham DR. The Brief Psychiatric Rating Scale. *Psychol Rep.* 1962; 10:799-812.

56. Andreasen NC, Olsen S. Negative vs positive schizophrenia: definition and validation. *Arch Gen Psychiatry.* 1982;39:789-794.

57. National Institute of Mental Health. Abnormal Involuntary Movement Scale (AIMS). *Early Clin Drug Eval Unit Intercom.* 1975;4:3-6.

58. McGraw KO, Wong SP. Forming inferences about some intraclass correlation coefficients. *Psychol Methods.* 1996;1:30-46.

59. Jacobsen NS, Truax P. Clinical significance: a statistical approach to defining meaningful change in psychotherapy research. *J Consult Clin Psychol.* 1991;59:12-19.

60. Temkin NR, Heaton RK, Grant I, Dikmen SS. Detecting significant change in neuropsychological test performance: a comparison of four models. *J Int Neuropsychol Soc.* 1999;5:357-369.

61. Jeste DV, Wyatt RJ. *Understanding and Treating Tardive Dyskinesia.* New York, NY: Guilford Press Inc; 1982.

62. de Leon J, Canuso C, White AO, Simpson GM. A pilot effort to determine benztropine equivalents of anticholinergic medications. *Hosp Community Psychiatry.* 1994;45:606-607.

63. Schooler N, Kane JM. Research diagnoses for tardive dyskinesia. *Arch Gen Psychiatry.* 1982;39:486-487.

64. Waddington JL. Tardive dyskinesia in schizophrenia and other disorders: associa-tions with aging, cognitive dysfunction and structural brain pathology in relation to neuroleptic exposure. *Hum Psychopharmacol.* 1987;2:11-22.

65. Harvey PD, White L, Parrella M, Putnam KM, Kincaid MM, Powchik P, Mohs RC, Davidson M. The longitudinal stability of cognitive impairment in schizophrenia: Mini-Mental State scores at one- and two-year follow-ups in geriatric in-patients. *Br J Psychiatry.* 1995;166:630-633.

66. Wechsler D. *Wechsler Adult Intelligence Scale, 3rd Edition: Administration and Scoring Manual.* San Antonio, Tex: Psychological Corp; 1997.

67. Ivnik RJ, Smith GE, Malec JF, Petersen RC, Tangalos JF. Long-term stability and intercorrelations of cognitive abilities in older persons. *Psychol Assess.* 1995; 7:155-161.

68. Cohen CI, Cohen GD, Blank K, Gaitz C, Katz IR, Leuchter A, Maletta G, Meyers B, Sakauye K, Shamoian C. Schizophrenia and older adults, an overview: directions for research and policy. *Am J Geriatr Psychiatry.* 2000;8:19-28.

69. Jeste DV, Alexopoulos GS, Bartels SJ, Cummings JL, Gallo JJ, Gottlieb GL, Halpain MC, Palmer BW, Patterson TL, Reynolds CF III, Lebowitz BD. Consensus statement on the upcoming crisis in geriatric mental health: research agenda for the next two decades. *Arch Gen Psychiatry.* 1999;56:848-853.

70. Palmer BW, Simjee McClure F, Jeste DV. Schizophrenia in late-life: findings challenge traditional concepts. *Harvard Rev Psychiatry.* 1999;56:781-787.

71. Andreasen NC. A unitary model of schizophrenia: Bleuler's "fragmented phrene" as schizencephaly. *Arch Gen Psychiatry.* 1999;56:781-787.

72. Buchanan RW, Strauss ME, Kirkpatrick B, Holstein C, Breier A, Carpenter WT. Neuropsychological impairments in deficit vs nondeficit forms of schizophrenia. *Arch Gen Psychiatry.* 1994;51:804-811.

73. Palmer BW, Heaton RK, Paulsen JS, Kuck J, Braff D, Harris MJ, Zisook S, Jeste DV. Is it possible to be schizophrenic yet neuropsychologically normal? *Neuropsychology.* 1997;11:437-446.

74. Palmer BW, Heaton RK, Jeste DV. Older patients with schizophrenia: challenges in the coming decades. *Psychiatr Serv.* 1999;50:1178-1183.

75. Wyatt RJ, Henter ID. The effects of early and sustained intervention on the long-term morbidity of schizophrenia. *J Psychiatr Res.* 1998;32:169-177.

76. Dwork AJ, Susser ES, Keilp JG, Waniek C, Lieu D, Kaufman M, Zemishlany Z, Prohovnik I. Senile degeneration and cognitive impairment in chronic schizophrenia. *Am J Psychiatry.* 1998;155:1536-1543.

106

Predictors of Relapse Following Response From a First Episode of Schizophrenia or Schizoaffective Disorder

Delbert Robinson, MD; Margaret G. Woerner, PhD; Jose Ma. J. Alvir, DrPH; Robert Bilder, PhD;
Robert Goldman, PhD; Stephen Geisler, MD; Amy Koreen, MD; Brian Sheitman, MD;
Miranda Chakos, MD; David Mayerhoff, MD; Jeffrey A. Lieberman, MD

Background: We examined relapse after response to a first episode of schizophrenia or schizoaffective disorder.

Methods: Patients with first-episode schizophrenia were assessed on measures of psychopathologic variables, cognition, social functioning, and biological variables and treated according to a standardized algorithm. The sample for the relapse analyses consisted of 104 patients who responded to treatment of their index episode and were at risk for relapse.

Results: Five years after initial recovery, the cumulative first relapse rate was 81.9% (95% confidence interval [CI], 70.6%-93.2%); the second relapse rate was 78.0% (95% CI, 46.5%-100.0%). By 4 years after recovery from a second relapse, the cumulative third relapse rate was 86.2% (95% CI, 61.5%-100.0%). Discontinuing antipsychotic drug therapy increased the risk of relapse by almost 5 times (hazard ratio for an initial relapse, 4.89 [99% CI, 2.49-9.60]; hazard ratio for a second relapse, 4.57 [99% CI, 1.49-14.02]). Subsequent analyses controlling for antipsychotic drug use showed that patients with poor premorbid adaptation to school and premorbid social withdrawal relapsed earlier. Sex, diagnosis, obstetric complications, duration of psychotic illness before treatment, baseline symptoms, neuroendocrine measures, methylphenidate hydrochloride challenge response, neuropsychologic and magnetic resonance imaging measures, time to response of the initial episode, adverse effects during treatment, and presence of residual symptoms after the initial episode were not significantly related to time to relapse.

Conclusions: There is a high rate of relapse within 5 years of recovery from a first episode of schizophrenia and schizoaffective disorder. This risk is diminished by maintenance antipsychotic drug treatment.

Arch Gen Psychiatry. 1999;56:241-247

From the Departments of Psychiatry, Hillside Hospital, Long Island Jewish Medical Center, Glen Oaks, and the Albert Einstein College of Medicine, New York, NY (Drs Robinson, Woerner, Alvir, Bilder, Goldman, and Geisler) and University of North Carolina, Chapel Hill (Drs Sheitman, Chakos, and Lieberman); and Nassau County Medical Center, East Meadow, NY (Dr Mayerhoff). Dr Koreen is in private practice in Huntington, NY.

P ATIENTS WITH first-episode schizophrenia usually respond well to treatment,[1-5] but relapse is frequent during the first years of the illness and may be associated with clinical deterioration.[6] Previous studies have used different definitions of relapse, employed a variety of treatments and have reported a range of relapse rates. Despite this variability, some general trends are evident. In the first year, relapse rates in published studies[7-9] are relatively low. The largest rate was 41% in patients taking placebo (n = 17)[8]; only 17% of patients relapsed during 15 months in the study[9] with the largest sample size (n = 69). After the first year, relapse rates[8,10-15] rise substantially, with published rates of between 35% after 18 months[15] and 74% after 5 years of follow-up.[12]

Relapse prevention is a major challenge in the care of patients with schizophrenia. Our opportunity to study relapse and its predictors arose in the context of a long-term study of first-episode schizophrenia and schizoaffective disorder. Our patients had extensive clinical and biological assessments at baseline, were treated according to a specific medication algorithm, and were followed up prospectively with standardized assessments. This design allowed us to closely monitor symptom recurrences and to examine the association of clinical and biological variables and medication status with relapse.

RESULTS

PATIENTS

One hundred eighteen patients were treated in the study. The sample for the analyses presented consists of the 104 patients who were followed up for a minimum of 2 months after responding to treatment and thus were at risk for relapse. The sample included an equal number of men and women; their mean ± SD age at study

PATIENTS, MATERIALS, AND METHODS

STUDY DESIGN

The study design and methods have been described previously.[16,17] The study began in 1986; this report includes data collected until June 1, 1996. All patients were recruited from Hillside Hospital, Glen Oaks, NY; the study was conducted according to guidelines of the Long Island Jewish Medical Center, Glen Oaks, institutional review board. Written informed consent for the study was obtained from patients and, if available, from family members. Inclusion criteria were (1) a Research Diagnostic Criteria[18]–defined diagnosis of schizophrenia or schizoaffective disorder based on a Schedule for Affective Disorders and Schizophrenia[19] interview, (2) total lifetime exposure to antipsychotic medications of 12 weeks or less, (3) a rating of 4 (moderate) or more on at least 1 psychotic symptom item on the Schedule for Affective Disorders and Schizophrenia Change Version With Psychosis and Disorganization Items rating scale (SADS-C+PD),[20] (4) no medical contraindications to treatment with antipsychotic medications, and (5) no neurologic or endocrine disorder or neuromedical illness that could affect diagnosis or the biological variables in the study.

Initially, we did not limit the length of study participation. Later we established a maximum study time of 5 years and terminated the participation of patients who had been in the protocol longer (the longest duration of study participation was 475 weeks).

ASSESSMENTS AND MEASURES

Assessments included the following. (1) Psychopathologic variables: SADS-C+PD[20] and the Clinical Global Impression (CGI) Scale[21] at baseline and every 2 weeks during acute treatment and every 4 weeks at other times and the Scale for the Assessment of Negative Symptoms[22] at baseline and every 4 weeks. (2) Adverse effects/motor symptoms: the Simpson-Angus Extrapyramidal Symptom (SAEPS) Scale[23] at baseline and every 2 weeks during short-term treatment and every 4 weeks at other times and the Modified Simpson Dyskinesia Scale[24] at baseline and every 8 weeks. (3) Premorbid social adjustment: the Premorbid Adjustment Scale (PAS)[25] was completed at baseline using information from patients and family members. "Premorbid" was defined as the period ending 6 months before the first psychiatric contact or hospitalization or 6 months before any evidence of florid psychotic symptoms. Individual PAS item ratings were averaged to provide mean scores for childhood, early adolescence, late adolescence, and adulthood. (4) Obstetric history: obtained from mothers by questionnaire and interview and from birth records when available, and scored using the McNeil-

Sjöström scale.[26] (5) Neuropsychologic (NP) assessments: done when patients recovered from the initial episode or reached a stable plateau. The NP battery included 38 tests from which variables were selected to provide scores in 6 scales (language, memory, attention, executive, motor, and visuospatial function)[27] and a weighted global summary score for NP performance. For scale construction, raw scores were converted to standard scores (z scores) relative to the performance of a healthy control group (n = 36). Patients also underwent an abbreviated NP battery assessing attention and motor function before starting antipsychotic drug therapy. For the purpose of analysis, raw scores were converted to factor scores on the basis of principal components analysis. (6) Magnetic resonance imaging brain scans were obtained during the index episode using a 1.0-T whole-body magnetic resonance imaging system (Magnetom; Siemens, Erlangen, Germany). Images acquired by a 3-dimensional gradient echo sequence (fast low angle shot) (coronal acquisition, 3.1-mm-thick contiguous slices, with a 256 × 256 matrix in a 24-cm field of view; number of excitations = 1; repeat time = 40 milliseconds; echo time = 15 milliseconds; and flip angle = 50°) were used for morphometric analysis.[28] A semiautomated mensuration system was used for assessing whole brain, ventricular, caudate, superior temporal gyrus, and hippocampal volumes (methods described previously[16,27,29,30]). Presence of a septum pellucidum abnormality was rated as absent, questionable, or present using previously reported methods.[31]

During the initial study years, patients were rated for psychotic symptom activation in response to intravenous methylphenidate hydrochloride before starting antipsychotic treatment.[16] Homovanillic acid[32] and baseline and apomorphine hydrochloride–stimulated growth hormone[16] levels were also obtained for a subgroup of patients by indwelling catheter serial sample collection.

DEFINITIONS OF PREDICTOR VARIABLES

For analyses of relapse predictors, some variables required additional specification beyond that described above. Obstetric complications present equaled 1 or more complications rated 5 (potentially greatly harmful/relevant) on the McNeil-Sjöström scale; baseline hallucinations and delusions equaled the mean of the ratings for severity of delusions and severity of hallucinations on the SADS-C+PD; baseline disorganization equaled the mean of the SADS-C+PD ratings for bizarre behavior, inappropriate affect, and a composite measure of thought disorder consisting of the mean of the impaired understandability, derailment, and illogical thinking items; baseline negative symptoms equaled the mean of the global ratings for affective flattening, alogia, avolition-apathy, and anhedonia-asociality on the Scale for the Assessment of Negative Symptoms; baseline depressive symptoms equaled the Hamilton Depression scale total score extracted from the SADS-C+PD[33]; baseline

entry was 25.6 ± 6.3 years (range, 14-44 years); 40% were white, 37% were African American, 12% were Hispanic, 8% were Asian, and 3% were of mixed background. Fifty percent had some education beyond high school. Seventy-eight percent had never married. Patients had been ill for an extended period before study entry: the onset of the first behavioral changes related to the illness preceded

study entry by a mean ± SD of 119 ± 181 weeks, and the first psychotic symptoms began 64 ± 146 weeks before study entry. Patients were severely ill at baseline. Their mean ± SD CGI Severity Scale score was 5.4 ± 0.94 and their mean ± SD Global Assessment Scale score was 27.6 ± 8.6. Research Diagnostic Criteria–defined diagnoses of the index episode were schizophrenia (n = 71;

extrapyramidal signs present equaled a score of 1 (mild) or more on rigidity, cogwheel rigidity, akinesia, or brady-kinesia on the SAEPS; parkinsonism present equaled a rating of 3 or more on rigidity or 2 or more on cogwheeling and rigidity on the SAEPS; and akathisia present equaled a rating of 2 or greater on akathisia on the SAEPS. To examine the effect of interepisode residual symptoms, patients were classified as having no residual symptoms, residual symptoms without prominent negative symptoms, and residual symptoms with prominent negative symptoms using the DSM-IV[34] schizophrenia course specifiers.

TREATMENT PROTOCOL

Patients were treated openly according to a standard algorithm, progressing from one phase of the algorithm to the next until they met response criteria. The sequence was initial treatment with fluphenazine, up to 20 mg/d; after 6 weeks, the dose for nonresponders was increased to 40 mg/d for an additional 4 weeks. Patients nonresponsive to fluphenazine therapy were switched to haloperidol therapy, 20 mg/d, for 6 weeks, which was raised to 40 mg/d for 4 additional weeks if needed. Patients who were still unresponsive, and a trial of a neuroleptic agent from a different biochemical class—either molindone hydrochloride, up to 300 mg/d, or loxapine, up to 150 mg/d, was the next strategy (because of a protocol change during the study, lithium augmentation was not used for all eligible patients). Patients who were still treatment resistant were treated with clozapine, up to 900 mg/d. Benztropine mesylate, 2 to 6 mg/d, was given if extrapyramidal symptoms developed, and lorazepam, 1 to 3 mg/d, or propranolol, 10 to 60 mg/d, was prescribed for akathisia. Mood stabilizers were prescribed if needed. Patients who remained unresponsive were treated as clinically indicated by the research team.

DEFINITION OF TREATMENT RESPONSE AND RELAPSE

Treatment response was operationally defined as a CGI global improvement scale rating of "much improved" or "very much improved" and a rating of 3 (mild) or less on all of the following SADS-C+PD psychosis items: severity of delusions, severity of hallucinations, impaired understandability, derailment, illogical thinking, and bizarre behavior. To be classified as responders, patients had to maintain this level of improvement for 8 consecutive weeks; treatment response was dated from the time response criteria were first met, ie, the beginning of this 8 weeks.

Responders continued taking the successful medication; if clinically appropriate, the dose was lowered by up to 50% in the maintenance phase of treatment. Patients who were clinically stable for 1 year were given the option of discontinuing use of the antipsychotic medication while continuing to be followed up by the study team. Patients who had symptom exacerbations after discontinuing medication use were given the antipsychotic drug that had been successful for them in the past. Continuous antipsychotic medication therapy was prescribed for the remainder of the study for all patients who developed signs of relapse. Whenever possible, we continued to follow up and assess patients who discontinued treatment against our advice; these patients were restarted on antipsychotic drug therapy if they later agreed to treatment.

The following rating scale criteria were used to define a relapse: at least "moderately ill" on the CGI Severity of Illness Scale, "much worse" or "very much worse" on the CGI Improvement Scale, and at least "moderate" on 1 or more of the SADS-C+PD psychosis items listed above; these criteria had to be sustained for a minimum of 1 week. Date of relapse was defined as the first day of this period. Patients who had nonpsychotic symptom exacerbations (eg, affective symptoms) were not classified as relapsed.

DATA ANALYSIS

Because of the longitudinal nature of the study, length of follow-up (and the period at risk for relapse) varied among study patients. Survival analysis, which adjusts for differences in length of follow-up, was used to estimate the cumulative rate of relapse and to test the effects of potential predictors of relapse. Cumulative rates of relapse were estimated using life-table methods, with 95% confidence intervals (CIs) to indicate the precision of these relapse rate estimates.

Analyses that estimated the effects of single and multiple potential risk factors were done using Cox proportional hazards regression. To ensure that the proportional hazards assumption of Cox regression was met, we ran additional analyses incorporating the interaction terms of individual risk factors with time into the models. Because of the number of risk factors included in the Cox regression analysis, we defined statistical significance as $P<.01$. We thus used 99% CIs to indicate the precision of the hazard ratios from these analyses.

Cox proportional hazards regression was run with neuroleptic medication status (taking drugs vs not taking drugs) entered as a time-dependent covariate. A lag of 7 days was incorporated into the medication status time-dependent variable so that a patient was considered to be taking medication until a week after stopping medication use and considered to be not taking medication until a week after restarting medication use. These lags were instituted to model the time needed for medications to wear off after discontinuation or build up when resumed and to account for the possibility that stopping medication use constituted part of the relapse process. Additional Cox regression models examining other potential predictors of relapse controlled for medication status as a time-dependent covariate.

82% paranoid, 11% undifferentiated, 6% disorganized, and 1% catatonic subtypes) and schizoaffective disorder (n = 33).

Patients were followed up for a mean ± SD of 207 ± 101 weeks. The mean ± SD antipsychotic drug dose in fluphenazine equivalents during acute treatment was 24 ± 15 mg/d. Twenty-eight patients received some treatment that did not conform to the standard medication algorithm. Nine patients were in initial pilot protocols and began treatment with conventional antipsychotic medications other than fluphenazine. Nineteen patients began treatment with fluphenazine but subsequently received medications not specified in the algorithm for a variety of clinical reasons.

109

Table 1. Cumulative Relapse Rates by Episode of Illness

Year*	Relapse Rate (95% Confidence Interval)	Patients Remaining at Risk at End of Year, No.
	First Relapse—104 Patients at Risk	
1	16.2 (8.9-23.4)	80
2	53.7 (43.4-64.0)	39
3	63.1 (52.7-73.4)	22
4	74.7 (64.2-85.2)	9
5	81.9 (70.6-93.2)	4
	Second Relapse—63 Patients at Risk	
1	19.1 (8.4-29.9)	36
2	48.7 (33.6-63.9)	17
3	56.0 (43.2-80.2)	10
4	56.0 (43.2-80.2)	3
5	78.0 (46.5-100.0)	1
	Third Relapse—20 Patients at Risk	
1	12.5 (0-28.7)	10
2	31.1 (4.8-57.4)	7
3	72.4 (41.0-100.0)	2
4	86.2 (61.5-100.0)	1

Refers to year(s) after recovery from the previous episode.

Magnetic resonance imaging, NP, and obstetric measures were not obtained on all patients because of clinical condition or patient or family member refusal.

RELAPSE RATES

Relapse rates are presented in **Table 1**. The cumulative rate for first relapse for the 104 patients was 81.9% (95% CI, 70.6%-93.2%) by the end of the 5-year follow-up. For the 63 patients who recovered after the first relapse, cumulative rate for a second relapse was 78.0% (95% CI, 46.5%-100%) after 5 years. Similarly, the cumulative rate for a third relapse was 86.2% (95% CI, 61.5%-100%) by the end of 4 years among 20 patients who were at risk after recovery from the second relapse.

A survival analysis of relapse using medication status as a time-dependent covariate indicated that the risk for a first and second relapse was almost 5 times greater when not taking than when taking medication (hazard ratio for first relapse, 4.89 [99% CI, 2.49-9.60]; hazard ratio for the second relapse, 4.57 [99% CI, 1.49-14.02]). Survival analyses for the third relapse produced high but unstable estimates because of the small number of patients at risk.

Thirteen stable patients who had discontinued antipsychotic drug therapy dropped out of the study (5 patients had been followed up for ≥2 years after recovery from the initial episode, 4 patients were at risk for relapse for 1-2 years, and 4 patients were at risk for relapse for <1 year). These were categorized as censored observations at the time they dropped out. This raised the possibility that our hazard ratios were biased upward because they would not reflect the possibility that these patients might have remained stable without taking medication after they dropped out. To assess this possibility, we reran our analyses assuming that these 13 patients continued not taking antipsychotic drugs and did not relapse from the time they dropped out of the study

until either the June 1, 1996, cutoff date for our analyses or the date that would have marked their completion of 5 years in the study. For the first relapse, the hazard ratio estimating the effect of not taking antipsychotic medications was 3.31 (99% CI, 1.66-6.61) in these analyses. Thus, even given these extreme assumptions, stopping antipsychotic drug therapy had a large effect on relapse.

Given the strong association between medication discontinuation and relapse, we next examined the possibility that antipsychotic drug therapy discontinuation was an early phase of the relapse process rather than a precipitant, ie, patients who are becoming psychotic might lose insight and stop taking medication. If this were the case, relapse onset and antipsychotic discontinuation should be temporally close; a long period between stopping antipsychotic drug use and relapse onset would not be consistent with this hypothesis. One way to examine this issue was to lengthen the lag period in our analyses during which patients were classified as taking medication after administration of their last actual medication dose. If stopping antipsychotic drug therapy occurred at or just before the time of relapse, lengthening these lag periods would cause patients in our analyses to be considered as taking medication at the time of relapse and thereby decrease the relapse risk associated with not taking antipsychotic drugs. In subsequent analyses using longer lag periods, antipsychotic drug therapy discontinuation continued to be associated with a substantial relapse risk; this suggests that stopping antipsychotic drug use was not just an early manifestation of relapse. For example, the hazard ratios associated with not taking medication for the first relapse were 4.49 (99% CI, 2.31-8.75) using a 14-day lag, 4.16 (99% CI, 2.15-8.06) using a 28-day lag, and 4.41 (99% CI, 2.27-8.57) using a 56-day lag.

PREDICTORS

Because antipsychotic medication status was such a strong predictor of relapse, the time-dependent covariate measuring medication status (using a 7-day lag period) was controlled for in analyses of other predictor variables. Analyses of predictors of the first relapse are presented in **Table 2**. Early adolescent premorbid adjustment was the only variable significantly related to first relapse; late adolescent premorbid adjustment and hippocampal volume were trend level predictors (P<.05). Results of subsequent analysis of individual PAS items indicated that shorter time to first relapse was significantly associated with social withdrawal in late adolescence (hazard ratio, 1.29; 99% CI, 1.09-1.61) and poor adaptation to school in early adolescence (hazard ratio, 1.38; 99% CI, 1.06-1.81); relapse was also associated at a trend level (P<.05) with poor school adaptation in childhood (hazard ratio, 1.41; 99% CI, 0.96-2.05) and late adolescence (hazard ratio, 1.17; 99% CI, 0.96-1.44).

To demonstrate the clinical relevance of our premorbid adjustment findings, the **Figure** presents the predicted cumulative relapse rates for patients in the 25th and 75th percentiles of early adolescent global PAS scores (PAS scores = 0.8 and 1.7, respectively). Predicted rates

Table 2. Predictors of First Relapse*

Characteristic	HR (99% CI)
Female	1.02 (0.53-1.98)
Diagnosis of initial episode (schizoaffective vs schizophrenia)	0.68 (0.33-1.40)
Obstetric complications (n = 53)†	0.73 (0.22-2.40)
Childhood PAS score	1.37 (0.89-2.11)
Early adolescence PAS score	1.57‡ (1.02-2.40)
Late adolescence PAS score	1.34§ (0.99-1.83)
Adulthood PAS score	1.12 (0.86-1.47)
Duration of psychotic symptoms before study entry of >1 y†	1.28 (0.56-2.90)
Baseline hallucinations and delusions	1.15 (0.82-1.61)
Baseline disorganization	1.22 (0.88-1.69)
Baseline negative symptoms	0.90 (0.57-1.42)
Baseline depressive symptoms	0.97 (0.92-1.02)
Baseline extrapyramidal symptoms†	1.16 (0.34-3.98)
Parkinsonism during the first 16 wk of treatment†	1.64 (0.77-3.50)
Akathisia during the first 16 wk of treatment†	1.12 (0.52-2.39)
Dystonia during the first 16 wk of treatment†	0.94 (0.47-1.87)
Baseline homovanillic acid level, ng/mL (n = 56)	1.02 (0.93-1.12)
Growth hormone	
Baseline, ng/mL (n = 55)	0.98 (0.85-1.13)
Mean response to apomorphine therapy, ng/mL (n = 43)	0.98 (0.90-1.06)
Psychotic symptom activation to methylphenidate (n = 61)†	0.72 (0.29-1.84)
Magnetic resonance imaging measures (n = 95)	
Whole-brain volume, cm³	1.00 (1.00-1.00)
Lateral ventricular volume, cm³	0.99 (0.94-1.05)
Caudate volume, cm³	1.23 (0.81-1.87)
Superior temporal gyrus volume, cm³	0.98 (0.92-1.05)
Hippocampal volume, cm³	1.23§ (0.95-1.60)
Presence of cavum septum‖	1.56 (0.48-5.09)
Neuropsychologic measures	
Baseline attention (n = 45)	1.20 (0.64-2.23)
Baseline motor (n = 45)	1.24 (0.65-2.35)
Global neuropsychologic functioning after response to initial episode (n = 74)	1.22 (0.75-1.99)
Time to treatment response of initial episode, wk	1.00 (0.99-1.02)
Interepisode residual symptoms	1.25 (0.58-2.68)

*All analyses included neuroleptic medication status (taking vs not taking) as a time-varying covariate. Analyses involving ventricular, caudate, superior temporal gyrus, and hippocampal volume controlled for whole-brain volume. HR indicates hazard ratio; CI, confidence interval; and PAS, Premorbid Adjustment Scale.
†Present vs absent.
‡P<.01.
§P<.05.
‖0 indicates absent; ½, questionable; and 1, present.

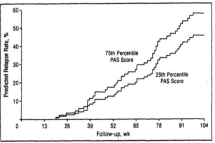

Predicted cumulative relapse rates for patients in the 25th and 75th percentiles for early adolescent global Premorbid Adjustment Scale (PAS) scores (PAS scores = 0.8 and 1.7, respectively) based on Cox proportional hazards regression. The drug status time-varying covariate was set at 0.5 (midway between taking and not taking drugs).

COMMENT

We found that most patients who recover from a first episode of schizophrenia or schizoaffective disorder experience psychotic relapse within 5 years. Furthermore, patients who recover from a first relapse have high rates of second and third relapses despite careful monitoring by a dedicated research treatment team.

Our study offered stable patients the option of discontinuing antipsychotic medication after 1 year of treatment. Those who did so were carefully monitored and treated at the first sign of symptom exacerbation. This conformed to clinical practice at our center when the study began and is consistent with the recently published "American Psychiatric Association Practice Guideline for the Treatment of Patients With Schizophrenia,"[35] which recommends at least 1 year of maintenance antipsychotic medication treatment for remitted first-episode patients. Our data show that medication discontinuation substantially increases relapse risk. This is consistent with earlier findings[8,10] and argues strongly for maintenance medication therapy for first-episode patients with schizophrenia and schizoaffective disorder.

How long should maintenance treatment last? A definitive answer requires systematic medication discontinuation studies, but our data provide some suggestions. The almost 5-fold increase in relapse risk associated with stopping antipsychotic drug use in our analyses was based on the entire follow-up for each patient; our ability to make inferences about a particular period depends on the number of patients who relapsed during that period. We had enough patients who relapsed within 2 years (n = 50) to be confident that medication use should be continued at least this long. Is maintenance medication therapy needed for first-episode patients who have been stable for longer than 2 years? We had only 15 patients who relapsed for the first time after 2 years of stability; 8 of these patients had discontinued medication use when they relapsed, suggesting the continued importance of maintenance medication treatment.

Aside from medication status, premorbid social adjustment was the only predictor of relapse in our study. Kane et al[8] found a significant association between so-

were based on Cox proportional hazards regression; antipsychotic drug status was set at 0.5 (midway between taking and not taking drugs), the approximate mean for this variable. At 1 year, the relapse rate for patients in the 75th percentile was 43% larger than that for patients in the 25th percentile, but both had little absolute difference because both had low relapse rates (17.3% [99% CI, 6.2%-27.1%] and 12.9% [99% CI, 3.1%-20.2%] for patients in the 75th and 25th percentiles, respectively). With the substantial increase in overall relapse rate at 2 years of follow-up, the difference in relapse between patients in the 75th and 25th percentiles was potentially large enough (57.8% [99% CI, 39.6%-70.5%] vs 44.3% [99% CI, 26.0%-58.1%], respectively) to be clinically important.

111

cial isolation in childhood and adolescence as measured by the Premorbid Asocial Adjustment Scale[36] and relapse in first-episode patients taking placebo but not in patients taking antipsychotic drugs for maintenance. Our results, based on a larger sample, indicate that premorbid social isolation predicts initial relapse independent of medication status and that poor adaptation to school also predicts relapse in first-episode patients. Thus, specific behaviors that are present long before the expression of overt psychotic symptoms predict some aspects of the course of psychotic symptoms once they develop. This raises the possibility of a subtype of patients with schizophrenia and schizoaffective disorder characterized by poor early adjustment and a severe, relapsing course.

Few of our predictor variables have been examined in other first-episode samples. Our failure to find an association between sex and relapse is consistent with previous studies.[8,10] Crow et al[10] found that relapse was more common in patients who had an illness onset of 1 year or longer before starting antipsychotic drug use; we did not confirm this, although this variable was associated with initial treatment response in our sample. Study differences in the treatments given and in the definitions of relapse used may have contributed to these divergent findings. Furthermore, illness duration before medication use averaged 2.8 months in the study by Crow et al vs 16.0 months in our study, suggesting differences between the studies in patient clinical characteristics, illness definition, or both. Additional studies are required to clarify the effects of illness duration before treatment on relapse.

In the 5-year follow-up of a subsample of the Northwick Park cohort, Geddes et al[11] found that depressive delusions at baseline were associated with lower risk of readmission. Neither the severity of baseline depressive symptoms nor the presence of affective symptoms sufficient to warrant a schizoaffective diagnosis was related to relapse in our sample. We did, however, find a possible relationship between affective symptoms and relapse. Review of clinical profiles of the 8 patients in our sample who survived 1 year or longer without taking antipsychotic drugs and without relapse revealed that affective symptoms were prominent in this small subgroup who were relatively "invulnerable" to discontinuation of antipsychotic drug therapy.

The failure of most of our candidate variables to predict relapse is interesting given that many of them predicted treatment response to the initial episode in our sample.[1,32,37-40] This suggests either that the pathologic mechanisms of relapse differ from those of acute treatment response or—if common mechanisms initially underlie treatment response and relapse—that the pathologic process changes over time because of a deteriorative component, the effects of prolonged antipsychotic medication exposure, or both.

Our findings have some potential limitations. Our study used a standardized treatment algorithm; this allowed patients to be taking different antipsychotic drugs and different doses depending on their response to treatment. This may have introduced confounds between treatment variables and outcome that would not have been present if we had provided treatment with a set dose of only 1 antipsychotic medication. On the other hand, the treatment algorithm strategy more closely follows optimal clinical practice and thus our findings may be more generalizable to "real world" settings than would a single antipsychotic drug design. Our study preceded the widespread availability of the new generation of antipsychotic medications. Whether use of these agents as first-line treatments will produce different results is an open and important, question.

Although many studies have addressed maintenance treatment in schizophrenia and schizoaffective disorder, relatively few studies have examined relapse in the early years of illness. The high rate of relapse we found and the salience of its relationship to medication discontinuation strongly argues for an increased attention to maintenance treatment issues in the initial stages of schizophrenia and schizoaffective disorder from a clinical and scientific perspective. The fact that so many of our patients refused maintenance antipsychotic drug therapy—even after experiencing 1 or more relapses and despite vigorous patient and family educational efforts—highlights the need for developing strategies to enhance compliance at this early illness stage.

Accepted for publication November 18, 1998.

This study was supported by grant MH41646 and Research Scientist Development Award MH00537 from the National Institute of Mental Health, Bethesda, Md, and grant MH41960 from the Hillside Mental Health Clinical Research Center for the Study of Schizophrenia, Glen Oaks, NY.

Magnetic resonance image analysis was performed in association with the Brain Morphometry and Image Analysis Center of the Long Island Jewish Medical Center, New Hyde Park, NY, supported by a grant from the Helen and Irving Schneider Family, New York, NY.

Reprints: Delbert Robinson, MD, Department of Psychiatry, Hillside Hospital, 266th Street and 76th Avenue, Glen Oaks, NY 11004 (e-mail: robinson@lij.edu).

REFERENCES

1. Lieberman J, Jody D, Geisler S, Alvir J, Loebel A, Szymanski S, Woerner M, Borenstein M. Time course and biologic correlates of treatment response in first-episode schizophrenia. Arch Gen Psychiatry. 1993;50:369-376.
2. Wing JK. Five-year outcome in early schizophrenia. Proc R Soc Med. 1966;59: 17-18.
3. Bland RC, Newman SC, Orn H. Schizophrenia: lifetime co-morbidity in a community sample. Acta Psychiatr Scand. 1987;75:383-391.
4. Macmillan JF, Gold A, Crow TJ, Johnson AL, Johnstone EC. Expressed emotion and relapse. Br J Psychiatry. 1986;148:133-143.
5. Scottish Schizophrenia Research Group. The Scottish First Episode Schizophrenia Study V: one-year follow-up. Br J Psychiatry. 1988;152:470-476.
6. McGlashan TH. A selective review of recent North American long-term follow up studies of schizophrenia. Schizophr Bull. 1988;14:515-542.
7. Rabiner CJ, Wegner JT, Kane JM. Outcome study of first-episode psychosis, I: relapse rates after 1 year. Am J Psychiatry. 1986;143:1155-1158.
8. Kane JM, Rifkin A, Quitkin F, Nayak D, Ramos Lorenzi J. Fluphenazine vs placebo in patients with remitted, acute first-episode schizophrenia. Arch Gen Psychiatry. 1982;39:70-73.
9. Linszen DH, Dingemans PM, Lenior ME. Cannabis abuse and the course of recent-onset schizophrenic disorders. Arch Gen Psychiatry. 1994;51:273-279.
10. Crow TJ, Macmillan JF, Johnson AL, Johnstone EC. A randomised controlled trial of prophylactic neuroleptic treatment. Br J Psychiatry. 1986;148:120-127.
11. Geddes J, Mercer G, Frith CD, MacMillan F, Owens DGC, Johnstone EC. Predic-

tion of outcome following a first episode of schizophrenia: a follow-up study of Northwick Park first episode study subjects. *Br J Psychiatry.* 1994;165:664-668.

12. Scottish Schizophrenia Research Group. The Scottish First Episode Schizophrenia Study VIII: five-year follow-up: clinical and psychosocial findings. *Br J Psychiatry.* 1992;161:496-500.

13. Rajkumar S, Thara R. Factors affecting relapse in schizophrenia. *Schizophr Res.* 1989;2:403-409.

14. Leff J, Wig NN, Bedi H, Menon DK, Kuipers L, Korten A, Ernberg G, Day R, Sartorius N, Jablensky A. Relatives' expressed emotion and the course of schizophrenia in Candigarh: a two-year follow-up of a first-contact sample. *Br J Psychiatry.* 1990;156:351-356.

15. Zhang M, Wang M, Li J, Phillips MR. Randomised-control trial of family intervention for 78 first-episode male schizophrenia patients: an 18-month study in Suzhou, Jiangsu. *Br J Psychiatry.* 1994;165(suppl 24):96-102.

16. Lieberman JA, Jody D, Alvir JM, Ashtari M, Levy D, Bogerts B, Degreef G, Mayerhoff D, Cooper T. Brain morphology, dopamine, and eye-tracking abnormalities in first-episode schizophrenia: prevalence and clinical correlates. *Arch Gen Psychiatry.* 1993;50:357-368.

17. Lieberman JA, Alvir JM, Woerner M, Degreef G, Bilder R, Ashtari M, Bogerts B, Mayerhoff DI, Loebel A, Levy D, Hinrichsen G, Szymanski S, Chakos M, Borenstein M, Kane JM. Prospective study of psychobiology in first-episode schizophrenia at Hillside Hospital. *Schizophr Bull.* 1992;18:351-371.

18. Spitzer RL, Endicott J, Robins E. *Research Diagnostic Criteria (RDC) for a Selected Group of Functional Disorders.* New York, NY: New York Biometrics Research Division; 1977.

19. Endicott J, Spitzer RL. A diagnostic interview: the Schedule for Affective Disorders and Schizophrenia. *Arch Gen Psychiatry.* 1978;35:837-844.

20. Spitzer RL, Endicott J. *Schedule for Affective Disorders and Schizophrenia—Change Version.* 3rd ed. New York: New York State Psychiatric Institute; 1978.

21. Guy W. *ECDEU Assessment Manual for Psychopharmacology.* Washington, DC: US Government Printing office; 1976:217-222. Department of Health, Education and Welfare publication ABM 76-338.

22. Andreasen NC, Olsen S. Negative vs positive schizophrenia: definition and validation. *Arch Gen Psychiatry.* 1982;39:789-794.

23. Simpson GM, Angus JW. A rating scale for extrapyramidal side effects. *Acta Psychiatr Scand Suppl.* 1970;212:11-19.

24. Simpson GM, Lee JH, Zoubok B, Gardos G. A rating scale for tardive dyskinesia. *Psychopharmacology.* 1979;64:171-179.

25. Cannon-Spoor HE, Potkin SG, Wyatt RJ. Measurement of premorbid adjustment in chronic schizophrenia. *Schizophr Bull.* 1982;8:470-484.

26. McNeil TF, Cantor-Graae E, Sjöström K. Obstetric complications as antecedents

of schizophrenia: empirical effects of using different obstetric complication scales. *J Psychiatr Res.* 1994;28:519-530.

27. Bilder RM, Bogerts B, Ashtari M, Wu H, Alvir JM, Jody D, Reiter G, Bell L, Lieberman JA. Anterior hippocampal volume reductions predict frontal lobe dysfunction in first episode schizophrenia. *Schizophr Res.* 1995;17:47-58.

28. Ashtari M, Zito JL, Gold BI, Lieberman JA, Borenstein MT, Herman PG. Computerized volume measurement of brain structure. *Invest Radiol.* 1990;25:798-805.

29. Degreef G, Ashtari M, Bogerts B, Bilder RM, Jody DN, Alvir JMJ, Lieberman JA. Volumes of ventricular system subdivisions measured from magnetic resonance images in first-episode schizophrenic patients. *Arch Gen Psychiatry.* 1992; 49:531-537.

30. Chakos MH, Lieberman JA, Bilder RM, Lerner G, Bogerts B, Degreef G, Wu H, Ashtari M. Increase in caudate nuclei volumes of first-episode schizophrenic patients taking antipsychotic drugs. *Am J Psychiatry.* 1994;151:1430-1436.

31. Degreef G, Lantos G, Bogerts B, Ashtari M, Lieberman J. Abnormalities of the septum pellucidum on MR scans in first-episode schizophrenic patients. *AJNR Am J Neuroradiol.* 1992;13:835-840.

32. Koreen AR, Lieberman J, Alvir J, Mayerhoff D, Loebel A, Chakos M, Amin F, Cooper T. Plasma homovanillic acid levels in first-episode schizophrenia: psychopathology and treatment response. *Arch Gen Psychiatry.* 1994;51:132-138.

33. Endicott J, Cohen J, Nee J, Fleiss J, Sarantakos S. Hamilton Depression Rating Scale: extracted from regular and change versions of the Schedule for Affective Disorders and Schizophrenia. *Arch Gen Psychiatry.* 1981;38:98-103.

34. American Psychiatric Association. *Diagnostic and Statistical Manual of Mental Disorders,* Fourth Edition. Washington, DC: American Psychiatric Association; 1994.

35. American Psychiatric Association practice guideline for the treatment of patients with schizophrenia. *Am J Psychiatry.* 1997;154(suppl 4):1-63.

36. Gittelman-Klein R, Klein DF. Premorbid asocial adjustment and prognosis in schizophrenia. *J Psychiatr Res.* 1969;7:35-53.

37. Szymanski S, Lieberman JA, Alvir JMJ, Mayerhoff D, Loebel A, Geisler S, Chakos M, Koreen A, Jody D, Kane JM, Woerner M, Cooper T. Gender differences in onset of illness, treatment response, course, and biologic indexes in first-episode schizophrenic patients. *Am J Psychiatry.* 1995;152:698-703.

38. Lieberman JA, Koreen AR, Chakos M, Sheitman B, Woerner M, Alvir JMJ, Bilder R. Factors influencing treatment response and outcome of first-episode schizophrenia: implications for understanding the pathophysiology of schizophrenia. *J Clin Psychiatry.* 1996;57:5-9.

39. Lieberman JA, Alvir JM, Koreen A, Geisler S, Chakos M, Sheitman B, Woerner M. Psychobiologic correlates of treatment response in schizophrenia. *Neuropsychopharmacology.* 1996;14(suppl):13S-21S.

40. Bogerts B, Ashtari M, Degreef G, Alvir JM, Bilder RM, Lieberman JA. Reduced temporal limbic structure volumes on magnetic resonance images in first episode schizophrenia. *Psychiatry Res.* 1990;35:1-13.

Progressive Cortical Change During Adolescence in Childhood-Onset Schizophrenia

A Longitudinal Magnetic Resonance Imaging Study

Judith L. Rapoport, MD; Jay N. Giedd, MD; Jonathan Blumenthal, MA; Susan Hamburger, MA, MS; Neal Jeffries, PhD; Tom Fernandez; Rob Nicolson, MD; Jeff Bedwell; Marge Lenane, MSW; Alex Zijdenbos, PhD; Tomás Paus, MD, PhD; Alan Evans, PhD

Background: Adolescence provides a window to examine regional and disease-specific late abnormal brain development in schizophrenia. Because previous data showed progressive brain ventricular enlargement for a group of adolescents with childhood-onset schizophrenia at 2-year follow-up, with no significant changes for healthy controls, we hypothesized that there would be a progressive decrease in volume in other brain tissue in these patients during adolescence.

Methods: To examine cortical change, we used anatomical brain magnetic resonance imaging scans for 15 patients with childhood-onset schizophrenia (defined as onset of psychosis by age 12 years) and 34 temporally yoked, healthy adolescents at a mean (SD) age of 13.17 (2.73) years at initial baseline scan and 17.46 (2.96) years at follow-up scan. Cortical gray and white matter volumes were obtained with an automated analysis system that classifies brain tissue into gray matter, white matter, and cerebrospinal fluid and separates the cortex into anatomically defined lobar regions.

Results: A significant decrease in cortical gray matter

volume was seen for healthy controls in the frontal (2.6%) and parietal (4.1%) regions. For the childhood-onset schizophrenia group, there was a decrease in volume in these regions (10.9% and 8.5%, respectively) as well as a 7% decrease in volume in the temporal gray matter. Thus, the childhood-onset schizophrenia group showed a distinctive disease-specific pattern (multivariate analysis of variance for change × region × diagnosis: F, 3.68; $P = .004$), with the frontal and temporal regions showing the greatest between-group differences. Changes in white matter volume did not differ significantly between the 2 groups.

Conclusions: Patients with very early-onset schizophrenia had both a 4-fold greater decrease in cortical gray matter volume during adolescence and a disease-specific pattern of change. Etiologic models for these patients' illness, which seem clinically and neurobiologically continuous with later-onset schizophrenia, must take into account both early and late disruptions of brain development.

Arch Gen Psychiatry. 1999;56:649-654

From the Child Psychiatry Branch, National Institute of Mental Health (Drs Rapoport, Giedd, and Nicolson, Messrs Blumenthal, Fernandez, and Bedwell, and Mss Hamburger and Lenane), and Biometry Branch, National Institute of Neurological Disorders and Stroke (Dr Jeffries), Bethesda, Md; and the Montreal Neurological Institute, McGill University, Montreal, Quebec (Drs Zijdenbos, Paus, and Evans).

THE neurodevelopmental hypothesis of schizophrenia suggests that a brain "lesion" is present early in life but does not manifest itself until late adolescence or early adulthood.[1-3] Compelling clinical support for this model comes from numerous demonstrations of subtle but consistent abnormalities in cognitive and behavioral development noted years before the onset of psychosis.[4-6] In addition, the postmortem neuropathological findings in schizophrenia can be viewed as consistent with an early nonprogressive event.[2]

The lack of progressive change in longitudinal brain imaging studies of patients with adult-onset schizophrenia is also cited as support for the "fixed-lesion" neurodevelopmental hypothesis. Of the 5 prospective longitudinal anatomi-

cal brain magnetic resonance imaging (MRI) studies of adult-onset schizophrenia that compared patients with temporally yoked controls, only 2 found greater progression for their schizophrenic group as a whole.[7-9] Others found either no progression[10] or evidence of progression for only a subgroup.[11,12]

Childhood-onset schizophrenia (COS) (defined as onset of psychosis by age 12 years) is a rare, usually severe manifestation of the disorder that has been shown to be continuous with the adult-onset disorder with respect to clinical and neurobiological characteristics, including brain MRI pattern.[13-16] There is also continuity in the pattern of associated risk factors, such as early developmental language and speech abnormalities years before the onset of psychosis,[17] cytogenetic abnormalities,[18] and various psychopatho-

115

SUBJECTS AND METHODS

Subjects included 15 children and adolescents who had been recruited to the National Institute of Mental Health study of COS. Recruiting and diagnostic methods have been described elsewhere.[26-28] Briefly, children were sought via national recruiting who met unmodified DSM-III-R criteria for schizophrenia, with onset of psychotic symptoms by age 12 years. From more than 1000 referrals, approximately 250 patients and their families were screened in person, using both clinical examination and structured interviews over a daylong evaluation. The clinical diagnosis of schizophrenia for this group showed good reliability.[27] Fifty-four patients received the diagnosis of COS; 47 had participated in the study at the time of this report. As patients were also participating in a clozapine treatment trial,[28] they were refractory to treatment with typical neuroleptics.

All subjects returned at regular intervals, at which time clinical reevaluation and MRI follow-up scans were carried out. Of the 47 subjects studied to date, valid baseline scans could not be obtained for 2. Of the remaining 45, 28 had returned for a follow-up scan; 18 were rescanned after 3 to 5 years while they were still in adolescence, and 3 of these 18 had 1 scan each that could not be processed by the automated system. Most of the remaining subjects who had not been rescanned were not yet due for their 4-year (approximate) follow-up scan. Thus, only 3 eligible cases were truly unavailable to our team for MRI reevaluation. The 15 cases in the present study did not differ significantly with respect to any clinical or demographic measure from the remainder of the sample.

A temporally yoked, age- and sex-matched healthy control group of 46 adolescents was selected by a systematic evaluation process[29]; 34 with processable scans served as the contrast group for this report. Controls were free of lifetime medical or psychiatric disorders as determined by clinical examination and standardized interview. Psychiatric illness in a first-degree relative was also exclusionary. The combined groups had a mean (SD) age of 13.17 (2.73) years at the time of initial scan, and returned after 4.28 (0.63) years for follow-up scans. Characteristics of patients and control subjects at baseline and follow-up scan are shown in **Table 1**.

As shown in Table 1, patients were severely ill, with a mean ± SD age of onset of psychotic symptoms at 10.3 ± 2.0 years. The patient group received a considerable amount of medication prior to initial scan, and at follow-up, all but 2 were taking medication. The scan intervals did not differ for the 2 groups. Moreover, while at first scan, the medications were primarily typical neuroleptics, at follow-up, 11 of the 15 patients were receiving atypical neuroleptics, with 2 receiving both a typical and an atypical agent. All met the criteria for schizophrenia (4 were in remission while taking clozapine) at the follow-up scan. None of these young subjects had a history of substance abuse. Thus, while patients were matched for age, sex, and time of scan, they differed significantly with respect to ethnicity, socioeconomic status, IQ score, exposure to medication, and weight at follow-up scan.

The study was approved by the National Institute of Mental Health Institutional Review Board. Parents gave written consent, and minor volunteers and patients gave verbal assent for this study.

MRI ACQUISITION AND ANALYSIS

All images were acquired on the same 1.5-T Signa scanner (General Electric, Milwaukee). The scan was done at the National Institutes of Health Clinical Center, Bethesda, Md. A 3-dimensional spoiled gradient-recalled echo in the steady-state sequence designed to optimize discrimination between gray matter, white matter, and cerebrospinal fluid was used to acquire 124 contiguous 1.5-mm-thick slices

logic conditions, including schizophrenia and/or "spectrum" disorders, smooth-pursuit eye movement abnormalities, and/or cognitive abnormalities in the close relatives of the COS patients.[14,19]

An ongoing National Institute of Mental Health study of COS included brain MRI rescans at regular intervals as part of the follow-up examination. A previous report documented an increase in brain ventricular volume between mean ages 14 and 16 years for this group that was more striking and consistent than that reported for adult-onset cases.[20] The study also found a trend for differential decrease in total brain volume for adolescents with schizophrenia, but regional cortical volumes were not examined.

The present report is of regional cortical gray and white matter volumes for a group of patients with COS scanned at initial contact (mean age, 13.9 years) and at 3- to 5-year follow-up (mean age, 18.1 years). To carry out this examination, an automated segmentation system developed at the Montreal Neurological Institute, Montreal, Quebec, was used.[21-25] Because of our earlier brain ventricular data and the smaller total brain and temporal lobe volumes with greater loss of gray matter characteristic of adults with schizophrenia, we hypoth-

esized that there would be commensurate differential changes in other brain tissue, including cortical gray matter, with patients with COS showing a greater and more regionally selective decline than seen for healthy controls.

RESULTS

Both absolute baseline and follow-up scan values and percentage change for total and regional gray and white volumes are shown in **Table 2** for COS patients and healthy controls.

WITHIN-GROUP CHANGE

For the 34 healthy controls, there was a significant (1.3%) decrease in total cerebral volume that was accounted for by a decrease in gray matter volume (1.98%) ($t = 2.12$, $P = .04$). As seen in Table 2, the regional gray matter changes also showed a statistically significant selective regional pattern (MANOVA Wilks λ: F, 19.1; $P<.001$), with the greatest change in the frontal and parietal gray matter and the smallest change in the occipital and temporal gray matter regions.

116

in the axial plane and 124 contiguous 2.0-mm-thick slices in the coronal plane. Imaging parameters were as follows: time to echo, 5 milliseconds; time to repeat, 24 milliseconds; flip angle, 45°; acquisition matrix, 256 × 192; number of excitations, 1; and field of view, 24 cm.

Three vitamin E capsules, 1 placed in the meatus of each ear and 1 taped to the left lateral inferior orbital ridge, were used to standardize head placement across individuals. The vitamin E capsules showed up brightly on the scans, and an axial-localizing sequence was acquired to assess whether the 3 capsules were visible in the same axial plane. This served to ensure brain coverage and minimize partial volume losses. If this criterion was not met the subject's head was repositioned. The subject's nose was aligned at the 12-o'clock position to assist standardization within the axial plane. Foam padding was placed around the head to minimize scanner noise and help steady the head position. Subjects were scanned in the evening to promote natural sleep. Sedation with chloral hydrate (0.5-2.0 g) or lorazepam (0.5-2.0 mg) was used for 20% of the COS subjects. No controls were sedated.

Gray matter, white matter, and cerebrospinal fluid segmentation was performed via a 3-part automated image analysis process.[21-25,31] First, the images are corrected for regional intensity nonuniformities resulting from magnetic field inhomogeneities inherent in the image acquisition process. Next, the images are transformed to a standardized stereotactic (Talairach) space using a 9-parameter linear process.[21] The images are then registered in a nonlinear way to a template brain for which anatomical regions have been manually defined. The nonlinear registration of each subject's MRI with the anatomically defined template brain allows each voxel to be assigned a tissue type and an anatomical structure of which it is a part.[22,23,32]

The lobar boundaries were defined as in a standard atlas.[33] The central sulcus was used to separate the frontal lobe from the parietal lobe, which was bounded inferiorly by the lateral fissure and a line extending the lateral fissure to the occipital lobe. The temporal lobe was bounded superiorly by the lateral fissure and an extension of the lateral fissure to the occipital lobe. The occipital lobe was bounded by a curved line extending from the parieto-occipital fissure to the temporo-occipital incisure.

This information was merged with information from an artificial neural network classification technique that assigns a gray matter, white matter, or cerebrospinal fluid designation based on voxel intensity.

STATISTICAL ANALYSIS

Demographic characteristics of patients and controls were compared using t tests or χ^2 tests where appropriate.

Subtracting the baseline MRI value from the follow-up value and then dividing by the baseline measurement value created change scores for total and regional gray and white matter. These percentage change scores were then used in all statistical analyses. Group differences were examined with 1-way analysis of variance (ANOVA), repeated-measures ANOVA, or multivariate ANOVA (MANOVA) using the Wilks λ result. Post hoc testing determined significant differences.

For the control group, regional regression slopes for individual change over time were examined, using absolute values of the region, in relation to sex, socioeconomic status, and the Wechsler Intelligence Scale for Children Vocabulary and Block Design scores. For the patients with schizophrenia, these slopes were examined in relation to sex, ethnicity, age of onset, weight gain while taking neuroleptics, and neuroleptic exposure (typical and atypical separately). The results were expressed as standard regression β coefficients.

The SPSS 9.0 statistical package for Windows (SPSS Inc, Chicago, Ill) was used for all analyses, with a 2-tailed α level of .05.

For the 15 COS patients, there was a significant (5.5%) decrease in total cerebral volume that was accounted for by a decrease in gray matter (8.0%). The regional gray matter change also differed selectively for COS patients (MANOVA Wilks λ: F, 11.2; P = .001), with 7% to 10% decreases for frontal, parietal, and temporal gray matter volume and no significant change in the occipital region.

BETWEEN-GROUP COMPARISONS

As shown in Table 2, the percentage change differed strikingly between the groups for gray matter, with the COS group showing an exaggerated and unique pattern (MANOVA Wilks λ: F, 3.72; P = .002 overall; F, 3.68; P = .004 for regional × diagnosis interaction). The diagnostic differences were most striking for temporal (P<.001) and frontal (P = .001) gray matter volumes. There was no significant difference between the groups with respect to white matter change.

The disease-specific change in brain development is seen most clearly in the **Figure**, showing the difference in the percentage and pattern of decline between the COS and healthy control groups.

CLINICAL AND DEMOGRAPHIC RELATIONSHIPS

Boys had more robust decreases in gray matter than did girls (P = .05), and this difference was more pronounced for the COS group (ANOVA: F, 4.09; P = .05 for diagnosis × sex). For the healthy controls, there was no significant relationship between full-scale IQ score, socioeconomic status, or ethnicity and slope of change for any region. For the COS group, those with higher baseline Brief Psychiatric Rating Scale scores had a greater rate of volume decrease for temporal, parietal, and frontal gray matter (t, 2.6-3.5; P<.01). There was no significant relationship between weight gain or drug exposure and slope for any region. Further clinically relevant analyses were precluded by missing data and small sample size.

―――――――――――――― **COMMENT** ――――――――――――――

Within a 4-year mid-adolescent period, a significant decline in cortical gray matter volume was seen for the healthy controls. The frontal gray and white matter and parietal gray matter volumes decreased, while white matter volumes in the parietal temporal and occipital regions increased. These data support previous cross-

117

Table 1. Demographic Data for Patients With Childhood-Onset Schizophrenia and Healthy Controls*

	Patients (n = 15)		Controls (n = 34)		Diagnosis at Baseline, t Test	P
	Baseline	Follow-up	Baseline	Follow-up		
Age, y† (range)	13.9 ± 2.3 (9.2-17.9)	18.1 ± 2.7 (13.3-23.3)	12.8 ± 2.9 (8.2-17.8)	17.2 ± 3.1 (11.8-21.8)	1.66	.21
Follow-up interval, y† (range)	4.2 ± 0.7 (3.1-5.5)		4.3 ± 0.6 (3.1-5.4)		0.79	.38
Male/female, No.	6/9		17/17		0.42‡	.52
White/black/other, No.	5/7/3		33/0/1		25.03‡	<.001
SES†§	76.0 ± 34.5		32.2 ± 14.5		39.82	<.001
Height, cm†	160.8 ± 8.6	167.9 ± 8.1	156.9 ± 16.8	169.2 ± 11.1	0.68	.42
Weight, kg†	58.0 ± 14.3	81.3 ± 21.5	46.8 ± 14.5	62.2 ± 11.7	6.27	.02
Right-handed/left-handed/mixed, No.	11/3/1		30/4/0		3.04‡	.22
WISC Block Design score†	6.2 ± 2.8		14.4 ± 2.8		78.04	<.001
WISC Vocabulary score†	4.5 ± 3.4		14.0 ± 2.0		128.17	<.001
Full-scale IQ score†∥	70.4 ± 12.9		124.5 ± 12.9		135.88	<.001
Familial schizophrenia/spectrum disorders, No. (%)	7 (47)					
Age at onset of psychosis, y†	10.3 ± 2.0					
Motor or speech abnormalities, No. (%)	10 (67)					
Atypical neuroleptics, No.	4	11¶				
BPRS score†	53 ± 10	38 ± 9#				
SANS score†	68 ± 19	53 ± 29#				
SAPS score†	56 ± 17	26 ± 18#				

*SES indicates socioeconomic status; WISC, Wechsler Intelligence Scale for Children; BPRS, Brief Psychiatric Rating Scale; SANS, Scale for Assessment of Negative Symptoms; and SAPS, Scale for Assessment of Positive Symptoms.
†Values are mean ± SD.
‡χ² analysis.
§Rated using the Hollingshead 2-factor index.[30]
∥The estimated full-scale IQ score for 26 subjects was used; IQ scores were not available for 5 patients.
¶Two additional patients were given both typical and atypical neuroleptics.
#Follow-up BPRS, SANS, and SAPS scores were missing for 2 patients.

Table 2. Anatomical Brain Magnetic Resonance Imaging Measures and Percentage Changes at Baseline and 3- to 5-Year Follow-up During Adolescence for Patients With Childhood-Onset Schizophrenia and Healthy Controls*

Region	Patients (n = 15)†			Controls (n = 34)†			Diagnosis	
	Baseline	Follow-up	Percentage Change, %‡	Baseline	Follow-up	Percentage Change, %‡	F₄,₄₄	P
Gray and white matter	1050.91 ± 140.17	990.12 ± 121.71	−5.53 ± 5.15	1116.34 ± 117.00	1103.81 ± 127.33	−1.19 ± 3.25	12.81	.001
Gray matter§	666.72 ± 106.02	608.99 ± 82.88	−8.01 ± 8.17∥	725.10 ± 68.50	710.43 ± 71.78	−1.99 ± 4.67	5.79	.001
Frontal lobe	203.83 ± 33.30	180.27 ± 26.77	−10.92 ± 9.15¶	226.53 ± 20.35	219.26 ± 20.88	−3.11 ± 5.39		
Parietal lobe	109.55 ± 17.44	99.54 ± 14.28	−8.51 ± 8.51#	121.49 ± 11.48	116.36 ± 12.55	−4.24 ± 4.72		
Temporal lobe	173.39 ± 29.52	160.25 ± 24.65	−7.02 ± 7.68¶	183.11 ± 17.98	183.58 ± 17.44	0.42 ± 5.47		
Occipital lobe	60.46 ± 11.99	59.32 ± 10.05	−0.74 ± 11.90	65.50 ± 9.54	67.67 ± 11.12	3.52 ± 10.66		
White matter§	384.19 ± 40.95	381.14 ± 46.06	−0.83 ± 4.98	391.24 ± 57.24	393.38 ± 62.30	0.45 ± 3.21	0.78	.54
Frontal lobe	143.12 ± 15.94	137.20 ± 16.46	−4.05 ± 6.06	148.86 ± 22.06	145.55 ± 23.16	−2.28 ± 4.32		
Parietal lobe	76.27 ± 7.63	76.60 ± 8.08	0.55 ± 6.24	77.13 ± 11.18	79.00 ± 12.51	2.31 ± 3.92		
Temporal lobe	80.15 ± 10.78	80.87 ± 11.92	0.91 ± 5.42	80.54 ± 12.22	83.24 ± 13.43	3.32 ± 4.49		
Occipital lobe	34.83 ± 5.28	35.21 ± 5.56	1.32 ± 7.62	33.31 ± 6.58	34.25 ± 7.12	2.88 ± 7.83		

*Values are mean ± SD.
†Values are in cubic centimeters.
‡Values were calculated as follows: ([follow-up − baseline]/baseline) × 100.
§Multivariate analysis of variance was used for gray matter vs white matter: $F_{4,44}$, 6.23; P = .004.
∥Post hoc results for diagnostic differences: P = .003.
¶Post hoc results for diagnostic differences: P = .001.
#Post hoc results for diagnostic differences: P = .04.

sectional studies of clinically referred children and adolescents[34] and healthy prescreened controls,[35] which found age-related decreases in cortical gray matter.[35] Most recently, Sowell et al[36,37] found similar and striking age-related decreases in frontal and parietal gray matter for 35 healthy children and adolescents for whom statistical mapping of subtraction images was carried out. Brain regions do not normally mature in parallel, and the re-

gional changes seen here are more robust than generally seen in young adults.[12]

These longitudinal data for middle and late adolescence show that frontocortical gray matter volume is decreasing. While it is tempting to ascribe these developmental brain changes to peripubertal events, this is clearly not the case. Evidence from cross-sectional studies,[29,34,35,38,39] shows that the trend for decrease in gray mat-

118

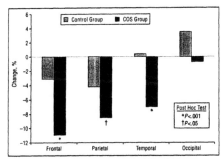

Change in regional cortical gray matter volumes during adolescence (between mean ages 13 and 18 years) by brain magnetic resonance imaging for healthy volunteers (n = 34) and patients with childhood-onset schizophrenia (COS) (n = 15) (multivariate analysis of variance for gray matter volume by diagnosis: F, 3.68; P = .004).

ter volume and continued myelination occurs across a wide age range. Previous postmortem[40,41] data also show decreases in occipital cortex volume during the first decade of life.

The adolescents with schizophrenia showed an exaggerated pattern of brain changes similar in part to that of the controls, with a significantly more robust decrease in volume for the frontal and parietal gray matter and no significant change in occipital gray matter. The significant decrease in temporal lobe volume was, however, unique to the schizophrenic group. The selective regional decline in frontal and temporal gray matter is consistent with the MRI findings in adult-onset schizophrenia, for which the greatest regional difference is found in the frontal and temporal areas.[42] These data are also consistent with evidence suggesting that abnormalities in frontal and temporal lobe connectivity underlie the symptoms of schizophrenia.[43] Thus, a specific pattern in keeping with MRI findings for adults with schizophrenia develops across the adolescent years. The presumed changes underlying this differential progression would include excessive synaptic and dendritic pruning, and probably also trophic glial and vascular decreases, compatible with the neuropathological findings of Selemon et al,[44] Rajkowska et al,[45] and Selemon and Goldman-Rakic[46] showing increased neuronal density and possible trophic glial changes in the schizophrenic cortex.

Adolescence is a period of marked change in brain anatomy and metabolism.[47-49] Because neuropathological observations of normal development are based on very meager data sets since death during childhood and adolescence of otherwise healthy individuals is rare, brain MRI studies provide a unique and noninvasive way to study brain development in healthy children.[29] This study extends our earlier cross-sectional data with the first longitudinal brain MRI study of healthy adolescents; surprisingly robust changes are seen during this limited period between ages 13 and 18 years.

This study of diagnostic differences in brain development is limited by many factors. The samples are not matched for socioeconomic status, race, IQ score, or exposure to neuroleptic medication. Moreover, several COS

patients were switched to therapy with newer atypical antipsychotics at follow-up. In addition, COS patients represent a severely ill, treatment-refractory population; "episodes" of illness were virtually unknown and fluctuations in clinical state were regrettably few. Thus, it might be argued that these differences in progression reflect the course of a subgroup of subjects with poor outcomes described in previous studies of patients with adult-onset schizophrenia. This seems unlikely, however, given that as our patients reach their early adult years, the rate of ventricular enlargement slows and does not differ from that of healthy controls.[50] Thus, the lack of progression seen in most studies of adult patients was also observed in our subjects after they passed through adolescence.

In theory, the late progressive brain changes might reflect some unique interaction between adolescent brain development and the illness, including stress and drastically altered environmental exposure and/or treatments, not seen in schizophrenia at other ages. This possibility cannot be addressed by these data. An ongoing longitudinal MRI study of our patients' siblings may shed further light on a familial genetic basis for these progressive events. It is unlikely, however, that the patients' differential weight gain affected our findings; after age was taken into account, neither weight nor body mass index was significantly related to any brain measure or to these progressive changes.

The differential changes seen in our COS patients are not directly relevant to the issue of "triggers" for psychosis. Our patients had a mean age of onset of psychotic symptoms of 10.3 years (Table 1), while their mean age at first scan was 14 years. These data do, however, indirectly support models of schizophrenia postulating[51,52] later abnormalities of brain development.

Finally, this study does not undermine the neurodevelopmental model of schizophrenia. In fact, the early developmental histories of our group show more striking impairments in language and motor development than reported for patients with adult-onset schizophrenia. However, it is already evident that genes known to influence prenatal brain development may also play a role in later maturation.[53] These findings do indicate that etiologic models of schizophrenia, whether genetic or environmental, need to take into account both early and late neurodevelopmental events.

Accepted for publication March 30, 1999.

Reprints: Judith L. Rapoport, MD, Child Psychiatry Branch, National Institute of Mental Health, Bldg 10, Room 3N202, 10 Center Dr, MSC 1600, Bethesda, MD 20892-1600 (e-mail: rapoport@helix.nih.gov).

REFERENCES

1. Weinberger DR. Implications of normal brain development for the pathogenesis of schizophrenia. Arch Gen Psychiatry. 1987;44:660-669.
2. Weinberger D. From neuropathology to neurodevelopment. Lancet. 1995;346:552-557.
3. Murray R. Neurodevelopmental schizophrenia: the rediscovery of dementia praecox. Br J Psychiatry. 1994;165:6-12.
4. Jones P, Rodgers B, Murray R, Marmot, M. Child developmental risk factors for adult schizophrenia in the British 1946 birth cohort. Lancet. 1994;344:1398-1402.

119

5. Done D, Crow T, Johnstone E, Sacker A. Childhood antecedents of schizophrenia and affective illness: social adjustment at ages 7 and 11. *BMJ*. 1994;309: 699-703.

6. Walker E, Lewine R. Predictions of adult onset schizophrenia from childhood home movies of the parents. *Am J Psychiatry*. 1990;147:1052-1056.

7. Mathalon DH, Sullivan EV, Lim KO, Pfefferbaum A. Longitudinal analysis of MRI brain volumes in schizophrenia. *Schizophr Res*. 1997;24:152.

8. DeLisi LE, Tew W, Xie S, Hoff AL, Sakuma M, Kushner M, Lee G, Shadlock K, Smith AM, Grimson R. A prospective follow-up study of brain morphology and cognition in first-episode schizophrenic patients: preliminary findings. *Biol Psychiatry*. 1995;38:349-360.

9. DeLisi LE, Sakuma M, Tew W, Kushner M, Hoff AL, Grimson R. Schizophrenia as a chronic active brain process: a study of progressive brain structural change subsequent to the onset of schizophrenia. *Psychiatry Res*. 1997;74:129-140.

10. DeLisi LE, Stritzke P, Riordan H, Holan V, Boccio A, Kushner M, McClelland J, Van Eyl O, Anand A. The timing of brain morphological changes in schizophrenia and their relationship to clinical outcome. *Biol Psychiatry*. 1992;31:241-254.

11. Nair TR, Christensen JD, Kingsbury SJ, Kumar NG, Terry WM, Garver DL. Progression of cerebroventricular enlargement and the subtyping of schizophrenia. *Psychiatry Res*. 1997;74:141-150.

12. Gur RE, Cowell P, Turetsky BI, Gallacher F, Cannon T, Bilker W, Gur RC. A follow-up magnetic resonance imaging study of schizophrenia: relationship of neuroanatomical changes to clinical and neurobehavioral measures. *Arch Gen Psychiatry*. 1998;55:145-152.

13. Asarnow J. Annotation: childhood onset schizophrenia. *J Child Psychol Psychiatry*. 1994;35:1345-1371.

14. Asarnow R, Brown W, Strandburg R. Children with a schizophrenic disorder: neurobehavioral studies. *Eur Arch Psychiatry Clin Neurosci*. 1995;245:70-79.

15. Frazier JA, Giedd JN, Hamburger SD, Albus KE, Kaysen D, Vaituzis AC, Rajapakse JC, Lenane MC, McKenna K, Jacobsen LK, Gordon CT, Breier A, Rapoport J. Brain anatomic magnetic resonance imaging in childhood-onset schizophrenia. *Arch Gen Psychiatry*. 1996;53:617-624.

16. Jacobsen L, Rapoport J. Childhood-onset schizophrenia: implications of clinical and neurobiological research. *J Child Psychol Psychiatry*. 1998;39:101-113.

17. Alaghband-Rad J, McKenna K, Gordon C, Albus K, Hamburger S, Rumsey J, Lenane M, Rapoport J. Childhood onset schizophrenia: the severity of premorbid course. *J Am Acad Child Adolesc Psychiatry*. 1995;43:1273-1283.

18. Kumra S, Wiggs E, Krasnewich D, Meck J, Smith A, Bedwell J, Fernandez T, Jacobsen L, Rapoport J. Association of sex chromosome anomalies with childhood onset psychotic disorder. *J Am Acad Child Adolesc Psychiatry*. 1998;37: 292-296.

19. Nicolson R, Rapoport J. Childhood-onset schizophrenia: what can it teach us? In: Rapoport J, ed. *Childhood Onset of Adult Psychopathology: Clinical and Research Advances*. Washington, DC: American Psychiatric Press Inc. In press.

20. Rapoport JL, Giedd J, Kumra S, Jacobsen L, Smith A, Lee P, Nelson J, Hamburger S. Childhood-onset schizophrenia: progressive ventricular change during adolescence. *Arch Gen Psychiatry*. 1997;54:897-903.

21. Collins DL, Neelin P, Peters TM, Evans AC. Automatic 3D intersubject registration of MR volumetric data in standardized Talairach space. *J Comput Assist Tomogr*. 1994;18:192-205.

22. Collins DL, Holmes C, Peters TM, Evans AC. Automatic 3D segmentation of neuroanatomical structures from MRI. *Hum Brain Mapping*. 1995;3:190-208.

23. Zijdenbos A, Evans A, Riahi F, Sled J, Chui H-C, Kollokian, V. Automatic quantification of multiple sclerosis lesion volume using stereotaxic space. In: Hohne KH, Kikinis R, eds. *Proceedings of the Fourth International Conference on Visualization in Biomedical Computing (VBC)*. New York, NY: Springer Publishing Co Inc; 1996:439-448.

24. Evans AC, Collins DL, Holmes CJ. Automatic 3D regional MRI segmentation and statistical probability anatomy maps. In: Uemura K, Jones T, Lassen NA, Kanno I, eds. *Quantification of Brain Function: Tracer Kinetics and Image Analysis in Brain PET*. New York, NY: Excerpta Medica; 1995:123-130.

25. Sled JG, Zijdenbos AP, Evans AC. A non-parametric method for automatic correction of intensity non-uniformity in MRI data. *IEEE Trans Med Imaging*. 1998; 17:87-97.

26. Gordon CT, Frazier JA, McKenna K, Giedd J, Zametkin A, Zahn, T, Hommer D, Hong W, Kaysen D, Albus KE. Childhood-onset schizophrenia: an NIMH study in progress. *Schizophr Bull*. 1994;20:697-712.

27. McKenna K, Gordon CT, Lenane M, Kaysen D, Fahey K, Rapoport J. Looking for childhood onset schizophrenia: the first 71 cases screened. *J Am Acad Child Adolesc Psychiatry*. 1994;33:636-644.

28. Kumra S, Frazier JA, Jacobsen LK, McKenna K, Gordon CT, Lenane MC, Hamburger SD, Smith AK, Albus KE, Alaghband-Rad J, Rapoport JL. Childhood-onset schizophrenia: a double-blind clozapine-haloperidol comparison. *Arch Gen Psychiatry*. 1996;53:1090-1097.

29. Giedd JN, Snell JW, Lange N, Rajapakse JC, Casey BJ, Kozuch PL, Vaituzis AC, Vauss YC, Hamburger SD, Kaysen D, Rapoport JL. Quantitative magnetic resonance imaging of human brain development: ages 4-18. *Cereb Cortex*. 1996;6: 551-560.

30. Hollingshead AB. *Four Factor Index of Social Status*. New Haven, Conn: Yale University Department of Sociology;1975.

31. Collins DL, Evans AC. Animal: validation and applications of non-linear registration-based segmentation. *Int J Pattern Recognition Artif Intell*. 1997;11:1271-1294.

32. Zijdenbos A, Forghani R, Evans AC Automatic quantification of MS lesions in 3D MRI brain data sets: validation of INSECT. In: Delp S, Wells WM, Colchester A, eds. *Medical Image Computing and Computer-Assisted Intervention—MICCAI '98: First International Conference, Cambridge, MA, USA, October 11-13, 1998, Proceedings*. New York, NY: Springer-Verlag NY Inc; 1998:439-448.

33. Duvernoy HM. *The Human Brain: Surface, Three-Dimensional Sectional Anatomy With MRI and Blood Supply*. New York, NY: Springer-Verlag NY Inc; 1991.

34. Pfefferbaum A, Mathalon DH, Sullivan EV, Rawles JM, Zipursky RB, Kim KO. A quantitative magnetic resonance imaging study of changes in brain morphology from infancy to late adulthood. *Arch Neurol*. 1994;51:874-887.

35. Reiss A, Abrams M, Singer H, Ross J, Denckla M. Brain development, gender, and IQ in children: a volumetric imaging study. *Brain*. 1996;119:1763-1774.

36. Sowell E, Thompson P, Holmes C, Jernigan TR, Barth R, Naravan S, Toga A. Statistical parametric mapping of structural brain changes between childhood and adolescence. Presented as poster 43.3 at the 28th Annual Meeting of the Society for Neurosciences; November 7-12, 1998; Los Angeles, Calif.

37. Sowell E, Jernigan T. Further MRI evidence of late brain maturation: limbic volume increases and changing asymmetries during childhood and adolescence. *Dev Neuropsychol*. In press.

38. Benes F, Turtle M, Khan Y, Faroi P. Myelenization of a key relay zone in the hippocampal formation occurs in the human brain during childhood, adolescence, and adulthood. *Arch Gen Psychiatry*. 1994;51:477-484.

39. Jernigan T, Tallal P. Late childhood changes in brain morphology observable with MRI. *Dev Med Child Neurol*. 1990;32:379-385.

40. Huttenlocher P, DeCourten C. The development of synapses in striate cortex of man. *Hum Neurobiol*. 1987;6:1-9.

41. Sauer B, Kammradt I, Krauthausen G, Kretchmann H, Lange H, Wingert F. Qualitative and quantitative development of the visual cortex in man. *J Comp Neurol*. 1983;214:441-450.

42. Cannon TD, van Erp TG, Huttunen M, Lonnqvist J, Salonen O, Valanne L, Poutanen VP, Standertskjold-Nordenstam CG, Gur RE, Yan M. Regional gray matter, white matter, and cerebrospinal fluid distributions in schizophrenic patients, their siblings, and controls. *Arch Gen Psychiatry*. 1998;55:1084-1091.

43. Weinberger D, Berman K, Suddath R, Torrey E. Evidence of dysfunction of a prefrontal-limbic network in schizophrenia: a magnetic resonance imaging and regional cerebral blood flow study of discordant monozygotic twins. *Am J Psychiatry*. 1992;149:890-897.

44. Selemon LD, Rajkowska G, Goldman-Rakic PS. Abnormally high neuronal density in the schizophrenic cortex: a morphometric analysis of prefrontal area 9 and occipital area 17. *Arch Gen Psychiatry*. 1995;52:805-818.

45. Rajkowska G, Selemon LD, Goldman-Rakic PS. Neuronal and glial somal size in the prefrontal cortex: a postmortem morphometric study of schizophrenia and Huntington disease. *Arch Gen Psychiatry*. 1998;55:215-224.

46. Selemon LD, Goldman-Rakic PS. The reduced neuropil hypothesis: a circuit-based model of schizophrenia. *Biol Psychiatry*. 1999;45:17-25.

47. Huttenlocher PR. Synaptic density in human frontal cortex—developmental changes and effects of aging. *Brain Res*. 1979;163:195.

48. Huttenlocher PR, Dabholkar AS. Regional differences in synaptogenesis in human cerebral cortex. *J Comp Neurol*. 1997;387:167-178.

49. Chugani H, Phelps M, Mazziotta JC. Positron emission tomography study of human brain functional development. *Ann Neurol*. 1987;22:487-497.

50. Giedd J, Jeffries N, Nicolson R, Hamburger SD, Nelson J, Vaituzis AC, Lenane M, Rapoport JL. Differential progression of MRI ventricular and temporal lobe structure during adolescence for childhood onset schizophrenics. *Biol Psychiatry*. In press.

51. Feinberg I. Schizophrenia: caused by a fault in programmed synaptic elimination during adolescence? *J Psychiatr Res*. 1982;17:317-334.

52. Feinberg I, Thode HC Jr, Chugani HT, March JD. Gamma distribution model describes maturational curves for delta wave amplitude, cortical metabolic rate and synaptic density. *J Theor Biol*. 1990;142:149-161.

53. Irwin SA, Swain RA, Christion FA, Chakravarti A, Galvez R, Greenough WT. Behavioral alteration of fragile X mental retardation protein expression. Presented as poster 171.7 at: 28th Annual Meeting of the Society for Neurosciences; November 7-12, 1998; Los Angeles, Calif.

120

Mapping adolescent brain change reveals dynamic wave of accelerated gray matter loss in very early-onset schizophrenia

Paul M. Thompson*[†], Christine Vidal*, Jay N. Giedd[‡], Peter Gochman[‡], Jonathan Blumenthal[‡], Robert Nicolson[‡], Arthur W. Toga*, and Judith L. Rapoport[‡]

*Laboratory of Neuro Imaging, Department of Neurology, Division of Brain Mapping, 4238 Reed Neurology, University of California School of Medicine, Los Angeles, CA 90095-1761; and [‡]Child Psychiatry Branch, National Institute of Mental Health, National Institutes of Health, Bethesda, MD 20892-1600

Edited by Solomon H. Snyder, Johns Hopkins University School of Medicine, Baltimore, MD, and approved July 18, 2001 (received for review May 16, 2001)

Neurodevelopmental models for the pathology of schizophrenia propose both polygenetic and environmental risks, as well as early (pre/perinatal) and late (usually adolescent) developmental brain abnormalities. With the use of brain mapping algorithms, we detected striking anatomical profiles of accelerated gray matter loss in very early-onset schizophrenia; surprisingly, deficits moved in a dynamic pattern, enveloping increasing amounts of cortex throughout adolescence. Early-onset patients were rescanned prospectively with MRI, at 2-year intervals at three time points, to uncover the dynamics and timing of disease progression during adolescence. The earliest deficits were found in parietal brain regions, supporting visuospatial and associative thinking, where adult deficits are known to be mediated by environmental (nongenetic) factors. Over 5 years, these deficits progressed anteriorly into temporal lobes, engulfing sensorimotor and dorsolateral prefrontal cortices, and frontal eye fields. These emerging patterns correlated with psychotic symptom severity and mirrored the neuromotor, auditory, visual search, and frontal executive impairments in the disease. In temporal regions, gray matter loss was completely absent early in the disease but became pervasive later. Only the latest changes included dorsolateral prefrontal cortex and superior temporal gyri, deficit regions found consistently in adult studies. These emerging dynamic patterns were (i) controlled for medication and IQ effects, (ii) replicated in independent groups of males and females, and (iii) charted in individuals and groups. The resulting mapping strategy reveals a shifting pattern of tissue loss in schizophrenia. Aspects of the anatomy and dynamics of disease are uncovered, in a changing profile that implicates genetic and nongenetic patterns of deficits.

L ittle is known about the profile of brain change in adolescence and its modulation in diseases with adolescent onset. Schizophrenia, for example, has typical onset in late adolescence or early adulthood. Cases occurring in childhood or early adolescence, however, present unique opportunities to study disease development during adolescence. Childhood-onset schizophrenia (COS) is a severe form of the disorder that appears to be clinically and neurobiologically continuous with the later onset illness (1). The causes of schizophrenia are not known, but it is increasingly considered a neurodevelopmental disorder (2, 3). Both early (pre-natal) and later abnormalities of brain development have been proposed (4–6). However, neither the anatomical pattern nor the timing of these developmental events has been established.

In response to these challenges, we designed a brain mapping strategy to uncover deficit patterns as they emerged in populations imaged longitudinally through adolescence for 5 years. Because gray matter is implicated in schizophrenia and is also known to occur in adolescence (7–15), we set out to create detailed spatio-temporal maps of these loss processes. Their timing and anatomical profile are fundamental to understanding how the disease emerges; so far it has been difficult to test hypotheses about genetic and environmental triggers of schizophrenia because the topography and dynamics of the disease, especially at the cortex, are not well understood. In a recent cross-sectional genetic study based on a

cohort of 80 adult twins discordant for schizophrenia,[§] we isolated a genetic continuum in which cortical deficits were found in gradually increasing degrees, in individuals with increasing genetic affinity to a patient. By controlling for common genotype, we isolated discrete regions of cortex whose deficits were attributable to genetic and to nongenetic factors, although the emergence and timing of these deficits could not be evaluated.

The current study was intended to chart the emergence of these deficits in a severely affected cohort followed for 5 years, revealing an unsuspected developmental trajectory in these schizophrenic adolescents. This technique uncovered a dynamic wave of accelerated gray matter loss, spreading from parietal cortices at disease onset to encompass temporal and frontal regions later in the disease. The rates and temporal sequencing of cortical gray matter loss was mapped in the teenage years and was found to be greatly accelerated in diseased relative to healthy teenagers matched for age, gender, and demographics. The final profile was consistent with the loss pattern in adult schizophrenia. We also correlated loss rates with symptom severity and controlled for potential medication and IQ effects. Local changes were examined in relation to genetic and nongenetic deficit patterns found in adults. This study is therefore a three-dimensional visualization of the timing, rates, and anatomical distribution of brain structure changes in adolescents with schizophrenia. It suggests a dynamic structural basis for early prodromal symptoms and for the positive and negative deficit symptoms observed clinically (16).

Methods

Summary. Three-dimensional maps of brain change were derived from high-resolution magnetic resonance images (MRI scans) acquired repeatedly from the same subjects over a 5-year time span. Twelve schizophrenic subjects (aged 13.9 ± 0.8 years at first scan) and a parallel group of 12 healthy adolescents (aged 13.5 ± 0.7 years at initial scan) were imaged repeatedly for 4.6 years (the combined groups were scanned every 2.3 years ± 1.4 months (SD); for clarity this is referred to as 5 years). Patients and controls were matched for age, gender, and demographics

This paper was submitted directly (Track II) to the PNAS office.

Abbreviations: NOS, not otherwise specified; SAPS/SANS, Scales for the Assessment of Positive and Negative Symptoms; COS, childhood-onset schizophrenia.

[†]To whom reprint requests should be addressed at: Laboratory of Neuro Imaging, Department of Neurology, Reed Neurological Research Center, Room 4238, University of California School of Medicine, 710 Westwood Plaza, Los Angeles, CA 90095-1769. E-mail: thompson@loni.ucla.edu.

[§]Cannon, T. D., Thompson, P. M., van Erp, T. G. M., Toga, A. W., Huttunen, M., Lönnqvist, J. & Standertskjöld-Nordenstam, C.-G., A Probabilistic Atlas of Cortical Gray Matter Changes in Monozygotic Twins Discordant for Schizophrenia, Proceedings of the International Congress on Schizophrenia Research, Whistler, Canada, April 28–May 2, 2001 (available at http://www.loni.ucla.edu/~thompson/HBM2001/ty_HBM2001.html).

The publication costs of this article were defrayed in part by page charge payment. This article must therefore be hereby marked "advertisement" in accordance with 18 U.S.C. §1734 solely to indicate this fact.

122

A

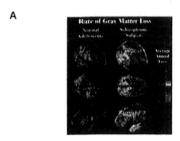

B

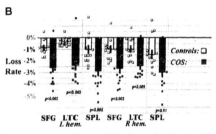

SFG LTC SPL   SFG LTC SPL
  L hem.   *R hem.*

Fig. 1. Average rates of gray matter loss in normal adolescents and in schizophrenia. (*A*) Three-dimensional maps of brain changes, derived from high-resolution magnetic resonance images (MRI scans) acquired repeatedly from the same subjects, reveal profound, progressive gray matter loss in schizophrenia (*Right*). Average rates of gray matter loss from 13 to 18 years of age are displayed on average cortical models for the group. Severe loss is observed (red and pink; up to 5% annually) in parietal, motor, and temporal cortices, whereas inferior frontal cortices remain stable (blue; 0–1% loss). Dynamic loss is also observed in the parietal cortices of normal adolescents, but at a much slower rate. (*B*) Average gray matter loss rates were computed for all 24 subjects in superior frontal gyri (SFG), lateral temporal cortices (LTC), and superior parietal lobules (SPL) in both brain hemispheres. Error bars indicate the standard error of the sample means, by region, in controls and patients. Individual loss rates (in percent per year) are plotted (■, patients; □, controls), showing significant group separation, despite some outliers.

and were scanned identically on the same scanner at exactly the same ages and intervals. The three-dimensional distribution of gray matter in the brain was computed, as in previous studies of Alzheimer's disease (17), and was compared from one scan to the next with the use of a computational cortical pattern matching strategy that aligns corresponding locations on the cortical surface, across time and across subjects. This procedure allowed us to pool maps of individual gray matter loss over time. Average rates of gray matter loss were computed for each region and compared across corresponding regions of cortex (Fig. 1), before a more detailed analysis of nonlinear and age-dependent effects. The amount of loss and the rate of loss were evaluated. Findings were also examined in relation to genetic and nongenetic patterns found in recent studies of adult patients.

Subjects and Imaging. Subjects were recruited as part of an ongoing National Institute of Mental Health study of schizophrenia. Twelve patients (six males and six females) and 12 healthy volunteers (six males and six females), as well as an additional medication-matched group (see below), were followed longitudinally. All

patients satisfied DSM-III-R diagnostic criteria for schizophrenia (18), with onset of psychotic symptoms by age 12. All patients had a history of poor response to, or intolerance of, at least two typical neuroleptics. They had a mean full-scale IQ at study entry of 70.4 ± 12.9 SD and no other active neurological or medical disease. Diagnosis was determined from clinical and structured interviews with the adolescents and their parents based on portions of the Schedule for Affective Disorders and Schizophrenia for School-Age Children–Epidemiologic Version (19) and of the Diagnostic Interview for Children and Adolescents Revised (20), as well as from previous records. Psychopathological symptoms were evaluated with the use of the Scales for the Assessment of Positive and Negative Symptoms (SAPS/SANS) (21) and the Brief Psychiatric Rating Scale (22) (see ref. 1 for details). Normal adolescent controls were screened for medical, neurologic, and psychiatric illness and learning disabilities as described (1). We rigorously matched the cohorts for age (see below), gender, follow-up interval (which was identical), social background, and height.

Medication and IQ-Matched Group. Medication effects were assessed by analyzing a second group of nonschizophrenic medication-matched subjects. The 10 age- and gender-matched psychosis patients not otherwise specified (NOS) (1, 23) received the same medication as the schizophrenic group and follow-up but did not satisfy DSM-III-R criteria for schizophrenia. They were also IQ-matched with the COS patients (mean IQ: 76 ± 10 SD) and matched for age, gender, and demographics with the healthy controls. These children had very transient psychotic symptoms, emotional lability, poor interpersonal skills, normal social interest, and multiple deficits in information processing (1). They were less severely impaired than the COS group but continued with a mixture of mood and behavior problems. None at follow-up was schizophrenic but rather exhibited chronic mood disturbance and lack of behavioral control; they were treated with neuroleptics for these symptoms (at doses similar to that used for COS; see below), which were quite effective in controlling these behaviors.

Of the 10 psychosis NOS patients, two patients received 300 and 450 mg clozapine (mean dose 375 mg/day), six received risperidone (2–8 mg; mean dose 5.25 ± 2.4 mg/day) [four in combination with valproic acid (mean 1,025 mg/day) and one in combination with olanzapine (20 mg/day)], and two were drug-free.

Magnetic Resonance Imaging. Three-dimensional (256² × 124 resolution) T₁-weighted fast SPGR (spoiled gradient) MRI volumes were acquired from all 34 subjects. All images were acquired with the same 1.5-T Signa scanner (General Electric) located at the National Institutes of Health Clinical Center (Bethesda, MD). Imaging parameters were as follows: time to echo, 5 ms; time to repeat, 24 ms; flip angle, 45°; and field of view, 24 cm. The same set of 12 healthy controls was scanned at baseline (aged 13.5 ± 0.7 years) and ultimately after a 5-year interval (mean interval: 4.6 ± 0.2 years; age: 18.0 ± 0.8 years). In parallel, the 12 age- and gender-matched schizophrenic subjects were identically scanned at the exact same ages and intervals (mean age at first scan: 13.9 ± 0.8 years; 18.6 ± 1.0 years at final scan; mean interval: 4.6 ± 0.3 years). All subjects (controls, schizophrenic subjects, and the medication controls) were scanned three times, first at baseline, then a mean of 2.3 years later, and then again 4.6 years later. The combined groups were scanned every 2.3 years ± 1.4 months (SD).

Image Processing and Analysis. For each scan pair, a radiofrequency bias field correction algorithm eliminated intensity drifts due to scanner field inhomogeneity. The initial scan was then rigidly aligned (registered) to the target (24) and a supervised tissue classifier generated detailed maps of gray matter, white matter, and cerebrospinal fluid (25). A nearest-neighbor tissue classifier then assigned each image voxel to a particular

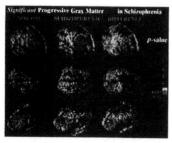

Fig. 2. Significance of dynamic gray matter loss in normal adolescents and in schizophrenia. Highly significant progressive loss occurs in schizophrenia in parietal, motor, supplementary motor, and superior frontal cortices. Broad regions of temporal cortex, including the superior temporal gyrus, experience severe gray matter attrition. By comparison of the average rates of loss in disease (middle column) with the loss pattern in normal adolescents (first column), the normal variability in these changes can also be taken into account, and the significance of disease-specific change can be established (last column).

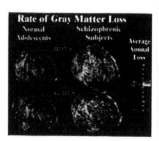

Fig. 3. Dynamic changes in male and female teenagers with schizophrenia. A consistent pattern of progressive gray matter loss, in parietal, frontal, and temporal cortices, is observed in independent groups of males and female patients. A single pattern is observable in both boys and girls, supporting the anatomical specificity of the findings.

tissue class (gray, white, or cerebrospinal fluid) or to a background class (15). Gray matter maps were retained for subsequent analysis.

Three-Dimensional Cortical Maps. To compare and pool cortical data across subjects, a high-resolution surface model of the cortex was automatically extracted for each subject and time point. Based on the cortical models we created for each subject at different time points, a three-dimensional deformation vector field was computed that captured the shape change in the brain surface across the time interval. This method allows us to accommodate any brain shape changes when comparing cortical gray matter within a subject across time. Given that the deformation maps associate cortical locations with the same relation to the primary folding pattern across subjects, a local measurement of gray matter density was made in each subject and averaged across equivalent cortical locations. To quantify local gray matter, we used a measure termed gray matter density (15, 17, 26, 27). This method measures the proportion of gray matter in a small region of fixed radius (5 mm) around each cortical point. Given the large anatomic variability in some cortical regions, high-dimensional elastic matching of cortical patterns (17, 28) was used to associate measures of gray matter density from homologous cortical regions across subjects and across time. Annualized four-dimensional maps of gray matter loss rates within each subject were elastically realigned for averaging and comparison across diagnostic groups. Statistical maps were generated that indicated locally the degree to which gray matter loss rates were statistically linked with diagnosis, gender, and positive or negative symptoms (SAPS/SANS) (21). The P value describing the significance of this linkage was plotted at each point on the cortex with a color code to produce a statistical map (e.g., Fig. 2). A null distribution was developed for the area of the average cortex with statistics above a fixed threshold in the significance maps (17, 29), so the significance of the loss patterns could be assessed after the appropriate correction for multiple comparisons.

Results

In schizophrenic patients, a striking accelerated loss of gray matter (peak values > 5% loss/year; Fig. 1A) was observed in a broad anatomical region encompassing frontal eye fields and supplementary motor, sensorimotor, parietal, and temporal cortices in both brain hemispheres (see Fig. 1). Average loss rates were significantly

faster in patients in superior parietal lobules (left hemisphere mean ± standard error: 2.9 ± 0.5%/year, right hemisphere: 2.9 ± 0.5%/year; in controls: 1.1 ± 0.4 and 1.4 ± 0.5; group difference: $P < 0.005$ and 0.01), in superior frontal cortices (L/R: 2.6 ± 0.5 and 2.7 ± 0.4 in patients; 0.9 ± 0.3 and 1.0 ± 0.3 in controls; group difference: $P < 0.003$ and 0.002), and in lateral temporal cortices (L/R: 2.3 ± 0.9 and 2.4 ± 0.4 in patients; 0.7 ± 0.2 and 1.1 ± 0.3 in controls; group difference: $P < 0.003$ and 0.005). Subtle but significant changes were detected in normal adolescents (0.9–1.4% average loss per year; all regions showed significant loss, at $P < 0.02$). The schizophrenia group exhibited a region of intense, severely progressive loss, terminating anteriorly in the frontal eye fields and encompassing the temporal cortices.

Significance of the Progressive Loss. To understand whether these changes could be normal fluctuations, the variability in both the anatomical distribution and loss rates for gray matter were computed locally across the cortex, and the significance of the changes was established. Again, schizophrenic subjects underwent a significant, pervasive, and unrelenting loss of gray matter ($P < 0.00002$, all P values corrected), with progressive deficits throughout superior frontal, motor, and parietal brain regions, and a separate loss pattern observed in temporal cortices. Normal adolescents also lost tissue ($P < 0.05$, in parietal regions) even after normal variability was accounted for (Fig. 2A). A subtraction map was created to emphasize the fundamental loss pattern specific to the disease (Fig. 2C). Regions of progressive loss, in both anterior frontal and temporal cortices, were anatomically circumscribed in both the percentage loss and significance maps and appeared to terminate anteriorly in the frontal eye fields (Figs. 1 and 2). These figures show regions where tissue loss is faster in diseased than in normal adolescents. The same anatomically specific, dynamic profiles of tissue loss were replicated in independent samples of male and female schizophrenic patients (Fig. 3), suggesting that a similar profile and degree of progressive gray matter loss may operate in schizophrenia, irrespective of gender.

Nonlinear Loss. We further hypothesized that loss rates would be relatively greater in younger patients, possibly reflecting a more severe neurodevelopmental abnormality that may have led to an earlier illness onset and/or a disease-related exaggeration of nonlinear normal developmental processes. Right parietal and sensorimotor cortices (Fig. 4) underwent significantly faster loss in the younger adolescents, consistent with recent findings of overall volume reductions specific to parietal lobes in younger patients (30). In other brain regions, the rates of gray matter loss were not

124

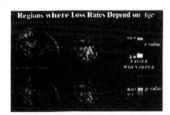

Fig. 4. Mapping nonlinear brain changes and age effects. Dependencies between the rate of gray matter loss and the patient's age are mapped locally and visualized. Parietal regions lose gray matter faster in younger patients (red; $r > 0.8$; $P < 0.001$), consistent with an earlier timing of deficits and a slowing of the rates of progression as adolescence continues.

strongly affected by age, corroborating the use of annual averages to describe the dynamic pattern. Although nonlinear effects in other brain regions may be detectable in a much larger cohort, similar annual rates of loss were observed consistently in subjects throughout our sample, and across independent samples (Fig. 3).

Early Deficits. Because of the apparent sparing of inferior frontal cortices in the dynamic maps (Figs. 1 and 2) and their appearance in our recent cross-sectional studies of adult schizophrenia,[§] we were concerned that earlier (perinatal or prepubertal) nonprogressive maldevelopment may not have been observed in the dynamic maps, as these maps only capture loss that intensifies over time. To detect earlier loss, we compared gray matter profiles across all 24 subjects at their first scan (Fig. 5 *Upper*) and at their last scan 4.6 years later (Fig. 5 *Lower*). Two striking features emerged. First, the severe progressive lateral temporal and dorsolateral prefrontal cortex deficit observed later was not apparent at age 13, even at a mean of 3 years after the onset of psychotic symptoms. These deficits, which are characteristic of adult and childhood schizophrenia (1, 31), were severely progressive after illness onset (on average 5% lateral temporal attrition per year) but were absent in the early phase of the disease. In evaluating the power of the approach, we would have been likely to detect an early temporal and dorsolateral prefrontal cortex deficit, if present, but the near identity (to within 0–1%) of average normal and patient gray matter distribution at first scan, combined with the high rate of progression and significant deficit observed later (Fig. 5*B*), jointly suggest that the process of temporal and prefrontal gray matter attrition is a later develop-

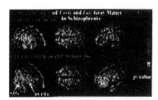

Fig. 5. Mapping early and late deficits in schizophrenia. Deficits occurring during the development of schizophrenia are detected by comparing average profiles of gray matter between patients and controls at their first scan (age 13; *Upper*) and their last scan 5 years later (age 18; *Lower*). Although parietal, motor, and diffuse frontal loss has already occurred (*Upper*) and subsequently continues (Figs. 1 and 2), the temporal and dorsolateral prefrontal loss characteristic of adult schizophrenia is not found until later in adolescence (*Lower*), where a process of fast attrition occurs over the next 5 years. The color code shows the significance of these effects.

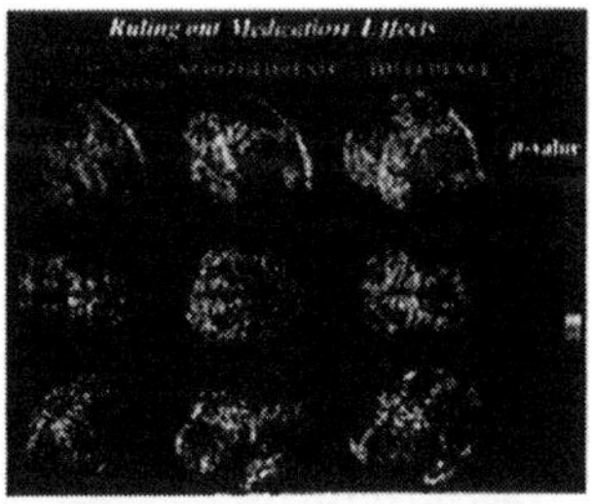

Fig. 6. Mapping brain change in medication-matched subjects not satisfying criteria for schizophrenia. No temporal lobe deficits are found, suggesting that the progression of the deficits into the temporal lobe is specific to schizophrenia, regardless of medication (and regardless of gender; Fig. 3). Nonetheless, these patients share some symptoms with schizophrenics, exhibiting frontal deficits in a similar anatomical pattern. These frontal deficits (i.e., gray matter loss rates) are statistically significant relative to healthy controls but significantly smaller in magnitude than the greatly accelerated loss rates in schizophrenia.

mental event. Second, parietal and motor cortices showed a severe early deficit (up to 20% loss; $P < 0.0005$) with diffuse loss in other (but not temporal) cortical regions. This early (prepubertal) parietal deficit is consistent with the faster parietal loss found in younger patients (Fig. 4), whereas the dynamics of loss in other regions is more uniform with age. The initial parietal deficit, which is also progressive (Fig. 1), also occurs in regions where normal adolescents lose gray matter, although in disease this loss process is significantly accelerated (Fig. 2). Although it is unclear whether the normal and aberrant processes have a similar mechanism or are independent, the parietal and motor cortical deficits are progressive and are the earliest to develop. We recently found that the parietal regions, specifically, are also in deficit in adult patients relative to genetically identical controls (their monozygotic discordant twins). This finding indicates that environmental and not purely genetic factors are implicated in triggering this deficit, at least in adults.[§] In the present study, a dynamic wave of progression from parietal cortices occurs later, into superior frontal, dorsolateral prefrontal, and temporal cortices (including superior temporal gyri; Fig. 5). These regions comprise a specific band of cortical territory in which adult deficits are thought to be strongly influenced by genetic factors (32),[§] as deficits here (i) are found in unaffected relatives and (ii) significantly covary with an individual's degree of genetic affinity to a patient. In our adolescent cohort, the temporal and dorsolateral prefrontal cortex deficits were among the most severe but began in late adolescence and were observed only after symptom onset (Fig. 5).

Medication-Matched Subjects. To address the possibility that neuroleptic exposure and/or lower IQ could have determined differential gray matter loss in the schizophrenics, we mapped 10 serially imaged subjects referred to the childhood schizophrenia study who did not meet diagnostic criteria for schizophrenia [labeled psychosis NOS, in DSM (18) terms] (23). These subjects received medication identical to that of the patients in this study through adolescence, primarily for control of aggressive outbursts, and at follow-up, none had progressed to schizophrenia (33) but all continued to exhibit chronic mood and behavior disturbance. Although medication is unlikely to be responsible for a loss profile that moves across the brain, clozapine, for example, may increase Fos immunoreactivity in the thalamus (34) and might, logically, modulate rates of cortical change. (In addition, brain regions important for motor function,

125

Table 1. Clinical severity of the schizophrenic and medication-controlled groups

		Schizophrenics (COS)	Medication/IQ controls (psychosis NOS)
SAPS	Baseline	58.3 ± 5.3	18.4 ± 5.1
	Follow-up	18.2 ± 4.3	20.2 ± 5.4
SANS	Baseline	73.8 ± 4.7	19.3 ± 3.9
	Follow-up	49.8 ± 8.5	28.4 ± 5.8
CGAS	Baseline	37.4 ± 5.7	43.0 ± 6.5
	Follow-up	30.8 ± 3.4	41.9 ± 3.8

SANS and SAPS tests (22) of positive and negative symptom severity (as well as the Children's Global Assessment of Functioning Scale, CGAS) (58) were administered both at baseline and every 2.3 years at follow-up. Mean scores and standard errors are given for both groups, at study entry and at the follow-up 4.6 years later. SAPS and SANS scores improved in the COS group ($P < 3 \times 10^{-6}$ and $P < 0.005$, respectively), partly as a result of neuroleptic treatment. However, the COS group's positive and negative symptoms were initially much more severe than the medication/IQ controls ($P < 2 \times 10^{-5}$ and $P < 10^{-7}$ for SAPS and SANS, respectively), and they were more impaired in global functioning at follow-up (group difference: $P < 0.05$).

including the basal ganglia, show increased volumes in response to some older, conventional neuroleptics, although these effects are renormalized after treatment with the atypical antipsychotics used in this study.) As seen in Fig. 6, although the nonschizophrenic group did show some subtle but significant tissue loss, this loss was much less marked than for the schizophrenics. Moreover, no temporal lobe deficits were observed in the psychosis NOS group (Fig. 6), suggesting that the wave of disease progression into temporal cortices may be specific to schizophrenia, regardless of medication and gender or IQ. Intriguingly, the psychosis NOS subjects, who share some of the deficit symptoms but do not satisfy criteria for schizophrenia, exhibited significantly accelerated gray matter loss in frontal cortices relative to healthy controls, in approximately the same (but a less pervasive) region as schizophrenics (a significant loss of 1.9% ± 0.7%/year was detected in both left and right superior frontal gyri; $P < 0.03$). Groups of healthy controls, psychosis NOS, and schizophrenic patients therefore lost frontal gray matter at successively increasing rates, i.e., in a statistical hierarchy with loss rates significantly faster in the nonschizophrenic control group than in healthy controls, and even faster in schizophrenia. In the region where the medication controls were affected (superior frontal cortices), their deficits at follow-up averaged 7.5% ± 1.6% relative to healthy controls ($P < 0.006$). This deficit was significantly less severe ($P < 0.05$) than the 13.0% ± 3.2% deficit in the schizophrenic group ($P < 0.001$, relative to healthy controls), whose global functioning was more greatly impaired at follow-up ($P < 0.05$; compare Children's Global Assessment of Functioning Scale scores, Table 1).

Relationship to Clinical Deficits. We further evaluated the clinical specificity and functional correlates of these findings. The patient group deteriorated overall; their Children's Global Assessment of Functioning Scale scores, which provide a global assessment of function, deteriorated from 37.4 ± 5.7 at study entry to 30.8 ± 3.4 at follow-up ($P < 0.05$; Table 1). Meanwhile, the average scores for the IQ/medication control group remained stable (43.0 ± 6.5 at entry; 41.9 ± 3.8 at follow-up) and were higher (less impaired) than those of the schizophrenic patients at follow-up ($P < 0.05$). This finding suggests an overall deterioration of global functioning in COS, consistent with the progressive deterioration of structure.

At an individual level, rates of temporal loss correlated strongly with a SAPS total score at final scan (21) ($P < 0.015$, left hemisphere; $P < 0.004$, right hemisphere; all p values corrected). Faster loss in both the superior temporal gyri and the entire temporal cortices was significantly associated with a more severe

clinical profile of positive symptoms (e.g., hallucinations or delusions). Although tissue loss rates were not significantly linked with the rate of change in SAPS scores from baseline ($P > 0.05$), and SAPS scores were not linked with the amount of tissue at baseline ($P > 0.05$), loss rates were a good predictor of positive symptoms at follow-up, i.e., the remaining symptoms that were refractory to medication. In addition, those with the least overall tissue deficit had the best cognitive performance in terms of full-scale IQ at follow-up, and those with the worst deficit on MRI had the lowest full-scale IQ at follow-up ($r = 0.62$; $P < 0.016$). Gray matter quantity at initial scan was also a good predictor of full-scale IQ in the patient group at follow-up ($r = 0.52$; $P < 0.042$). At baseline, this linkage did not reach significance ($r = 0.44$; $P = 0.077$), but a change in correlations between baseline and follow-up was not significant ($r_2 - r_1 = 0.18$; $z = 0.54$; $P = 0.3$). Faster loss rates in frontal cortex were also strongly correlated with more severe negative symptoms (e.g., flat affect, poverty of speech; $P < 0.038$ for total SANS score at final scan). This linkage is consistent with the physiological hypothesis that negative symptoms of schizophrenia may depend on reduced dopaminergic activity in frontal cortices (35). The tight linkage between the deficit symptoms of schizophrenia and the pervasive loss of cortical tissue suggests a disease mechanism that may only be partially opposed by neuroleptics (36).

Discussion

During the development of schizophrenia in these early adolescent subjects, a dynamic wave of gray matter loss occurred, starting in parietal association cortices and proceeding frontally to envelop dorsolateral prefrontal cortex and temporal cortices, including the superior temporal gyri. The deficits spread and intensified, in the same subjects, over 5 years of disease progression and eventually engulfed parietal, motor and supplementary motor, temporal (including primary auditory), and prefrontal cortices. The dynamic pattern is intriguing, as it begins in brain regions where deficits, at least in adults, appear to be mediated by environmental (nongenetic) factors (parietal cortices).[§] It then progresses over a multiyear time frame into frontal and temporal regions where deficits appear, from our twin and other familial studies, to be strongly mediated by genetic factors (32).

Relation to Prior Findings. The dynamic pattern of loss may also suggest a structural basis for the prodromal and chronic neuromotor, sensory, and associative deficits observed clinically and in studies of the functional and metabolic integrity of the cortex. Glucose metabolism is reduced in frontal cortices in chronic childhood and adult schizophrenics both at rest and during the performance of tasks that increase frontal lobe metabolism, such as the Continuous Performance Test (38). COS patients also display significantly increased metabolic rates in inferior frontal gyri, with marked decreases in superior and middle frontal gyri. This profile may mirror, to some degree, the discrete pattern of accelerated gray matter loss identified here (Fig. 1). Whether or not this increased metabolism represents an adaptive or compensatory response to cell loss in superior frontal systems, a similar underlying pathophysiology may underlie these structural, metabolic, and functional impairments as the disease develops.

The early parietal deficits observed here are consistent with recent functional MRI studies in adult patients showing marked parietal activation deficits in working memory tasks (38). Recent functional imaging studies with positron emission tomography (39, 40) and functional MRI (41) also show a diminished activation of the sensorimotor cortex and supplementary motor area during motor tasks (finger-to-thumb opposition) in schizophrenia. Implication of cortical motor systems is also consistent with preceding motor impairments, consistently noted in studies of COS. In frontal cortices, regions of the fastest progressive gray matter loss terminated anteriorly in the frontal eye fields. Visual search tasks are thought to tap a key attentional dysfunction in schizophrenia (42),

126

namely a deficit in the ability to hone in on the most important elements in a picture and a tendency to stare instead of engaging in active visual search. By studying exploratory eye movements during scene perception, impairments have been observed in schizophrenic adolescents in the basic control of exploratory eye movements, suggesting that they stared more and had difficulty in the top-down control of selective attention and visual search. Continuous attrition of gray matter in frontal eye fields may underlie some of the deficit symptoms in visual attention. The marked anterior limit of the loss pattern around the anterior limit of the frontal eye fields (Brodmann area 8) may indicate an anatomically specific progression that has a direct impact on the systems supporting attentional dysfunction.

Recent neuropathological studies (43), evaluating regional neuronal density postmortem, have found altered cell packing of pyramidal and nonpyramidal neurons in the schizophrenic cortex, with a disproportionate reduction in layer V of prefrontal area 9. Pathologic and in vivo MRI studies jointly suggest that neuronal atrophy may be one anatomic substrate for deficient information processing in schizophrenia. Altered laminar density of cells in the schizophrenic cortex and moderate reductions in cortical thickness may be major contributors to the intense dynamic processes of gray matter loss that are imaged here in vivo and mapped as they spread from parietal to frontal and temporal regions.

Developmental Implications. Neurodevelopmental theories of the onset of schizophrenia posit disturbances, either pre- or postnatal, in the processes of neuronal migration (3, 44), or in synaptic pruning, which intensifies around the age of 5 years (15, 45–47). Our data indicate that structural changes clearly progress after

psychosis onset and well into adolescence, consistent with earlier reports of ventricular expansion and overall lobar reduction (7, 9, 48). Cross-sectional studies of this COS population have also found a failure of normal maturation in neurological test performance during adolescence (49). This level of performance is also consistent with several recent brain structure studies showing more subtle but significant progressive cortical gray matter loss in adult-onset schizophrenia (8, 11, 50, 51). Perhaps surprisingly in this cohort, whereas parietal and frontal/motor deficits precede puberty, temporal deficits do not. It is probable that early neurodevelopmental abnormalities and later gray matter loss are related, as genes affecting prenatal development may also have roles in later brain maturation (45, 52, 53). Intriguingly, the earliest deficits occur in a region of parietal cortices where progressive cortical change occurs significantly both in healthy and schizophrenic subjects in the teenage years. In adults, parietal deficits appear to be mediated by environmental (nongenetic) factors, as the mathematical pattern of these deficits distinguishes schizophrenic adult twins from their healthy, genetically identical, monozygotic co-twins. Finally, the frontal and temporal territories, which were spared when our cohort was first scanned, are later engulfed by the wave of tissue loss. In these regions, deficits in adult patients appear to be highly heritable (32). By dissociating early brain structure deficits that predate psychosis onset, those that progress, and those that begin in adolescence, dynamic and genetic brain mapping may shed light on the triggers of schizophrenia. These findings are consistent with the notion that activation of some nongenetic trigger contributes to the onset and initial progression of the illness (54, 55).

Grant support was provided by P41 RR13642, National Institutes of Health intramural funding, LM/MH05639, NS38753, and P20 MH/DA52176.

1. Jacobsen, L. K. & Rapoport, J. L. (1998) *J. Child Psychol. Psychiatry* **39**, 101–113.
2. Feinberg, I. (1982) *J. Psychiatr. Res.* **17**, 319–334.
3. Weinberger, D. R. (1995) in *Schizophrenia*, eds. Hirsch, S. R. & Weinberger, D. R. (Blackwood, London), pp. 294–323.
4. Baromdas, S. H., Alberts, B. M., Andreasen, N. C., Bargmann, C., Benes, F., Goldman-Rakic, P., Gottesman, I., Heinemann, S. F., Jones E. G., Kirschner, M., *et al.* (1997) *Proc. Natl. Acad. Sci. USA* **94**, 1612–1614.
5. McGlashan, T. H. & Hoffman, R. E. (2000) *Arch. Gen. Psychiatry* **57**, 637–648.
6. Selemon, L. D. & Goldman-Rakic, P. S. (1999) *Biol. Psychiatry* **45**, 17–25.
7. Rapoport, J. L., Giedd, J., Kumra, S., Jacobsen, L., Smith, A., Lee, P., Nelson, J. & Hamburger, S. (1997) *Arch. Gen. Psychiatry* **54**, 897–903.
8. DeLisi, L. E., Sakuma, M., Ge, S. & Kushner, M. (1998) *Psychiatry Res.* **84**, 75–88.
9. Giedd, J. N., Jeffries, N. O., Blumenthal, J., Castellanos, F. X., Vaituzis, A. C., Fernandez, T., Hamburger, S. D., Liu, H., Nelson, J., Bedwell, J., *et al.* (1999) *Biol. Psychiatry* **46**, 892–898.
10. Giedd, J. N., Blumenthal, J., Jeffries, N. O., Castellanos, F. X., Liu, H., Zijdenbos, A., Paus, T., Evans, A. C. & Rapoport, J. L. (1999b) *Nat. Neurosci.* **2**, 861–863.
11. Mathalon, D. H., Sullivan, E. V., Lim, K. O. & Pfefferbaum, A. (2001) *Arch. Gen. Psychiatry* **58**, 148–157.
12. Yakovlev, P. I. & Lecours, A. R. (1967) in *Regional Development of the Brain in Early Life*, ed. Minkowski, A. (Davis, Philadelphia), pp. 3–65.
13. Jernigan, T. L. & Tallal, P. (1990) *Dev. Med. Child Neurol.* **32**, 379–385.
14. Pfefferbaum, A., Mathalon, D. H., Sullivan, E. V., Rawles, J. M., Zipursky, R. B. & Lim, K. O. (1994) *Arch. Neurol.* **51**, 874–887.
15. Sowell, E. R., Thompson, P. M., Holmes, C. J., Jernigan, T. L. & Toga, A. W. (1999) *Nat. Neurosci.* **2**, 859–861.
16. McCarley, R. W., Wible, C. G., Frumin, M., Hirayasu, Y., Levitt, J. J., Fischer, I. A. & Shenton, M. E. (1999) *Biol. Psychiatry* **45**, 1099–1119.
17. Thompson, P. M., Mega, M. S., Woods, R. P., Zoumalan, C. I., Lindshield, C. J., Blanton, R. E., Moussai, J., Holmes, C. J., Cummings, J. L. & Toga, A. W. (2001) *Cereb. Cortex* **11**, 1–16.
18. American Psychiatric Association (1987) *Diagnostic and Statistical Manual of Mental Disorders* (Am. Psychiatric Assoc., Washington, DC), 3rd Ed. revised.
19. Puig-Antich, J., Orvaschel, H., Tabrizi, M. A. & Chambers, W. (1980) *Schedule for Affective Disorders and Schizophrenia for School-Age Children: Epidemiologic Version* (New York State Psychiatric Institution, New York, and Yale Univ. School of Medicine, New Haven, CT).
20. Reich, W., Welner, Z. & Herjanic, B. (1990) *Diagnostic Interview for Children and Adolescents Revised—Computer Program: Child/Adolescent Version and Parent Version* (Multi-Health Systems, North Tonawanda, NY).
21. Andreasen, N. C. (1983) *Scale for the Assessment of Positive Symptoms (SAPS) and Scale for the Assessment of Negative Symptoms (SANS)* (Univ. of Iowa College of Medicine, Iowa City).
22. Overall, J. E. & Gorham, D. R. (1962) *Psychol. Rep.* **10**, 799–812.
23. Kumra, S., Briguglio, C., Lenane, M., Goldhar, L., Bedwell, J., Venuchekov, J., Jacobsen, L. K. & Rapoport, J. L. (1999) *Am. J. Psychiatry* **156**, 1065–1068.
24. Woods, R. P., Cherry, S. R. & Mazziotta, J. C. (1992) *J. Comput. Assist. Tomogr.* **16**, 620–633.
25. Zijdenbos, A. P. & Dawant, B. M. (1994) *Crit. Rev. Biomed. Eng.* **22**, 401–465.
26. Wright, I. C., McGuire, P. K., Poline, J. B., Travere, J. M., Murray, R. M., Frith, C. D., Frackowiak, R. S. & Friston, K. J. (1995) *NeuroImage* **2**, 244–252.
27. Ashburner, J. & Friston, K. J. (2000) *NeuroImage* **11**, 805–821.
28. Thompson, P. M., Woods, R. P., Mega, M. S. & Toga, A. W. (2000) *Hum. Brain Mapp.* **9**, 81–92.
29. Thompson, P. M., Mega, M. S., Narr, K. L., Sowell, E. R., Blanton, R. E. & Toga, A. W. (2000) in *SPIE Handbook on Medical Image Analysis*, ed. Fitzpatrick, M. (Soc. Photo-Optical Instrumentation Engineers, Bellingham, WA), pp. 1063–1131.
30. Gogate, N., Giedd, J. N., Jansen, K. & Rapoport, J. L. (2001) *Clin. Neurosci. Res.* **1**, 283–290.
31. Lawrie, S. M. & Abukmeil, S. S. (1998) *Br. J. Psychiatry* **172**, 110–120.
32. Cannon, T. D., Huttunen, M. O., Lonnqvist, J., Tuulio-Henriksson, A., Pirkola, T., Glahn, D., Finkelstein, J., Hietanen, M., Kaprio, J. & Koskenvuo, M. (2000) *Am. J. Hum. Genet.* **67**, 369–382.
33. Nicolson, R., Lenane, M., Brookner, F., Gochman, P., Kumra, S., Spechler, L., Giedd, J. N., Thaker, G. K., Wudarsky, M. & Rapoport, J. L. (2001) *Comprehensive Psychiatry* **42**, 319–325.
34. Cohen, B. M. & Wan, W. (1996) *Am. J. Psychiatry* **153**, 104–106.
35. Melis, M., Diana, M. & Gessa, G. L. (1999) *Eur. J. Pharmacol.* **366**, R11–R13.
36. Goldberg, T. E. & Weinberger, D. R. (1996) *J. Clin. Psychiatry* **57**, 62–65.
37. Jacobsen, L. K., Hamburger, S. D., Van Horn, J. D., Vaituzis, A. C., McKenna, K., Frazier, J. A., Gordon, C. T., Lenane, M. C., Rapoport, J. L. & Zametkin, A. J. (1997) *Psychiatry Res.* **75**, 131–144.
38. Menon, V. V., Anagnoson, R. T., Mathalon, D. H., Glover, G. H. & Pfefferbaum, A. (2001) *NeuroImage* **13**, 433–446.
39. Günther, W., Brodie, J. D., Bartlett, E. J., Dewey, S. L., Henn, F. A., Volkow, N. D., Alper, K., Wolkin, A., Cancro, R. (1994) *Eur. Arch. Psychiatry Clin. Neurosci.* **244**, 115–125.
40. Spence, S. A., Brooks, D. J., Hirsch, S. R., Liddle, P. F., Meehan, J. & Grasby, P. M. (1997) *Brain* **120**, Part 11, 1997–2011.
41. Schroder, J., Essig, M., Baudendistel, K., Jahn, T., Gerdsen, I., Stockert, A., Schad, L. R. & Knopp, M. V. (1999) *NeuroImage* **9**, 81–87.
42. Karatekin, C. & Asarnow, R. F. (1999) *J. Abnormal Child Psychol.* **27**, 35–49.
43. Selemon, L. D., Rajkowska, G. & Goldman-Rakic, P. S. (1998) *Arch. Gen. Psychiatry* **52**, 805–820.
44. Cannon, T. D., Mednick, S. A. & Parnas, J. (1989) *Arch. Gen. Psychiatry* **46**, 883–889.
45. Huttenlocher, P. R. (1979) *Brain Res.* **163**, 195–205.
46. Feinberg, I. (1990) *Schizophr. Bull.* **16**, 567–570.
47. Huttenlocher, P. R. & Dabholkar, A. S. (1997) *J. Comp. Neurol.* **387**, 167–178.
48. Lim, K. O., Harris, D., Beal, M., Hoff, A. L., Minn, K., Csernansky, J. G., Faustman, W. O., Marsh, L., Sullivan, E. V. & Pfefferbaum, A. (1996) *Biol. Psychiatry* **39**, 4–13.
49. Karp, B. I., Garvey, M., Jacobsen, L. K., Frazier, J. A., Hamburger, S. D., Bedwell, J. S. & Rapoport, J. L. (2001) *Am. J. Psychiatry* **158**, 118–122.
50. Mathalon, D. H., Alvir, J. M., Woerner, M. G. & Pfefferbaum, A. (1996) *Neuropsychopharmacology* **14**, 13S–21S.
51. Gur, R. E., Cowell, P., Turetsky, B. I., Gallacher, F., Cannon, T., Bilker, W. & Gur, R. C. (1998) *Arch. Gen. Psychiatry* **55**, 145–152.
52. Burrows, R. C., Levitt, P. & Shors, T. J. (2000) *Neuroscience* **96**, 825–836.
53. Mirnics, K., Middleton, F. A., Marquez, A., Lewis, D. A. & Levitt, P. (2000) *Neuron* **28**, 53–67.
54. Karlsson, H., Bachmann, S., Schröder, J., McArthur, J., Fuller Torrey, E. & Yolken, R. H. (2001) *Proc. Natl. Acad. Sci. USA* **98**, 4634–4639.
55. Lewis, D. A. (2001) *Proc. Natl. Acad. Sci. USA* **98**, 4293–4294.
56. Shaffer, D., Gould, M. S., Brasic, J., Ambrosini, P., Fisher, P., Bird, H. & Aluwahlia, S. (1983) *Arch. Gen. Psychiatry* **40**, 1228–1231.

127

Lamina-Specific Alterations in the Dopamine Innervation of the Prefrontal Cortex in Schizophrenic Subjects

Mayada Akil, M.D., Joseph N. Pierri, M.S., M.D., Richard E. Whitehead, B.S., Christine L. Edgar, B.S., Carrie Mohila, B.S., Allan R. Sampson, Ph.D., and David A. Lewis, M.D.

Objective: Abnormalities in dopamine neurotransmission in the prefrontal cortex have been implicated in the pathophysiology of schizophrenia. However, the integrity of the dopamine projections to the prefrontal cortex in this disorder has not been directly examined. **Method:** The authors employed immunocytochemical methods and antibodies against tyrosine hydroxylase, the rate-limiting enzyme in dopamine biosynthesis, and the dopamine membrane transporter to examine dopamine axons in the dorsomedial prefrontal cortex (area 9) from 16 pairs of schizophrenic and matched control subjects. **Results:** Compared to the control subjects, the total length of tyrosine hydroxylase-immunoreactive axons was unchanged in the superficial and middle layers of the schizophrenic subjects but was reduced by an average of 33.6% in layer 6. The total length of tyrosine hydroxylase-positive axons in layer 6 was decreased in 13 of the schizophrenic subjects compared to their control subjects. Axons immunoreactive for the dopamine membrane transporter showed a similar pattern of change. In contrast, axons labeled for the serotonin transporter did not differ between schizophrenic and control subjects in any layer examined. In addition, the density of tyrosine hydroxylase-containing axons did not differ between monkeys chronically treated with haloperidol and matched control animals. **Conclusions:** These findings reveal that schizophrenia is associated with an altered dopamine innervation of prefrontal cortex area 9 that is lamina- and neurotransmitter-specific and that does not appear to be a consequence of pharmacological treatment. Together, these data provide direct evidence for a disturbance in dopamine neurotransmission in the prefrontal cortex of schizophrenic subjects.

(Am J Psychiatry 1999; 156:1580–1589)

In its original formulation, the dopamine hypothesis of schizophrenia posited that the psychotic symptoms of this disorder were due to a hyperdopaminergic state (1, 2). This hypothesis has undergone substantial revi-

Presented in part at the 22nd annual meeting of the Society for Neuroscience, Nov. 11–16, 1996. Received Nov. 24, 1998; revision received March 26, 1999; accepted April 12, 1999. From the Departments of Psychiatry, Neuroscience, and Statistics, University of Pittsburgh. Address reprint requests to Dr. Lewis, Western Psychiatric Institute and Clinic, University of Pittsburgh, Biomedical Science Tower, W1651, 3811 O'Hara St., Pittsburgh, PA 15213; lewisda@msx.upmc.edu (e-mail).

Supported by a Young Investigator Award from the National Alliance for Research on Schizophrenia and Depression (Dr. Akil) and by NIMH grants MH-00519, MH-45156, and MH-43784 (Dr. Lewis).

The authors thank Drs. Gretchen Haas, Carol Sue Johnston, Matcheri Keshavan, and Nina Schooler for their participation in the diagnostic conferences; Ms. Sungyoung Auh and Ms. Katia Charland for statistical computations; and Ms. Mary Brady for photographic assistance.

sions as a result of recent advances in our understanding of the complexity of dopamine systems and of the pathophysiology of schizophrenia. For example, perturbations of the dopamine system in schizophrenia have been suggested to be in opposite directions in different brain regions (3), such that a hyperdopaminergic state in subcortical structures coexists with a deficit in dopamine neurotransmission in the prefrontal cortex. The former has been proposed to account for the psychotic symptoms, and the latter has been proposed to contribute to the cognitive deficits and negative symptoms, that are characteristic of schizophrenia (4, 5).

The normal function of the prefrontal cortex clearly depends on an intact dopamine innervation (6–8), and several lines of evidence suggest that the dopamine innervation of the prefrontal cortex may be abnormal in schizophrenia. For example, schizophrenic subjects have been shown to have altered levels of expression of the mRNAs for some classes of dopamine receptors in the prefrontal cortex (9, 10). In addition, drug-naive schizophrenic subjects were reported to exhibit a decreased density of dopamine D₁-like receptors in the prefrontal cortex, and the density of receptors was directly associated with performance on a cognitive task, the Wisconsin Card Sorting Test (11), that is dependent on the function of the prefrontal cortex. This notion of a hypodopaminergic state in the prefrontal cortex of schizophrenic subjects is also supported by the observation that dopamine agonists increase prefrontal cortex blood flow and that these metabolic changes are associated with improved performance on the Wisconsin Card Sorting Test (12, 13). Finally, chronic administration of phencyclidine, which mimics some symptoms of schizophrenia in humans, produces cognitive deficits and hypofunction of prefrontal cortex dopamine in monkeys (14). However, despite the substantial interest in the role of prefrontal cortex dopamine in the pathophysiology of schizophrenia, the integrity of dopamine afferents from the mesencephalon to the prefrontal cortex has not previously been examined in schizophrenic subjects.

We and others have previously described the dopamine innervation of the primate prefrontal cortex by using immunocytochemical methods and antibodies directed against dopamine, the dopamine membrane transporter, or tyrosine hydroxylase, the rate-limiting enzyme in catecholamine biosynthesis (15–19). In both monkeys and humans, dopamine afferents innervate all regions of the prefrontal cortex, with labeled axons being particularly dense in the dorsomedial region, area 9. In the present study, we used a similar approach to evaluate the relative density and laminar distribution of dopamine axons in postmortem specimens of area 9 from matched pairs of schizophrenic and normal control subjects.

METHOD

Human Tissue Specimens

Postmortem tissue specimens from 32 human brains were obtained during autopsies conducted at the Allegheny County Coroner's Office. Written informed consent for brain donation and diagnostic interviews was obtained from the next of kin. These procedures were approved by the University of Pittsburgh's Institutional Review Board for Biomedical Research.

Neuropathological examination revealed abnormalities in four subjects. In three (subjects 207, 213, and 313), occasional neuritic plaques were identified in the neocortex. However, the density of plaques was insufficient to meet the diagnostic criteria for Alzheimer's disease, and none of the subjects had a clinical history of dementia. The cause of death involved brain damage in two subjects (subject 207: subdural hematoma in the left parietal region; subject 517: vascular malformation and hemorrhage confined to the right temporal lobe), but no neuropathological abnormalities were detected in either subject in the region of interest for this study.

Consensus DSM-III-R diagnoses were made by an independent panel of experienced clinicians, who used information obtained from clinical records and structured interviews with one or more surviving relatives of each subject (20). Sixteen of the subjects had a diagnosis of schizophrenia or schizoaffective disorder (table 1). One

of the schizophrenic subjects (subject 234) had never been medicated; three (subjects 537, 621, and 207) had not taken neuroleptics for 10 months, 8 years, and 10 years, respectively, before death; and another subject (subject 185) was known to have been noncompliant with prescribed medications. The absence of medication in these subjects was confirmed by toxicology screens conducted on all subjects at the time of death. Two schizophrenic subjects (subjects 428 and 517) were being treated with the atypical antipsychotic agent clozapine at the time of death, and the remaining nine schizophrenic subjects were receiving typical neuroleptics.

As shown in table 1, each schizophrenic subject was matched to one control subject for gender (the ratio of men to women was 10:6 in both groups) and race (with the exception of pair 16). Subjects were also matched as closely as possible for age and postmortem interval. The schizophrenic and control subjects did not differ in mean age (53.8 years, SD=9.4, and 54.6 years, SD=9.2, respectively) or postmortem interval (9.4 hours, SD=3.9, and 9.2 hours, SD=4.7, respectively). One control subject (subject 245) had a history of alcohol dependence. The remaining 15 control subjects had no known neurological, psychiatric, or substance abuse histories.

Tissue Preparation and Immunocytochemical Procedures

The left frontal lobe of each brain was cut into 1.0-cm-thick coronal blocks. Blocks were immersed in cold 4% paraformaldehyde in phosphate buffer for 48 hours and then stored in a cryoprotectant at –30°C (20). Mean tissue storage time in cryoprotectant did not significantly differ between schizophrenic (51.0 months, SD=21.9) and control (43.4 months, SD=28.9) subjects. In addition, previous studies have demonstrated that tissue storage under these conditions does not alter immunoreactivity for the antigens examined in this study (21). Blocks were sectioned coronally at 40 µm, and every 10th section was stained for Nissl substance with thionin. These sections were used to identify the location of area 9 on the superior frontal gyrus through use of the cytoarchitectonic criteria (20).

Floating tissue sections were processed for tyrosine hydroxylase or serotonin transporter immunoreactivity by using the avidin-biotin procedure and the Vectastain ABC Elite kit (Vector Laboratories, Burlingame, Calif.), as previously described (22), or for dopamine membrane transporter immunoreactivity by using a modification of the biotin amplification procedure (23). Tissue sections from each matched pair of schizophrenic and control subjects were always processed together. All slides were coded to conceal the subject number and diagnosis. The following antibodies were used in this study. 1) An affinity-purified IgG1 antibody (supplied by Dr. J. Haycock, Louisiana State University, New Orleans), raised against tyrosine hydroxylase purified from rat pheochromocytoma (24), was used at a concentration of 0.7 µg/ml. 2) A rat antibody (Chemicon, Temecula, Calif.), raised against a fusion protein containing the N-terminus of the human dopamine membrane transporter protein (25), was used at a dilution of 1:2,000. 3) A rabbit antibody, raised against a fusion protein containing the carboxy-terminus of the human serotonin transporter (provided by Dr. Randy Blakely, Vanderbilt University, Nashville, Tenn.), was used at a dilution of 1:10,000. The specificity of each antibody has been demonstrated in immunoblot, immunoprecipitation, and immunocytochemical studies (19, 26–28).

Pharmacological Treatment and Tissue Preparation in Monkeys

To assess the possible influence of antipsychotic medications on the measures of interest in the human studies, we studied four male cynomolgus (Macaca fascicularis) monkeys, each of whom was treated chronically with the typical antipsychotic agent haloperidol decanoate, and four control animals matched for sex, age, and weight. Animals were stabilized with daily doses of haloperidol that produced 8-hour trough serum concentrations of 4–8 ng/ml, and then that dose was multiplied by 15 to obtain the dose of haloperidol decanoate to be administered intramuscularly every 4 weeks. The mean dose of haloperidol decanoate was 16.0 mg/kg (SD=2.11). Trough serum levels obtained just before the next dose averaged 4.3 ng/ml (SD=1.1); these levels have been shown to be associated with

129

TABLE 1. Characteristics of Schizophrenic and Matched Normal Control Subjects in Postmortem Study

Pair	Case	DSM-III-R Diagnosis	Sex	Age (years)	Postmortem Interval (hours)	Race	Storage Time (months)	Cause of Death
					Schizophrenic Subjects			
1	207	Chronic undifferentiated schizophrenia[a]	M	72	3.8	White	65.0	Subdural hematoma
2	317	Chronic undifferentiated schizophrenia	M	48	8.3	White	48.0	Broncho-pneumonia
3	322	Chronic undifferentiated schizophrenia	M	40	8.5	White	47.6	Suicide by combined drug overdose
4	377	Chronic undifferentiated schizophrenia[b]	M	52	10.0	White	39.3	Gastrointestinal bleeding
5	398	Schizoaffective disorder	F	41	10.3	White	33.9	Pulmonary embolism
6	422	Chronic paranoid schizophrenia	M	54	11.0	White	27.9	Atherosclerotic coronary vascular disease
7	428	Schizoaffective disorder[c]	F	67	9.0	White	25.8	Chronic obstructive pulmonary disease
8	131	Chronic undifferentiated schizophrenia[c]	M	62	3.9	Black	101.2	Pneumonia
9	185	Chronic undifferentiated schizophrenia[a,b]	M	64	8.6	White	87.2	Atherosclerotic coronary vascular disease
10	517	Chronic disorganized schizophrenia[b]	F	48	3.7	White	22.1	Intracerebral hemorrhage
11	341	Chronic undifferentiated schizophrenia[d]	F	47	14.5	White	65.2	Suicide by chlorpromazine overdose
12	537	Schizoaffective disorder[a]	F	37	14.5	White	19.8	Suicide by hanging
13	234	Chronic paranoid schizophrenia[a]	M	51	12.8	White	80.5	Cardiomyopathy
14	621	Chronic undifferentiated schizophrenia[a]	M	83	16.0	White	9.8	Accidental asphyxiation
15	640	Chronic paranoid schizophrenia	M	49	5.2	White	7.4	Pulmonary embolism
16	597	Schizoaffective disorder	F	46	10.1	White	14.1	Pneumonia

[a] Subject was not taking antipsychotic medication at time of death.   [c] Also met the criteria for alcohol abuse, in remission, at time of death.
[b] Also met the criteria for alcohol dependence, current, at time of death. [d] Also met the criteria for alcohol abuse, current, at time of death.

a therapeutic response in humans (29). Consistent with our attempt to mimic the clinical model of neuroleptic threshold dosing (30), all haloperidol-treated animals developed extrapyramidal symptoms that were effectively controlled with maintenance administration of benztropine mesylate. After 9–12 months of treatment, each animal was euthanized with an overdose of pentobarbital, and the brain was retrieved. Following a 45-minute postmortem interval, coronal tissue blocks from the left hemisphere were fixed by immersion in 4% paraformaldehyde and processed for tyrosine hydroxylase immunocytochemistry in a manner identical to that described earlier for the human subjects. All procedures were approved by the University of Pittsburgh's Institutional Animal Care and Use Committee.

Qualitative and Quantitative Assessments of Tyrosine Hydroxylase-, Dopamine Membrane Transporter-, and Serotonin Transporter-Labeled Axons

Coded sections from matched pairs of human and monkey subjects were independently examined by three investigators (M.A., D.A.L... and J.N.P.) who were blind to subject number and group. Qualitative assessments of the relative density and laminar distribution of tyrosine hydroxylase-, dopamine membrane transporter-, and serotonin transporter-immunoreactive axons were rated for each subject, and differences, if evident, were used to rank order subjects within a pair. Assessments of three-way interrater agreement (Light's kappa estimates [31]) for the four sets of comparisons were as follows: tyrosine hydroxylase-immunoreactive axons in humans, 0.88; dopamine membrane transporter-immunoreactive axons in humans, 0.83; serotonin transporter immunoreactive axons in humans, 0.79; and tyrosine hydroxylase-immunoreactive axons in monkeys, 1.0. For the small number of cases in which the raters' independent assessments did not agree, slides were reviewed together in order to achieve consensus.

Quantitative studies were conducted by investigators (R.E.W., C.L.F., and C.M.) who were blind to subject number and group and who had not previously examined the tissue sections. Because the density of dopamine axons has previously been shown to be greater in medial than lateral area 9 (15, 16), quantitative studies were focused on the portion of area 9 located on the medial surface of the superior frontal gyrus. To obtain quantitative measures of axon length in the same laminar locations across brains, measurements of the distance from the pial surface to the borders of layers 1–2, 3–4, and 6–white matter were determined on the Nissl-stained sections

from each brain. The ratios of the depth of each laminar border to the total cortical thickness were then used to identify the same borders in the adjacent sections processed for immunocytochemistry. In order to examine the laminar specificity of any changes in dopamine axons in schizophrenia, we sampled cortical layers 1, deep 3, and 6. These layers were selected for analysis because they contain the highest densities of dopamine axons in monkeys and humans (15–18) and because the substantial differences in the extrinsic connectivity of these three layers provide a means for interpreting the possible functional significance of any laminar-specific alterations in dopamine innervation.

Square sampling frames (10,000 μm^2) were randomly placed in each of these three laminar locations on each tissue section with one axis of the sampling frame oriented parallel to the pial surface. Labeled processes were visualized under brightfield optics at a magnification of 600x, and the Eutectic Neuron Reconstruction System was used to reconstruct in three dimensions all labeled processes. The summed length of all reconstructed axons (total axon length) in each frame was determined and expressed as μm axon length/10,000 μm^2. These procedures have been previously used to characterize differences in tyrosine hydroxylase- and dopamine membrane transporter-immunoreactive axons across experimental conditions in animals, and they have been externally validated by comparisons with biochemical measures in both developmental and lesion studies (21, 32, 33). Similar procedures were used in both human and monkey studies. The adequacy of the sampling procedures was assessed by calculations of the coefficient of error across sampling frames within each layer of each subject. The mean coefficient of error was 0.20 (SD=0.11) for the human studies and 0.07 (SD=0.04) for the monkey studies.

Statistical Analyses

For the human studies, the sample frames yielded three identifiable measurements in each of the three laminar locations on each tissue section. For the statistical analyses of axon length, the response variable was treated as a three-variate, multivariate observation of axon length. Within each laminar location, multivariate analysis of variance (MANOVA) was employed to analyze the multivariate axon length variable. The main effect in this MANOVA was the diagnosis variable (indicating whether the subject was schizophrenic or control), with blocking on the pairing of subjects and controlling for the covariates age, postmortem interval, and tissue storage time.

130

				Control Subjects		
Case	Sex	Age (years)	Postmortem Interval (hours)	Race	Storage Time (months)	Cause of Death
200	M	79	3.8	White	65.7	Trauma
344	M	50	6.8	White	45.1	Atherosclerotic coronary vascular disease
395	M	42	12.3	White	34.3	Pericardial tamponade
245[b]	M	46	6.3	White	58.7	Trauma
253	F	46	4.5	White	56.7	Trauma
178	M	48	7.8	White	68.5	Atherosclerotic coronary vascular disease
390	F	72	11.0	White	36.3	Atherosclerotic coronary vascular disease
270	M	62	3.3	Black	74.6	Atherosclerotic coronary vascular disease
313	M	60	11.0	White	68.6	Atherosclerotic coronary vascular disease
449	F	47	4.3	White	36.7	Accidental carbon monoxide poisoning
452	F	40	14.3	White	36.3	Atherosclerotic coronary vascular disease
567	F	46	15.0	White	14.6	Mitral valve prolapse
451	M	48	12.0	White	36.4	Atherosclerotic coronary vascular disease
213	M	83	19.0	White	88.2	Tuberculosis
278	M	50	4.5	White	78.0	Atherosclerotic coronary vascular disease
575	F	55	11.3	Black	`17.5	Atherosclerotic coronary vascular disease

The resulting F test for diagnosis compared schizophrenic and control subjects on the basis of the axon length measures, resulting in the F statistic having three degrees of freedom in the numerator. The same MANOVA model was used to assess the possible effects of the covariates beyond that controlled by pairing. Data summaries of axon length are based on the mean of the measures within each laminar location for each subject. For the monkey studies, paired t tests were used to assess differences between control and haloperidol-treated animals.

RESULTS

Tyrosine Hydroxylase- and Dopamine Membrane Transporter-Immunoreactive Axons in the Prefrontal Cortex of Schizophrenic and Control Subjects

Qualitative analyses conducted by investigators who were blind to diagnosis for each pair of subjects revealed that each control subject exhibited the regional and laminar patterns of distribution of tyrosine hydroxylase-immunoreactive axons characteristic of area 9 (15, 18), although the overall density of labeled axons differed across subjects. In 10 of the schizophrenic subjects, the density of tyrosine hydroxylase-immunoreactive axons was clearly reduced relative to that of their matched control subjects, and in some cases, this reduction was quite striking (figure 1, parts A and B). In four of these schizophrenic subjects, the reduction in density of tyrosine hydroxylase-immunoreactive axons was present across all cortical layers, whereas in the other six subjects, the difference was evident only in the deep layers. Two of the schizophrenic subjects appeared to have an increase in tyrosine hydroxylase-immunoreactive axon density, and the remaining four subjects were judged to be similar to their matched control subjects.

Although the intensity of axon labeling was usually less robust with the dopamine membrane transporter antibody than with the tyrosine hydroxylase antibody in the same subject, the overall patterns of regional and laminar distribution of labeled axons were the same with both antibodies. Compared to control subjects, the density of dopamine membrane transporter-immunoreactive axons was rated as decreased in 10 schizophrenic subjects, increased in one, and unchanged in five. In some schizophrenic subjects, the decrease in density of dopamine membrane transporter-immunoreactive axons was marked, especially in the deep layers (figure 2). With one exception, the difference in dopamine membrane transporter-immunoreactive axon density between a matched pair of subjects paralleled the difference in tyrosine hydroxylase-immunoreactive axon density.

Quantitative Analysis of Tyrosine Hydroxylase-Immunoreactive Axons in Schizophrenic and Control Subjects

To determine the magnitude of these differences, we measured the innervation density of tyrosine hydroxylase-immunoreactive axons because of the higher quality of labeling obtained with the anti-tyrosine hydroxylase antibody. The mean total length of tyrosine hydroxylase-immunoreactive axons in medial area 9 was decreased by 10.8% and 13.8% in layers 1 and 3, respectively, of the schizophrenic subjects compared to the control subjects (figure 3). However, these differences in layers 1 and 3 did not achieve statistical significance (F=0.74 and 1.45, respectively, df=3, 10, p>0.30, MANOVA). In contrast, mean total axon length (per 10,000 μm^2) in layer 6 of the schizophrenic

FIGURE 1. Dark-Field Photomicrographs of Tyrosine Hydroxylase-Immunoreactive (A, B) and Serotonin Transporter-Immunoreactive (C, D) Axons in Prefrontal Cortex Area 9 From a Schizophrenic (B, D) and Matched Control (A, C) Subject in Postmortem Study[a]

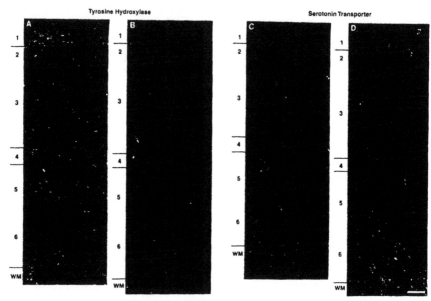

Tyrosine Hydroxylase   Serotonin Transporter

[a] Pair 7; see table 1. Note the marked decrease in the density of tyrosine hydroxylase-immunoreactive axons across all cortical layers in the schizophrenic subject compared to the matched control subject, whereas the density of serotonin transporter-immunoreactive axons in adjacent sections does not appear to differ between subjects. Numerals indicate cortical layers, and WM indicates white matter. Calibration bar=200 µm and applies to all panels.

FIGURE 2. Dark-Field Photomicrographs of Dopamine Membrane Transporter-Immunoreactive Axons in Prefrontal Cortex Area 9 From a Control Subject (A) Matched to a Schizophrenic Subject (B)[a]

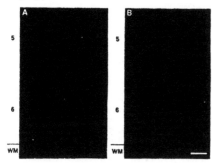

[a] Pair 3; see table 1. Numerals indicate cortical layers, and WM indicates white matter. Calibration bar=200 µm.

subjects was significantly decreased, by 33.6%, compared to the matched control subjects (276.8 µm, SD= 206.4, and 416.3 µm, SD=174.0, respectively) (F= 5.23, df=3, 10, p=0.02, MANOVA). Comparison of individual matched pairs of subjects revealed that in 13 of the 16 schizophrenic subjects, the mean total axon length in layer 6 was less than that in the matched control subjects (figure 4).

Serotonin Transporter-Immunoreactive Axons in Prefrontal Cortex of Schizophrenic and Control Subjects

In order to determine whether this reduction in the relative density of labeled axons in layer 6 of schizophrenic subjects was specific to dopamine axons or representative of a more generalized alteration in monoamine-containing afferents to the prefrontal cortex, we examined serotonin transporter-immunoreactive axons in the same 16 pairs of subjects. Both the relative density and laminar distribution of these fibers appeared unaltered in schizophrenic subjects. For example, qualitative evaluations did not reveal any apparent differences in

FIGURE 3. Mean Total Length of Tyrosine Hydroxylase-Immunoreactive Axons in Layers 1, 3, and 6 of Prefrontal Cortex Area 9 in Schizophrenic and Control Subjects in Postmortem Study[a]

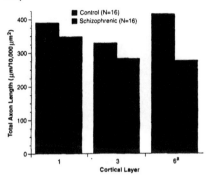

[a] F=5.23, df=3, 10, p=0.02 (MANOVA).

FIGURE 4. Percent Difference in Total Length of Tyrosine Hydroxylase-Immunoreactive Axons in Layer 6 of Prefrontal Cortex Area 9 for Each of 16 Matched Pairs of Schizophrenic and Control Subjects[a]

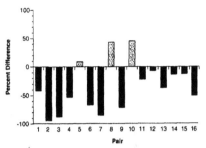

[a] Pair numbers are the same as those used in table 1. Note that the total length of tyrosine hydroxylase-immunoreactive axons is reduced in 13 of the schizophrenic subjects. Bars above 0 indicate pairs in which total axon length was increased in schizophrenic subjects, and bars below 0 indicate pairs in which total axon length was reduced in schizophrenic subjects relative to the matched control subjects.

serotonin transporter-immunoreactive axons between the same matched pair of schizophrenic and control subjects (figure 1, parts C and D) that showed a marked reduction in tyrosine hydroxylase-immunoreactive axons (figure 1, parts A and B). Quantitative studies confirmed that the total length of serotonin transporter-immunoreactive axons did not differ between the schizophrenic and control subjects in any layer (F=0.56, df=3, 10, p>0.40). In layer 6, the mean total length of serotonin transporter-immunoreactive axons for each schizophrenic subject was within the range of that of all control subjects (figure 5, part B), whereas for eight of the schizophrenic subjects, mean total length of tyrosine hydroxylase-immunoreactive axons was lower than that of all control subjects (figure 5, part A). It should also be noted that the total length of serotonin transporter-immunoreactive axons was less than that of tyrosine hydroxylase-immunoreactive axons in the control subjects (figure 5). This finding is consistent with previous comparisons of the relative density of dopamine and serotonin axons in medial area 9 of the primate prefrontal cortex (34).

Assessment of Influence of Other Variables

Each schizophrenic subject was matched to a control subject to minimize the possible influence of gender, race, age, and postmortem interval on the measures of interest. When the pairing of subjects is taken into account, there were no significant effects of these variables, or of tissue storage time, on any measures of axon length. Correlational analyses also failed to detect any association between the magnitude of the decrease in tyrosine hydroxylase-immunoreactive axons in layer 6 of the schizophrenic subjects and age at onset or duration of illness (r<0.056, df=1, 14, p>0.84).

As shown in figure 6, total length of tyrosine hydroxylase-immunoreactive axons in layers 1, 3, and 6 did not differ between monkeys treated chronically with the antipsychotic agent haloperidol and their matched control subjects.

DISCUSSION

The results of this study demonstrate a significant reduction in the relative density of axons immunoreactive for tyrosine hydroxylase and dopamine membrane transporter, two proteins that play a critical role in dopamine neurotransmission, in layer 6 of prefrontal cortex area 9 in subjects with schizophrenia. In contrast, cortical afferents immunoreactive for the serotonin transporter, a central protein in serotonin neurotransmission, did not differ between schizophrenic and control subjects. Furthermore, chronic treatment with haloperidol and benztropine did not alter the density of tyrosine hydroxylase-immunoreactive axons in the monkey prefrontal cortex; this suggests that our findings are not likely to be a consequence of the typical treatments used in schizophrenic subjects. Together, these findings provide evidence that the pathophysiology of schizophrenia includes a lamina- and neurotransmitter-specific alteration in the dopamine innervation of the prefrontal cortex.

Specificity of Alterations to Dopamine Innervation of the Prefrontal Cortex in Schizophrenia

The dopamine membrane transporter and tyrosine hydroxylase antibodies used in this study have both

FIGURE 5. Mean Total Length of Tyrosine Hydroxylase-Immunoreactive (A) and Serotonin Transporter-Immunoreactive (B) Axons in Layer 6 of Prefrontal Cortex Area 9 in Schizophrenic and Control Subjects[a]

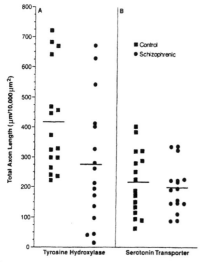

[a] Horizontal lines indicate group means. Note that the total length of tyrosine hydroxylase-immunoreactive axons is decreased in the schizophrenic subjects compared to control subjects, whereas the total length of serotonin transporter-immunoreactive axons does not differ across groups.

FIGURE 6. Mean Total Length of Tyrosine Hydroxylase-Immunoreactive Axons in Layers 1, 3, and 6 of the Prefrontal Cortex in Haloperidol-Treated and Matched Control Monkeys[a]

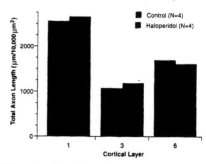

[a] Group values did not differ in any layer (t<0.89, df=3, p>0.44, two-tailed test).

been shown to specifically label dopamine axons in the primate neocortex. The mRNA for the dopamine membrane transporter is expressed selectively in dopamine neurons, and the protein is confined to the cell bodies, dendrites, and axonal projections of these neurons (25). Although tyrosine hydroxylase is expressed in all catecholamine-containing neurons, multiple lines of evidence indicate that antibodies against tyrosine hydroxylase predominantly label dopamine axons in the primate neocortex (22). In both monkeys and humans, the distribution and morphology of cortical tyrosine hydroxylase-immunoreactive axons differ from those of axons immunolabeled for dopamine-beta-hydroxylase, a marker of noradrenergic structures (18, 35), and few cortical axons exhibit both tyrosine hydroxylase and dopamine-beta-hydroxylase immunoreactivity (36, 37). In contrast, direct comparisons of tyrosine hydroxylase-immunoreactive axons and those labeled with an anti-dopamine antibody revealed identical patterns of distribution in the monkey cortex (17, 37), and over 95% of all tyrosine hydroxylase-immunoreactive axons in the monkey prefrontal cortex are also dopamine membrane transporter-immunoreactive (19).

While our findings of a reduced density of tyrosine hydroxylase- and dopamine membrane transporter-immunoreactive axons are indicative of an alteration in dopamine afferents, they do not preclude the possibility of a concomitant reduction in other afferent systems to the prefrontal cortex in schizophrenia. Indeed, the magnitude of the reported decrease in synaptophysin (20, 38), a marker of axon terminals, in the prefrontal cortex of schizophrenic subjects cannot be accounted for solely by reductions in dopamine afferents. However, the absence of a difference between schizophrenic and control subjects in serotonin transporter-immunoreactive axons in the present study indicates that the observed change in dopamine axons does not reflect a nonspecific alteration in all monoaminergic projections to the prefrontal cortex in schizophrenia. These observations are also consistent with previous radioligand binding studies that found similar levels of serotonin uptake sites in the prefrontal cortex of schizophrenic and control subjects (39, 40).

Specificity of Alterations to the Disease Process of Schizophrenia

Several lines of evidence suggest that the findings of this study directly reflect the pathophysiology of the disease process and do not represent an epiphenomenon of its treatment or other factors. The absence of a change in serotonin transporter-immunoreactive axons in concert with the laminar-specific reduction in dopamine axons argues against the possibility that the present findings are a consequence of differences in the quality of the tissue between the two groups of subjects. In addition, previous investigations that included many of the subjects in the present study failed to find differences between the schizophrenic and control subjects in other immunocytochemical markers (41, 42). Most of the schizophrenic subjects included in the present study, but none of the control subjects, had been treated at some point in their lives with antipsychotic agents. However, the available evidence suggests that our findings are not the result of treatment with these agents, or of the anticholinergic drugs that are frequently used to treat the side effects of antipsychotic medications. First, our study included one schizophrenic subject who was never medicated and four subjects who were not receiving medications at the time of death. In each of these subjects, the density of tyrosine hydroxylase-immunoreactive axons in layer 6 was reduced compared to that in the matched control subjects (see pairs 1, 9, and 12–14 in figure 4). Second, chronic treatment of monkeys with haloperidol and benztropine did not alter the relative density of tyrosine hydroxylase-immunoreactive axons in the prefrontal cortex. The absence of an effect of antipsychotic medications on the measures used in this study is supported by a recent report that chronic haloperidol administration in the rat did not affect tyrosine hydroxylase immunoreactivity in neurons of the mesocortical dopamine system, although it did decrease tyrosine hydroxylase immunoreactivity in the nigrostriatal system (43).

The possible influence of other clinical factors frequently associated with schizophrenia on tyrosine hydroxylase and dopamine membrane transporter immunoreactivity must also be considered. In the present study, six of the schizophrenic subjects had a history of alcohol abuse or dependence (table 1). However, nine of the 10 schizophrenic subjects without any history of alcohol abuse or dependence also had a reduced density of tyrosine hydroxylase-immunoreactive axons in layer 6 compared to the matched control subjects (compare table 1 and figure 4). In addition, in one of the pairs of subjects (pair 4 in table 1 and figure 4), both the schizophrenic and the control subject had a history of alcohol dependence, and yet the density of tyrosine hydroxylase-immunoreactive fibers was still decreased in the schizophrenic subject.

Pathophysiological Significance

The finding of a relative decrease in innervation density of both tyrosine hydroxylase- and dopamine membrane transporter-immunoreactive axons in the prefrontal cortex of schizophrenic subjects suggests that either 1) the concentrations of both proteins are reduced in a subpopulation of dopamine axons, such that these axons are no longer detectable by immunocytochemical techniques, or 2) the dopamine axons containing these proteins are decreased in number. Although the first possibility cannot be excluded, we are not aware of any data that would directly support this interpretation. On the other hand, a reduced number of cortical dopamine axons might be expected to be associated with alterations in the dopamine neurons of the ventral tegmental area, which furnish many of the dopamine afferents to the prefrontal cortex. In the only study that has examined dopamine neurons in

schizophrenic subjects, the number of neuromelanin-containing cells in the medial mesencephalon was reported to be decreased by 16%, although this difference was not significant (44). However, the somal volume of pigmented neurons was significantly reduced in the schizophrenic subjects. The latter findings could reflect a reduction in the size of the axon arbor of cortically projecting dopamine neurons, since somal size and total axon length tend to be positively correlated (45, 46).

Either reduced amounts of tyrosine hydroxylase and dopamine membrane transporter in dopamine axons or the presence of fewer dopamine axons could be associated with diminished dopamine neurotransmission in the prefrontal cortex of schizophrenic subjects. This possibility is consistent with the interpretation of other studies (see introduction) suggesting that schizophrenia is associated with a hypodopaminergic state in the prefrontal cortex. In addition, animal studies suggest that even relatively modest reductions in the density of dopamine axons in the prefrontal cortex can be associated with a substantial decrease in indices of dopamine neurotransmission. For example, in contrast to the nigrostriatal dopamine system in which residual dopamine terminals can compensate for the loss of the majority of axons in this projection (47), partial lesions of the dopamine mesocortical projection result in significantly decreased extracellular levels of dopamine in the prefrontal cortex (33). We do not know whether the magnitude of the decrease in prefrontal cortex dopamine axons observed in the present study of schizophrenia is sufficient to produce the types of cognitive impairments previously associated with reductions of prefrontal cortex dopamine in nonhuman primates (6–8). However, the similarities in cognitive deficits observed in these animal studies and in subjects with schizophrenia (48) suggest that the decrease in markers of prefrontal cortex dopamine axons observed in the present study could contribute to prefrontal cortex dysfunction in schizophrenia.

On the other hand, our findings of decreased tyrosine hydroxylase- and dopamine membrane transporter-immunoreactive axons do not necessarily provide evidence for a hypodopaminergic state in the prefrontal cortex of schizophrenic subjects. In fact, the complete absence of dopamine membrane transporter and reductions of 90% in tyrosine hydroxylase levels are associated with a markedly hyperdopaminergic state in the dopamine membrane transporter knockout mouse (49). Some studies have indicated that prefrontal cortex function may be impaired by either a deficiency or an excess of stimulation at prefrontal cortex dopamine D_1 receptors (7, 50–52). Layer 6 of the primate prefrontal cortex contains a high density of dopamine D_1-like receptors (53), and the density of these receptors has been reported to be decreased in drug-naive schizophrenic subjects (11). Since the symptoms of schizophrenia are frequently worsened by stress, which increases prefrontal cortex dopamine release (54), it is possible that decreases in pre- and postsynaptic dopamine markers in the prefrontal cortex represent a homeostatic response to minimize the impact of excessive levels of prefrontal cortex dopamine induced by environmental stress.

Although our findings reveal a lamina- and neurotransmitter-specific alteration in the dopamine innervation of the prefrontal cortex, other data suggest that these changes are likely to represent only one component of a more extensive set of alterations in prefrontal cortex circuitry in schizophrenia. For example, imaging and postmortem studies suggest that the mediodorsal thalamic nucleus, which furnishes the principal thalamic projection to the prefrontal cortex, may be reduced in size and contain fewer neurons in subjects with schizophrenia (55, 56). In addition, findings from other studies support the notion that the thalamic projections to the middle layers of the prefrontal cortex are decreased in schizophrenia (57, 58). Interestingly, the feedback projections from the prefrontal cortex to the mediodorsal thalamus originate from pyramidal neurons located in layers 5 and 6 (59), and the prefrontal cortex projections to the mediodorsal thalamus appear to play a prominent role in regulating thalamic activity (see reference 60 for a review). Since the dendritic shafts and spines of pyramidal cells are the principal synaptic target of dopamine axon terminals (61), and dopamine appears to play a critical role in regulating the influence of other inputs on pyramidal cell activity (62, 63), a shift in dopamine neurotransmission in prefrontal cortex layer 6 could reflect a change in the modulation of corticothalamic feedback in response to abnormal thalamocortical drive in schizophrenia.

REFERENCES

1. Snyder SH: Catecholamines in the brain as mediators of amphetamine psychosis. Arch Gen Psychiatry 1972; 27:169–179

2. Carlsson A, Lindquist M: Effect of chlorpromazine and haloperidol on formation of 3-methoxytyramine and normetanephrine in mouse brain. Acta Pharmacol Toxicol 1963; 20:140–144

3. Goldstein M, Deutch AY: Dopaminergic mechanisms in the pathogenesis of schizophrenia. FASEB J 1992; 6:2413–2421

4. Grace AA: Phasic versus tonic dopamine release and the modulation of dopamine system responsivity: a hypothesis for the etiology of schizophrenia. Neuroscience 1991; 41:1–24

5. Davis KL, Kahn RS, Ko G, Davidson M: Dopamine in schizophrenia: a review and reconceptualization. Am J Psychiatry 1991; 148:1474–1486

6. Brozoski TJ, Brown RM, Rosvold HE, Goldman PS: Cognitive deficit caused by regional depletion of dopamine in prefrontal cortex of rhesus monkeys. Science 1979; 205:929–932

7. Sawaguchi T, Goldman-Rakic PS: D1 dopamine receptors in prefrontal cortex: involvement in working memory. Science 1991; 251:947–950

8. Arnsten AFT, Cai JX, Murphy BL, Goldman-Rakic PS: Dopamine D1 receptor mechanisms in the cognitive performance of young adult and aged monkeys. Psychopharmacology (Berl) 1994; 116:143–151

9. Meador-Woodruff JH, Haroutunian V, Powchik P, Davidson M, Davis KL, Watson SJ: Dopamine receptor transcript expression in striatum and prefrontal occipital cortex. Arch Gen Psychiatry 1997; 54:1089–1095

10. Stefanis NC, Bresnik JN, Kerwin RW, Schofield WN, McAllister G: Elevation of D4 dopamine receptor mRNA in postmortem schizophrenic brain. Mol Brain Res 1998; 53:112–119

11. Okubo Y, Suhara T, Suzuki K, Kobayashi K, Inoue O, Terasaki O, Someya Y, Sassa T, Sudo Y, Matsuchima E, Iyo M, Tateno Y, Toru M: Decreased prefrontal dopamine D1 receptors in schizophrenia revealed by PET. Nature 1997; 385:634–636

12. Daniel DG, Weinberger DR, Jones DW, Zigun JR, Coppola R, Handel S, Bigelow LR, Goldberg TE, Berman KF, Kleinman JE: The effect of amphetamine on regional cerebral blood flow during cognitive activation in schizophrenia. J Neurosci 1991; 11:1907–1917

13. Daniel DG, Berman KF, Weinberger DR: The effect of apomorphine on regional cerebral blood flow in schizophrenia. J Neuropsychiatry 1989; 1:377–384

14. Jentsch JD, Redmond DE Jr, Elsworth JD, Taylor JR, Youngren KD, Roth RH: Enduring cognitive deficits and cortical dopamine dysfunction in monkeys after long-term administration of phencyclidine. Science 1997; 277:953–955

15. Lewis DA: The catecholaminergic innervation of primate prefrontal cortex. J Neural Transm 1992; 36:179–200

16. Lewis DA, Foote SL, Goldstein M, Morrison JH: The dopaminergic innervation of monkey prefrontal cortex: a tyrosine hydroxylase immunohistochemical study. Brain Res 1988; 449:225–243

17. Williams SM, Goldman-Rakic PS: Characterization of the dopaminergic innervation of the primate frontal cortex using a dopamine-specific antibody. Cereb Cortex 1993; 3:199–222

18. Gaspar P, Berger B, Fabvret A, Vigny A, Henry JP: Catecholamine innervation of the human cerebral cortex as revealed by comparative immunohistochemistry of tyrosine hydroxylase and dopamine-beta-hydroxylase. J Comp Neurol 1989; 279:249–271

19. Lewis DA, Sesack SR, Levey AI, Rosenberg DR: Dopamine axons in primate prefrontal cortex: specificity of distribution, synaptic targets, and development, in Advances in Pharmacology. Edited by Goldstein D, Eisenhofer G, McCarty R. San Diego, Academic Press, 1998, pp 703–706

20. Glantz LA, Lewis DA: Reduction of synaptophysin immunoreactivity in the prefrontal cortex of subjects with schizophrenia: regional and diagnostic specificity. Arch Gen Psychiatry 1997; 54:943–952

21. Erickson SL, Akil M, Levey AI, Lewis DA: Postnatal development of tyrosine hydroxylase- and dopamine transporter-immunoreactive axons in monkey rostral entorhinal cortex. Cereb Cortex 1998; 8:415–427

22. Akil M, Lewis DA: The distribution of tyrosine hydroxylase-immunoreactive fibers in the human entorhinal cortex. Neuroscience 1994; 60:857–874

23. Adams JC: Biotin amplification of biotin and horseradish peroxidase signals in histochemical stains. J Histochem Cytochem 1992; 40:1457–1463

24. Renfroe JB, Chronister RB, Haycock JW, Waymire JC: The localization of tyrosine hydroxylase-like immunoreactivity in the central nervous system: methodological considerations. Brain Res Bull 1984; 13:109–126

25. Ciliax BJ, Heilman C, Demchyshyn LL, Pristupa ZB, Ince E, Hersch SM, Niznik HB, Levey AI: The dopamine transporter: immunochemical characterization and localization in brain. J Neurosci 1995; 15:1714–1723

26. Lewis DA, Melchitzky DS, Haycock JW: Four isoforms of tyrosine hydroxylase are expressed in human brain. Neuroscience 1993; 54:477–492

27. Miller GW, Staley JK, Heilman CJ, Perez JT, Mash DC, Rye DB, Levey AI: Immunochemical analysis of dopamine transporter protein in Parkinson's disease. Ann Neurol 1997; 41:530–539

28. Qian Y, Melikian HE, Rye DB, Levey AI, Blakely RD: Identification and characterization of antidepressant-sensitive serotonin transporter proteins using site-specific antibodies. J Neurosci 1995; 15:1261–1274

29. Janicak PG, Davis JM, Preskorn SH, Ayd FJ: Principles and Practice of Psychopharmacotherapy. Baltimore, Williams & Wilkins, 1993

30. McEvoy JP, Schooler NR, Wilson WH: Predictors of therapeutic response to haloperidol in acute schizophrenia. Psychopharmacol Bull 1991; 27:97–101

31. Light RJ: Measures of response agreement for qualitative data: some generalizations and alternatives. Psychol Bull 1971; 76:356–377

32. Rosenberg DR, Lewis DA: Postnatal maturation of the dopaminergic innervation of monkey prefrontal and motor cortices: a tyrosine hydroxylase immunohistochemical analysis. J Comp Neurol 1995; 358:383–400

33. Venator DK, Lewis DA, Finlay JM: Effects of partial dopamine loss in the medial prefrontal cortex on local baseline and stress-evoked extracellular dopamine concentrations. Neuroscience (in press)

34. Lewis DA, Hayes TL, Lund JS, Oeth KM: Dopamine and the neural circuitry of primate prefrontal cortex: implications for schizophrenia research. Neuropsychopharmacology 1992; 6: 127–134

35. Lewis DA, Campbell MJ, Foote SL, Goldstein M, Morrison JH: The distribution of tyrosine hydroxylase-immunoreactive fibers in primate neocortex is widespread but regionally specific. J Neurosci 1987; 7:279–290

36. Noack HJ, Lewis DA: Antibodies directed against tyrosine hydroxylase differentially recognize noradrenergic axons in monkey neocortex. Brain Res 1989; 500:313–324

37. Akil M, Lewis DA: The dopaminergic innervation of monkey entorhinal cortex. Cereb Cortex 1993; 3:533–550

38. Perrone-Bizzozero NI, Sower AC, Bird ED, Benowitz LI, Ivins KJ, Neve RL: Levels of the growth-associated protein GAP-43 are selectively increased in association cortices in schizophrenia. Proc Natl Acad Sci USA 1996; 93:14182–14187

39. Dean B, Hayes W, Opeskin K, Naylor L, Pavey G, Hill C, Keks N, Copolov DL: Serotonin 2 receptors and the serotonin transporter in the schizophrenic brain. Behav Brain Res 1996; 73: 169–175

40. Gurevich EV, Joyce JN: Alterations in the cortical serotonergic system in schizophrenia: a postmortem study. Biol Psychiatry 1997; 42:529–545

41. Woo T-U, Miller JL, Lewis DA: Schizophrenia and the parvalbumin-containing class of cortical local circuit neurons. Am J Psychiatry 1997; 154:1013–1015

42. Woo T-U, Whitehead RE, Melchitzky DS, Lewis DA: A subclass of prefrontal gamma-aminobutyric acid axon terminals are selectively altered in schizophrenia. Proc Natl Acad Sci USA 1998; 95:5341–5346

43. Levinson AJ, Garside S, Rosebush PI, Mazurek MF: Haloperidol induces persistent down-regulation of tyrosine-hydroxylase immunoreactivity in substantia nigra but not ventral tegmental area in the rat. Neuroscience 1998; 84:201–211

44. Bogerts B, Hantsch J, Herzer M: A morphometric study of the dopamine-containing cell groups in the mesencephalon of normals, Parkinson patients, and schizophrenics. Biol Psychiatry 1983; 18:951–969

45. Lund JS, Lund RD, Hendrickson AE, Bunt AH, Fuchs AF: The origin of efferent pathways from the primary visual cortex, area 17, of the macaque monkey as shown by retrograde transport of horseradish peroxidase. J Comp Neurol 1975; 164:287–304

46. Gilbert CD, Kelly JP: The projections of cells in different layers of the cat's visual cortex. J Comp Neurol 1975; 63:81–106

47. Snyder GL, Keller RW, Zigmond MJ: Dopamine efflux from striatal slices after intracerebral 6-hydroxydopamine: evidence for compensatory hyperactivity of residual terminals. J Pharmacol Exp Ther 1990; 253:867–876

48. Park S, Holzman PS: Schizophrenics show spatial working memory deficits. Arch Gen Psychiatry 1992; 49:975–982

49. Giros B, Jaber M, Jones SR, Wightman RM, Caron MG: Hyperlocomotion and indifference to cocaine and amphetamine in mice lacking the dopamine transporter. Nature 1996; 379: 606–612

50. Murphy BL, Arnsten AFT, Goldman-Rakic PS, Roth RH: Increased dopamine turnover in the prefrontal cortex impairs spatial working memory performance in rats and monkeys. Proc Natl Acad Sci USA 1996; 93:1325–1329

51. Arnsten AFT, Goldman-Rakic PS: Noise stress impairs prefrontal cortical cognitive function in monkeys: evidence for a hyperdopaminergic mechanism. Arch Gen Psychiatry 1998; 55:362–369

52. Williams GV, Goldman-Rakic PS: Modulation of memory fields by dopamine D1 receptors in prefrontal cortex. Nature 1995; 376:572–575

53. Goldman-Rakic PS, Lidow MS, Gallagher DW: Overlap of dopaminergic, adrenergic, and serotoninergic receptors and complementarity of their subtypes in primate prefrontal cortex. J Neurosci 1990; 10:2125–2138

54. Thierry A-M, Tassin JP, Blanc G, Glowinski J: Selective activation of the mesocortical DA system by stress. Nature 1976; 263:242–244

55. Andreasen NC, Arndt S, Swayze V II. Cizadlo T, Flaum M, O'Leary D, Ehrhardt JC, Yuh WTC: Thalamic abnormalities in schizophrenia visualized through magnetic resonance image averaging. Science 1994; 266:294–298

56. Pakkenberg B: Pronounced reduction of total neuron number in mediodorsal thalamic nucleus and nucleus accumbens in schizophrenics. Arch Gen Psychiatry 1990; 47:1023–1028

57. Glantz LA, Lewis DA: Prefrontal cortical pyramidal neurons exhibit decreased dendritic spine density in subjects with schizophrenia. Arch Gen Psychiatry (in press)

58. Pierri JN, Edgar CL, Lewis DA: Somal size of prefrontal cortical pyramidal neurons in the thalamic recipient zone of subjects with schizophrenia. Abstracts of the Society for Neuroscience 1998; 24:987

59. Goldman-Rakic PS, Porrino LJ: The primate mediodorsal (MD) nucleus and its projection to the frontal lobe. J Comp Neurol 1985; 242:535–560

60. Guillery RW, Feig SL, Lozsádi DA: Paying attention to the thalamic reticular nucleus. Trends Neurosci 1998; 21:28–32

61. Goldman-Rakic PS, Leranth C, Williams SM, Mons N, Geffard M: Dopamine synaptic complex with pyramidal neurons in primate cerebral cortex. Proc Natl Acad Sci USA 1989; 86: 9015–9019

62. Yang CR, Seamans JK: Dopamine D1 receptor actions in layers V–VI rat prefrontal cortex neurons in vitro: modulation of dendritic-somatic signal integration. J Neurosci 1996; 16: 1922–1935

63. Penit-Soria J, Audinat E, Crépel F: Excitation of rat prefrontal cortical neurons by dopamine: an in vitro electrophysiological study. Brain Res 1987; 425:263–274

137

Absence of Neurodegeneration and Neural Injury in the Cerebral Cortex in a Sample of Elderly Patients With Schizophrenia

Steven E. Arnold, MD; John Q. Trojanowski, MD, PhD; Raquel E. Gur, MD, PhD; Peter Blackwell; Li-Ying Han, MS; Catherine Choi

Background: The cognitive and functional deterioration that is observed in many "poor-outcome" patients with schizophrenia suggests a neurodegenerative process extending into late life. Previous diagnostic studies have excluded known neurodegenerative diseases as explanations for this dementia. However, we hypothesized that relatively small accumulations of age- or disease-related neurodegenerative lesions occurring in an otherwise abnormal brain could result in deterioration in schizophrenia.

Methods: Postmortem studies were conducted using 23 prospectively accrued elderly persons with chronic schizophrenia for whom clinical ratings had been determined before death, 14 elderly control patients with no neuropsychiatric disease, and 10 control patients with Alzheimer disease. Immunohistochemistry and unbiased stereological counting methods were used to quantify common neurodegenerative lesions (ie, neurofibrillary tangles, amyloid plaques, and Lewy bodies) and cellular reactions to a variety of noxious stimuli (ubiquitinated dystrophic neurites, astrocytosis, and microglial infil-

trates) in the ventromedial temporal lobe and the frontal and the calcarine (primary visual) cortices.

Results: No statistically significant differences were found between the patients with schizophrenia and the control patients without neuropsychiatric disease for the densities of any of the markers, while both groups exhibited fewer lesions than did the control group with Alzheimer disease. Correlation analyses in the schizophrenia sample failed to identify significant correlations between cognitive and psychiatric ratings and densities of any of the neuropathologic markers.

Conclusions: No significant evidence of neurodegeneration or ongoing neural injury in the cerebral cortex was found in this sample of elderly persons with schizophrenia. Furthermore, the behavioral and cognitive deterioration observed in late life did not correlate with age-related degenerative phenomena.

Arch Gen Psychiatry. 1998;55:225-232

A HISTORICALLY important hypothesis about the pathogenesis of schizophrenia is that it is due to a process of neural injury or neurodegeneration. This was first suggested by Emil Kraepelin,[1] who emphasized the chronic deteriorating course of dementia praecox. Subsequent longitudinal studies have shown heterogeneity of outcome in schizophrenia; the conditions of some patients deteriorate, while the conditions of others improve or stabilize.[2-5] Recent life-span studies of schizophrenia in late life have revealed frequent severe cognitive and functional impairments among elderly patients who are chronically institutionalized.[6,7] However, not all investigators find cognitive decline over time,[8-10] so further clinical and neurobiological study of this possibility, as well as its presumed neurodegenerative substrate, is warranted.

Arnold et al,[6] and Davidson et al[7] have found that as many as two thirds of institutionalized elderly patients with schizophrenia meet the *DSM-IV*[11] criteria for an additional diagnosis of dementia and that

the neuropsychological profile of this dementia resembles that seen in Alzheimer disease (AD).[12] However, to date, neuropathologic studies have identified no abnormalities to explain the dementia in the overwhelming majority of patients.[6,13-15] This is remarkable because postmortem studies of community populations consistently show that approximately 50% to 60% of elderly patients with dementia have AD, 20% to 30% have vascular dementia or mixed AD-vascular dementia, and 10% to 20% have dementia due to various other neurodegenerative, structural, or metabolic causes.[16] Thus, the neurobiological basis for the dementia in "poor-outcome" patients with schizophrenia remains unknown.

A number of common alterations in the cellular and molecular composition of the brain occur with neurodegenerative diseases or as nonspecific responses to neural injury.

From the Departments of Psychiatry (Drs Arnold and Gur, Mr Blackwell, and Mss Han and Choi), Neurology (Drs Arnold and Gur), and Pathology and Laboratory Medicine (Dr Trojanowski), University of Pennsylvania School of Medicine, Philadelphia.

This article is also available on our Web site: www.ama-assn.org/psych.

139

PATIENTS AND METHODS

PATIENTS

Autopsies were performed on 23 patients with schizophrenia (group 1), 14 age-compatible control patients with no neuropsychiatric disease (group 2), and 10 patients with AD who served as "positive" controls (group 3); **Table 1** and **Table 2**. All patients with schizophrenia were prospectively accrued from 8 state hospitals in Pennsylvania and were clinically assessed and diagnosed according to the *DSM-IV*[12] criteria by research psychiatrists of the University of Pennsylvania Schizophrenia Mental Health Clinical Research Center, Philadelphia (under the direction of R.E.G.), as previously described.[6] Of the 23 patients in group 1, 16 met the criteria for an additional diagnosis of dementia. Clinical features were characterized with standard research psychiatric rating instruments before death for correlation with the postmortem findings. These included the Mini-Mental State Examination,[22] the Brief Psychiatric Rating Scale,[23] the Scale for the Assessment of Positive Symptoms,[24] the Scale for the Assessment of Negative Symptoms,[25] the Abnormal Involuntary Movement Scale,[26] and the activities of daily living subscale of the Physical Self-Maintenance Scale (Functional Assessment Scale).[27] The mean (±SD) interval between testing and death was 10.0±6.7 months (range, 1-24 months). While there was a broad range, the mean values for the patients in group 1 characterized them as having moderate to severe dementia, moderate to severe global psychopathologic disease, marked negative symptomatology, questionable to mild positive symptomatology, rare tardive dyskinesia, and a need for assistance with basic activities of daily living.

Brain tissues from patients in groups 2 and 3 were obtained through the University of Pennsylvania Alzheimer Disease Center Core, Philadelphia. While none of these patients had undergone antemortem assessments, a review of their clinical histories found no evidence of major psychiatric illness. Most patients in group 3 had end-stage dementia. There were no differences among patients in the 3 groups for age ($F_{2,44}=1.67$; $P=20.$), sex ($\chi^2=0.72$; $df=2$; $P=.70$), or postmortem interval (PMI; $F_{2,44}=0.50$; $P=.61$).

Gross and microscopic diagnostic neuropathologic examinations, which included examination of multiple cortical and subcortical regions, were performed for all patients. No neuropathologic abnormalities relevant to mental status were found in groups 1 and 2. Minor abnormalities were noted in 3 patients in group 1 (lacunar infarcts in 2 and posterior fossa meningioma in 1) and 2 patients in group 2 (lacunar infarcts in 1 and small bitemporal contusions in 1). Aside from abundant NFTs and APs, no other abnormalities were found in group 3. The diagnosis of AD was based on established consensus criteria.[28]

TISSUE PROCESSING AND IMMUNOHISTOCHEMISTRY

Blocks from the ventromedial temporal lobe, the middle frontal gyrus, the straight gyrus, and the calcarine sulcus were dissected at autopsy, fixed in ethanol (ethyl alcohol, 70%; sodium chloride concentration, 150 mmol/L) for 24 hours, paraffin embedded, and cut into 20-µm-thick sections. Pathologic markers were immunohistochemically identified with the following antibodies: PHF-1[20] for NFTs, 2332[30] for APs, RMO32[31] for Lewy bodies, Ubi-1 (Zymed Labs Inc, South San Francisco, Calif) for ubiquitinated dystrophic neurites, 2.2B10[32] for glial fibrillary acidic protein (GFAP) in astrocytes, and CD68 (DAKO Corp, Carpinteria, Calif) for resting and active microglia. For the monoclonal antibodies (PHF-1, Ubi-1, 2.2B10, and RMO32), immunocytochemistry was performed using a previously described peroxidase-antiperoxidase procedure,[33] and for the polyclonal antibodies (2332 and CD68), the avidin-biotin-complex method (Vector Laboratories Inc, Burlingame, Calif) was used. For each antibody and region, all cases were included in single, precisely timed runs.

SELECTION OF REGIONS AND NEUROPATHOLOGIC MARKER DENSITY ESTIMATION

Six regions were delineated: entorhinal cortex (Brodmann area [BA] 28), subiculum and CA1 of the hippocampus, midfrontal cortex (BAs 9 and 46), orbitofrontal cortex (BA 11), and calcarine cortex (BA 17). The entorhinal and hippocampal sections were obtained from the anterior portion of the main body of the hippocampus. Regional boundaries were cytoarchitecturally determined in comparison with adjacent Nissl-stained sections.[34,35] Neurons in these subfields are especially vulnerable to the accumulation of pathologic lesions in AD[36] and other neurodegenerative diseases (eg, Pick disease, amyotrophic lateral sclerosis–dementia complex).[17] Midfrontal and orbitofrontal cortices were identified topographically and cytoarchitecturally.[37] They are also vulnerable in various neurodegenerative diseases.[36,38] The calcarine cortex (primary visual cortex) was chosen as an internal control region that is relatively resistant to the accumulation of neurodegenerative lesions.[36,39]

After codification of slides for blind measurements, the densities of NFTs, Lewy bodies, ubiquitinated dystrophic

---

For instance, neurofibrillary tangles (NFTs) and amyloid plaques (APs) are relatively specific features of AD,[17] and Lewy bodies are typical of Parkinson disease and related conditions.[18] More general indicators of neural injury include reactive astrocytosis, microglial proliferation, and accumulations of ubiquitin (an 8.6-kd heat shock protein induced by a variety of noxious stimuli) in neurons, neuronal processes, and glia.[19-21]

The present study was designed to test the hypotheses that abnormal neurodegeneration or neu-ral injury occurs in the brains of elderly poor-outcome patients with schizophrenia and that the quantities of neurodegenerative lesions correlate with deterioration of their clinical conditions. While not representative of schizophrenia at large, our sample is particularly well suited for these studies because of its severity, chronicity, and advanced age. Thus, if accumulated degenerative pathology is an aspect of schizophrenia, it should be more evident in this sample than in a younger or better-functioning groups.

neurites, astrocytes, and microglia were determined by using computer-assisted microscopy, systematic sampling, and nonbiased stereological object counting software[40] (StereoInvestigator, MicroBrightField Inc, Colchester, Vt). Slides from the 47 patients underwent analyses in random order by either of 2 trained operators (C.C. or L.-Y.H.). Preliminary studies indicated high interrater and intrarater reliability for the stereological counting method with an intraclass correlation coefficient greater than 0.80 for the markers. Briefly, after the region was delimited at low power, a grid of predetermined size was randomly placed over the entire region by the software program. The objective was raised to ×40, and the program was engaged to direct the motorized stage on the microscope to stop at each intersection point of the grid for sampling. The fields were visualized on the video monitor with a superimposed counting frame, and objects were counted by using the optical fractionator and optical dissector.[40,41] The counting frame remained superimposed on the image as the operator focused through a fixed depth of 10 µm in the section. All new objects coming into focus were counted if they were within the frame or touching either of the 2 inclusion lines and as long as they did not touch the exclusion lines of the box.

The NFTs were counted after identification by their immunoreactivity for PHF-1 and their characteristic appearance. Ubiquitinated dystrophic neurites were identified by their appearance as "dots" of various sizes. The GFAP astrocytes were identified by the presence of a visible nucleus and characteristic processes. Finally, the criteria for CD68 resting and activated microglia included small size, round or elongated nuclei, and scant cytoplasm (**Figure 1** through **Figure 5**).

For APs, we measured the total area occupied by amyloid deposits within 3 systematically selected ×20 fields in each of the regions of interest in each case using image analysis software (NIH Image, version 1.59, W. Rasband, National Institutes of Health, Bethesda, Md). This method obviated the inherent difficulty in counting individual plaques that may be contiguous or overlapping. The amyloid-laden area was determined in layers II and III of the entorhinal cortex, the pyramidal cell layer of subiculum and CA1, and layer V of midfrontal and orbitofrontal cortices. These layers were chosen because they are especially vulnerable to the accumulation of APs and other neurodegenerative lesions.[36] In the calcarine cortex, layer IVb was chosen because of its particular resistance to neurodegenerative lesions. After standardizing the threshold, the total area of amyloid deposition within each captured field was determined automatically and expressed as a percentage of the area for the field.

DATA ANALYSIS AND STATISTICS

Normal aging and PMI effects were assessed for correlations with each neuropathologic measure within the nonneuropsychiatric control group (group 2). Correlations for these variables also were conducted for the schizophrenia group (group 1) with the consideration that an interaction between the disease state and the aging process could affect the accumulation of neurodegenerative lesions. In addition, the possible effect of antipsychotic medication was assessed with correlations between the medication dosage 1 month before death (expressed as chlorpromazine milligram equivalents) and each neuropathologic measure in each region of the brain that was studied. Because all of the markers we studied are considered to be age-related phenomena, we included age as a regressor in the analyses. Significant correlations for the other potentially confounding variables prompted their inclusion as regressors in subsequent analyses as well.

For analyses of between-group differences, we collapsed the 6 individual regions into 3: hippocampal, frontal, and calcarine. This was done to generate a meaningful neural system–density value and to avoid overweighting the 3 ventromedial temporal regions in comparison with the 2 frontal regions and the 1 visual region. The mean hippocampal score was the average of the density values for the entorhinal cortex, subiculum, and CA1. Similarly, midfrontal and orbitofrontal cortices were combined into a "frontal" mean. Group differences for each neuropathologic measure were analyzed in analyses of covariance (ANCOVA), with the diagnostic group as the independent variable, marker densities in the 3 regions as the repeated-measures dependent variable, and age as the regressor. These were followed by post hoc Scheffé S tests to assess between-group differences in each region. To further assess possible region-specific differences, individual ANCOVAs were similarly performed. Analyses were conducted using statistical software (Statview 4.1 and SuperANOVA, Abacus Concepts Inc, Berkeley, Calif). An α level of .05 was used to determine significance.

Whether or not patients in group 1 had excessive amounts of neurodegenerative lesions compared with patients in group 2, we also considered the possibility that a person with an otherwise abnormal brain may be more vulnerable to the neuropsychological impact of any "normal" age-related neurodegenerative changes. We explored this by determining correlations between the summary scores for each of our clinical measures and the density values for each of the neuropathologic markers.

───────── **RESULTS** ─────────

EFFECTS OF AGE, SEX, PMI, AND ANTIPSYCHOTIC MEDICATION AS POTENTIAL CONFOUNDING VARIABLES

Within group 2, we found significant correlations between age and NFT density in the hippocampal region ($r=0.545$, $P<.05$), between age and astrocytosis in the hippocampal region ($r=0.58$, $P<.03$), and

between age and microglial density in all regions (hippocampal, $r=0.79$, $P<.001$; frontal, $r=0.52$, $P=.05$; and calcarine, $r=0.52$, $P=.05$), but we found no significant correlations between age and AP deposition or ubiquitinated dystrophic neurite densities. We found no significant correlations between age and pathologic markers in group 1 or between PMI and markers in groups 1 and 2 for any region. There were no sex differences. Within group 1, we found negative correlations between the dosage of antipsychotic medication

141

Table 1. Demographic Data*

	Group		
	1 (n=23)	2 (n=14)	3 (n=10)
Age, y	79.8 (8.2)	75.3 (12.1)	81.8 (6.6)
Sex, M/F	8/15	6/8	5/5
Postmortem interval, h	11.0 (3.1)	11.4 (5.3)	9.8 (3.8)
Brain weight, g	1192 (156)	1223 (193)	1141 (173)

Group 1, patients with schizophrenia; group 2, control patients with no neuropsychiatric disease; and group 3, "positive" control patients with Alzheimer disease. Data, except for sex, are given as mean (SD).

Table 2. Clinical Data for Subjects With Schizophrenia(n=23)*

	Mean	SD	Range
Age at onset, y	24.7	5.6	16-39
Duration of illness, y	55.1	9.2	38-76
Antipsychotic dosage, CPZ mg	225	291	0-900 (7 drug free)
MMSE	12.3	8.6	0-28
BPRS	59.0	21.1	20-87
SANS	2.69	1.34	0.33-4.65
SAPS	0.91	0.58	0.0-2.19
FAS	2.04	0.75	1.0-3.0
AIMS	1.70	1.15	1-5

CPZ mg indicates chlorpromazine milligram equivalents; MMSE, Mini-Mental State Examination; BPRS, Brief Psychiatric Rating Scale; SANS, Scale for the Assessment of Negative Symptoms; SAPS, Scale for the Assessment of Positive Symptoms; FAS, the Functional Assessment Scale of the Physical Self-Maintenance Scale; and AIMS; Abnormal Involuntary Movement Scale.

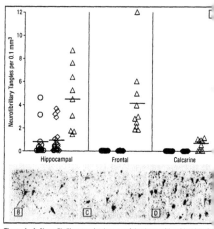

Figure 1. A, Neurofibrillary tangles in group 1 (patients with schizophrenia) group 2 (control patients with no neuropsychiatric disease), and group 3 ("positive" control patients with Alzheimer disease). There was a significant main effect of diagnosis ($F_{2,1,43}$=47.53, P =.001), with group 3 differing from each of the other diagnostic groups overall and in individual regional analyses. The subiculum in an 80-year-old woman from group 1 (B), an 81-year-old woman from group 2 (C), and a 79-year-old woman from group 3 (D) (B-D, immunohistochemical stain with PHF-1, original magnification ×200). Diamonds indicate group 1; circles, group 2; and triangles, group 3.

and astrocyte density in the frontal region (r=-0.49, P<.04) and microglia in the hippocampal region (r=-0.56, P<.02).

MARKERS OF NEURODEGENERATION AND NEURAL INJURY

We found significant between-group differences for the densities of NFTs, APs, ubiquitinated dystrophic neurites, GFAP astrocytes, and microglia, with group 3 having much higher density values than the other 2 groups, as expected (**Table 3** and Figures 1-5). Analyses of individual regions revealed no differences between groups 1 and 2 for any marker. No RMO32 immunoreactive Lewy bodies were observed in any cortical region in any of the cases.

Ubiquitin-immunoreactive dots of varying sizes, which represent degenerating axons, dendrites, and, perhaps, other cellular debris, were found freestanding in the cortices and in association with APs but not NFTs. Because of this association, we also performed an ANCOVA using the percentage area of AP as an additional regressor. This failed to diminish the between-group differences in the repeated-measures ANCOVA ($F_{2,1,1,42}$=25.20, P<.001) or for individual regions in post hoc analyses.

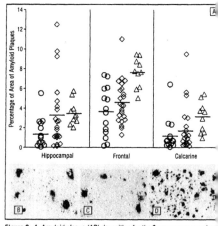

Figure 2. A, Amyloid plaque (AP) deposition for the 3 groups expressed as the percentage of the microscopic field occupied by 2332 immunoreactive amyloid plaque deposits. There was a significant effect of diagnosis for AP deposition overall ($F_{2,1,43}$=7.05, P =.002) and regionally in the hippocampal and frontal regions but not the calcarine cortex, with group 3 greater than groups 1 and 2 in the frontal region, but only group 2 in the hippocampal region. Scattered amyloid deposition in layer V of the orbitofrontal cortex in the patients in groups 1 (B) and 2 (C) and heavy amyloid deposition in the patient in group 3 (D) (B-D, immunohistochemical stain with 2332,[30] original magnification ×200) . See the legend to Figure 1 for the definitions of the groups and descriptions of the patients represented in the photomicrographs. Diamonds indicate group 1; circles, group 2; and triangles, group 3.

142

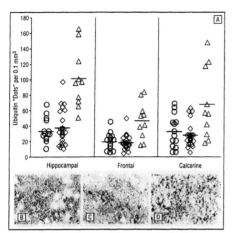

Figure 3. *A, Ubi-1 ubiquitin-immunoreactive dystrophic neurites. There was a significant between-group difference ($F_{2,1,43}=33.14$, P<.001) with post hoc comparisons showing differences between group 3 and each of the other diagnostic groups overall and in regional analyses. Scattered ubiquitinated neurites in layer III of the midfrontal cortex in the patients in groups 1 (B) and 2 (C) and dense accumulation of ubiquitinated neurites in the patient in group 3 (D) (B-D, immunohistochemical stain with Ubi-1, original magnification ×400). See the legend to Figure 1 for the definitions of the groups and descriptions of the patients represented in the photomicrographs. Diamonds indicate group 1; circles, group 2; and triangles, group 3.*

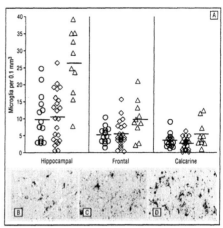

Figure 5. *A, CD68-immunoreactive microglia. Between-group differences were significant overall ($F_{2,1,43}=13.16$, P<.001). Regional analyses of covariance demonstrated higher microglial cell densities in group 3 compared with groups 1 and 2 in all regions except the calcarine cortex, in which the mean value for group 1 was significantly lower than for group 3, but was not significantly different between groups 2 and 3. CA1 in the hippocampus demonstrate scattered microglia in the patients from groups 1 (B) and 2 (C) and more dense infiltration in the patient from group 3 (D) (B-D, immunohistochemical stain with CD68, original magnification ×400). See the legend to Figure 1 for the definitions of the groups and descriptions of the patients represented in the photomicrographs. Diamonds indicate group 1; circles, group 2; and triangles, group 3.*

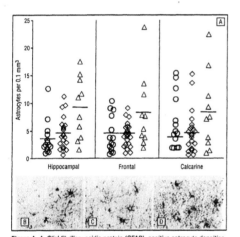

Figure 4. *A, Glial fibrillary acidic protein (GFAP)–positive astrocyte densities. The GFAP-immunoreactive astrocytosis also showed a between-group difference ($F_{2,1,43}=5.14$, P<.01) with density values for group 3 that were significantly greater than for groups 1 and 2 overall and in each region. The GFAP-positive astrocytes in the the entorhinal cortex in patients from groups 1 (B), 2 (C), and 3 (D). In the patient from group 3, the astrocytes were more numerous, larger, and more intensely decorated than in the patients from groups 1 and 2 (B-D, immunohistochemical stain with 2.2B10, original magnification ×200). See the legend to Figure 1 for the definitions of the groups and descriptions of the patients represented in the photomicrographs. Diamonds indicate group 1; circles, group 2; and triangles, group 3.*

CLINICOPATHOLOGIC CORRELATIONS

Although there were no differences between groups 1 and 2 for any of the neuropathologic markers studied, we determined the extent to which the clinical features correlated with neuropathologic findings. This was prompted by our hypothesis that the accumulation of any neurodegenerative lesions might affect cognition or psychiatric status in persons with schizophrenia if their illness caused them to be less resilient to the toxic effects of such lesions. No significant correlations were observed between clinical variables and any neuropathologic markers for any region.

COMMENT

In this series, we used a panel of highly sensitive and molecularly specific antibodies to identify diverse pathologic features of the most common neurodegenerative diseases, as well as general responses to neural injury, in a sample of elderly poor-outcome patients with schizophrenia. The temporal and frontal regions that we evaluated are found to be preferentially vulnerable to aging, neurodegenerative disease, and other types of neural injury.[17,19,36,42] Furthermore, these regions have been invoked as abnormal in schizophrenia.[43,44] We found no differences between patients with schizophrenia and control patients with no neuropsychiatric disease for any marker in any region. Therefore, the hypothesis that neurodegenerative disease processes or postmaturational neu

143

Table 3. Mean (SD) Density Values
for Neuropathologic Markers*

Antibody and	Group		
Lesion/Region	1 (n=23)	2 (n=14)	3 (n=10)
PHF-1 neurofibrillary tangles			
Entorhinal	0.76 (0.11)	0.55 (0.10)	3.23 (2.45)
Subiculum	0.67 (0.11)	0.48 (0.99)	5.98 (4.79)
CA1	0.63 (0.85)	0.96 (2.22)	4.03 (2.18)
Midfrontal	0 (0)	0 (0)	5.20 (3.82)
Orbitofrontal	0 (0)	0 (0)	2.93 (2.55)
Calcarine	0 (0)	0 (0)	0.52 (4.72)
2332 for amyloid plaques			
Entorhinal	4.15 (3.89)	2.12 (2.57)	4.18 (2.24)
Subiculum	1.11 (1.41)	1.14 (1.70)	2.64 (1.57)
CA1	1.17 (1.74)	0.92 (1.36)	3.58 (1.39)
Midfrontal	4.30 (3.57)	3.52 (2.84)	6.63 (3.33)
Orbitofrontal	4.89 (4.08)	3.73 (3.48)	8.55 (1.85)
Calcarine	1.72 (2.29)	1.20 (1.66)	3.04 (1.58)
Ubi-1† for ubiquitinated dystrophic neurites			
Entorhinal	24.5 (1.3)	19.6 (1.1)	106.1 (42.7)
Subiculum	46.6 (34.8)	50.7 (19.4)	101.6 (42.4)
CA1	40.5 (33.4)	31.2 (3.5)	92.4 (51.5)
Midfrontal	20.2 (9.5)	27.2 (18.2)	55.0 (35.8)
Orbitofrontal	16.5 (10.7)	12.2 (8.3)	38.2 (16.9)
Calcarine	28.0 (15.8)	32.7 (21.2)	67.7 (46.2)
2.2B10 for GFAP in astrocytes			
Entorhinal	5.02 (4.61)	3.69 (4.27)	9.97 (5.63)
Subiculum	5.36 (4.67)	4.54 (4.48)	10.02 (7.98)
CA1	2.66 (2.39)	2.00 (1.61)	7.16 (5.49)
Midfrontal	4.75 (2.92)	5.28 (4.47)	7.64 (5.55)
Orbitofrontal	3.75 (2.57)	3.18 (2.63)	8.72 (9.12)
Calcarine	4.60 (3.79)	6.49 (4.86)	8.35 (6.98)
CD68 for resting and active microglia			
Entorhinal	8.01 (5.93)	6.95 (4.93)	21.98 (7.00)
Subiculum	11.52 (9.13)	11.32 (8.94)	31.82 (14.51)
CA1	11.83 (9.10)	11.47 (8.64)	24.49 (14.81)
Midfrontal	4.99 (4.33)	5.24 (3.31)	9.18 (5.91)
Orbitofrontal	5.67 (4.59)	4.96 (2.86)	10.71 (7.11)
Calcarine	2.62 (1.75)	3.41 (2.08)	5.39 (3.85)

*Group 1, patients with schizophrenia; group 2, control patients with no neuropsychiatric disease; and group 3, positive control patients with Alzheimer disease. Values are given per 0.1 mm³ execpt 2332 for amyloid plaques, which is expressed as a percentage of the area for the microscopic field. GFAP indicates glial fibrillary acidic protein.
†Zymed Labs Inc, South San Francisco, Calif.

ral injury are active in the cerebral cortex in schizophrenia in late life is not supported.

METHODOLOGICAL CONSIDERATIONS

Our study was designed to overcome many of the methodological limitations that have beset postmortem research in schizophrenia. Among these have been the uncertainties inherent in using diagnoses from the medical record or retrospective application of diagnostic criteria to review of the medical record; inconsistencies in tissue handling, preparation, and fixation; inconsistencies in the selection of regions of interest; limited sensitivity and specificity of classic histological stains; and the lack

or inadequacy of quantitative methods of analysis to detect subtle brain abnormalities. All of our patients were accrued prospectively and underwent antemortem assessments that included clinical rating scales that could be used for clinicopathologic correlation. The postmortem intervals between death and autopsy were short, and autopsies were performed uniformly with tissue fixation and processing protocols optimized to preserve the antigens of interest. Regions of interest were defined using cytoarchitectural criteria, and we identified the neuropathologic markers using immunohistochemistry with well-characterized molecule-specific antibodies. Finally, we used computer-assisted random systematic sampling and stereological counting methods for reliable and unbiased counts.

Some potential limitations in our design should be recognized. One concerns the regions we chose to study. We selected the cortical regions because of their known vulnerability to neurodegenerative processes. A broader array of cortical and subcortical regions were surveyed in diagnostic neuropathologic examinations that preceded our quantitative analyses, and no pertinent abnormalities were identified. Nevertheless, subtle but important neurodegenerative abnormalities could still occur in subcortical or other cortical regions. Another limitation is our choice of neuropathologic markers. We studied the most important and common disease-specific and non–disease-specific markers that reflect diverse mechanisms of cell death. Programmed cell death is another mode of cell death that is not necessarily accompanied by an elevation of the neurodegenerative markers we studied, and, thus, it warrants future study. A third limitation is the relatively small sample available for correlation analyses; caution is warranted in drawing firm conclusions from the negative findings. Finally, we cannot rule out extremely remote, occult, or indolent neurodegenerative processes. All of the markers we studied are dynamic and persist only to varying degrees after neural injury. Thus, we can say for certain only that we found no evidence for ongoing or recent neurodegeneration or neural injury in schizophrenia in late life.

COMPARISON WITH PREVIOUS STUDIES

Previous studies of AD-related pathology in schizophrenia have been controversial. For example, some studies of archival specimens reported an increased prevalence of AD among patients with schizophrenia.[45,46] However, other studies that used better-characterized specimens and quantitative methods found no increase in AD-related lesions,[13,15,47,48] and we confirm this finding in the present study.

Investigations of astrocytosis in schizophrenia have figured prominently in discussions of neurodevelopmental vs postmaturational neural injury hypotheses for schizophrenia, but the results also have been controversial. Studies using the traditional Holzer stain have reported subcortical fibrillary gliosis, particularly in periventricular, periaqueductal, and basal forebrain regions.[47,49] In contrast, numerous other studies using Nissl stains or GFAP immunohistochemistry have failed to find astrocytosis in patients with schizophrenia com

144

pared with persons with no neuropsychiatric disease.[50-55] Methodological issues have been raised with a number of these studies, chiefly the sensitivities and specificities of staining methods and the type and duration of fixation before staining.[56] We found no difference in GFAP-immunoreactive astrocytosis between groups with and without schizophrenia, similar to results in another cohort from our registry.[50]

To our knowledge, there has been only 1 previous study of ubiquitin in schizophrenia. Horton et al[57] found no increase in ubiquitin in the prefrontal cortex of patients with schizophrenia, although the mean postmortem interval before tissue fixation in that study was 105 hours. We focused on ubiquitinated dystrophic neurites as a general index of neuronal degeneration that is present in a host of neurodegenerative diseases, as well as in normal aging and age-associated cognitive impairment.[58] Our negative results in the group with schizophrenia with this sensitive marker provide further strong evidence against there being neural injury in the disease.

Finally, microglia have been found to be increased in a number of pathologic conditions[21] but have not been studied previously in schizophrenia. Of special relevance to the consideration that microglia might be increased in schizophrenia are several reports of the abnormal lymphocyte production of immunoregulatory cytokines, including interleukin 2 and interleukin 6, that have been related to clinical and medication status.[59-61] We were particularly interested in whether these immunologic abnormalities might be reflected in abnormal microglial density in the brain. Again, no abnormality was found.

OTHER CONSIDERATIONS TO EXPLAIN THE DEMENTIA OF SCHIZOPHRENIA IN LATE LIFE

Without evidence of conventional neurodegenerative pathologic changes in schizophrenia, other factors must be considered to explain the dementia. It remains possible that the effects of normal age-related changes are amplified in the presence of presumably abnormal neural circuitry in schizophrenia. This is especially pertinent given the topographic similarities between the brain regions in which neuroanatomic abnormalities have been reported and those that are most vulnerable in aging and the common neurodegenerative diseases. For instance, abnormalities in cytoarchitecture, neuron density, and innervation have been described in the entorhinal cortex in schizophrenia.[52,62-67] Most of these have been presumed to result from aberrant development of the fetal brain. From a neurodegenerative perspective, the entorhinal cortex is the first region in the brain to accumulate NFTs in aging and AD and is the most severely affected,[68] and, along with the prefrontal cortices, it is severely affected in various other dementias, such as diffuse Lewy body disease, Pick disease, amyotrophic lateral sclerosis–dementia, and non-Alzheimer frontal lobe dementia. We postulate that the effects of any neurodegenerative lesions occurring in already dysfunctional neural systems might be great enough to cause dementia. We sought a correlation between dementia (and other clinical features) and neurodegenerative markers and did not

find one. As an alternative, we speculate that there is a correlation between the "baseline" severity of developmentally based abnormalities and clinical features, including dementia, in late life. The task remains to better delineate the nature of such abnormalities.

Other possible mechanisms should be considered to explain the deterioration in the conditions of patients with schizophrenia in late life. Beyond a contribution from psychosocial factors, such as chronic institutionalization or the effects of long-term use of antipsychotic medication, other cellular and subcellular neurobiological mechanisms might include disease and age-related regressive changes in dendritic arborization or axonal plexi, neuronal atrophy, nucleolar shrinkage and changes in RNA content, changes in protein metabolism, increased vulnerability to oxidative or excitotoxic damage, slowed axoplasmic transport, alterations in the neuronal cytoskeleton, and altered synaptic integrity and synaptic transmission. The study of these aspects of neuron structure and function in the context of the clinical expression of schizophrenia over the life span may further elucidate the basis of this severe illness.

Accepted for publication September 4, 1997.

Reprints: Steven E. Arnold, MD, Center for Neurobiology and Behavior, University of Pennsylvania, 142 Clinical Research Bldg, 415 Curie Blvd, Philadelphia, PA 19104 (e-mail: alveus@mail.med.upenn.edu).

REFERENCES

1. Kraepelin E. Dementia Praecox and Paraphrenia. Edinburgh, Scotland: E & S Livingstone; 1919.
2. Bleuler M. A 23-year longitudinal study of 208 schizophrenics and impressions in regard to the nature of schizophrenia. In: Rosenthal D, Kety SS, eds. The Transmission of Schizophrenia. New York, NY: Pergamon Press Inc; 1968:3-12.
3. Ciompi L. Catamnestic long-term study on the course of life and aging of schizophrenics. Schizophr Bull. 1980;6:606-618.
4. Carpenter WT, Kirkpatrick B. The heterogeneity of the long-term course of schizophrenia. Schizophr Bull. 1988;14:515-542.
5. Winokur G, Pfohl B, Tsuang M. A 40-year follow-up of hebephrenic-catatonic schizophrenia. In: Miller N, Cohen G, eds. Schizophrenia and Aging. New York, NY: Guilford Press; 1987:52-60.
6. Arnold SE, Gur RE, Shapiro RM, Fisher KR, Moberg PJ, Gibney MR, Gur RC, Blackwell P, Trojanowski JQ. Prospective clinicopathological studies of schizophrenia: accrual and assessment. Am J Psychiatry. 1995;152:731-737.
7. Davidson M, Harvey PD, Powchik P, Parella M, White L, Knobler HY, Losonczy MF, Keefe RSE, Katz S, Frecska E. Severity of symptoms in chronically institutionalized geriatric schizophrenic patients. Am J Psychiatry. 1995;152:197-207.
8. Goldberg TE, Hyde TM, Leinman JE, Weinberger DR. Course of schizophrenia: neuropsychological evidence for a static encephalopathy. Schizophr Bull. 1993; 19:797-804.
9. Chen EY, Lam LC, Chen RY, Nguyen DG, Chan CK. Prefrontal neuropsychological impairment and illness duration in schizophrenia: a study of 204 patients in Hong Kong. Acta Psychiatr Scand. 1996;93:144-150.
10. Hyde TM, Nawroz S, Goldberg TE, Bigelow LB, Strong D, Ostrem JL, Weinberger DR, Kleinman JE. Is there cognitive decline in schizophrenia? a cross-sectional study. Br J Psychiatry. 1994;164:494-500.
11. American Psychiatric Association. Diagnostic and Statistical Manual of Mental Disorders, Fourth Edition. Washington, DC: American Psychiatric Association; 1994.
12. Moberg PJ, Mahr R, Gibney M, Arnold SE, Shapiro R, Kumar A, Gottlieb G, Gur RE. Neuropsychological functioning in elderly patients with schizophrenia and Alzheimer's disease. J Int Neuropsychol Soc. 1995;1:132. Abstract.
13. Arnold SE, Franz BR, Trojanowski JQ. Elderly patients with schizophrenia exhibit infrequent neurodegenerative lesions. Neurobiol Aging. 1994;15:299-303.
14. Haroutunian V, Davidson M, Kanof PD, Perl DP, Powchik P, Losonezy M, McCrystal J, Purohit DP, Bierer LM, Davis KL. Cortical cholinergic markers in schizophrenia. Schizophr Res. 1994;12:137-144.

145

15. Purohit DP, Davidson M, Perl DP, Powchik P, Haroutunian VH, Bierer LM, McCrystal J, Losonsczy M, Davis KL. Severe cognitive impairment in elderly schizophrenic patients: a clinicopathological study. *Biol Psychiatry*. 1993;33:255-260.

16. Larson EB, Reifler BV, Featherstone HJ, English DR. Dementia in elderly outpatients: a prospective study. *Ann Intern Med*. 1984;100:417-423.

17. Tomlinson BE. Ageing and the dementias. In: Adams JH, Duchen LW, eds. *Greenfield's Neuropathology*. 5th ed. New York, NY: Oxford University Press Inc; 1992:1284-1410.

18. Lowe J. Lewy bodies. In: Calne DB, ed. *Neurodegenerative Diseases*. Philadelphia, Pa: WB Saunders Co; 1993:51-69.

19. Duchen LW. General pathology of neurons and neuroglia. In: Adams JH, Duchen LW, eds. *Greenfield's Neuropathology*. 5th ed. New York, NY: Oxford University Press Inc; 1992:1-68.

20. Lowe J, Mayer RJ, Landon M. Ubiquitin in neurodegenerative diseases. *Brain Pathol*. 1993;3:55-65.

21. Nakajima K, Kohsaka S. Functional roles of microglia in the brain. *Neurosci Res*. 1993;17:187-203.

22. Folstein MF, Folstein S, McHugh PR. Mini-mental state: a practical method for grading the cognitive state of patients for the clinician. *J Psychiatr Res*. 1975; 12:189-198.

23. Overall JE, Gorham DR. The Brief Psychiatric Rating Scale. *Psychol Rep*. 1962; 10:799-812.

24. Andreasen NC. *The Scale for the Assessment of Positive Symptoms (SAPS)*. Iowa City, Iowa: The University of Iowa; 1984.

25. Andreasen NC. *The Scale for the Assessment of Negative Symptoms (SANS)*. Iowa City, Iowa: The University of Iowa; 1983.

26. Guy W, ed. *ECDEU Assessment Manual for Psychopharmacology*. Washington, DC: US Dept of Health, Education and Welfare; 1976. US Dept of Health, Education and Welfare publication ADM76-338.

27. Lawton MP, Brody EM. Physical Self-Maintenance Scale (Functional Assessment). *Gerontologist*. 1969;9:179-186.

28. Khachaturian ZS. Diagnosis of Alzheimer's disease. *Arch Neurol*. 1985;42:1097-1105.

29. Greenberg SG, Davies P. A preparation of Alzheimer paired helical filaments that displays distinct tau proteins by polyacrylamide gel electrophoresis. *Proc Natl Acad Sci U S A*. 1990;87:5827-5831.

30. Schmidt ML, DiDario AG, Lee VM-Y, Trojanowski JQ. An extensive network of PHF-t-rich dystrophic neurites permeates neocortex and nearly all neuritic and diffuse amyloid plaques in Alzheimer disease. *FEBS Lett*. 1994;344:69-73.

31. Schmidt ML, Murray J, Lee VM-Y, Hill WD, Wertkin A, Trojanowski JQ. Epitope map of neurofilament protein domains in cortical and peripheral nervous system Lewy bodies. *Am J Pathol*. 1991;139:53-65.

32. Trojanowski JQ, Gordon D, Obrocka M, Lee VM-Y. The developmental expression of neurofilament and glial filament proteins in the human pituitary gland: an immunohistochemical study with monoclonal antibodies. *Dev Brain Res*. 1984; 13:229-239.

33. Arai H, Lee VM-Y, Messinger ML, Greenberg BD, Lowery DE, Trojanowski JQ. Expression patterns of beta-amyloid precursor protein (beta-APP) in neural and nonneural human tissues from Alzheimer's disease and control subjects. *Ann Neurol*. 1991;30:686-693.

34. Amaral DG, Insausti R. Hippocampal formation. In: Paxinos G, ed. *The Human Nervous System*. San Diego, Calif: Academic Press Inc; 1990:711-755.

35. Insausti R, Tunon T, Sobreviela T, Insausti AM, Gonzalo LM. The human entorhinal cortex: a cytoarchitectonic analysis. *J Comp Neurol*. 1995;355:171-198.

36. Arnold SE, Hyman BT, Flory J, Damasio AR, Hoesen GWV. The topographical and neuroanatomical distribution of neurofibrillary tangles and neuritic plaques in the cerebral cortex of patients with Alzheimer's disease. *Cereb Cortex*. 1991;1:103-116.

37. Rajkowska G, Goldman-Rakic PS. Cytoarchitectonic definition of prefrontal areas in the normal human cortex, I: remapping of areas 9 and 46 using quantitative criteria. *Cereb Cortex*. 1995;5:307-322.

38. Arnold SE. Cellular and molecular pathology of the frontal lobe dementias. In: Trojanowski JQ, Clark CM, eds. *Neurodegenerative Dementia: Clinical and Pathological Mechanisms*. New York, NY: McGraw-Hill Book Co. In press.

39. Carey J. Visual system. In: Paxinos G, ed. *The Human Nervous System*. San Diego, Calif: Academic Press Inc; 1990:945-977.

40. West MJ. New stereological methods for counting neurons. *Neurobiol Aging*. 1993;14:287-293.

41. Gundersen HJG, Bendtsen TF, Korbo L, Marcussen N, Moller A, Nielsen K, Nyengaard JN, Pakkenberg B, Sorenson FB, Vesterby A, West MJ. Some new, simple and efficient stereological methods and their use in pathological research and diagnosis. *APMIS*. 1988;96:379-394.

42. Mann DMA. Vulnerability of specific neurons to aging. In: Calne DB, ed. *Neurodegenerative Diseases*. Philadelphia, Pa: WB Saunders Co; 1994:15-31.

43. Gur RE, Pearlson GD. Neuroimaging in schizophrenia research. *Schizophr Bull*. 1993;19:337-353.

44. Arnold SE, Trojanowski JQ. Recent advances in defining the neuropathology of schizophrenia. *Acta Neuropathol*. 1996;92:217-231.

45. Buhl L, Bojsen-Moller M. Frequency of Alzheimer's disease in a postmortem study of psychiatric patients. *Dan Med Bull*. 1988;35:288-290.

46. Prohovnik I, Dwork AJ, Kaufman MA, Wilson N. Alzheimer-type neuropathology in elderly schizophrenia patients. *Schizophr Bull*. 1993;19:805-816.

47. Bruton CJ, Crow TJ, Frith CD, Johnstone EC, Owens DGC, Roberts GW. Schizophrenia and the brain: a prospective clinico-neuropathological study. *Psychol Med*. 1990;20:285-304.

48. Powchik P, Davidson M, Nemeroff CB, Haroutunian V, Purohit DP, Losonczy M, Bissette G, Perl D, Ghanbari H, Miller B, Davis K. Alzheimer's-disease-related protein in geriatric schizophrenic patients with cognitive impairment. *Am J Psychiatry*. 1993;150:1726-1727.

49. Stevens JR. Neuropathology of schizophrenia. *Arch Gen Psychiatry*. 1982;39: 1131-1139.

50. Arnold SE, Franz BR, Trojanowski JQ, Moberg PJ, Gur RE. Glial fibrillary acidic protein immunoreactive astrocytosis in elderly patients with schizophrenia and dementia. *Acta Neuropathol*. 1996;91:269-277.

51. Benes FM, Davidson J, Bird ED. Quantitative cytoarchitectural studies of the cerebral cortex of schizophrenics. *Arch Gen Psychiatry*. 1986;43:31-35.

52. Falkai P, Bogerts B, Rozumek M. Limbic pathology in schizophrenia: the entorhinal region: a morphometric study. *Biol Psychiatry*. 1988;24:515-521.

53. Roberts GW, Colter N, Lofthouse R, Johnstone EC, Crow TJ. Is there gliosis in schizophrenia? investigation of the temporal lobe. *Biol Psychiatry*. 1987;22: 1459-1468.

54. Stevens CD, Altshuler LL, Bogerts B, Falkai P. Quantitative study of gliosis in schizophrenia and Huntington's chorea. *Biol Psychiatry*. 1988;24:697-700.

55. Selemon LD, Rajkowska G, Goldman-Rakic PS. Abnormally high neuronal density in the schizophrenic cortex: a morphometric analysis of prefrontal area 9 and occipital area 17. *Arch Gen Psychiatry*. 1995;52:805-818.

56. Stevens JR, Casanova M, Poltorak M, Germain L, Buchan GC. Comparison of immunocytochemical and Holzer's methods for detection of acute chronic gliosis in human postmortem material. *J Neuropsychiatry Clin Neurosci*. 1992;4: 168-173.

57. Horton K, Forsyth CS, Sibtain N, Ball S, Bruton CJ, Royston MC, Roberts GW. Ubiquitination as a probe for neurodegeneration in the brain in schizophrenia: the prefrontal cortex. *Psychiatry Res*. 1993;48:145-152.

58. Dickson DW, Wertkin A, Kress Y, Ksiezak-Reging H, Yen S-H. Ubiquitin-immunoreactive structures in normal brains: distribution and developmental aspects. *Lab Invest*. 1990;63:87-99.

59. Ganguli R, Zang Z, Shurin G, Chengappa KN, Brar JS, Gubbi AV, Rabin BS. Serum interleukin-6 concentration in schizophrenia: elevation associated with duration of illness. *Psychiatry Res*. 1994;51:1-10.

60. McAllister CG, van Kammen DP, Rehn TJ, Miller AL, Gurklis J, Kelley ME, Yao J, Peters JL. Increases in CSF levels of IL-2 in schizophrenia: effects of recurrence of psychosis and medication status. *Am J Psychiatry*. 1995;152:1291-1297.

61. Ganguli R, Brar JS, Chengappa KR, DeLeo M, Yang ZW, Shurin G, Rabin BS. Mitogen-stimulated interleukin-2 production in never-medicated first-episode schizophrenic patients: the influence of age at onset and negative symptoms. *Arch Gen Psychiatry*. 1995;52:668-672.

62. Arnold SE, Hyman BT, Hoesen GWV, Damasio AR. Some cytoarchitectural abnormalities of the entorhinal cortex in schizophrenia. *Arch Gen Psychiatry*. 1991; 48:625-632.

63. Arnold SE, Han L-Y, Ruschainsky DD. Further evidence of cytoarchitectural abnormalities of the entorhinal cortex in schizophrenia using spatial point pattern analyses. *Biol Psychiatry*. 1997;42:639-647.

64. Jakob H, Beckmann H. Prenatal developmental disturbances in the limbic allocortex in schizophrenics. *J Neural Transm*. 1986;65:303-326.

65. Krimer LS, Herman MM, Saunders RC, Boyd JC, Kleinman JE, Hyde TM, Weinberger DR. Qualitative and quantitative analysis of the entorhinal cortex cytoarchitectural organization in schizophrenics. *Soc Neurosci Abstr*. 1995;21:239.

66. Longson D, Deakin JFW, Benes FM. Increased density of entorhinal glutamate-immunoreactive vertical fibers in schizophrenia. *J Neural Transm*. 1996;103: 503-507.

67. Akil M, Lewis DA. The catecholaminergic innervation of the human entorhinal cortex: alterations in schizophrenia. *Soc Neurosci Abstr*. 1995;21:238.

68. Braak H, Braak E. Neuropathological staging of Alzheimer-related changes. *Acta Neuropathol*. 1991;82:239-259.

146

Selective Deficits in Prefrontal Cortex Function in Medication-Naive Patients With Schizophrenia

Deanna M. Barch, PhD; Cameron S. Carter, MD; Todd S. Braver, PhD; Fred W. Sabb, BA; Angus MacDonald III, MA; Douglas C. Noll, PhD; Jonathan D. Cohen, MD, PhD

Background: Previously we proposed that dorsolateral prefrontal cortex (PFC) supports a specific working memory (WM) subcomponent: the ability to represent and maintain context information necessary to guide appropriate task behavior. By context, we mean prior task-relevant information represented in such a form that it supports selection of the appropriate behavioral response. Furthermore, we hypothesized that WM deficits in schizophrenia reflect impaired context processing due to a disturbance in dorsolateral PFC. We use functional magnetic resonance imaging to examine PFC activation in medication-naive, first-episode patients with schizophrenia during a WM, task-isolating context processing.

Methods: Fourteen first-episode, medication-naive patients with schizophrenia and 12 controls similar in age, sex, and parental education underwent functional magnetic resonance imaging during performance of an A-X version of the Continuous Performance Test.

Results: Patients with schizophrenia demonstrated deficits in dorsolateral PFC activation in task conditions requiring context processing but showed intact activation of posterior and inferior PFC. In addition, patients demonstrated intact activation of the primary motor and somatosensory cortex in response to stimulus processing demands.

Conclusions: These results demonstrate selectivity in dorsolateral PFC dysfunction among medication-naive first-episode patients with schizophrenia, suggesting that a specific deficit in PFC function is present at illness onset, prior to the administration of medication or the most confounding effects of illness duration. Furthermore, these results are consistent with the hypothesis that WM deficits in patients with schizophrenia reflect an impairment in context processing due to a disturbance in dorsolateral PFC function.

Arch Gen Psychiatry. 2001;58:280-288

D ISTURBANCES in prefrontal cortex (PFC) functioning have long been implicated in schizophrenia and have been linked to working memory (WM) deficits.[1] Working memory is typically defined as the ability to temporarily maintain and manipulate information on-line.[2] Several lines of research support a link between PFC and WM dysfunction in schizophrenia[3-19] (for contrasting evidence, see the articles by Manoach et al[17] and Fletcher et al[20]). However, many studies have examined large areas of PFC, combining subregions that may be functionally distinct.[9,13,15,16] Thus, it is not clear whether all or only certain subregions of PFC show disturbed patterns of cognition-related activation in schizophrenia. Additionally, most functional imaging studies have chosen tasks based on their sensitivity to frontal lobe dysfunction (eg, Wisconsin Card Sorting Test)[16,19] or used tasks that tap multiple components of

WM,[9,14,15] making it difficult to determine which specific processes are disturbed in schizophrenia.

Considerable controversy exists about what functions specific regions of PFC carry out in support of WM. Several researchers have argued that ventral regions (ie, Brodmann area [BA] 44, BA 45, and BA 47) subserve pure maintenance functions, whereas dorsolateral (DL) PFC (ie, DLPFC; BA 46, BA 9) is involved in manipulating the contents of WM.[21-23] In contrast, Goldman-Rakic[24] has argued that DLPFC supports the maintenance of information. Our hypothesis regarding DLPFC function combines elements of both views. Specifically, we have proposed that DLPFC supports a subcomponent of WM: the ability to represent and maintain context information necessary to guide appropriate task behavior.[25,26] By context, we mean prior task-relevant information represented in a form that supports selection of the appropriate re-

From the Department of Psychology, Washington University, St Louis, Mo (Drs Barch and Braver); Department of Psychiatry, University of Pittsburgh, Pittsburgh, Pa (Drs Carter and Cohen and Mr MacDonald); Department of Psychology, Princeton University, Princeton, NJ (Mr Sabb and Dr Cohen); and the Department of Biomedical Engineering, University of Michigan, Ann Arbor (Dr Noll).

148

PATIENTS AND METHODS

PARTICIPANTS

Participants were 12 healthy controls and 14 medication-naive first-episode patients with schizophrenia. Controls were recruited through advertisements and evaluated using the nonpatient version of the Structured Clinical Interview for DSM-III-R.[33] All patients were neuroleptic naive and recruited if they were experiencing any type of psychotic symptom (ie, hallucination, delusion, thought disorder) and it was their first psychiatric hospitalization or contact with outpatient psychiatric services. Patients were scanned as soon as possible after initial contact, typically within 1 to 2 days. Patients were followed longitudinally and confirmed to have a diagnosis of schizophrenia 6 months after their participation in this study. Diagnoses were confirmed by diagnostic conference, including information from the Structured Clinical Interview for DSM-III-R,[33] administered by trained research personnel, and thorough medical record review. In addition, the Brief Psychiatric Rating Scale,[34] the Global Assessment Scale, and the Scales for the Assessment of Positive and Negative Symptoms were used to evaluate symptom severity (**Table 1**). Ratings were completed by trained research team personnel, blind to task performance, who regularly participated in evaluation sessions to insure reliability. All ratings were made within 1 week of testing.

Participants were excluded for (1) age (older than 50 years or younger than 14 years); (2) Wechsler Adult Intelligence Scale–Revised full scale IQ lower than 70; (3) non-English native language; (4) lifetime diagnosis of substance dependence or substance abuse within 1 month of testing; (5) neurologic disorders or family history of hereditary neurologic disorder; or (6) pregnancy. Potential controls were excluded if they had (1) lifetime history of axis I disorder or first order family history of a psychotic disorder or (2) treatment with any psychotropic medication within 6 months of testing. Controls were similar to patients regarding age, sex, race, and father's education (as a proxy for socioeconomic status). t Tests indicated that controls did not differ from patients with schizophrenia on any of these variables (Table 1). All participants were right-handed and signed informed consent forms in accordance with the University of Pittsburgh, Pittsburgh, Pa, institutional review board.

COGNITIVE TASK

Single letters were presented centrally on a visual display. Trials lasted 10 seconds and included a cue, a delay period, a probe, and an intertrial interval (ITI). Cue and probe durations were 0.5 seconds. In long delay trials, the cue-probe interval was 8 seconds, and the ITI was 1 second. In short delay trials this was reversed, with a 1-second cue-probe interval and an 8-second ITI to control general pace of the task). Subjects responded to every stimulus with their dominant hand, pressing one button for targets and an adjacent button for nontargets. Eleven patients and 8 controls performed the task continuously for blocks made up of 10 trials. The remaining 3 patients and 4 controls performed the task continuously for blocks of 12 trials. Between each block there was a brief delay, allowing the subject to rest, and the hemodynamic response to recover. Six blocks were run for each of the 2 delay conditions, pseudorandomly ordered to control for the confounding effects of time on task, head movement, and scanner drift.

IMAGE ACQUISITION

Scanning took place using a whole-body scanner (1.5T GE Signa; General Electric Medical Systems, Milwaukee, Wis) and standard head coil in the University of Pittsburgh Medical School, Pittsburgh, Pa, MR Research Center. Sixteen slices (3.75 mm³ voxels) were acquired parallel to the anterior commissure-posterior commissure (AC-PC) line. Functional scans were acquired using a spiral-scan pulse sequence.[35] In 11 patients and 8 controls, we used a 2-shot spiral sequence (TR [time to repetition], 1250 milliseconds; TE [time to echo], 35 milliseconds; flip, 40°; field of view, 24 cm), with scanning synchronized with stimulus presentation so that a set of 16 slices was acquired 4 times during each 10-second trial (Figure 1). In the other 3 patients and 4 controls, we used a 4-shot spiral sequence (TR, 640 milliseconds; TE, 35 milliseconds; flip, 40°; field of view, 24 cm); which allowed 8 slices to be acquired every 2.5 seconds. Scanning was again synchronized with stimulus presentation so that 4 scans of 8 slice locations were acquired during each 10-second trial (Figure 1). A first set of 8 locations was scanned for 3 trials, followed by 2 additional sets of 8 different locations, each scanned for 3

Continued on next page

sponse. Context representations can include instructions, specific prior stimuli, or the result of processing a sequence of prior stimuli (eg, a sentence). Thus, we believe that DLPFC plays a role in manipulation by recoding information into context representations. However, we believe that context representations are also actively maintained in DLPFC, a hypothesis supported by prior imaging work.[27] We have also hypothesized that WM deficits in schizophrenia reflect impaired context processing due to disturbed DLPFC function.[26] In behavioral studies, we have observed a highly selective pattern of schizophrenic deficits in task conditions sensitive to context processing.[28-30] However, we have not yet determined whether context processing deficits in schizophrenia are associated with a selective disturbance in DLPFC function.

The current study, using functional magnetic resonance imaging (fMRI), examined PFC activation in medication-naive first-episode patients with schizophrenia during a WM task-isolating context processing: a version of the A-X Continuous Performance Test (AX-CPT).[25,27,29,30] In the AX-CPT, subjects are presented with a sequence of letters and instructed to respond to a prespecified probe (X) only if it follows a particular contextual cue (A). Target (A-X) trials occur frequently (70%), producing (1) a prepotent tendency to make a target response to an X, and (2) an expectancy to make a target response following an A. Thus, context processing can be selectively probed in 2 types of nontarget trials, B-X and A-Y (B and Y refer to the letters used other than A and X). In B-X trials, context is required to inhibit the prepotent tendency to make a target response to the X. In A-Y trials, the context creates an trials. Slice acquisition order was counterbalanced across subjects and blocks. Individual subject analyses did not indicate differences between results with the 2- and 4-shot sequences, so data from these 2 sequences were combined in the analyses presented in the "Imaging Data" section. T1-weighted structural scans were performed in the same planes as the functional scans for anatomic localization and coregistration of images across subjects.

IMAGE ANALYSIS

Images were movement corrected using a 6-parameter rigid body translation, coregistered to a common reference brain using a 12-parameter algorithm[36] and smoothed using a 3-dimensional Gaussian filter (8-mm full with half maximum) to accommodate between-subject differences in anatomy.

DATA ANALYSIS

Reaction time (RT) and accuracy (normalized using an arcsine transformation[37]) for behavioral data acquired during scanning were analyzed using analyses of variance (ANOVAs) with group as a between-subject factor and trial type and delay as within-subject factors. We also examined a more specific measure of sensitivity to context, referred to as d'-context, which computes d'[38] from A-X hits and B-X false alarms. Since d'-context compares responses to X in the presence of contextual cues indicating a target response (A-X) with a nontarget response (B-X), it provides a more focused measure of sensitivity to context.

For the fMRI data, we conducted group analyses using voxel-wise ANOVAs with subject as a random factor, group as a between-subject factor (control vs patients), and both scan (scans 1-4 within each trial) and delay (short vs long) as within-subject factors. In theory, one could examine all possible main effects and interactions in this design. However, our a priori hypotheses focused on regions demonstrating 1 of the following 4 patterns. (1) The first pattern was a main effect of delay, designed to identify regions responding to the context memory manipulation, by identifying voxels demonstrating greater activity in the longer-than short-delay condition. If a region demonstrated a main effect of delay, planned contrasts were conducted to confirm that this effect was significant for both controls and patients. (2) The second pattern was a group × delay

interaction. If a region demonstrated such an interaction, planned contrasts were conducted to confirm that the interaction reflected a significant delay effect in at least 1 of the groups. (3) The third pattern was a main effect of scan. This effect was designed to identify regions showing significant responses to motor and sensory processes, which should be transient events with a specific hemodynamic response shape. Thus, we only examined regions showing a main effect of scan, the activity of which also demonstrated an event-related time course that reflected greater signal during scans 2 and 3 than scans 1 and 4 (taking into account the well-characterized lag in hemodynamic response that results in peak activation occurring approximately 5 seconds after stimulus onset[39,40]). To identify such time courses, we conducted planned contrasts on voxels showing a main effect of scan using inverse quadratic contrast weights (-1, 1, 1, -1). The signal values for each of 4 scans are multiplied by their corresponding contrast weights and then summed for each subject. If activity during scans 2 and 3 is significantly greater than activity during scans 1 and 4, then the summed value is significantly greater than 0 (tested using a t test against 0).[41] As with the main effect of delay, additional planned contrasts were then conducted on any such region to confirm that the inverse quadratic effects of a scan were significant in both patients and controls. (4) The fourth pattern was a group × scan interaction, with planned contrasts conducted to confirm that the interaction reflected a significant scan effect in at least 1 of the groups. Voxel-wise statistical maps were generated for each pattern and then thresholded for significance using a cluster-size algorithm[42] that protects against an inflation of the false-positive rate with multiple comparisons. A cluster-size threshold of 8 voxels and a per-voxel α of .01 was chosen, corresponding to a corrected image-wise false-positive rate of 0.01. Regions showing such effects were overlaid onto the reference structural image and transformed to standard stereotactic space using computer software (Analysis of Functional Neuroimages; R.W. Cox, Medical College of Wisconsin, Milwaukee).[43] We also conducted individual subject analyses (using ANOVAs treating trial as a random factor) to locate regions showing a main effect of delay, using the same significance threshold as the group analyses. These analyses were conducted to insure that any failures to obtain PFC activation in the group analyses among patients did not reflect increased heterogeneity of the location of activation in PFC.

expectancy that an X will occur next, leading to a tendency to false alarm to the probe. Thus, the same failure to represent and maintain context should manifest as an increase in B-X false alarms but no change, or even a decrease, in A-Y false alarms. The B-Y trials serve as a control since performance is unaffected by context processing. We manipulated contextual memory demands by varying the delay between the cue and probe (**Figure 1**).[25,27,29,30] Our task design allowed us to provide internal activation standards among patients,[15] which are needed to establish the validity of fMRI findings in schizophrenia. Specifically, we used event-related methods to track the dynamics of activation during each trial (Figure 1) and identify sensory and motor regions that exhibited transient activation associated with stimulus presentation and/or response execution.

Based on prior work,[25,29,30] we first predicted that patients would show behavioral evidence of selective cognitive deficits involving the active maintenance of context. Second, we predicted that cognitive deficits in patients would manifest in the neuroimaging data as a failure to show increased activity in DLPFC during the long delay.[27] In contrast, we predicted that patients would show intact delay-related activation of posterior and inferior PFC (ie, BA 44, BA 45). This latter hypothesis was based on findings suggesting that patients with schizophrenia are not impaired while performing short-term memory tasks that primarily require verbal rehearsal of items,[29,31] a process commonly associated with the function of BA 44 and BA 45.[32] Lastly, we predicted that patients would show normal activation in motor and somatosensory regions associated with response demands, providing evidence of intact basic somatosensory and motor processing.

RESULTS

BEHAVIORAL DATA

The accuracy of ANOVA (**Table 2**) did not reveal significant main effects of group ($F_{1,24}=2.18$, $P=.11$) or delay ($F_{1,24}=0.3$, $P>.10$) but did indicate a significant trial type main effect ($F_{3,72}=4.6$, $P=.005$), which was moderated by a group $\times$ trial type interaction ($F_{3,72}=3.49$, $P=.02$). As predicted, planned contrasts indicated that this interaction reflected (1) worse performance on B-X trials ($t_{24}=2.65$, $P=.01$) and (2) better performance on A-Y trials for patients ($t_{24}=2.96$, $P=.007$); and (3) no B-Y differences ($t_{24}=0.92$, $P=.37$). The RT ANOVA (Table 2) indicated main effects of group ($F_{1,24}=6.5$, $P=.02$; patients slower than controls), delay ($F_{1,24}=8.9$, $P=.006$; long delay slower), and trial type ($F_{3,72}=26.8$, $P<.001$). Again, the trial type main effect was moderated by a group $\times$ trial type interaction ($F_{3,72}=3.8$, $P<.01$). Planned contrasts indicated that this interaction reflected (1) slower B-X RTs for patients ($t_{24}=2.2$, $P=.037$), (2) no significant differences on A-Y RTs ($t_{24}=1.6$, $P=.12$), (3) slower B-X than A-Y RTs in patients ($t_{24}=2.6$, $P=.016$), and (4) slower A-Y than B-X RTs in controls ($t_{24}=2.6$, $P=.47$). The group $\times$ trial type $\times$ delay interactions for accuracy and RT did not reach significance. However, we did find the predicted interaction with delay in d'-context (Table 2). The d'-context ANOVA indicated main effects of group ($F_{1,24}=5.4$, $P=.029$) and delay ($F_{1,24}=18.1$, $P<.001$) and a group $\times$ delay interaction ($F_{1,24}=4.1$, $P=.05$). Planned contrasts indicated no significant differences between patients and controls at the short delay ($t_{24}=1.0$, $P=.33$) but significantly decreased d'-context among patients at the long delay ($t_{24}=3.2$, $P=.004$).

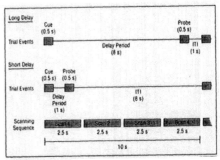

Figure 1. Experimental design. This diagram shows a timeline of the events occurring in each trial in the short and long delay blocks and the timing of scan acquisitions. ITI indicates intertrial interval.

Table 2. Behavioral Data*				
	Normal Controls (n = 12)		Patients With Schizophrenia (n = 14)	
Behavior†	Short Delay	Long Delay	Short Delay	Long Delay
Errors				
A-X	2.6 (4.0)	8.3 (11.6)	1.6 (3.8)	22.3 (29.5)
A-Y	12.2 (17.5)	8.0 (10.0)	11.0 (16.9)	0
B-X	5.3 (8.0)	4.2 (7.5)	16.1 (29.2)	16.9 (15.0)
B-Y	2.8 (6.5)	0	2.1 (5.4)	1.2 (4.5)
Reaction time				
A-X	470 (110)	523 (143)	554 (156)	621 (111)
A-Y	632 (113)	686 (146)	722 (121)	779 (147)
B-X	587 (225)	609 (250)	828 (205)	802 (197)
B-Y	497 (157)	571 (160)	623 (121)	652 (122)
d'-Context	3.7 (0.4)	3.4 (0.6)	3.4 (1.0)	2.5 (0.7)

*Values given as mean (SD).
†Working memory task-isolating context processing conducted using a version of the A-X Continuous Performance Test.[25,27,29,30]

IMAGING DATA

We first examined regions showing a main effect of delay. In the group analysis, we observed a network of WM-related regions[21] showing this effect (**Table 3**). Planned contrasts indicated that most of these regions demonstrated significant delay effects in both groups, including bilateral inferior/posterior frontal cortex (**Figure 2**), right parietal cortex, and the anterior cingulate. The 2 right temporal regions demonstrated significant delay effects in patients but marginally significant effects in controls ($P<.10$). Individual subject analyses provided similar results (Table 3). Most patients and controls displayed delay-related activity in anterior cingulate, bilateral inferior frontal, and right parietal cortex, though fewer individual subjects displayed significant activity in the temporal regions.

As predicted, only 1 brain region displayed a significant group $\times$ delay interaction. This was located in DLPFC (Table 3 and **Figure 3**), and planned contrasts revealed significantly greater activity in the long compared with short delay among controls ($t_{11}=3.6$, $P<.005$)

151

Table 3. Regions Exhibiting Significant Delay-Related Activity

Regions of Interest	Brodmann Area	X*	Y*	Z*	Region of Interest, F	Volume, mm³†	No. (%), Healthy Controls‡ (n = 12)	No. (%), Patients With Schizophrenia‡ (n = 14)
Main effect of delay								
Anterior cingulate/supplementary motor area	32, 24	7	17	33	10.88	2844	9 (75)	8 (57)
Right inferior frontal cortex	44, 6	46	11	34	20.88	5520	10 (83)	10 (71)
Left inferior frontal cortex	44, 6	-48	7	20	10.84	1060	10 (83)	11 (79)
Right parietal cortex	40	40	-49	46	17.97	5356	11 (92)	12 (86)
Right temporal cortex	22	61	-39	16	9.32	2492	6 (50)	8 (57)
Right temporal cortex	39	38	-74	18	7.20	645	5 (42)	4 (29)
Group × delay interaction								
Left dorsolateral prefrontal cortex	46, 9	-34	25	26	11.24	472	10 (83)	6 (50)

*X, Y, and Z are coordinates in a standard stereotactic space⁴⁴ in which positive values refer to regions right of (X), anterior to (Y), and superior to (Z) the anterior commissure.

†Volume refers to the number of voxels (converted to cubic millimeters) that reached statistical significance in each region of interest.

‡The number of healthy controls and patients with schizophrenia who displayed significant activity in this region in the individual subject analyses.

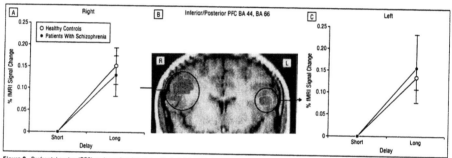

Figure 2. Prefrontal cortex (PFC) regions showing main effect of delay. The functional magnetic resonance image (fMRI) shows PFC regions active in long delay relative to short delay blocks with significant effects in both controls and patients. Insets plot the signal for healthy controls (n = 12) and patients with schizophrenia (n = 14) separately as a percent change from the short delay condition. BA indicates Brodmann area.

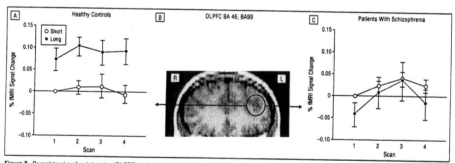

Figure 3. Dorsolateral prefrontal cortex (DLPFC) region showing group × delay interaction. Functional magnetic resonance image (fMRI) shows DLPFC region demonstrating group × delay interaction. Insets plot the signal for healthy controls (n = 12) and patients with schizophrenia (n = 14) separately as a percent change from the first scan of the short delay condition. BA indicates Brodmann area.

but not in patients ($t_{13} = 1.6$, $P > .10$). Moreover, among controls, the temporal dynamics of activity indicated a sustained response over the delay period (manifested as no main effect of scan in the long delay condition, $F_{3,33} = 1.81$, $P > .15$), consistent with the interpretation that this region is actively maintaining the context information provided by the cue. One possibility for this is that patients with schizophrenia did demonstrate DLPFC activation in response to the delay manipulation but simply in a different area than controls. However, no other

152

(REPRINTED) ARCH GEN PSYCHIATRY/VOL 58, MAR 2001 WWW.ARCHGENPSYCHIATRY.COM

Table 4. Regions Exhibiting Significant Scan-Related Activity

Regions of Interest (N = 26)	Brodmann Area	X*	Y*	Z*	Region of Interest, F	Volume, mm³†
Main effect of scan within trial						
Left motor cortex	4	-37	-13	42	53.85	13 772
Right motor cortex	4	49	6	34	31.08	5106
Anterior cingulate/supplemental motor area	32, 8	1	3	43	37.80	8332
Left inferior frontal cortex	44, 6	-51	-18	20	44.87	1728
Left parietal cortex	40, 7	-23	-57	45	12.12	2028
Right parietal cortex	40, 7	32	-57	43	7.17	1412
Group × scan interaction						
Left inferior frontal	44, 6	-52	8	37	5.81	460
Right inferior frontal	44	47	14	29	6.35	576
Posterior cingulate	23	7	-30	24	6.19	1356

*X, Y, and Z are coordinates in a standard stereotactic space[44] in which positive values refer to regions right of (X), anterior to (Y), and superior to (Z) the anterior commissure.
†Volume refers to the number of voxels (converted to cubic millimeters) that reached statistical significance in each region of interest.

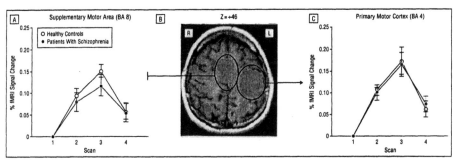

Figure 4. Representative regions demonstrating significant effects of functional magnetic resonance imaging (fMRI) within trial. Insets plot the signal for healthy controls (n = 12) and patients with schizophrenia (n = 14) separately as a percent change from the first scan. BA indicates Brodmann area.

regions anywhere in the brain demonstrated a group × delay interaction with a significant delay effect in patients. Furthermore, analyses examining delay effects in patients with schizophrenia alone did not reveal any significant activity in DLPFC, though they did reveal activation in the bilateral inferior/posterior frontal cortex, parietal cortex, anterior cingulate, and temporal cortex, consistent with the main effect of delay analyses presented in the section. In addition, individual subject analyses indicated that 10 of 12 controls displayed significantly greater activity in the long compared with short delay in DLPFC, while only 6 of 14 patients did (Table 3).

We did not predict that DLPFC activity would interact with trial type, even though we did predict and find such interactions in the behavioral data. This is because we believe that the behavioral trial type interaction reflects the fact that the same deficit in maintaining context information can lead to worse (eg, more B-X errors) and better performance (eg, fewer A-Y errors). Thus, reduced DLPFC activation should be present during all trial types at the long delay, even though its behavioral manifestations may differ across trial types. We were able to examine trial type effects in those individuals scanned with the 2-shot spiral sequence (n = 19), though the AX-CPT design provided only a small number of trials for

each nontarget trial type. Consistent with our predictions, the DLPFC did not show a further interaction with trial type (P>.25).

We next examined regions showing significant effects of scan within trial. As given in **Table 4** and **Figure 4**, controls and patients showed response-related activation of motor and somatosensory cortex, with similar amplitude and dynamics. Three additional regions showed a group × scan interaction (Table 4). One region (left posterior frontal cortex) demonstrated significant inverse quadratic effects of scan within trial among patients but not controls, while the other 2 (right inferior frontal and posterior cingulate) showed such effects among controls but not patients.

A potential criticism of fMRI studies in schizophrenia is that increased movement among patients creates artifacts that impair the detection of cortical activation. To explore this possibility, we analyzed the 12 estimated movement parameters (pitch, roll, yaw, X, Y, and Z for absolute and image-to-image movement). Patients differed significantly from controls only on average absolute pitch (t_{24}=2.03, P=.05) due primarily to increased movement in 2 patients. When these patients were removed, no significant group differences in movement remained (P>.10 for all parameters), but the behavioral (eg, d'-context group × delay interaction; $F_{1,22}$=4.6,

285

$P = .04$) and imaging effects (eg, DLPFC group $\times$ delay interaction; $F_{1,22} = 14.7$, $P = .001$) remained significant. We also examined signal-to-noise ratios in each slice of the imaging data. There were significant signal-to-noise ratio reductions among patients but only in more inferior slices (ie, slices 11-14, $Z = +7$-18 mm), well below the regions of interest in either PFC or parietal cortex.

A second criticism of fMRI studies in schizophrenia is that the poorer behavioral performance on the part of patients confounds the interpretation of observed activation differences.[9,17] To address this concern we looked at DLPFC activation in a subset of 8 controls and 8 patients roughly matched for performance based on d'-context at the long delay (mean [SD]: controls, 3.14 [0.62]; patients, 3.10 [0.41]). The DLPFC group $\times$ delay interaction remained significant in this subset of patients and controls ($F_{1,16} = 11.25$, $P = .004$).

The pattern of results obtained in the current study were consistent with our hypothesis that patients with schizophrenia have a specific impairment in the ability to actively represent and maintain context information due to an underlying neurophysiological disturbance in DLPFC. Specifically, patients with schizophrenia demonstrated a specific pattern of both better (fewer A-Y errors) and worse behavioral performance (more B-X errors), suggestive of a deficit in the ability to actively represent and maintain context information. In addition, patients with schizophrenia demonstrated a selective deficit in the ability to appropriately activate DLPFC in response to demands for the maintenance of context. Our results suggested that the observed differences between controls and patients were not due to increased movement or reduced signal-to-noise ratios in the patient data. Since this study was conducted in first-episode medication-naive patients, we can conclude that DLPFC deficits are present at the onset of the first acute exacerbation in this illness and are not due to current or previous medication effects. More importantly, our findings suggest that PFC disturbances among patients with schizophrenia, at least first-episode medication-naive patients, may be somewhat anatomically specific. In particular, we found that more posterior and inferior regions of PFC, such as BA 44, were relatively functionally intact in our sample of patients with schizophrenia, providing critical "internal activation standards" against which to interpret decreased DLPFC activation among patients with schizophrenia. Patients also showed intact response-related activation of motor and somatosensory cortex, with amplitude and dynamics similar to controls.

Such results raise the question of the functional significance of activation in DL vs inferior regions of PFC and have implications for normal cognitive function as well as for the nature of cognitive impairments in schizophrenia. Activation of BA 44 is frequently found in neuroimaging studies of language and verbal WM.[32,45-47] This activity has typically been interpreted as reflecting articulatory planning and covert rehearsal processes.[32,47-49] As such, normal activation in BA 44 among patients is consistent with prior research, suggesting that patients are not impaired while performing tasks for which explicit rehearsal is sufficient to drive performance (eg, span tasks).[31,50] However, the AX-CPT is qualitatively different from some traditional WM tasks. In many such tasks, an articulatory or phonologically based representation of stimuli may be sufficient for correct performance. For example, in the digit-span task, the representation of the digits must be actively maintained in a form that allows them to be correctly repeated back without error. Thus, an ideal representation for this task would be an articulatory or phonologically based one. In contrast, in the AX-CPT, such articulatory or phonologically based representations may be useful or even necessary but not sufficient for correct performance. Instead, performance is critically dependent on transforming the cue into a representational form that carries information regarding the cue's implications for future stimulus evaluation and response, which we refer to as a *context representation*. For example, following a B cue, representing the stimulus in a phonological or articulatory form may not be sufficient. What is also needed is an interpretation of a B cue as indicating that a subsequent X should be associated with a nontarget rather than a target response. It is the representation and maintenance of information in this contextual code that we feel best characterizes the function of DLPFC[25] and which we believe is a key function that is impaired in schizophrenia.[26]

Although our results suggested impaired DLPFC activation but relatively intact activation of BA 44 in patients with schizophrenia, we should note that some prior studies have found disturbed activation of BA 44 in this illness. In particular, a recent study by Stevens et al[51] using word and tone span tasks found hypoactivation of a number of inferior/posterior PFC regions, such as BA 44, BA 6, and BA 45. There are a number of differences between the current study and the study of Stevens and colleagues that may have contributed to the differences in our results. First, and perhaps most importantly, the patients in the study by Stevens and coauthors had received long-term medication, while ours were medication-naive first-episode patients. As such, in future research, it will be important to determine whether illness duration and/or medication effects influence the integrity of BA 44 and BA 45 in schizophrenia. Second, the tasks used in the study by Stevens et al[51] placed a heavy demand on covert rehearsal, as noted by the authors themselves, and may not have strongly tapped the context processing component of WM. Consistent with this task analysis, Stevens and colleagues did not find activation of DLPFC among controls in their study. In contrast, the AX-CPT task used in the current study was specifically designed to tap context processing and may have only placed a moderate demand on covert rehearsal. Thus, another possibility is that the magnitude of BA 44 and BA 45 dysfunction demonstrated by patients with schizophrenia is related to the degree to which the task taxes or is critically dependent on covert rehearsal, a hypothesis that can be investigated in future cognitive and neuroimaging studies. Although we believe our results are consistent with the hypotheses outlined in the introduction, we should also note some limitations of the current study. First, our patients were experiencing their first contact with the psychiatric system and had not yet experienced any potential confounding effects of antipsychotic medications or repeated hospitalizations. However, prodromal symptoms of schizophrenia can sometimes appear years before the onset of the first acute psychotic episode. Thus, we cannot rule out the possibility that our results may have been influenced by subtle effects of this prodromal period. Second, we did not match our patients and controls on variables such as IQ. This was a deliberate choice, as it has been argued that the development of schizophrenia itself may influence IQ and that matching groups on IQ can lead to nonrepresentative groups of both patients and controls.[52] Nonetheless, in future work it will be important to determine how variables such as IQ are related to both context-processing deficits and DLPFC dysfunction in schizophrenia. Lastly, we have interpreted the results of our study as reflecting disturbances in the ability to represent and maintain context. However, the results of this study itself cannot rule out an alternative interpretation, namely that patients have a deficit in actively maintaining any type of information, not just context representations, over a delay. This alternative hypothesis is consistent with the proposals of Goldman-Rakic[1,24] regarding the function of DLPFC and with data showing deficits on delayed matched to sample tasks among patients with schizophrenia.[6,53] To arbitrate between these alternatives, future research will need to directly compare the role of DLPFC in the maintenance of contextual vs noncontextual information and determine the critical parameters influencing WM deficits in schizophrenia.

Accepted for publication September 25, 2000.

This work was supported by grants from the National Institute of Mental Health (NIMH), Bethesda, Md, and NIMH center grant 2 P50 MH45156-09 (Dr Cohen).

Presented in part at the International Congress on Schizophrenia Research, Albuquerque, NM, April, 1999, and the Society for Neurosciences Conferences, Miami, Fla, September, 1999.

We thank Judy Johnstonbaugh, BA, Brittany Lourea, BA, Grace Nah, BA, and Greg Nickliss, BA, for their invaluable assistance in the conduct of this study.

Corresponding author and reprints: Deanna M. Barch, PhD, Department of Psychology, Campus Box 1125, 1 Brookings Dr, Washington University, St Louis, Mo 63130 (e-mail: dbarch@artsci.wustl.edu).

REFERENCES

1. Goldman-Rakic PS. Prefrontal cortical dysfunction in schizophrenia: the relevance of working memory. In: Carroll BJ, Barrett JE, eds. *Psychopathology and the Brain.* New York, NY: Raven Press Ltd; 1991:1-23.
2. Baddeley A, Della Sala S. Working memory and executive control. *Philos Trans R Soc Lond B Biol Sci.* 1996;351:1397-1404.
3. Malmo HP. On frontal lobe functions: psychiatric patient controls. *Cortex.* 1974; 10:231-237.
4. Abramczyk RR, Jordan DE, Hegel M. "Reverse" Stroop effect in the performance of schizophrenics. *Percept Mot Skills.* 1983;56:99-106.
5. Cornblatt BA, Keilp JG. Impaired attention, genetics, and the pathophysiology of schizophrenia. *Schizophr Bull.* 1994;20:31-62.
6. Park S, Holzman PS. Schizophrenics show spatial working memory deficits. *Arch Gen Psychiatry.* 1992;49:975-982.
7. Buchsbaum MS, Haier RJ, Potkin SG, Nuechterlein K, Bracha HS, Katz M, Lohr J, Wu J, Lottenberg S, Jerabek PA, et al. Frontrostriatal disorder of cerebral metabolism in never-medicated schizophrenics. *Arch Gen Psychiatry.* 1992;49:935-942.
8. Weinberger DR, Bigelow LB, Kleinman JE, Klein ST, Rosenblatt JE, Wyatt RJ. Cerebral ventricular enlargement in chronic schizophrenia. *Arch Gen Psychiatry.* 1980;37:11-13.
9. Callicott JH, Ramsey NF, Tallent K, Bertolino A, Knable MB, Coppola R, Goldberg T, van Gelderen P, Mattay VS, Frank JA, Moonen CT, Weinberger DR. Functional magnetic resonance brain mapping in psychiatry: methodological issues illustrated in a study of working memory in schizophrenia. *Neuropsychopharmacology.* 1998;18:186-196.
10. Fletcher PC, McKenna PJ, Frith CD, Grasby PM, Friston KJ, Dolan RJ. Brain activation in schizophrenia during a graded memory task studied with functional neuroimaging. *Arch Gen Psychiatry.* 1998;55:1001-1008.
11. Andreasen NC, Rezai K, Alliger R, Swayze VW 2d, Flaum M, Kirchner P, Cohen G, O'Leary DS. Hypofrontality in neuroleptic-naive patients and in patients with chronic schizophrenia: assessment with xenon 133 single photon emission computed tomography and the tower of london. *Arch Gen Psychiatry.* 1992;49:943-958.
12. Berman KF, Zec RF, Weinberger DR. Physiological dysfunction of dorsolateral prefrontal cortex in schizophrenia, II: role of neuroleptic treatment, attention and mental effort. *Arch Gen Psychiatry.* 1986;43:126-135.
13. Weinberger DR, Berman KF, Illowsky BP. Physiological dysfunction of the dorsolateral prefrontal cortex, III: a new cohort and evidence for a monoaminergic mechanism. *Arch Gen Psychiatry.* 1988;45:609-615.
14. Carter C, Perlstein W, Ganguli R, Brar J, Mintun M, Cohen J. Functional hypofrontality and working memory dysfunction in schizophrenia. *Am J Psychiatry.* 1998;155:1285-1287.
15. Weinberger DR, Mattay V, Callicott J, Kotria K, Santha A, van Gelderen P, Duyn J, Moonen C, Frank J. fMRI applications in schizophrenia research. *Neuroimage.* 1996;4:S118-S126.
16. Volz HP, Gaser C, Hager F, Rzanny R, Mentzel HJ, Kreitschmann-Andermahr I, Kaiser WA, Sauer H. Brain activation during cognitive stimulation with the Wisconsin Card Sorting Test: a functional MRI study on healthy volunteers and schizophrenics. *Psychiatry Res.* 1997;75:145-157.
17. Manoach DS, Press DZ, Thangaraj V, Searl MM, Goff DC, Halpern E, Saper CB, Warach S. Schizophrenia subjects activate dorsolateral prefrontal cortex during a working memory task, as measured by fMRI. *Biological Psychiatry.* 1999;45:1128-1137.
18. Berman KF, Torrey F, Daniel DG, Weinberger DR. Regional cerebral blood flow in monozygotic twins discordant and concordant for schizophrenia. *Arch Gen Psychiatry.* 1992;49:927-934.
19. Weinberger DR, Berman KF, Zec RF. Physiological dysfunction of dorsolateral prefrontal cortex in schizophrenia, I: regional cerebral blood flow evidence. *Arch Gen Psychiatry.* 1986;43:114-124.
20. Fletcher PC, Frith CD, Grasby PM, Friston KJ, Dolan RJ. Local and distributed effects of apomorphine on fronto-temporal function in acute unmedicated schizophrenia. *J Neurosci.* 1996;16:7055-7062.
21. D'Esposito M, Aguirre GK, Zarahn E, Ballard D, Shin RK, Lease J. Functional MRI studies of spatial and nonspatial working memory. *Brain Res Cogn Brain Res.* 1998;7:1-13.
22. Owen AA, Evans AC, Petrides M. Evidence for a two-stage model of spatial working memory processing within the lateral frontal cortex: a positron emission tomography study. *Cereb Cortex.* 1996;6:31-38.
23. Petrides M. Lateral frontal cortical contribution to memory. *Semin Neurosci.* 1996; 8:57-63.
24. Goldman-Rakic PS. Circuitry of primate prefrontal cortex and regulation of behavior by representational memory. In: Plum F, Mountcastle V, eds. *Handbook of Physiology: The Nervous System V.* Vol 5. Bethesda, Md: American Physiological Society; 1987:373-417.
25. Braver TS, Barch DM, Cohen JD. Cognition and control in schizophrenia: a computational model of dopamine and prefrontal function. *Biol Psychiatry.* 1999;46: 312-328.
26. Cohen JD, Servan-Schreiber D. Context, cortex and dopamine: a connectionist approach to behavior and biology in schizophrenia. *Psychol Rev.* 1992;99:45-77.
27. Barch DM, Braver TS, Nystrom L, Forman SD, Noll DC, Cohen JD. Dissociating working memory from task difficulty in human prefrontal cortex. *Neuropsychologia.* 1997;35:1373-1380.
28. Barch DM, Braver TS, Cohen JD, Servan-Schreiber D. In reply to: Stratta P, Daneluzzo E, Bustini M, Casacchia M, Rossi A. Schizophrenic deficits in the processing of context. *Arch Gen Psychiatry.* 1998;55:186-188.

155

29. Cohen JD, Barch DM, Carter CS, Servan-Schreiber D. Schizophrenic deficits in the processing of context: converging evidence from three theoretically motivated cognitive tasks. *J Abnorm Psychol.* 1999;108:120-133.
30. Servan-Schreiber D, Cohen JD, Steingard S. Schizophrenic deficits in the processing of context: a test of a theoretical model. *Arch Gen Psychiatry.* 1996;53:1105-1112.
31. Rushe TM, Woodruff PWR, Murray RM, Morris RG. Episodic memory and learning in patients with chronic schizophrenia. *Schizophr Res.* 1998;35:85-96.
32. Paulesu E, Frith CD, Frackowiak RSJ. The neural correlates of the verbal component of working memory. *Nature.* 1993;362:342-345.
33. Spitzer RL, Williams JB, Gibbon M, First MB. *Structured Clinical Interview for DSM-III-R–Patient Edition (SCID-P Version 1.0).* Washington, DC: American Psychiatric Press; 1990.
34. Overall JE. The Brief Psychiatric Rating Scale in psychopharmacology research. In: Pichot P, ed. *Psychological Measurements in Psychopharmacology: Modern Problems in Pharmacopsychiatry.* Vol 7. Paris, France: Karger; 1974.
35. Noll DC, Cohen JD, Meyer CH, Schneider W. Spiral K-space MR imaging of cortical activation. *J Magn Reson Imaging.* 1995;5:49-56.
36. Woods RP, Cherry SR, Mazziotta JC. Rapid automated algorithm for aligning and reslicing PET images. *J Comput Assist Tomogr.* 1992;16:620-633.
37. Neter J, Wasserman W, Kutner MH. *Applied Linear Statistical Models.* Boston, Mass: Irwin Press; 1990.
38. Swets JA, Sewall ST. Invariance of signal detectability over stages of practice and levels of motivation. *J Exp Psychol.* 1963;66:120-126.
39. Kwong KK, Belliveau JW, Chesler DA, Goldberg IE, Weisskoff RM, Poncelet BP, Kennedy DN, Hoppel BE, Cohen MS, Turner R, et al. Dynamic magnetic resonance imaging of human brain activity during primary sensory stimulation. *Proc Natl Acad Sci U S A.* 1992;89:5675-5679.
40. Woods RP, Cherry SR, Mazziotta JC. Non-linear temporal aspects of the BOLD response in fMRI. *Proc Int Soc Magn Reson Med.* 1996;4th meeting:1765.
41. Rosenthal R, Rosnow RL. *Contrast Analysis.* Cambridge, England: Cambridge University Press; 1985.
42. Forman SD, Cohen JD, Fitzgerald M, Eddy WF, Mintun MA, Noll DC. Improved assessment of significant activation in functional magnetic resonance imaging (fMRI): use of a cluster-size threshold. *Magn Reson Med.* 1995;33:636-647.
43. Cox RW. AFNI: software for analysis and visualization of functional magnetic resonance neuroimages. *Comput Biomed Res.* 1996;29:162-173.
44. Talairach J, Tournoux P. *Co-planar Stereotaxic Atlas of the Human Brain.* New York, NY: Thieme; 1988.
45. Fiez JA, Raife EA, Balota DA, Schwarz JP, Raichle ME, Petersen SE. A positron emission tomography study of the short-term maintenance of verbal information. *J Neurosci.* 1996;16:808-822.
46. Frackowiak RSJ. Functional mapping of verbal memory and language. *Trends Neurosci.* 1994;17:109-115.
47. Zatorre RJ, Meyer E, Gjedde A, Evans AC. PET studies of phonetic processes in speech perception: review, replication, and re-analysis. *Cereb Cortex.* 1996;6:21-30.
48. Gathercole SE. Neuropsychology and working memory: a review. *Neuropsychology.* 1994;8:494-505.
49. Awh E, Jonides J, Smith EE, Schumacher EH, Koeppe R, Katz S. Dissociation of storage and rehearsal in verbal working memory: evidence from PET. *Psychol Sci.* 1996;7:25-31.
50. Cohen JD, Barch DM, Carter C, Servan-Schreiber D. Context-processing deficits in schizophrenia: converging evidence from three theoretically motivated cognitive tasks. *J Abnorm Psychol.* 1999;108:120-133.
51. Stevens AA, Goldman-Rakic PS, Gore JC, Fulbright RK, Wexler BE. Cortical dysfunction in schizophrenia during auditory word and tone working memory demonstrated by functional magnetic resonance imaging. *Arch Gen Psychiatry.* 1998;55:1097-1103.
52. Meehl PE. High school yearbooks: a reply to Schwarz. *J Abnorm Psychol.* 1971;77:143-148.
53. Park S, Holzman PS. Association of working memory deficit and eye tracking dysfunction in schizophrenia. *Schizophr Res.* 1993;11:55-61.

156

Thalamic Volumes in Patients With First-Episode Schizophrenia

Andrew R. Gilbert, M.D.

David R. Rosenberg, M.D.

Keith Harenski, B.S.

Stephen Spencer, B.S.

John A. Sweeney, Ph.D.

Matcheri S. Keshavan, M.D.

Objective: The thalamus, a highly evolved sensory and motor gateway to the cortex, has been implicated in the pathophysiology of several illnesses, including schizophrenia. Several studies have suggested thalamic volume differences in patients with schizophrenia, although only a few studies have examined thalamic structure in new-onset patients.

Method: The authors used magnetic resonance imaging to measure thalamic volumes in previously untreated patients with first-episode schizophrenia (N=16) relative to those of healthy comparison subjects (N=25). The age range of the patients and comparison subjects was 15 to 45 years of age. Thalamic volumes in the right and left hemispheres were segmented and analyzed, both separately and as total thalamic volume, by a rater blind to clinical data. The thalamus was further segmented into regions that roughly reflected individual thalamic nuclei. Analysis of covariance was used to control for intracranial volume.

Results: Right, left, and total thalamic volumes of the patients with schizophrenia were significantly smaller than those of the comparison subjects. Significantly smaller volumes were found in the left central medial subdivision of the patients as well as a smaller volume in the right central medial subdivision that approached significance. These regions primarily comprised the dorsomedial nucleus, a thalamic nucleus thought to be an important component of aberrant circuitry in schizophrenia. Significant volume differences were also seen in the left anterior, right anterior, and right posterior medial subdivisions.

Conclusions: These findings suggest significant thalamic volumetric differences between patients with newly diagnosed schizophrenia and healthy comparison subjects. Future analysis of individual thalamic nuclei may reveal important, specific relationships between thalamic abnormalities and schizophrenia.

(Am J Psychiatry 2001; 158:618–624)

Schizophrenia is a complex disease, the pathogenesis of which remains to be elucidated. Alterations in cortical-subcortical circuitry and the components of these pathways may contribute to positive and negative symptoms and executive function deficits and may result from abnormal brain development (1–6). Examination of the early course of the disease may reveal important characteristics of schizophrenic brains that may underlie disease evolution and progression.

Several studies have demonstrated morphological and functional changes in the thalamus of patients with schizophrenia. The thalamus is the vital relay station to the cortex and is important for consciousness, perception, and the integration of thought processes (6). An aberrant thalamus could contribute to the perceptual and motor dysfunction of schizophrenia (7). It has been postulated that abnormal prefrontal-thalamic-cerebellar circuitry may contribute to the cognitive impairment characteristic of the disease (5, 8). Cell loss and reduced tissue volume of the thalamus have been described in several studies of schizophrenic brains (9–13). Furthermore, imaging studies have consistently revealed smaller thalamic volumes in

patients with schizophrenia as well as altered thalamic perfusion and metabolism (8, 14–22).

The most recent emphasis on the neurodevelopmental model of schizophrenia (1–6) points to the importance of first-episode schizophrenia research. Studies of first-episode patients may reveal the biological basis of psychotic disorders without the potential confounds of prior treatment and illness chronicity. Prospective studies of this population can clarify the impact of illness course and treatment on neurobiology (23). Because a specific thalamic role in schizophrenia remains unknown, and most structural and functional thalamic imaging studies have examined chronic, treated patients, we sought to measure thalamic volume in treatment-naive patients with first-episode schizophrenia. Furthermore, since the thalamus is composed of several nuclei, we conducted the first study to our knowledge that has measured subdivisions of the thalamus in this patient population. Our goal was to better understand the role of individual thalamic nuclei, particularly the dorsomedial nucleus and pulvinar, which have connections to brain regions previously implicated in the pathophysiology of schizophrenia (6). We hypothe-

618

sized that the regions mainly comprising the dorsomedial nucleus and pulvinar in patients with first-episode schizophrenia would differ from those of healthy comparison subjects.

Method

Subjects were 16 patients with schizophrenia and 25 healthy comparison subjects. The patients (15 with schizophrenia and one with schizoaffective disorder, depressed type) were diagnosed according to DSM-IV criteria at consensus conference meetings of senior diagnostic/clinical researchers approximately 1 month after entry into the study. All available clinical information and data gathered by using the Structured Clinical Interview for DSM-III-R Axis I disorders (SCID) (24) were incorporated. All diagnoses were ascertained as part of a longitudinal, prospective study and included a careful diagnostic rereview to ensure diagnostic stability (23). None of the subjects currently met criteria for DSM-IV psychoactive substance abuse or dependence; two subjects had a prior history of substance abuse and were dropped from the study. None of the patients had histories of significant head injury (with loss of consciousness of more than 10 minutes), neurological or medical illness, prior neuroleptic treatment, or mental retardation (IQ lower than 75). Illness duration was computed from the date of onset of prodromal symptoms to entry into the study. Clinical ratings were determined by using the Brief Psychiatric Rating Scale (BPRS) (25).

The healthy comparison subjects were recruited through advertisements in the same local neighborhoods and communities in which the patients resided. These subjects were free from any current or past axis I disorder (including substance abuse or dependence) as determined by the nonpatient version of the SCID. None had any prior exposure to any psychotropic medication within 6 months of the baseline assessment; a history of neurologic disorders or any other chronic medical problems with potential to influence neurological function; or mental retardation (IQ lower than 75). None reported a history of schizophrenia or major mood disorder in a first-degree relative. The comparison subjects were matched, as a group, with the schizophrenia patients for age, gender, race, and parental socioeconomic status (from the Hollingshead Four-Factor Index [26]). After an initial screening evaluation by telephone, these subjects were interviewed by a psychiatrist (M.S.K.) or clinical psychologist with the SCID (nonpatient version).

After complete description of the study to the subjects, written informed consent was obtained. The study was approved by the Biomedical Institutional Board of the University of Pittsburgh.

MRI Studies

All volumetric magnetic resonance imaging (MRI) scans were conducted at the University of Pittsburgh Medical Center (1.5-T Signa Whole Body Scanner, GE Medical Systems, Milwaukee). Image quality and clarity as well as patient head position were determined with a sagittal scout series. Total brain volume was measured with a three-dimensional spoiled gradient recalled acquisition in the steady state pulse sequence that obtained 124 1.5-mm thick contiguous coronal images (TE=5 msec, TR=25 msec, acquisition matrix=256 × 192, field of view=24 cm, flip angle=40°). In order to facilitate image orientation, coronal slices were obtained perpendicular to the anterior commissure-posterior commissure line. Axial proton density and T_2-weighted images were obtained for thalamic measurement and to exclude structural abnormalities on MRI scans. Image software (version 1.56) developed by the National Institutes of Health was used to measure brain anatomy (27). This technique yields valid and reliable neuroanatomic measurements of the regions of interest with a semi-

automated segmentation approach (28). None of the MRI scans in this data set showed motion or magnetic field inhomogeneity artifacts.

Neuroanatomic Measures

We measured the right and left hemispheres of the thalamus, their subdivisions, and total intracranial volume, which was used as a covariate. We also measured the volume of the dorsolateral prefrontal cortex in view of the implications of this structure in the pathophysiology of schizophrenia (3, 28) and its reciprocal connections with the thalamic nuclei (6). Neuroanatomic boundaries were determined by reference to standard neuroanatomical atlases (29, 30), and detailed definitions were adapted from previously published psychiatric neuroimaging studies of the thalamus (8, 15, 16, 31–33).

Thalamic Volume

Separate measurements were obtained for the left and right hemispheres of the thalamus by using a manual tracing technique. The mamillary body was used as the anterior boundary. The internal capsule was considered the lateral boundary, the third ventricle the medial boundary, and the inferior border of the third ventricle the inferior boundary. The posterior boundary was defined by where the hemispheres of the thalamus merged under the crux fornix. The superior boundary was the main body of the lateral ventricle (32). Measurements were made by a single well-trained and reliable rater (A.R.G.) who was blind to the study hypothesis, subject identification, and clinical data.

Thalamic Subdivisions

The thalamus was first divided into two distinct medial and lateral regions (axial view in Figure 1). The point of reference for the line that bisected the thalamus into medial and lateral regions was the emergence of the fourth ventricle as it appeared as a vertical line through the pons. A line drawn parallel to the lateral border of the midbrain, interhemispheric fissure, and cerebral aqueduct represented our line of vertical bisection of each thalamus (coronal view in Figure 1). This line was carried on through all thalamic slices to create a plane of bisection parallel to the interhemispheric fissure. We chose this approach because no significant differences have been seen between patients with schizophrenia and comparison subjects with regard to brainstem structures (34). Using the spoiled gradient recalled acquisition protocol, we measured contiguous coronal slices of the thalamus, dividing the regions into anterior, central, and posterior divisions. The anterior and central divisions each contained 40% of the total number of slices; the posterior division contained 20% of the total number of slices (axial and sagittal views in Figure 1). These divisions are based upon neuroanatomical atlases of the human brain as well as a previously published article examining the thalamus in schizophrenia (16, 29, 30). The divisions roughly reflect the individual nuclei that are located in these thalamic regions (axial view in Figure 1). Each individual subdivision was measured as a percentage of the total number of slices. Measurements were made by a single, well-trained, and reliable rater (A.R.G.) who was blind to the study hypothesis, subject identification, and clinical data.

Dorsolateral Prefrontal Cortical Volume

The dorsolateral prefrontal cortex was measured in the coronal plane by a method similar to that used by Seidman et al. (35). The most posterior part of the genu was located and used as the first slice in measuring the dorsolateral prefrontal cortex. The borders of the dorsolateral prefrontal cortex were first manually outlined, and the gray matter was then segmented. The superior boundary was the superior frontal sulcus, and the inferior boundary was the posterior lateral fissure and the horizontal ramus of the anterior

FIGURE 1. Axial, Coronal, and Sagittal Views of the Thalamic Regions Measured to Assess Volume Differences Between Patients With First-Episode Schizophrenia and Healthy Comparison Subjects[a]

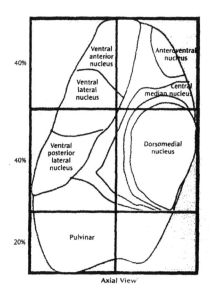

Axial View

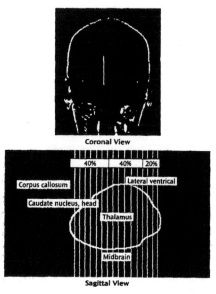

Coronal View

Sagittal View

[a] Approximate regions of specific thalamic nuclei are depicted in the representation of the axial view, which was adapted, with permission, from Buchsbaum et al. (16). The line drawn in the coronal view—which is parallel to the lateral border of the midbrain, interhemispheric fissure, and cerebral aqueduct—represents the line of vertical bisection of each thalamus. This line was carried on through all thalamic slices to create a plane of bisection parallel to the interhemispheric fissure. The average number of coronal slices composing the anterior, central, and posterior subdivisions of the thalamus is shown in the sagittal view.

lateral fissure. The lateral border was the edge of the cerebral cortex, and the medial border was created by connecting the deepest points on the superior frontal sulcus and the lateral fissure. Ten successive anterior slices were measured. The dorsolateral prefrontal cortex was segmented, and the gray matter and total volume were measured.

Intracranial Volume

Intracranial volume included the following volumes: total brain, dura, ventricular and extraventricular CSF, brainstem, and cerebellum; this was measured by manually outlining the outer limit of the tracing along the inner border of the inner table of skull. This measurement was made from the coronal slices. The intracranial volume was used as a covariate in comparison to volumetric measures of the aforementioned structures across diagnostic groups.

Statistical Analysis

The thalamic volumes and their subdivisions were compared between subjects by using analysis of covariance, with the intracranial volume as a covariate. The relations between thalamic volumes and subject characteristics (age, symptom severity) were examined by using Pearson correlation coefficients. Interrater (K.H., A.R.G.) reliabilities (intraclass correlations; N=10) for all measurements and intrarater reliabilities for measurements by the same rater (A.R.G.), conducted approximately 1 month apart on 10 scans, were all greater than 0.90.

Results

The two groups did not significantly differ with regard to age, gender, or handedness (Table 1). The right hemisphere, left hemisphere, and total thalamic volumes of the patient group were significantly smaller than those of the comparison subjects, after we controlled for intracranial volume (Table 2). Intracranial volume did not significantly differ between the groups. When only right-handed subjects (12 patients and 23 comparison subjects) were examined, there were continuing differences between the groups (left hemisphere: F=9.34, df=1, 33, p=0.004; right hemisphere: F=3.86, df=1, 33, p=0.06; total thalamus: F= 7.14, df=1, 33, p=0.01). There were no differences observed when we controlled for handedness.

No significant gender effect was seen for left-hemisphere thalamic volume (F=1.75, df=1, 36, p=0.19), but female subjects had smaller right-hemisphere thalamic volumes (F=4.18, df=1, 36, p=0.04). No gender-by-diagnosis interactions were seen for either structure. Right hemisphere, left hemisphere, and total thalamic volumes, after we controlled for intracranial volume, did not correlate

620

TABLE 1. Demographic and Clinical Characteristics of Patients With First-Episode Schizophrenia and Healthy Comparison Subjects

Characteristic	Patients With First-Episode Schizophrenia (N=16)		Healthy Comparison Subjects (N=25)		Analysis	
	Mean	SD	Mean	SD	$F (df=1, 39)$	p
Age (years)	26.56	7.30	23.60	4.66	2.53	0.12
Global Assessment of Functioning score	31.25	7.33				
BPRS score (18 items)	53.50	8.50				
	N	%	N	%	$\chi^2 (df=1)$	p
Gender					1.13	0.28
Male	11	68.75	13	52.00		
Female	5	31.25	12	48.00		
Handedness[a]					3.81	0.051
Right	12	75.00	23	95.83		
Left	4	25.00	1	4.17		

[a] Data were missing for one subject.

TABLE 2. Thalamic Volumes in Patients With First-Episode Schizophrenia and Healthy Comparison Subjects

	Volume (cm³)					
	Patients With First-Episode Schizophrenia (N=16)		Healthy Comparison Subjects (N=25)		Analysis	
Area	Mean	SD	Mean	SD	F (df=1, 40)	p
Thalamic region						
Right hemisphere	3.40	1.21	4.09	0.74	5.43	0.03
Left hemisphere	3.21	0.98	4.03	0.78	8.40	0.006
Total	6.62	2.00	8.12	1.41	7.74	0.008
Intracranial total[a]	1436.47	192.71	1440.64	133.86	0.01	0.94

[a] Measurement used as a covariate that included the following volumes: total brain, dura, ventricular and extraventricular CSF, brainstem, and cerebellum.

with age in either the patients (partial correlation coefficients<0.25, df=13, p>0.50) or the comparison subjects (partial correlation coefficients<0.25, df=22, p>0.50). In the patient group, thalamic volumes were not correlated with Global Assessment of Functioning scores (r<0.15, df=14, p>0.60) or total BPRS scores (r<0.15, df=14, p>0.60). When the patient with schizoaffective disorder was excluded, thalamic volume differences remained significant (left hemisphere: F=8.53, df=1, 37, p=0.006; right hemisphere: F=5.84, df=1, 37, p=0.02; total: F=8.08, df=1, 37, p=0.007). The number of coronal slices used to quantify the thalamus ranged from 13 to 21 slices, with an average of 17.5 slices. There were no significant differences between groups in the number of slices.

Thalamic Subdivisions

Measurements of thalamic subdivisions were conducted in 16 patients and 25 comparison subjects (Table 3). The 18% difference in volume for the left central medial subdivision was significant, and the 17% difference in volume for the right central medial subdivision approached significance. There was a highly significant difference in right posterior medial subdivision volume (43% smaller in the patient group). Significant volume differences were also found in the right and left anterior medial subdivisions (13% and 14%, respectively). There were no significant volume differences in the lateral subdivisions.

Dorsolateral Prefrontal Cortical Volume

The dorsolateral prefrontal cortex volumes (gray, white, total) did not differ significantly between patients and comparison subjects. However, the left dorsolateral prefrontal cortex gray matter volume was smaller in the patients than in the comparison subjects (mean=9.94 cm³ [SD=1.35] versus 10.56 cm³ [SD=1.13], respectively) (F= 2.86, df=1, 38, p<0.10). No significant correlations were seen between the thalamic and thalamic subdivision volumes on the one hand and the gray, white, and total dorsolateral prefrontal cortex volumes on the other (all partial correlations [after partialing out intracranial volume] <0.50, df=13, p>0.20).

Discussion

Consistent with the results of other early course as well as chronic schizophrenia studies, we have demonstrated significant thalamic volume differences in patients with first-episode schizophrenia relative to those of healthy comparison subjects. Furthermore, by examining treatment-naive, first-episode patients, we have eliminated the potentially confounding effects of prior treatment and illness chronicity.

Thalamic volume differences in patients with schizophrenia may reflect abnormal thalamic circuitry—a potential contributor to the cognitive dysfunction characteristic of schizophrenia. The thalamus is a recognized compo-

TABLE 3. Thalamic Subdivision Volumes in Patients With First-Episode Schizophrenia and Healthy Comparison Subjects

	Volume (cm³)					
	Patients With First- Episode Schizophrenia (N=16)		Healthy Comparison Subjects (N=25)		Analysis	
Thalamic Subdivision	Mean	SD	Mean	SD	F (df=1, 39)	p
Right hemisphere—medial region						
Anterior	0.88	0.18	1.01	0.23	4.34	0.04
Central	0.97	0.33	1.17	0.39	3.12	0.08
Posterior	0.16	0.08	0.28	0.15	8.91	0.01
Right hemisphere—lateral region						
Anterior	0.26	0.18	0.26	0.17	0.00	0.99
Central	0.85	0.32	0.83	0.37	0.04	0.84
Posterior	0.68	0.35	0.61	0.18	0.68	0.41
Left hemisphere—medial region						
Anterior	0.94	0.20	1.09	0.26	4.30	0.05
Central	1.01	0.27	1.23	0.30	5.47	0.03
Posterior	0.24	0.14	0.29	0.13	1.43	0.24
Left hemisphere—lateral region						
Anterior	0.23	0.18	0.31	0.27	1.29	0.26
Central	0.57	0.25	0.71	0.26	3.08	0.09
Posterior	0.45	0.12	0.51	0.16	2.07	0.16

nent of frontal, cerebellar, and limbic circuits (36–38). Lesions of thalamic nuclei have been reported to result in neuropsychological and behavioral disturbances similar to the deficits of executive function in patients with schizophrenia. Vascular and degenerative disorders affecting the thalamus are often indistinguishable from "frontal lobe"-type syndromes (36). With many cortical and subcortical connections, the thalamus is thought to filter sensory information before it reaches the cortex. Therefore, abnormal thalamic function could result in the inability to filter or "gate" sensory input to the cortex, creating the type of sensory overload often experienced by patients with schizophrenia (5, 39). Furthermore, an aberrant thalamic component to thalamocortical circuitry may contribute to or result from the frontal lobe dysfunction described in previous schizophrenia research (8). However, our inability to find a correlation between thalamic and dorsolateral prefrontal cortex volume alterations suggests that caution is warranted for such conclusions.

Thalamic volume differences in patients with schizophrenia, suggestive of aberrant thalamic circuitry, are consistent with previous structural and functional studies that have demonstrated abnormalities in other brain regions. Several postmortem studies have revealed differences in superior temporal gyrus cell and total cortical volumes as well as lower prefrontal and anterior cingulate cell densities in schizophrenic brains (40–43). Differences in cell number, density, and volume in the mediodorsal thalamic nucleus have been reported as well as lower cell volume in the globus pallidus (9, 13, 44). Imaging studies have revealed smaller thalamic volumes and less glucose metabolism and neuronal activity in patients with schizophrenia (15, 16, 20, 21). Furthermore, abnormal striatal (45, 46) as well as superior temporal gyral volumes (47) have been observed. Functional imaging studies have consistently demonstrated abnormal perfusion and metabolism in cortical and cerebellar regions of schizophrenic brains (8, 48–51). These findings support the concept of abnormal

cortical-subcortical circuitry underlying the pathophysiology of schizophrenia. A greater understanding of the thalamic components of these circuits is critical.

We have previously proposed that a developmentally mediated neural dysplasia in cortical-subcortical circuitry may be associated with the pathogenesis of schizophrenia. A substantial reorganization of cortical connections, involving a programmed synaptic pruning, takes place during human development (28). It has been suggested that in schizophrenia, aberrant migration or programmed cell death in the subplate zone of the developing cortex may impair normal patterns of synaptic connections in the overlying cortex and lead to compromised circuitry (6). Recent studies have revealed abnormal thalamic projections to the prefrontal cortex and other signs of impaired thalamocortical connectivity in schizophrenia (52, 53). The primary versus secondary nature of thalamic dysfunction in schizophrenia remains unclear; however, it is understood that neuronal loss in the thalamus is commonly a retrograde degeneration ensuing from pathology in the cerebral cortex that affects the axon terminations of thalamocortical relay cells. Furthermore, retrograde degeneration secondary to cortical damage in the developing brain is typically unaccompanied by gliosis (6). It is interesting to note that the lower neuronal density described in postmortem analysis of the thalamus occurred in the absence of gliosis, which suggests a neurodevelopmental rather than neurodegenerative process (8).

While smaller thalamic volumes in patients with schizophrenia has been a consistent finding in both in vivo and postmortem studies, the majority of this research has examined chronic or treated patients (9, 14, 15, 17, 20, 54, 55). We have demonstrated that caudate volumetric measurements may differ between neuroleptic-naive and treated schizophrenia patients, perhaps secondary to the effects of neuroleptic treatment (28). In light of these potential treatment-induced changes, we sought to examine patients with untreated schizophrenia. It is possible that,

622

162

similar to our caudate findings (28), volumetric measurements following 1 year of antipsychotic treatment may reveal significant treatment effects. A previous study (18) revealed no change in thalamic volumes, as compared to control subjects, in five schizophrenia patients following approximately 70 days of risperidone treatment, although higher doses of atypical neuroleptics were associated with larger thalamic volumes. It was suggested that medication-induced hypertrophy may have been responsible for the volumetric changes.

The inability to precisely measure discrete thalamic nuclei limits the interpretation of our findings. Our current measurements of thalamic subdivisions revealed significant and nearly significant volume differences in the regions primarily comprising the dorsomedial nucleus. As previously mentioned, postmortem analysis of schizophrenic brains has revealed a significant neuronal deficit in the dorsomedial nucleus. It is of interest that these changes appeared to be unaffected by treatment (9). Because of its connections to the prefrontal cortex, medial temporal cortex, and basal forebrain, all of which have been implicated in the pathophysiology of schizophrenia, the dorsomedial nucleus is thought to be an important component of aberrant circuitry (6). We also found significant volume differences in the right posterior medial subdivision, a thalamic region roughly reflecting the right medial half of the pulvinar. The pulvinar may also represent a critical thalamic nucleus in that it projects to temporal lobe regions reported to be abnormal in patients with schizophrenia and might be associated with altered visual perceptual functions (6, 42, 47).

It is important to note that our measurement of thalamic subdivisions has several limitations. We were unable to delineate and employ an intrathalamic marker as a consistent landmark for our regional subdivisions. Rather, we relied upon approximate percentage-based divisions of total thalamic area as a means of dividing the thalamus. It is possible that our approach may not account for thalamic volume loss that is inconsistent with these percentage-based divisions. Our approach assumes that all thalamic nuclei will be consistently represented by these rigid subdivisions. It is possible that some patients have thalamic nuclei that are not in proportion to the percentage-based parameters that we defined in this study. Furthermore, an enlarged third ventricle causing a mass-effect shift in thalamic volume could be misinterpreted as thalamic volume loss. Higher resolution imaging may allow for the delineation of an intrathalamic marker that may improve the reliability of our approach. Furthermore, by using more advanced imaging techniques, such as diffusion tensor imaging (56), it may be possible to delineate the white matter tracts that connect thalamic nuclei with their cortical projections and better understand the role of these circuits in schizophrenia.

Received May 8, 2000; revision received Oct. 31, 2000; accepted Nov. 2, 2000. From the Department of Psychiatry, Western Psychiatric Institute and Clinic; and the Department of Psychiatry, Wayne State University School of Medicine, Detroit. Address reprint requests to Dr. Keshavan, Western Psychiatric Institute and Clinic, 3811 O'Hara St., Pittsburgh, PA 15213-2593; keshavanms@msx.upmc.edu (e-mail).
Supported in part by NIMH grants MH-45203 and MH-45156 and a Scottish Rite grant.
The authors thank Dr. David Lewis for feedback, Drs. Gretchen L. Haas, Elizabeth D. Radomsky, and Nina Schooler for clinical characterization of the study subjects, and Ilana Mankowski for morphometric measurements.

References

1. Feinberg I: Schizophrenia: caused by a fault in programmed synaptic elimination during adolescence? J Psychiatr Res 1983; 17:319–334
2. Fish B: Neurological antecedents of schizophrenia in children: evidence for an inherited, congenital neurointegrative defect. Arch Gen Psychiatry 1977; 34:1297–1313
3. Weinberger DR: Implications of normal brain development for the pathogenesis of schizophrenia. Arch Gen Psychiatry 1987; 44:660–669
4. Murray RM, Lewis SW: Is schizophrenia a neurodevelopmental disorder? Br Med J 1987; 295:681–682
5. Andreasen NC: A unitary model of schizophrenia: Bleuler's "fragmented phrene" as schizencephaly. Arch Gen Psychiatry 1999; 56:781–787
6. Jones EG: Cortical development and thalamic pathology. Schizophr Bull 1997; 23:483–501
7. Scheibel AB: The thalamus and neuropsychiatric illness. J Neuropsychiatry Clin Neurosci 1997; 9:342–353
8. Andreasen NC: The role of the thalamus in schizophrenia. Can J Psychiatry 1997; 42:27–33
9. Pakkenberg B: Pronounced reduction of total neuron number in mediodorsal thalamic nucleus and nucleus accumbens in schizophrenia. Arch Gen Psychiatry 1990; 47:1023–1028
10. Pakkenberg B: The volume of the mediodorsal thalamic nucleus in treated and untreated schizophrenics. Schizophr Res 1992; 7:95–100
11. Fungfeld E: Pathological-anatomische untersuchungen bei Dementia praecox mit besonderer beruckischtigung des Thalamus opticus. Z Gesamte Neurol Psychiatrie 1925; 95:411–463
12. Baumer H: Veranderungen des Thalamus bei Schizophrenie. J Hirnforsch 1954; 1:157–172
13. Treff WM, Hempel KJ: Die zelidichte bei Schizophrenen und klinisch gesunden. J Hirnforsch 1958; 4:314–369
14. Andreasen NC, Ehrhardt JC, Swayze VW II, Alliger RJ, Yuh WT, Cohen G, Ziebell S: Magnetic resonance imaging of the brain in schizophrenia: the pathophysiologic significance of structural abnormalities. Arch Gen Psychiatry 1990; 47:35–44
15. Andreasen NC, Arndt S, Swayze V II, Cizadlo T, Flaum M, O'Leary D, Ehrhardt JC, Yuh WTC: Thalamic abnormalities in schizophrenia visualized through magnetic resonance image averaging. Science 1994; 266:294–298
16. Buchsbaum MS, Someya T, Teng CY, Abel L, Najafti A, Haier RJ, Wu J, Bunney WE Jr: PET and MRI of the thalamus in never-medicated patients with schizophrenia. Am J Psychiatry 1996; 153:191–199
17. Frazier JA, Giedd JN, Hamburger SD, Albus KE, Kaysen D, Vaituzis AC, Rajapakse JC, Lenane MC, McKenna K, Jacobsen LK, Gordon CT, Breier A, Rapoport JL: Brain anatomic magnetic resonance imaging in childhood-onset schizophrenia. Arch Gen Psychiatry 1996; 53:617–624

623

163

18. Gur RE, Maany V, Mozley PD, Swanson C, Bilker W, Gur RC: Subcortical MRI volumes in neuroleptic-naive and treated patients with schizophrenia. Am J Psychiatry 1998; 155:1711–1717

19. Rodriguez VM, Andree RM, Castejon MJ, Zamora ML, Alvaro PC, Delgado JL, Vila FJ: Fronto-striato-thalamic perfusion and clozapine response in treatment-refractory schizophrenic patients: a 99m Tc-HMPAQ study. Psychiatry Res 1997; 76:51–61

20. Holcomb HH, Cascella NG, Thaker GK, Medoff DR, Dannals RF, Tamminga CA: Functional sites of neuroleptic drug action in the human brain: PET/FDG studies with and without haloperidol. Am J Psychiatry 1996; 153:41–49

21. Heimberg C, Komoroski RA, Lawson WB, Cardwell D, Karson CN: Regional proton magnetic resonance spectroscopy in schizophrenia and exploration of drug effect. Psychiatry Res 1998; 83:105–115

22. Gunther W: MRI-SPECT and PET-EEG findings on brain dysfunction in schizophrenia. Prog Neuropsychopharmacol Biol Psychiatry 1992; 16:445–462

23. Keshavan MS, Schooler NR: First-episode studies in schizophrenia: criteria and characterization. Schizophr Bull 1992; 18:491–513

24. Spitzer RL, Williams JBW: Structured Clinical Interview for DSM-III-R (SCID). New York, New York State Psychiatric Institute, Biometrics Research, 1985

25. Overall JE, Gorham DR: The Brief Psychiatric Rating Scale. Psychol Rep 1962; 10:799–812

26. Hollingshead AB: Four-Factor Index of Social Status. New Haven, Conn, Yale University, Department of Sociology, 1975

27. Rasband W: NIH Image Manual. Bethesda, Md, National Institutes of Health, 1993

28. Keshavan MS, Anderson S, Pettegrew JW: Is schizophrenia due to excessive synaptic pruning in the prefrontal cortex? the Feinberg hypothesis revisited. J Psychiatr Res 1994; 28:239–265

29. Daniels DL, Haughton VM, Naidich TP: Cranial and Spinal Magnetic Resonance Imaging: An Atlas and Guide. New York, Raven Press, 1987

30. Talairach J, Tournoux P: Co-Planar Stereotaxic Atlas of the Human Brain. New York, Thieme Medical, 1988

31. Gilbert AR, Moore GJ, Keshavan MD, Paulson LD, Narula V, MacMaster FP, Stewart CM, Rosenberg DR: Decrease in thalamic volumes of pediatric obsessive compulsive disorder patients taking paroxetine. Arch Gen Psychiatry 2000; 57:449–456

32. Portas CM, Goldstein JM, Shenton ME, Hokama HH, Wible CG, Fischer I, Kikinis R, Donnino R, Jolesz FA, McCarley RW: Volumetric evaluation of the thalamus in schizophrenic male patients using magnetic resonance imaging. Biol Psychiatry 1998; 43:649–659

33. Staal WG, Pol HEH, Schnack H, van der Schot AC, Kahn RS: Partial volume decrease of the thalamus in relatives of patients with schizophrenia. Am J Psychiatry 1998; 155:1784–1786

34. Aylward EH, Reiss A, Barta PE, Tien A, Han W, Lee J, Pearlson GD: Magnetic resonance imaging measurement of posterior fossa structures in schizophrenia. Am J Psychiatry 1994; 151:1448–1452

35. Seidman LJ, Yurgelun-Todd D, Kremen WS, Woods BS, Goldstein JM, Faraone SV, Tsuang MT: Relationship of prefrontal and temporal lobe MRI measures to neuropsychological performance in chronic schizophrenia. Biol Psychiatry 1994; 35:235–246

36. Cummings JL: Frontal-subcortical circuits and human behavior. Arch Neurol 1993; 50:873–880

37. Alexander GE, Crutcher MD, DeLong MR: Basal ganglia-thalamo-cortical circuits: parallel substrates for motor, occulomotor, prefrontal and limbic functions, in Progress in Brain Research, vol 85. Edited by Uylins HBM, Van Eden CG, Corner MA, Feenstra MGP. Amsterdam, Elsevier, 1989, pp 119–146

38. Jones EG: The Thalamus. New York, Plenum, 1985

39. Braff DL, Swerdlow NR: Neuroanatomy of schizophrenia. Schizophr Bull 1997; 23:509–512

40. Pakkenberg B: Total nerve cell number in neocortex in chronic schizophrenics and controls estimated using optical disectors. Biol Psychiatry 1993; 34:768–772

41. Benes FM, McSparren J, San Giovanni JP, Vincent SL: Deficits in small interneurons in cingulate cortex of schizophrenics and schizoaffective patients. Arch Gen Psychiatry 1991; 48:996–1001

42. Akbarian S, Bunney WE, Potkin SG, Wigal SB, Hagman JO, Sandman CA, Jones EG: Altered distribution of nicotinamide-adenine-dinucleotide phosphate-diaphorase cells in frontal cortex of schizophrenics implies disturbances of cortical development. Arch Gen Psychiatry 1993; 50:169–177

43. Falkai P, Bogerts B, Schneider T, Greve B, Pfeiffer U, Pilz K, Gonsiorzcyk C, Majtenyi C, Ovary I: Disturbed planum temporale asymmetry in schizophrenia: a quantitative post-mortem study. Schizophr Res 1995; 14:161–176

44. Bogerts B, Falkai P, Haupts M, Greve B, Ernst S, Tapernon-Franz U, Heinzmann U: Post-mortem volume measurements of limbic system and basal ganglia structures in chronic schizophrenics: initial results from a new brain collection. Schizophr Res 1990; 3:295–301

45. Flaum M, Swayze VW II, O'Leary DS, Yuh WTC, Ehrhardt JC, Arndt SV, Andreasen NC: Effects of diagnosis, laterality, and gender on brain morphology in schizophrenia. Am J Psychiatry 1995; 152:704–714

46. Keshavan MS, Rosenberg D, Sweeney JA, Pettegrew JW: Decreased caudate volume in neuroleptic-naive psychotic patients. Am J Psychiatry 1998; 155:774–778

47. Keshavan MS, Haas GL, Kahn CE, Aguilar E, Dick EL, Schooler NR, Sweeney JA, Pettegrew JW: Superior temporal gyrus and the course of early schizophrenia: progressive, static, or reversible? J Psychiatr Res 1998; 32:161–167

48. Shihabuddin L, Buchsbaum MS, Hazlett EA, Haznedar MM, Harvey PD, Newman A, Schnur DB, Spiegel-Cohen J, Wei T, Machac J, Knesaurek K, Vallabhajosula S, Biren MA, Ciaravolo TM, Luu-Hsia C: Dorsal striatal size, shape, and metabolic rate in never-medicated and previously medicated schizophrenics performing a verbal learning task. Arch Gen Psychiatry 1998; 55:235–243

49. Berman KF, Illowsky BP, Weinberger DR: Physiological dysfunction of dorsolateral prefrontal cortex in schizophrenia, III: further evidence for regional and behavioral specificity. Arch Gen Psychiatry 1988; 45:616–622

50. Weinberger DR, Berman KF, Zec RF: Physiological dysfunction of dorsolateral prefrontal cortex in schizophrenia: regional cerebral blood flow (rCBF) evidence. Arch Gen Psychiatry 1986; 43:114–124

51. Gur RE, Mozley PD, Resnick SM, Mozley LH, Shtasel DL, Gallacher F, Arnold SE, Karp JS, Alavi A, Reivich M: Resting cerebral glucose metabolism in first-episode and previously treated patients with first episode schizophrenia relates to clinical features. Arch Gen Psychiatry 1995; 52:657–667

52. Lewis DA, Pierri JN, Volk DW, Melchitsky DS, Woo TU: Altered GABA neurotransmission and prefrontal cortical dysfunction in schizophrenia. Biol Psychiatry 1999; 46:616–626

53. Pierri JN, Chaudry AS, Woo T-UW, Lewis DA: Alterations in chandelier neuron axon terminals in the prefrontal cortex of schizophrenic subjects. Am J Psychiatry 1999; 156:1709–1719

54. Jeste DV, McAdams LA, Palmer BW, Braff D, Jernigan TL, Paulsen JS, Stout JC, Symonds LL, Bailey A, Heaton RK: Relationship of neuropsychological and MRI measures to age of onset of schizophrenia. Acta Psychiatr Scand 1998; 98:156–164

55. Corey-Bloom J, Jernigan T, Archibald S, Harris MJ, Jeste DV: Quantitative magnetic resonance imaging of the brain in late-life schizophrenia. Am J Psychiatry 1995; 152:447–449

56. Lim KO, Hedehus M, Moseley M, deCrespigny A, Sullivan EV, Pfefferbaum A: Compromised white matter tract integrity in schizophrenia inferred from diffusion tensor imaging. Arch Gen Psychiatry 1999; 56:367–374

164

ORIGINAL ARTICLE

Decreased Dendritic Spine Density on Prefrontal Cortical Pyramidal Neurons in Schizophrenia

Leisa A. Glantz, PhD; David A. Lewis, MD

Background: The pathophysiological characteristics of schizophrenia appear to involve altered synaptic connectivity in the dorsolateral prefrontal cortex. Given the central role that layer 3 pyramidal neurons play in corticocortical and thalamocortical connectivity, we hypothesized that the excitatory inputs to these neurons are altered in subjects with schizophrenia.

Methods: To test this hypothesis, we determined the density of dendritic spines, markers of excitatory inputs, on the basilar dendrites of Golgi-impregnated pyramidal neurons in the superficial and deep portions of layer 3 in the dorsolateral prefrontal cortex (area 46) and in layer 3 of the primary visual cortex (area 17) of 15 schizophrenic subjects, 15 normal control subjects, and 15 nonschizophrenic subjects with a psychiatric illness (referred to as psychiatric subjects).

Results: There was a significant effect of diagnosis on spine density only for deep layer 3 pyramidal neurons

in area 46 (P = .006). In the schizophrenic subjects, spine density on these neurons was decreased by 23% and 16% compared with the normal control (P = .004) and psychiatric (P = .08) subjects, respectively. In contrast, spine density on neurons in superficial layer 3 in area 46 (P = .09) or in area 17 (P = .08) did not significantly differ across the 3 subject groups. Furthermore, spine density on deep layer 3 neurons in area 46 did not significantly (P = .81) differ between psychiatric subjects treated with antipsychotic agents and normal controls.

Conclusion: This region- and disease-specific decrease in dendritic spine density on dorsolateral prefrontal cortex layer 3 pyramidal cells is consistent with the hypothesis that the number of cortical and/or thalamic excitatory inputs to these neurons is altered in subjects with schizophrenia.

Arch Gen Psychiatry. 2000;57:65-73

T HE DORSOLATERAL prefrontal cortex (DLPFC) appears to be a critical site of dysfunction in subjects with schizophrenia. For example, schizophrenic subjects perform poorly on cognitive tasks that are subserved by DLPFC circuitry,[1,2] and this performance deficit is correlated with diminished activation of the DLPFC.[2,3]

See also page 74

The results of structural imaging studies[4-8] suggest that DLPFC dysfunction in subjects with schizophrenia may be related to a decreased volume of this brain region. Findings of increased cell packing density,[9-11] without a change in neuronal number,[12,13] suggest that this volume reduction may be due to a decreased amount of DLPFC neuropil in subjects with schizophrenia.[14] Because the axon terminals and dendritic spines of the neuropil represent the major anatomical substrate for synapses, these findings suggest the presence of abnormalities in DLPFC connectivity in subjects with schizophrenia.

Consistent with this interpretation, magnetic resonance spectroscopic stud-

ies[15-18] have found decreased levels of N-acetylaspartate, a putative marker of neuronal and/or axonal integrity, in the DLPFC of schizophrenic subjects. Reports[19-21] of decreased phosphomonoesters, increased phosphodiesters, or both in the DLPFC of schizophrenic subjects have also been interpreted to reflect an increased breakdown of membrane phospholipids and, consequently, a decreased number of synapses.[22] Finally, levels of synaptophysin, a presynaptic terminal protein, are decreased in the DLPFC of schizophrenic subjects.[23-26] Although other interpretations are possible, each of these findings supports the hypothesis that DLPFC synaptic number is diminished in subjects with schizophrenia.

Understanding the pathophysiological significance of such alterations requires knowledge of the types of synapses that are affected and of their postsynaptic targets. Several findings suggest that schizophrenia may be associated with abnormalities in the excitatory inputs to layer 3 pyramidal neurons in the DLPFC. For example, the basilar dendritic spines of pyramidal cells in deep layer 3 are likely targets of projections from the mediodorsal thalamic nucleus,[27,28] and

From the Departments of Neuroscience (Drs Glantz and Lewis) and Psychiatry (Dr Lewis), University of Pittsburgh, Pittsburgh, Pa.

165

SUBJECTS AND METHODS

SUBJECT CHARACTERISTICS

Specimens from 45 human brains were obtained during autopsies conducted at the Allegheny County Coroner's Office, Pittsburgh, Pa (**Table 1**). Informed consent for brain donation was obtained from the next of kin. Neuropathological abnormalities were detected in 6 subjects. Subject 517 had a vascular malformation and hemorrhage confined to the right temporal lobe, and subject 622 had an acute infarction limited to the distribution of the right middle cerebral artery. However, the cortical regions of interest for the present study were not affected in either subject. In 4 subjects (subjects 532, 564, 609, and 632), thioflavine S staining revealed a few senile plaques without any neurofibrillary tangles. The density of plaques was insufficient to meet the diagnostic criteria for Alzheimer disease,[37] and there was no history of dementia in any subject.

Fifteen subjects with a diagnosis of schizophrenia or schizoaffective disorder were compared with 15 normal control subjects and 15 nonschizophrenic subjects with a psychiatric illness (referred to as psychiatric subjects) (Table 1). For each subject, an independent committee of experienced clinicians made consensus DSM-III-R[38] diagnoses using information obtained from clinical records and structured interviews conducted with surviving relatives of the subject.[23] One of the normal controls (subject 370) was later found to have a diagnosis of alcohol abuse, current at the time of death. Thirteen of the subjects in the psychiatric comparison group had a mood disorder, and 2 had other psychotic disorders. All of the schizophrenic subjects had a history of treatment with antipsychotic agents, and 9 of the psychiatric subjects had been treated with these medications. All procedures were approved by the Institutional Review Board for Biomedical Research at the University of Pittsburgh, Pittsburgh, Pa.

Subject groups did not differ significantly in sex, race, age, postmortem interval (PMI), tissue fixation time, or incidence of out-of-hospital deaths (**Table 2**). In addition, the schizophrenic and psychiatric subjects did not differ on the incidence of alcohol or other substance use disorders, mean age at onset of illness, or mean duration of illness. However, the number of deaths by suicide was significantly higher in the psychiatric subjects (Table 2).

PREPARATION OF TISSUE

From the left hemisphere of each brain, tissue blocks were cut from standardized locations in the DLPFC and primary visual cortex, immersed in 4% paraformaldehyde for longer than 4 weeks, and then processed by a previously described modification[39] of the rapid Golgi procedure.[40] Sections were cut at 90 µm and mounted onto coded slides so that investigators were not aware of subject number or diagnosis.

Area 46 of the DLPFC and area 17, primary visual cortex, were examined in this study. Area 17 was not available for 2 schizophrenic subjects (subjects 410 and 622) and 1 psychiatric subject (subject 637). Nissl-stained sections from tissue blocks immediately adjacent to those used for the Golgi procedure were examined to confirm that the Golgi material contained the cytoarchitectural features of areas 46 or 17.[9,41] The Nissl-stained sections were also used to determine the borders of layer 3 as a percentage of total cortical thickness. In area 46, the layer 2 to 3 border was located on average (±SD) 18.2% (±3.4%) and 20.8% (±2.8%) of the distance from the pial surface to the white matter for the schizophrenic and control subjects, respectively, and the layer 3 to 4 border was located at 53.6% (±3.1%) and 56.8% (±1.2%) of the total cortical thickness in these 2 subject groups, respectively. These findings are consistent with previous reports[11,42] that the relative thicknesses of cortical layers are similar in schizophrenic and control subjects. Consequently, Golgi-impregnated neurons located between 20%

---

the number of neurons in this nucleus appears to be decreased in subjects with schizophrenia.[29-31] In addition, excitatory inputs to layer 3 pyramidal cells decline substantially in number during late adolescence,[32-34] the typical age when the clinical features of schizophrenia become manifest.

Consequently, the purpose of this study was to test the hypothesis that schizophrenia is associated with a diminished complement of excitatory synapses onto DLPFC layer 3 pyramidal neurons. Because dendritic spines are the principal site of excitatory inputs to pyramidal neurons,[35] and reflect the number of these synapses,[35,36] we quantified dendritic spine density on the basilar dendrites of layer 3 pyramidal neurons in schizophrenic subjects and 2 groups of comparison subjects.

RESULTS

SPINE DENSITY ON LAYER 3 PYRAMIDAL NEURONS

The Golgi impregnation procedure clearly filled the basilar dendritic shafts and spines of layer 3 pyramidal neu-

rons. As shown in **Figure 2**, differences in spine density among neurons and across brains were sometimes quite evident.

In DLPFC area 46 (**Table 3**), the mean spine density on the basilar dendrites of pyramidal neurons in superficial layer 3 of the schizophrenic subjects was 15% lower than that of the normal controls and 13% lower than that of the psychiatric subjects (**Figure 3**, A). However, these differences did not achieve statistical significance ($F_{2,37} = 2.52, P = .09$).

In contrast, the spine density on the basilar dendrites of pyramidal neurons in deep layer 3 of area 46 did significantly differ ($F_{2,37} = 6.01, P = .006$) among the 3 subject groups (Table 3). There was also a main effect for age ($F_{1,37} = 8.49, P = .006$) on spine density, but reanalysis failed to reveal a significant age-by-diagnosis interaction ($F_{2,36} = 1.87, P = .17$). In addition, there was no effect of race, sex, PMI, or tissue fixation time ($F_{1,37} < 0.86, P > .47$) on spine density.

As shown in Figure 3, B, the mean spine density on pyramidal neurons in deep layer 3 was 23% lower (95% confidence interval, −42.3% to −6.7%) in the schizophrenic subjects than in the normal controls, a differ-

166

and 55% of the distance from the pial surface to the white matter in area 46 were considered to be located in layer 3. In Golgi-processed sections containing area 17, a dark band demarcated layer 4.[40] Therefore, sampled neurons were located superficially to this band or within 20% to 45% of the distance from the pial surface to the white matter.

NEURON RECONSTRUCTIONS

Golgi-impregnated pyramidal neurons were readily identified by their characteristic triangular somal shape, apical dendrite extending toward the pial surface, and numerous dendritic spines. The following criteria were used to select pyramidal neurons for reconstruction: (1) location of the cell soma in layer 3 and within the middle of the thickness (z-axis) of the section; (2) full impregnation of the neuron; (3) soma or dendrites not obscured by overlying opaque artifacts larger than 5 µm; (4) no morphologic changes attributable to PMI[43]; and (5) presence of at least 3 primary basilar dendritic shafts, each of which branched at least once. For each subject, 15 neurons were randomly sampled in each of 3 locations: (1) the superficial half of layer 3 (20%-37% of the total cortical depth) in area 46, (2) the deep half of layer 3 (38%-55% of the total cortical depth) in area 46, and (3) layer 3 of area 17. The adequacy of these sampling procedures for detecting differences in spine density has been previously demonstrated.[32,39,44]

For each neuron, the longest basilar dendrite, including all branches, was reconstructed in 3 dimensions with a tracing system (Neuron Tracing System; Eutectics Electronics Inc, Raleigh, NC) and a ×100 oil immersion objective (**Figure 1**). Only those portions of the dendritic tree within the same section as the cell soma were reconstructed. Because apical dendrites are frequently truncated during sectioning, these dendrites were not examined. Each dendritic branch was recorded as having either a natural end (gradual tapering of dendritic thickness with an end swelling, spine, or spine cluster) or an artificial end (cut dendrite).[39] For each basilar dendrite and its branches, the mean diameter and total length, the location and number of spines, the total number of dendritic segments (the portion of a dendrite located between either the soma or a dendritic bifurcation and either another bifurcation or the dendrite end), and the maximum branch order (highest numbered dendritic segment) of the dendrites were determined. The cross-sectional area of each cell body was determined by tracing its outline. All neurons were reconstructed by the same investigator (L.A.G.) without knowledge of the subject number or diagnostic group.

STATISTICAL ANALYSES

For each parameter measured, the results were analyzed using a multivariate analysis of covariance model with the independent variables of diagnostic group, sex, age, race, PMI, and tissue fixation time. The multiple observations per subject (15 neurons) for a particular parameter were treated as a multivariate observation. Because the measured parameters within a given subject were possibly correlated and were also exchangeable, they were modeled as repeated measures with a compound, symmetric covariance structure. To preserve degrees of freedom, the interactions with diagnostic group were only examined if the effect of a particular independent variable was significant ($P<.05$). For any neuron parameter in which the multivariate analysis of covariance test yielded a significant diagnostic group effect at the .05 level, post hoc simultaneous pairwise comparisons using the Bonferroni procedure at the .05 level were conducted to determine which of the groups' means differed significantly. Simultaneous 95% confidence intervals were also obtained for each pairwise comparison of diagnostic groups. Finally, paired t tests were used to compare spine density across layers within subject groups.

ence significant at $P = .004$ by post hoc comparisons. Furthermore, although spine density did not differ ($t = 0.52$, $P = .61$) between superficial and deep layer 3 pyramidal neurons in the normal controls (Table 3), spine density was significantly ($t = 3.65$, $P = .003$) decreased by 11% in deep layer 3 relative to superficial layer 3 in the subjects with schizophrenia. These comparisons confirm a laminar specificity to the spine density differences between schizophrenic and normal control subjects.

Compared with the psychiatric subjects, the mean spine density on deep layer 3 pyramidal neurons in the schizophrenic subjects was decreased by 16%. Although this difference did not achieve statistical significance ($P = .08$), the 95% confidence interval (−35.8% to 4.4%) was suggestive of a reduction in spine density in the schizophrenic subjects compared with the psychiatric subjects. In contrast, the mean spine density clearly did not differ ($P = .81$) between the psychiatric and control subjects.

In contrast to area 46, the spine density on layer 3 pyramidal neurons in area 17 (Figure 3, C), primary visual cortex, was decreased in the schizophrenic (13%) and psychiatric (11%) subjects relative to the normal controls (**Table 4**). However, these differences did not achieve statistical significance ($F_{2,34} = 2.70$, $P = .08$).

OTHER PARAMETERS OF LAYER 3 PYRAMIDAL NEURONS

In superficial layer 3 of area 46, only somal size significantly ($F_{2,37} = 3.84$, $P = .03$) differed among the 3 groups, and post hoc comparisons revealed that this difference was due to a smaller somal size in the psychiatric subjects compared with the normal controls (Table 3). In deep layer 3 of area 46, only total dendritic length (TDL) differed significantly ($F_{2,37} = 4.17$, $P = .02$) among the 3 groups. Post hoc comparisons revealed that the normal control group had a significantly ($P<.05$) greater TDL than the schizophrenic and psychiatric groups, which did not differ from each other. Interestingly, an analysis of covariance for spine density, controlling for TDL, in the schizophrenic and control groups revealed that the group difference in spine density on deep layer 3 pyramidal neurons was more highly significant ($F_{1,27} = 15.2$, $P<.001$) than that indicated by the initial analysis. In layer 3 of the primary visual cortex, TDL ($F_{2,34} = 4.11$, $P = .03$),

167

Table 1. Characteristics of Control, Schizophrenic, and Psychiatric Subjects[a]

Control Subjects				Schizophrenic Subjects					
Subject No./ Sex/Age, y	Race	PMI, h	Cause of Death	Subject No./ Sex/Age, y	Race	Diagnosis	PMI, h	Duration of Illness, y	Cause of Death
370/M/25[b]	W	5.3	Trauma	398/F/41	W	Schizoaffective disorder	10.3	20	Pulmonary embolism
390/F/72	W	11.0	ASCVD	410/M/30	B	Schizophrenia, chronic paranoia[d]	21.0	NA	Sickle-cell crisis
471/M/44	W	8.5	Hypertrophic cardiomyopathy	428/F/67	W	Schizoaffective disorder[e]	9.0	30	COPD
510/M/63	W	12.4	GI tract bleeding	450/M/48	B	Schizophrenia, chronic undifferentiated[d,e,h]	22.0	24	Suicide by jumping
516/M/20	B	14.0	Homicide by gun shot	466/M/48	B	Schizophrenia, chronic undifferentiated	19.0	NA	ASCVD
545/M/65	B	13.1	Pancreatic cancer	517/F/48	W	Schizophrenia, chronic disorganized[f]	3.7	20	Intracerebral hemorrhage
546/F/37	W	23.5	ASCVD	533/M/40	W	Schizophrenia, chronic undifferentiated	29.1	15	Accidental asphyxiation
551/M/61	W	16.4	Cardiac tamponade	537/F/37	W	Schizoaffective disorder[d]	14.5	8	Suicide by hanging
557/M/47	W	15.9	ASCVD	559/F/61	W	Schizoaffective disorder[f]	16.8	20	ASCVD
567/F/46	W	15.0	Mitral valve prolapse	566/M/63	W	Schizophrenia, chronic undifferentiated[e]	18.3	20	ASCVD
568/F/60	W	9.5	ASCVD	581/M/46	W	Schizophrenia, chronic paranoia[b,j]	28.1	30	Accidental combined drug overdose
575/F/55	B	11.3	ASCVD	587/F/38	B	Schizophrenia, chronic undifferentiated[e]	17.8	20	Myocardial hypertrophy
592/M/41	B	22.1	ASCVD	597/F/46	W	Schizoaffective disorder	10.1	25	Pneumonia
609/F/77	W	10.7	ASCVD	617/F/44	B	Schizophrenia, chronic undifferentiated	3.3	21	Amitriptyline hydrochloride toxicity
643/M/50	W	24.0	ASCVD	622/M/58	W	Schizophrenia, chronic undifferentiated[d]	16.0	16	Right MCA infarction

[a] PMI indicates postmortem interval; NA, data not available; ASCVD, atherosclerotic coronary vascular disease; COPD, chronic obstructive pulmonary disease; GI, gastrointestinal; and MCA, middle cerebral artery.
[b] Alcohol abuse, current at time of death.
[c] Other substance abuse, current at time of death.
[d] Subjects not taking antipsychotic medications at the time of death.
[e] Alcohol abuse, in remission at the time of death.
[f] Alcohol dependence, current at the time of death.
[g] Alcohol dependence, in remission at the time of death.
[h] Other substance dependence, in remission at the time of death.
[i] Other substance dependence, current at the time of death.
[j] Subjects treated with antipsychotic medications.
[k] Other substance abuse, in remission at the time of death.

number of branch segments ($F_{2,34} = 4.41$, $P = .02$), and maximum branch order ($F_{2,34} = 4.27$, $P = .02$) differed significantly among the diagnostic groups (Table 4). For each measure, the main effect was due to significantly lower values in the psychiatric subjects compared with the control and schizophrenic subjects.

EFFECT OF ANTIPSYCHOTIC MEDICATIONS ON SPINE DENSITY

To determine whether treatment with antipsychotic medications might account for the decreased spine density on DLPFC deep layer 3 pyramidal neurons in the schizophrenic subjects, we conducted a separate analysis of the 9 psychiatric subjects who had been treated with these medications (Table 1). The mean (±SD) spine density (measured as number of spines per micrometer) on deep

layer 3 pyramidal neurons in these subjects (0.30 ± 0.07) did not significantly differ from that of either the entire group of normal controls (0.33 ± 0.08, $F_{1,18} = 0.47$, $P = .50$) or a subset of 9 normal controls (0.31 ± 0.05, $F_{1,12} = 0.06$, $P = .81$) who, as a group, did not differ from the antipsychotic-treated psychiatric subjects in sex, age, or PMI.

COMMENT

These findings demonstrate that the density of basilar dendritic spines on deep layer 3 pyramidal neurons in the DLPFC area 46 of subjects with schizophrenia is significantly decreased in DLPFC area 46 of subjects with schizophrenia. This decrease does not appear to be a general correlate of having a psychiatric illness or a consequence of treatment with antipsychotic medications, suggesting that the decrease in spine density may be specific to the pathophysiological characteristics of schizophre-

168

Subject No./ Sex/Age, y	Race	Diagnosis	PMI, h	Duration of Illness, y	Cause of Death
453/M/37	W	Major depression[b,c]	11.0	NA	Suicide by gunshot
475/M/17	W	Major depression	23.0	1	Suicide by gunshot
505/M/57	W	Major depression[f]	12.8	18	Suicide by gunshot
513/M/24	W	Major depression with psychotic features[i]	13.1	8	Suicide by hanging
532/M/76	W	Mood disorder due to general medical condition with psychotic features[j]	13.9	0.3	Suicide by jumping
560/M/46	B	Alcohol-induced psychotic disorder[l,j]	10.6	2	GI bleeding
564/F/56	W	Major depression with psychotic features	16.6	1	Suicide by hanging
565/F/62	W	Major depression[b,h]	12.4	14	Suicide by gunshot
580/F/58	W	Major depression with psychotic features[i]	11.3	34	ASCVD
613/M/59	W	Major depression with psychotic features[*,j]	15.6	9	Suicide by gunshot
631/M/45	W	Major depression with psychotic features[b,j]	12.1	23	Suicide by thioridazine overdose
632/F/77	W	Delusional disorder[l]	17.4	36	ASCVD
637/M/34	W	Alcohol-induced mood disorder with psychotic features[l,k]	24.7	12	Suicide by chlorpromazine overdose
642/F/40	W	Bipolar disorder[l,j]	24.1	14	Acute alcohol intoxication
693/F/42	W	Major depression with psychotic features[l,j]	12.6	24	Suicide by propoxyphene hydrochloride overdose

nia. Because dendritic spine density directly reflects the number of excitatory inputs to pyramidal neurons,[35,36] these findings, in concert with those of a pilot study[45] that also reported decreased spine density on prefrontal layer 3 pyramidal neurons, support the hypothesis that schizophrenia is associated with diminished synaptic connectivity of the DLPFC.

In superficial layer 3 of area 46 and in layer 3 of area 17, pyramidal cells exhibited a trend toward decreased spine density in the schizophrenic subjects compared with the normal controls. Evidence suggestive of decreased cortical neuropil has been reported in both of these cortical regions.[10] However, in area 17, the psychiatric subjects also showed a trend toward decreased spine density on layer 3 pyramidal neurons. In addition, other measures of dendritic morphologic characteristics (TDL, number of branch segments, and maximum branch order) appeared to be altered in area 17 of the psychiatric sub-

jects, suggesting that a history of depression or death by suicide may be associated with altered neuronal morphologic characteristics in the primary visual cortex.

Interpretation of the pathophysiological significance of reduced spine density in the DLPFC requires a consideration of the potential influence of other factors. First, only a small percentage of neurons are labeled with the Golgi technique.[46] However, because the impregnation process is random, the cells reconstructed in this study are likely to be representative of the neuronal populations of interest. This interpretation is supported by our finding of a 9% to 12% decrease in mean somal size of layer 3 pyramidal neurons in the DLPFC of the schizophrenic subjects. Although these differences were not significant, perhaps because of sample size, their magnitude is consistent with that of other reports[47,48] that measured somal size in much larger samples of Nissl-stained neurons. Second, because the reaction product

169

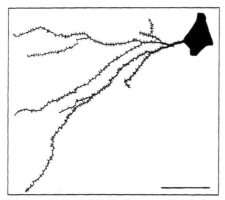

Figure 1. *Reconstruction of a basilar dendrite from a layer 3 pyramidal neuron in control subject 516. Fourth-order dendritic branches are present. For each neuron, calculation of dendritic spine density included the total length of the dendrite shown. The bar indicates 50 μm.*

Table 2. Summary of Subject Characteristics*

	Subject Group			
Characteristic	Control	Schizophrenic	Psychiatric	P†
Male-female ratio	9:6	7:8	9:6	.71
White-black ratio	11:4	10:5	14:1	.20
Age, y	50.9 ± 16.2	47.7 ± 10.5	48.7 ± 17.2	.84
PMI, h	14.2 ± 5.5	16.1 ± 7.7	15.4 ± 4.8	.73
Fixation time, mo	12.5 ± 10.1	10.7 ± 9.4	8.2 ± 6.6	.43
Alcohol disorder‡	1 (7)	7 (47)	8 (53)	.59
Other substance disorder	0 (0)	2 (13)	5 (33)	.17
Age at onset, y§	NA	28.6 ± 9.4	36.7 ± 18.3	.23
Duration of illness, y§	NA	20.7 ± 5.9	14.0 ± 11.8	.09
Out-of-hospital deaths	13 (87)	11 (73)	14 (93)	.19
Suicide	0 (0)	2 (13)	11 (73)	.005

Data are given as number (percentage) of subjects or mean ± SD. PMI indicates postmortem interval; NA, data not applicable.

†*Analyses were between all 3 groups for the following variables: sex, race, age, PMI, fixation time, and out-of-hospital deaths. Analyses were conducted only between the schizophrenic and psychiatric groups for the following variables: alcohol disorder, other substance disorder, age at onset, duration of illness, and suicide.*

‡*After the study was initiated, 1 control subject (subject 370) was determined to meet the criteria for alcohol abuse, current at the time of death.*

§*This information could not be reliably determined for 2 schizophrenic and 2 psychiatric subjects.*

of the Golgi impregnation procedure is opaque, some spines are hidden behind the dendritic shaft and are not counted. Consequently, the spine densities reported in this study are relative and not absolute. However, previous studies[49] have demonstrated that relative spine counts accurately reflect absolute numbers if comparisons are made between dendrites with similar shaft diameters, and, as shown in Tables 3 and 4, mean dendritic diameter did not differ across our subject groups. Third, the schizophrenic and psychiatric subjects available for this study were somewhat diagnostically heterogeneous. However, the mean (±SD) spine density in DLPFC deep layer 3 of the subjects with "pure" schizophrenia

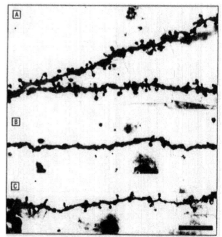

Figure 2. *Brightfield photomicrographs illustrating Golgi-impregnated basilar dendrites and spines on dorsolateral prefrontal cortex layer 3 pyramidal neurons from normal control subject 390 (A) and 2 subjects with schizophrenia (subjects 410 [B] and 466 [C]). The calibration bar equals 10 μm.*

(0.25 ± 0.06; n = 10) was 23% lower than that of the normal controls (0.32 ± 0.07; n = 14) and of the psychiatric subjects with major depression (0.33 ± 0.04; n = 10).

All of the schizophrenic subjects in this study had a history of treatment with antipsychotic agents. Studies addressing the effect of haloperidol on spine density in the rat prefrontal cortex have been inconclusive, with spine density reported to be decreased following high-dose, short-term treatment[50] but unchanged following long-term treatment at levels more consistent with clinical practice.[51] However, 3 lines of evidence suggest that antipsychotic medications do not account for the decreased dendritic spine density observed in the present study. First, the decrease in spine density exhibited regional and laminar specificity, an effect that is not readily explained by systemically administered agents. Second, the 4 schizophrenic subjects (subjects 410, 450, 537, and 622) who were not taking medications (for an average of 5.4 months) at the time of death actually had a lower spine density (0.24 ± 0.08) in deep layer 3 of area 46 than did the 11 subjects who were taking medications (0.26 ± 0.06). Finally, the 9 psychiatric subjects who had been treated with antipsychotic medications did not differ in spine density from normal controls. However, the lifetime exposure to antipsychotic medications is likely to have been lower in these psychiatric subjects than in the schizophrenic subjects.

Although decreased spine density represents a morphologic abnormality in the DLPFC of schizophrenic subjects, dendritic spines are relatively plastic structures. For example, spine number has been reported to change rapidly in certain brain regions of experimental animals under various conditions.[52-57] Although we cannot completely exclude the influence of such factors, their impact may have been minimized by the study design. For ex-

Table 3. Dendritic Parameters From Layer 3 Pyramidal Neurons in the DLPFC (Area 46)*

	Layer 3					
	Superficial			Deep		
Dendritic Parameter	Control Subjects	Schizophrenic Subjects	Psychiatric Subjects	Control Subjects	Schizophrenic Subjects	Psychiatric Subjects
Spine density, spines/µm†	0.34 ± 0.09	0.29 ± 0.10	0.33 ± 0.11	0.33 ± 0.10ᵃ	0.26 ± 0.10ᵇ	0.31 ± 0.09ᵃ,ᵇ
Somal area, µm²‡	355.2 ± 143.5ᵃ	312.1 ± 127.7ᵃ,ᵇ	300.4 ± 111.3ᵇ	350.9 ± 121.8	319 ± 126.5	308.9 ± 106.4
Total dendritic length, µm§	656.1 ± 308.9	566.8 ± 342.7	547.9 ± 308.5	707.7 ± 352.6ᵃ	576.6 ± 319.8ᵇ	557.4 ± 303.6ᵇ
Dendritic diameter, µm	0.44 ± 0.09	0.44 ± 0.1	0.42 ± 0.08	0.42 ± 0.08	0.47 ± 0.13	0.44 ± 0.08
No. of branch segments	10.8 ± 4.2	10.4 ± 4.8	10.6 ± 4.7	11.5 ± 4.8	10.4 ± 4.6	11.0 ± 4.5
Maximum branch order	4.4 ± 1.0	4.3 ± 1.1	4.3 ± 1.1	4.6 ± 1.1	4.3 ± 1.2	4.4 ± 1.1
No. of natural ends	3.3 ± 1.9	3.3 ± 2.0	3.1 ± 1.8	3.2 ± 1.9	3.1 ± 1.9	3.1 ± 1.9
No. of artificial ends	2.6 ± 1.9	2.4 ± 1.7	2.7 ± 2.0	3.0 ± 2.0	2.6 ± 2.0	2.9 ± 2.1

*Data are given as the mean ± SD. n = 15 for all subjects. DLPFC indicates dorsolateral prefrontal cortex.
†Group differences are significant in deep layer 3 only ($F_{2,37}$ = 6.01, P = .006). Within this row, values not sharing the same superscript letter are significantly different (P<.05) by pairwise post hoc analyses.
‡Group differences are significant in superficial layer 3 only ($F_{2,37}$ = 3.84, P = .03). Within this row, values not sharing the same superscript letter are significantly different (P<.05) by pairwise post hoc analyses.
§Group differences are significant in deep layer 3 only ($F_{2,37}$ = 4.17, P = .02). Within this row, values not sharing the same superscript letter are significantly different (P<.05) by pairwise post hoc analyses.

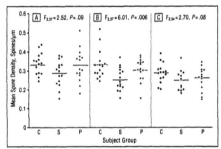

Figure 3. *Scatterplots illustrating mean spine densities for 15 pyramidal neurons per subject in the superficial (A) and deep (B) portions of layer 3 in dorsolateral prefrontal cortex area 46, and in area 17, primary visual cortex (C). Horizontal lines indicate group means; C, control subjects; S, schizophrenic subjects; and P, psychiatric subjects.*

Table 4. Dendritic Parameters From Layer 3 Pyramidal Neurons in the Primary Visual Cortex (Area 17)*

Dendritic Parameter	Control Subjects (n = 15)	Schizophrenic Subjects (n = 13)	Psychiatric Subjects (n = 14)
Spine density, spines/µm	0.29 ± 0.08	0.25 ± 0.09	0.26 ± 0.09
Somal area, µm²	190.9 ± 76.9	181.5 ± 70.0	174.2 ± 65.1
Total dendritic length, µm†	449.3 ± 227.9ᵃ	464.5 ± 325.0ᵃ	351.6 ± 178.5ᵇ
Dendritic diameter, µm	0.41 ± 0.11	0.43 ± 0.10	0.40 ± 0.10
Number of branch segments‡	9.3 ± 3.8ᵃ	9.1 ± 4.0ᵃ	8.2 ± 3.2ᵇ
Maximum branch order§	4.1 ± 1.0ᵃ	4.0 ± 1.1ᵃ,ᵇ	3.6 ± 0.9ᵇ
No. of natural ends	3.1 ± 1.7	3.0 ± 1.9	2.7 ± 1.6
No. of artificial ends	2.0 ± 1.6	2.1 ± 1.9	1.9 ± 1.5

*Data are given as the mean ± SD.
†Group differences are significant ($F_{2,34}$ = 4.11, P = .03). Within this row, values not sharing the same superscript letter are significantly different (P<.05) by pairwise post hoc analyses.
‡Group differences are significant ($F_{2,34}$ = 4.41, P = .02). Within this row, values not sharing the same superscript letter are significantly different (P<.05) by pairwise post hoc analyses.
§Group differences are significant ($F_{2,34}$ = 4.27, P = .02). Within this row, values not sharing the same superscript letter are significantly different (P<.05) by pairwise post hoc analyses.

ample, the comparison with subjects with mood or other psychotic disorders provides some assessment of the influence of environmental factors, such as hospitalizations, medications, and limitations in social and occupational activities, associated with being severely ill with a psychiatric disorder. In addition, spine density in deep layer 3 of area 46 was not associated with the duration of illness in either the schizophrenic (r = –0.358, P = .26) or psychiatric (r = –0.009, P = .98) subjects. However, the plasticity of dendritic spines suggests that the findings of this study, like many other observations in postmortem studies (alterations in gene expression or neurotransmitter receptor number), may not reflect a fixed lesion in the DLPFC of schizophrenic subjects.

Because the presynaptic and postsynaptic elements of axospinous synapses change in parallel,[35,54,58-60] the decreased spine density in schizophrenic subjects is likely to reflect a diminished number of excitatory synaptic inputs to DLPFC layer 3 pyramidal neurons. This interpretation is consistent with previous reports[10,11,23-25] of de-

creased synaptophysin protein and neuropil measures in the DLPFC of schizophrenic subjects. Interestingly, dendritic spine density on layer 3 pyramidal neurons undergoes a substantial decline during adolescence in primates.[32] In addition, the density of asymmetric (presumably excitatory) synapses changes in a similar manner in the monkey and human DLPFC.[33,34] These late developmental refinements in the excitatory circuitry of the DLPFC coincide with the age when the clinical manifestations of schizophrenia frequently first appear, suggesting that they may contribute to the pathophysiological characteristics of this disorder.[61] However, we cannot

171

determine from the present study whether the presynaptic terminals to DLPFC layer 3 pyramidal neurons never developed, were extensively pruned during adolescence, or were resorbed later in life.

The functional significance of a decrease in excitatory inputs depends on which population(s) of axon terminals is affected. Several lines of evidence suggest that the affected inputs may be from the mediodorsal thalamic nucleus. First, this nucleus has been reported to have fewer neurons in schizophrenic subjects.[29-31] Second, spine density was preferentially decreased on pyramidal neurons in deep layer 3 of the DLPFC. The basilar dendrites of these neurons typically extend through deep layer 3 and layer 4, the termination zone of afferents from the mediodorsal thalamic nucleus,[27] and dendritic spines appear to be the principal synaptic targets of thalamic projections.[28,62] Finally, decreased expression of the messenger RNA for GAD_{67}, the synthesizing enzyme for γ-aminobutyric acid, in the DLPFC of schizophrenic subjects[62,63] has been suggested to represent a compensatory response to diminished excitatory thalamic drive,[64] since decreased activity in thalamic inputs to sensory cortices produces a downregulation of GAD_{67} expression.[65,66]

However, the observations of this study may not be fully explained by a reduction in thalamic inputs to the DLPFC. For example, thalamocortical afferents appear to compose a small proportion ($<10\%$) of the total excitatory inputs to the targeted cortical neurons in the cat visual cortex.[67] If these findings can be extrapolated to the human DLPFC, then even a complete loss of thalamocortical afferents would not be sufficient to account for the observed 16% to 23% decrease in basilar dendritic spine density on deep layer 3 pyramidal cells in the schizophrenic subjects. Two other major sources of excitatory inputs to deep and superficial layer 3 DLPFC pyramidal neurons are intrinsic axon collaterals from other pyramidal neurons[68,69] and associational or callosal projections from other cortical regions.[69-71] Thus, given the trend for spine density to also be decreased on superficial layer 3 pyramidal cells, it may be that abnormalities in thalamocortical afferents to deep layer 3 have an additive effect to a disturbance in cortical axon terminals that are distributed across layer 3. However, our findings do not reveal the direction of the pathophysiological changes. For example, it is possible that the inputs to DLPFC layer 3 pyramidal cells are reduced not because of a more primary disturbance in the source of the inputs but because an abnormality intrinsic to these pyramidal cells renders them unable to support a normal complement of excitatory inputs.

In summary, our findings provide evidence for a decrease in excitatory inputs to DLPFC layer 3 pyramidal cells that may be most marked for pyramidal cells located in the thalamic recipient zone. Given the role of thalamic excitatory inputs in the mediation of working memory,[72,73] these findings may contribute to the pathophysiological basis for the disturbance of these cognitive abilities in subjects with schizophrenia.

Accepted for publication July 22, 1999.

This study was supported by grants MH00519 and MH45156 from the US Public Health Service, Bethesda, Md; and the Scottish Rite Schizophrenia Research Program N.M.J., Lexington, Mass.

We thank Allan Sampson, PhD, and Sungyoung Auh, MA, for statistical consultations; and Mary Brady for photographic assistance.

Reprints: David A. Lewis, MD, University of Pittsburgh, 3811 O'Hara St, W1650 Biomedical Science Tower Pittsburgh, PA 15213 (e-mail: lewisda@msx.upmc.edu).

REFERENCES

1. Park S, Holzman PS. Schizophrenics show spatial working memory deficits. Arc Gen Psychiatry. 1992;49:975-982.
2. Weinberger DR, Berman KF, Zec RF. Physiologic dysfunction of dorsolateral prefrontal cortex in schizophrenia, I: regional cerebral blood flow evidence. Arch Gen Psychiatry. 1986;43:114-124.
3. Steinberg JL, Devous MD, Paulman RG. Wisconsin card sorting activated regional cerebral blood flow in first break and chronic schizophrenic patients and normal controls. Schizophr Res. 1996;19:177-187.
4. Andreasen NC, Flashman L, Flaum M, Arndt S, Swayze V II, O'Leary DS, Ehrhardt JC, Yuh WTC. Regional brain abnormalities in schizophrenia measured with magnetic resonance imaging. JAMA. 1994;272:1763-1769.
5. Schlaepfer TE, Harris GJ, Tien AY, Peng LW, Lee S, Federman EB, Chase GA Barta PE, Pearlson GD. Decreased regional cortical gray matter volume in schizophrenia. Am J Psychiatry. 1994;151:842-848.
6. Shelton RC, Karson CN, Doran AR, Pickar D, Bigelow LB, Weinberger DR. Cerebral structural pathology in schizophrenia: evidence for a selective prefrontal cortical defect. Am J Psychiatry. 1988;145:154-163.
7. Sullivan EV, Lim KO, Mathalon D, Marsh L, Beal DM, Harris D, Hoff AL, Faustman WO, Pfefferbaum A. A profile of cortical gray matter volume deficits characteristic of schizophrenia. Cereb Cortex. 1998;8:117-124.
8. Zipursky RB, Lim KO, Sullivan EV, Brown BW, Pfefferbaum A. Widespread cerebral gray matter volume deficits in schizophrenia. Arch Gen Psychiatry. 1992: 49:195-205.
9. Daviss SR, Lewis DA. Local circuit neurons of the prefrontal cortex in schizophrenia: selective increase in the density of calbindin-immunoreactive neurons Psychiatry Res. 1995;59:81-96.
10. Selemon LD, Rajkowska G, Goldman-Rakic PS. Abnormally high neuronal density in the schizophrenic cortex: a morphometric analysis of prefrontal area 9 and occipital area 17. Arch Gen Psychiatry. 1995;52:805-818.
11. Selemon LD, Rajkowska G, Goldman-Rakic PS. Elevated neuronal density in prefrontal area 46 in brains from schizophrenic patients: application of a three-dimensional, stereologic counting method. J Comp Neurol. 1998;392:402-412.
12. Akbarian S, Kim JJ, Potkin SG, Hagman JO, Tafazzoli A, Bunney WE Jr, Jones EG. Gene expression for glutamic acid decarboxylase is reduced without loss of neurons in prefrontal cortex of schizophrenics. Arch Gen Psychiatry. 1995;52:258-266.
13. Thune JJ, Hofsten DE, Uylings HBM, Pakkenberg B. Total neuron numbers in the prefrontal cortex in schizophrenia. Soc Neurosci Abstracts. 1998;24:985.
14. Goldman-Rakic PS, Selemon LD. Functional and anatomical aspects of prefrontal pathology in schizophrenia. Schizophr Bull. 1997;23:437-458.
15. Bertolino A, Nawroz S, Mattay VS, Barnett AS, Duyn JH, Moonen CTW, Frank JA, Tedeschi G, Weinberger DR. Regionally specific pattern of neurochemical pathology in schizophrenia as assessed by multislice proton magnetic resonance spectroscopic imaging. Am J Psychiatry. 1996;153:1554-1563.
16. Bertolino A, Callicott JH, Nawroz S, Mattay VS, Duyn JH, Teclaschi G, Frank JA, Weinberger DR. Reproducibility of proton magnetic resonance spectroscopic imaging in patients with schizophrenia. Neuropsychopharmacology. 1998;18:1-9.
17. Pettegrew JW, Moore C, Long H, Larkin C, Thompson P, Mulvany F, Redmond O, Stack JP, Ennis JT, Waddington JL. 1H-magnetic resonance spectroscopy of the left temporal and frontal lobes in schizophrenia: clinical, neurodevelopmental, and cognitive correlates. Biol Psychiatry. 1994;36:792-800.
18. Deicken RF, Zhou L, Corwin F, Vinogradov S, Weiner MW. Decreased left frontal lobe N-acetylaspartate in schizophrenia. Am J Psychiatry. 1997;154:688-690.
19. Pettegrew JW, Keshavan MS, Panchalingam K, Strychor S, Kaplan DB, Tretta MG, Allen M. Alterations in brain high-energy phosphate and membrane phospholipid metabolism in first-episode, drug-naive schizophrenics. Arch Gen Psychiatry. 1991;48:563-568.
20. Shioiri T, Kato T, Inubushi T, Murashita J, Takahashi S. Correlations of phosphomonoesters measured by phosphorus-31 magnetic resonance spectroscopy in the frontal lobes and negative symptoms in schizophrenia. Psychiatr Res Neuroimaging. 1994;55:223-235.
21. Stanley JA, Williamson PC, Drost DJ, Carr TJ, Rylett RJ, Malla A, Thompson RT. An in vivo study of the prefrontal cortex of schizophrenic patients at different stages of illness via phosphorus magnetic resonance spectroscopy. Arch Gen Psychiatry. 1995;52:399-406.
22. Pettegrew JW, Keshavan MS, Minshew NJ. 31P nuclear magnetic resonance spectroscopy: neurodevelopment and schizophrenia. Schizophr Bull. 1993;19:35-53.
23. Glantz LA, Lewis DA. Reduction of synaptophysin immunoreactivity in the prefrontal cortex of subjects with schizophrenia: regional and diagnostic specificity. Arch Gen Psychiatry. 1997;54:943-952.

172

24. Karson CN, Mrak RE, Schluterman KO, Sturner WQ, Sheng JG, Griffin WST. Alterations in synaptic proteins and their encoding mRNAs in prefrontal cortex in schizophrenia: a possible neurochemical basis for "hypofrontality." *Mol Psychiatry*. 1999;4:39-45.

25. Perrone-Bizzozero NI, Sower AC, Bird ED, Benowitz LI, Ivins KJ, Neve RL. Levels of the growth-associated protein GAP-43 are selectively increased in association cortices in schizophrenia. *Proc Natl Acad Sci U S A*. 1996;93:14182-14187.

26. Honer WG, Falkai P, Chen C, Arango V, Mann JJ, Dwork AJ. Synaptic and plasticity-associated proteins in anterior frontal cortex in severe mental illness. *Neuroscience*. 1999;91:1247-1255.

27. Giguere M, Goldman-Rakic PS. Mediodorsal nucleus: areal, laminar, and tangential distribution of afferents and efferents in the frontal lobe of rhesus monkeys. *J Comp Neurol*. 1988;277:195-213.

28. Melchitzky DS, Sesack SR, Lewis DA. Parvalbumin-immunoreactive axon terminals in monkey and human prefrontal cortex: laminar, regional and target specificity of type I and type II synapses. *J Comp Neurol*. 1999;408:11-22.

29. Pakkenberg B. Pronounced reduction of total neuron number in mediodorsal thalamic nucleus and nucleus accumbens in schizophrenics. *Arch Gen Psychiatry*. 1990;47:1023-1028.

30. Manaye KF, Liang C-L, Hicks PB, German D, Young KA. Nerve cell numbers in thalamic anterior and mediodorsal nuclei are selectively reduced in schizophrenia. *Soc Neurosci Abstracts*. 1998;24:1236.

31. Popken GJ, Bunney WE Jr, Potkin SG, Jones EG. Neuron number and GABAergic and glutamatergic mRNA expression in subdivisions of the thalamic mediodorsal nucleus of schizophrenics. *Soc Neurosci Abstracts*. 1998;24:991.

32. Anderson SA, Classey JD, Condé F, Lund JS, Lewis DA. Synchronous development of pyramidal neuron dendritic spines and parvalbumin-immunoreactive chandelier neuron axon terminals in layer III of monkey prefrontal cortex. *Neuroscience*. 1995;67:7-22.

33. Bourgeois J-P, Goldman-Rakic PS, Rakic P. Synaptogenesis in the prefrontal cortex of rhesus monkeys. *Cereb Cortex*. 1994;4:78-96.

34. Huttenlocher PR, Dabholkar AS. Regional differences in synaptogenesis in human cerebral cortex. *J Comp Neurol*. 1997;387:167-178.

35. DeFelipe J, Farinas I. The pyramidal neuron of the cerebral cortex: morphological and chemical characteristics of the synaptic inputs. *Prog Neurobiol*. 1992; 39:563-607.

36. Peters A, Palay SL, Webster DF. *The Fine Structure of the Nervous System*. New York, NY: Oxford University Press; 1991.

37. Mirra SS, Heyman A, McKeel D, Sumi SM, Crain BJ, Brownlee LM, Vogel FS, Hughes JP, van Bell G. The Consortium to Establish a Registry for Alzheimer's Disease (CERAD), part II: standardization of the neuropathological assessment of Alzheimer's disease. *Neurology*. 1991;41:479-486.

38. American Psychiatric Association. *Diagnostic and Statistical Manual of Mental Disorders, Third Edition, Revised*. Washington, DC: American Psychiatric Association; 1987.

39. Hayes TL, Lewis DA. Magnopyramidal neurons in the anterior motor speech region: dendritic features and interhemispheric comparisons. *Arch Neurol*. 1996; 53:1277-1283.

40. Lund JS. Organization of neurons in the visual cortex, area 17, of the monkey (*Macaca mulatta*). *J Comp Neurol*. 1973;147:455-496.

41. Lewis DA, Campbell MJ, Terry RD, Morrison JH. Laminar and regional distributions of neurofibrillary tangles and neuritic plaques in Alzheimer's disease: a quantitative study of visual and auditory cortices. *J Neurosci*. 1987;7:1799-1808.

42. Woo T-U, Whitehead RE, Melchitzky DS, Lewis DA. A subclass of prefrontal γ-aminobutyric acid axon terminals are selectively altered in schizophrenia. *Proc Natl Acad Sci U S A*. 1998;95:5341-5346.

43. Williams RS, Ferrante RJ, Caviness VS Jr. The Golgi rapid method in clinical neuropathology: the morphologic consequences of suboptimal fixation. *J Neuropathol Exp Neurol*. 1978;37:13-33.

44. Jacobs B, Driscoll L, Schall M. Life-span dendritic and spine changes in areas 10 and 18 of human cortex: a quantitative Golgi study. *J Comp Neurol*. 1997; 386:661-680.

45. Garey LJ, Ong WY, Patel TS, Kanani M, Davis A, Mortimer AM, Barnes TRE, Hirsch SR. Reduced dendritic spine density on cerebral cortical pyramidal neurons in schizophrenia. *J Neurol Neurosurg Psychiatry*. 1998;65:446-453.

46. Pasternak JF, Woolsey TA. On the selectivity of the Golgi-Cox method. *J Comp Neurol*. 1975;160:307-312.

47. Pierri JN, Edgar CL, Lewis DA. Somal size of prefrontal cortical pyramidal neurons in the thalamic recipient zone of subjects with schizophrenia. *Soc Neurosci Abstracts*. 1998;24:987.

48. Rajkowska G, Selemon LD, Goldman-Rakic PS. Neuronal and glial somal size in the prefrontal cortex. *Arch Gen Psychiatry*. 1998;55:215-224.

49. Horner CH, Arbuthnott E. Methods of estimation of spine density: are spines evenly distributed throughout the dendritic field? *J Anat*. 1991;177:179-184.

50. Benes FM, Paskevich PA, Davidson J, Domesick VB. Synaptic rearrangements in medial prefrontal cortex of haloperidol-treated rats. *Brain Res*. 1985;348:15-20.

51. Vincent SL, McSparren J, Wang RY, Benes FM. Evidence for ultrastructural changes in cortical axodendritic synapses following long-term treatment with haloperidol or clozapine. *Neuropsychopharmacology*. 1991;5:147-155.

52. Brock JW, Prasad C. Alterations in dendritic spine density in the rat brain associated with protein malnutrition. *Dev Brain Res*. 1992;66:266-269.

53. Bryan GK, Riesen AH. Deprived somatosensory-motor experience in stumptailed monkey neocortex: dendritic spine density and dendritic branching of layer IIIb pyramidal cells. *J Comp Neurol*. 1989;286:208-217.

54. Horner CH. Plasticity of the dendritic spine. *Prog Neurobiol*. 1993;41:281-321.

55. Valverde F. Apical dendritic spines of the visual cortex and light deprivation in the mouse. *Exp Brain Res*. 1967;3:337-352.

56. Woolley CS, Gould E, Frankfurt M, McEwen BS. Naturally occurring fluctuation in dendritic spine density on adult hippocampal pyramidal neurons. *J Neurosci*. 1990;10:4035-4039.

57. Moser M-B, Trommald M, Andersen P. An increase in dendritic spine density on hippocampal CA1 pyramidal cells following spatial learning in adult rats suggests the formation of new synapses. *Proc Natl Acad Sci U S A*. 1994;91:12673-12675.

58. Parnavelas JG, Lynch G, Brecha N, Cotman CW, Globus A. Spine loss and regrowth in hippocampus following deafferentation. *Nature*. 1974;248:71-73.

59. Ingham CA, Hood SH, Taggart P, Arbuthnott GW. Plasticity of synapses in the rat neostriatum after unilateral lesion of the nigrostriatal dopaminergic pathway. *J Neurosci*. 1998;18:4732-4743.

60. Globus A, Scheibel AB. Synaptic loci on parietal cortical neurons: terminations of corpus callosum fibers. *Science*. 1967;156:1127-1129.

61. Lewis DA. Development of the prefrontal cortex during adolescence: insights into vulnerable neural circuits in schizophrenia. *Neuropsychopharmacology*. 1997; 16:385-398.

62. Kuroda M, Murakami K, Shinkai M, Ojima H, Kishi K. Electron microscopic evidence that axon terminals from the mediodorsal thalamic nucleus make direct synaptic contacts with callosal cells in the prelimbic cortex of the rat. *Brain Res*. 1995;677:348-353.

63. Volk DW, Austin MC, Lewis DA. Decreased expression of GAD₆₇ mRNA in a subpopulation of GABA neurons in the prefrontal cortex of schizophrenic subjects. *Soc Neurosci Abstracts*. 1998;24:986.

64. Lewis DA. Neural circuitry of the prefrontal cortex in schizophrenia. *Arch Gen Psychiatry*. 1995;52:269-273.

65. Jones EG. GABAergic neurons and their role in cortical plasticity in primates. *Cereb Cortex*. 1993;3:361-372.

66. Benson DL, Huntsman MM, Jones EG. Activity-dependent changes in GAD and preprotachykinin mRNAs in visual cortex of adult monkeys. *Cereb Cortex*. 1994; 4:40-51.

67. Ahmed B, Anderson JC, Douglas RJ, Martin KAC, Nelson JC. Polyneuronal innervation of spiny stellate neurons in cat visual cortex. *J Comp Neurol*. 1994; 341:39-49.

68. Levitt JB, Lewis DA, Yoshioka T, Lund JS. Topography of pyramidal neuron intrinsic connections in macaque monkey prefrontal cortex (areas 9 and 46). *J Comp Neurol*. 1993;338:360-376.

69. Pucak ML, Levitt JB, Lund JS, Lewis DA. Patterns of intrinsic and associational circuitry in monkey prefrontal cortex. *J Comp Neurol*. 1996;376:614-630.

70. Barbas H. Architecture and cortical connections of the prefrontal cortex in the rhesus monkey. *Adv Neurol*. 1992;57:91-115.

71. Goldman-Rakic PS, Schwartz ML. Interdigitation of contralateral and ipsilateral columnar projections to frontal association cortex in primates. *Science*. 1982; 216:755-757.

72. Goldman-Rakic PS. Cellular basis of working memory. *Neuron*. 1995;14:477-485.

73. Lewis DA, Anderson SA. The functional architecture of the prefrontal cortex and schizophrenia. *Psychol Med*. 1995;25:887-894.

173

The Emerging Role of Glutamate in the Pathophysiology and Treatment of Schizophrenia

Donald C. Goff, M.D.

Joseph T. Coyle, M.D.

Objective: Research has implicated dysfunction of glutamatergic neurotransmission in the pathophysiology of schizophrenia. This review evaluates evidence from preclinical and clinical studies that brain glutamatergic neurotransmission is altered in schizophrenia, may affect symptom expression, and is modulated by antipsychotic drugs.

Method: A comprehensive review of scientific articles published over the last decade that address the role of glutamate in the pathophysiology of schizophrenia was carried out.

Results: Glutamatergic neurons are the major excitatory pathways linking the cortex, limbic system, and thalamus, regions that have been implicated in schizophrenia. Postmortem studies have revealed alterations in pre- and postsynaptic markers for glutamatergic neurons in several brain regions in schizophrenia. The N-me-thyl-D-aspartic acid (NMDA) subtype of glutamate receptor may be particularly important as blockade of this receptor by the dissociative anesthetics reproduces in normal subjects the symptomatic manifestations of schizophrenia, including negative symptoms and cognitive impairments, and increases dopamine release in the mesolimbic system. Agents that indirectly enhance NMDA receptor function via the glycine modulatory site reduce negative symptoms and variably improve cognitive functioning in schizophrenic subjects receiving typical antipsychotics.

Conclusions: Dysfunction of glutamatergic neurotransmission may play an important role in the pathophysiology of schizophrenia, especially of the negative symptoms and cognitive impairments associated with the disorder, and is a promising target for drug development.

(Am J Psychiatry 2001; 158:1367–1377)

Because glutamate is ubiquitous in the brain as the primary excitatory neurotransmitter, a model positing generalized abnormalities of glutamatergic activity would be unlikely to account for the clinical characteristics of schizophrenia with any degree of specificity. However, specificity has been observed with pharmacological challenges, where antagonism of the glutamatergic N-methyl-D-aspartic acid (NMDA) receptor complex has produced behavioral and cognitive deficits in normal subjects that closely mimic schizophrenia (1), and in therapeutic trials, in which agents that enhance NMDA receptor activity have selectively improved symptoms in schizophrenia patients (2). In addition, postmortem studies have identified abnormalities of glutamate receptor density and subunit composition in the prefrontal cortex, thalamus, and temporal lobe (3–5), areas that exhibit impaired activation during performance of cognitive tasks in schizophrenia (6, 7). These findings suggest that glutamatergic dysregulation may occur in regionally specific subpopulations of glutamatergic receptors and so support the potential value of a glutamatergic model for guiding research into the pathophysiology and treatment of schizophrenia.

Although the relationship is speculative, glutamatergic receptor dysfunction could also play a role in neuroarchitectural abnormalities that have been described in schizophrenia, such as aberrant neuronal migration (8, 9) or reduced synaptic connections (10), because of the role of glutamatergic receptors in regulating neuronal migration, neurite outgrowth, synaptogenesis, and the "pruning" of supernumerary neurons by apoptosis (11–14). Neuronal excitotoxicity mediated by glutamatergic receptors has also been proposed as a consequence of dysregulated glutamatergic transmission in schizophrenia (15), but evidence for neurodegeneration from glutamate toxicity in the brain in schizophrenia remains poorly established. Because an extensive and functionally diverse range of glutamate receptor subtypes are genetically encoded and can interact with environmental stressors during brain development, the model of glutamatergic dysfunction may account for the interplay of genetic and environmental risk factors identified in schizophrenia. Furthermore, a proposed dysfunction of glutamatergic neuronal systems is not inconsistent with the dopamine hypothesis of schizophrenia, since reciprocal synaptic relationships between forebrain dopaminergic projections and glutamatergic systems have been well described (16), and dysregulation of one system by illness or pharmacological interventions would be expected to alter neurotransmission in the other.

This review will briefly summarize glutamate receptor physiology and evaluate the evidence for glutamatergic dysfunction in schizophrenia, focusing on postmortem findings, pharmacologic models, and clinical trials examining the effects of glutamatergic agents on the symptomatic manifestations of schizophrenia.

Glutamate Receptors

Glutamate and the structurally related acidic amino acid aspartate activate two families of receptors: ionotropic receptors, which gate cation channels, and metabotropic receptors, which are coupled to G-proteins that affect intracellular metabolic processes (17). The ionotropic receptors are designated by the potent glutamate analogues that selectively activate them: the kainate receptor, the α-amino-3-hydroxy-5-methyl-isoxazole-4-proprionic acid (AMPA) receptor, and the NMDA receptor. Electrophysiologic effects of all three ionotropic receptor families are mediated by the opening of cation channels permeable to Na^+ and, in a subtype-specific fashion, to Ca^{2+}, thereby depolarizing or "exciting" the neuron. AMPA and kainate receptors play the primary role in mediating fast excitatory postsynaptic potentials responsible for excitatory neurotransmission.

The NMDA receptor serves a different role. At resting membrane potential, its channel is blocked by Mg^{2+}. Upon depolarization caused by activation of the kainate and/or AMPA receptors, the Mg^{2+} block is removed, permitting glutamate to open the NMDA channel. The channel is permeable not only to Na^+ but also to Ca^{2+}, an important intracellular signaling ion that activates nitric oxide synthetase, among other enzymes (18). The NMDA receptor has a number of modulatory sites that affect its activity. Within the channel, there is a binding site for the dissociative anesthetics such as phencyclidine (PCP, "angel dust") and ketamine, which serve as noncompetitive antagonists (19). There is also a strychnine-insensitive binding site for the co-agonist glycine, which must be occupied in order for glutamate to open the ion channel (20). This site on the NMDA receptor is distinct from the strychnine-sensitive site associated with the inhibitory glycine receptor in the brainstem and spinal cord. Electrophysiologic studies indicate that the glycine modulatory site is not fully occupied under normal conditions (21–23).

Because the NMDA receptor is recruited only during periods of substantial neuronal depolarization, it appears to serve the purpose of a "coincidence" detector. In this way, the NMDA receptor plays a critical role in a major form of use-dependent synaptic plasticity known as long-term potentiation. In long-term potentiation, a brief period of high-intensity excitatory synaptic activity, which markedly depolarizes the neurons and recruits NMDA receptors, results in a subsequent persistent increase in synaptic efficacy. Long-term potentiation has been linked to memory formation (24).

Molecular cloning has revealed a family of eight genes encoding the metabotropic receptors (19). Four genes encode the peptides (GluR1–GluR4) that form the AMPA receptor. The molecular diversity of AMPA receptors is further enhanced by several splice variants, in which mRNA is constructed from different exons (coding regions of genes), resulting in a number of physiologically distinct receptor channels from the same gene, and from posttranscriptional processing of mRNA. Three genes encode the family of kainate receptors (GluR5–GluR7), whereas two additional genes encode polypeptides (KA1 and KA2) that alter the pharmacologic features of the kainate receptors. This rich receptor diversity in theory can account for significant differences in relative activity and potential toxicity of glutamate receptors and might permit selective pharmacologic manipulations of excitatory neurotransmission.

The glutamatergic ionotropic receptors are formed by the aggregation of four or five subunits, which transverse the cell membrane and form the receptor-ion channel complex. The subunits differ in important pharmacodynamic properties, including affinity for glutamate, threshold for channel opening, and permeability to Ca^{2+} ions. For example, the $GluR_2$ subunit reduces calcium permeability of the AMPA-gated channels; this effect is dependent on the posttranscriptional editing of the $GluR_2$ mRNA. AMPA receptors that lack the $GluR_2$ subunit produce channels permeable to Ca^{2+} influx, which promotes excitotoxic neuronal degeneration (25). Subunit composition may also differ according to the functional role of the receptor. For example, hippocampal inhibitory neurons preferentially express NMDA receptor subunits 2C and 2D (NR_{2C} and NR_{2D}), which are more sensitive to activation by glutamate, owing to a lower threshold for Mg^{2+} blockade, and are more sensitive to antagonists (25, 26). Subunit composition may also be modified by exposure to drugs such as alcohol, nicotine, and antipsychotics (27, 28).

Glutamate Markers and Schizophrenia

Kim et al. (29) reported reduced concentrations of glutamate in the CSF of patients with schizophrenia and first proposed that decreased glutamatergic activity may be an etiologic factor in the disorder. This finding was replicated by some (30, 31) but not all subsequent studies (32–34). Tsai et al. (35) examined eight regions in postmortem brains and found lower concentrations of glutamate and aspartate in the prefrontal cortex and a lower concentration of glutamate in the hippocampus of patients with schizophrenia than in comparison subjects. In addition, the concentration of N-acetyl-aspartyl glutamate (NAAG), an acidic dipeptide that acts as an antagonist at NMDA receptors (36), was increased in the hippocampus, and the activity of glutamate carboxypeptidase II (GCP II), the enzyme that cleaves NAAG to produce glutamate and N-acetyl aspartate (NAA), was selectively reduced in the frontal cortex, temporal cortex, and hippocampus in the schizophrenia brains. It is noteworthy that magnetic reso-

1368

nance spectroscopic studies in schizophrenic subjects have demonstrated significant reduction of NAA levels in these same regions (37). However, the factors that regulate brain NAA levels are complex (38). While these findings suggest diminished activity at glutamatergic receptors in relevant brain regions, it remains uncertain whether this represents a primary vulnerability factor or a compensatory response to a more proximal defect.

Ligand binding studies in postmortem brains from individuals with schizophrenia have revealed consistent increases in kainate receptors in the prefrontal cortex (39, 40) and decreased AMPA and kainate receptor binding in the hippocampus (41, 42) without consistent abnormalities in NMDA receptor density (3, 4). Immunocytochemical analyses have confirmed a decrease in AMPA receptors in the medial temporal lobe, although reductions in the hippocampus were not found in one study (3). Whereas ligands binding to the cation channel of the NMDA receptor complex ("PCP binding site") have not demonstrated consistent alterations in density (3), Ishimaru et al. (43, 44) reported increased binding to the glycine site of the NMDA receptor throughout the primary sensory cortex and related association fields. In addition, the binding of [^{3}H]-D-aspartate, which labels the transporters that remove synaptic glutamate, was increased in the frontal cortex and decreased in the striatum (39, 45).

The cloning of receptor subunits has facilitated the measurement of glutamate receptor expression in the brain. Most consistent has been the finding of a lower level of mRNA encoding AMPA receptor subunits in the hippocampus and parahippocampus of schizophrenia brains than in the brains of comparison subjects (3, 46, 47). In addition, Akbarian et al. (48) found a higher proportion (1% versus 0.1%) of unedited GluR$_2$ mRNA in the prefrontal cortex of patients with schizophrenia and Alzheimer's disease than in normal subjects, suggesting a higher level of permeability of AMPA receptors to calcium, which could increase the potential for neurotoxicity. Although less studied, the measurement of mRNA encoding kainate receptor subunits has demonstrated a similar pattern of lower density in the hippocampus and parahippocampus (3). Although ligand binding studies have generally failed to find altered NMDA receptor density in the brain in schizophrenia, two studies have found evidence of altered subunit composition of NMDA receptors. Akbarian et al. (48) found a relatively higher level of the NR$_{2D}$ subunit in the prefrontal cortex of schizophrenia subjects than in normal subjects and neuroleptic-treated comparison patients, suggesting increased potential responsiveness to glutamate. In contrast, Gao and colleagues (4) recently reported a relative decrease of the NR$_1$ subunit in the hippocampus of schizophrenia patients. The investigators demonstrated that this finding was unlikely to represent a medication effect since treatment with haloperidol for 6 months produced no effect on NMDA receptor subunit composition in the rat hippocampus (4). NMDA receptors

lacking an NR$_1$ subunit are nonfunctional; the relative lack of the NR$_1$ subunit in the brain in schizophrenia suggests less than normal pharmacodynamic responsiveness of NMDA receptors in the hippocampus. Mohn and colleagues (49) used recombinant DNA technology to develop transgenic mice expressing only 5% of the normal levels of NR$_1$; the NMDA receptor-deficient mice exhibited hyperactivity, stereotypies, and social isolation. The hyperactivity and stereotypies were ameliorated by treatment with haloperidol and clozapine, but only clozapine corrected the impairments in social behaviors. Finally, Ibrahim and colleagues (5) recently reported lower levels of mRNA expression for subunits composing NMDA, AMPA, and kainate receptors in the thalamus of schizophrenia patients, and lower levels of binding to the polyamine and glycine binding sites of thalamic NMDA receptors. Differences between schizophrenic and comparison subjects were most prominent in nuclei with reciprocal projections to limbic regions.

Dissociative Anesthetics

It has long been recognized that PCP produces a syndrome in normal individuals that closely resembles schizophrenia (50, 51) and exacerbates symptoms in patients with chronic schizophrenia (50, 52). At subanesthetic doses, PCP binds to a site within the ion channel of the NMDA receptor that blocks the influx of cations, thereby acting as a noncompetitive antagonist (19). After reports linking PCP to protracted psychosis, abuse, and neurotoxicity (for review see reference 53), PCP was abandoned as an anesthetic agent in humans. Ketamine, another cyclohexylamine anesthetic that has approximately a 10-to-50-fold lower affinity for the NMDA receptor, continues to be used as an anesthetic in children. It is interesting to note that psychotic reactions associated with exposure to ketamine are reported to occur less frequently in children than in adults, suggesting the similar age dependence in vulnerability to psychoses associated with NMDA antagonists and onset of schizophrenia.

When infused intravenously to normal subjects, ketamine produces an amotivational state characterized by blunted affect, withdrawal, and psychomotor retardation (54). Psychotic symptoms typically take the form of suspiciousness, disorganization, and visual or auditory illusions. Psychotomimetic and perceptual effects of PCP are diminished under conditions of sensory deprivation, suggesting that processing of sensory information, rather than perception, is disrupted (55). Dissociative symptoms are also prominent. Although dissociative symptoms are not typically associated with schizophrenia, depersonalization may be an important early feature of the schizophrenia prodrome (53). Finally, ketamine produces the characteristic cognitive deficits of schizophrenia, including impaired performance on the Wisconsin Card Sorting Test and on verbal declarative memory, delayed word recall, and verbal fluency tests, without evidence of global impairment on the Mini-Mental State Examination (54, 56, 57).

When administered to patients with schizophrenia who were stabilized with conventional neuroleptics, ketamine produces delusions, hallucinations, and thought disorder, consistent with the patient's typical pattern of psychotic relapse (58, 59). Cognitive functioning, particularly recall and recognition memory, are further impaired. It is noteworthy that treatment with clozapine but not with haloperidol attenuated ketamine's exacerbation of clinical symptoms (58, 59).

Jentsch and Roth (19) argued that repeated administration of the NMDA receptor antagonists provides a more valid model of schizophrenia than acute administration. Whereas psychotic symptoms resulting from single-dose infusions of ketamine in normal subjects tend to be mild and somewhat inconsistent, prolonged exposure in PCP abusers is associated with severe, persistent psychotic symptoms more typical of schizophrenia (19, 51). However, it is debated whether the experience of chronic abusers is a valid model for PCP effects on the normal brain (60). Acute administration of ketamine in normal subjects increased perfusion in the prefrontal cortex and anterior cingulate (61–64) and decreased hippocampal perfusion (62), whereas chronic PCP abusers displayed classical "hypofrontality" (65, 66). Compared with single-dose administration, chronic treatment with PCP produced in monkeys more perseveration and fewer nonspecific cognitive deficits and caused memory deficits that persisted after PCP was discontinued (67). These memory deficits were prevented by clozapine treatment.

In rodents, acute administration of NMDA receptor antagonists markedly increases the release of dopamine and glutamate in the prefrontal cortex and subcortical structures (68–70). Moghaddam et al. (71) demonstrated in rats that ketamine-induced augmentation of dopamine release in the prefrontal cortex was associated with impaired performance on a memory task sensitive to prefrontal cortical function; these alterations could be ameliorated by treatment with an AMPA/kainic acid receptor antagonist. Using single cell recordings from dopamine neurons of the ventral tegmental area in rats, Svensson et al. (72) demonstrated that NMDA antagonists increase the rate but decrease the variability of neuronal firing, thereby impairing the signal-to-noise ratio. Burst firing was increased in the ventral tegmental area dopamine neurons that projected to limbic regions but was decreased in dopamine neurons that projected to the prefrontal cortex, indicating regional specificity of effects. By using positron emission tomography to monitor the displacement of [^{11}C]raclopride binding in the striatum after acute administration of ketamine in normal volunteers, several groups have demonstrated increased dopamine release of a magnitude comparable to the effects of amphetamine; furthermore, raclopride displacement correlated with severity of psychotic symptoms (73–75). Microdialysis in

monkeys further revealed that increased striatal dopamine release was accompanied by increased reuptake, resulting in increased turnover but unchanged extracellular dopamine concentrations (76).

Whereas the acute administration of NMDA receptor antagonists enhances dopamine turnover in the prefrontal cortex, subchronic administration is associated with decreased dopamine turnover in the frontal cortex (67, 77), reflecting potentially persistent, compensatory effects. Jentsch et al. (77) found a reduction of approximately 75% in prefrontal dopamine utilization, as reflected by the ratio of 3,4-dihydroxyphenylacetic acid (DOPAC) to dopamine in brain tissue after daily administration of 10 mg/kg of PCP in rats for 7 days. Jentsch et al. (78) also demonstrated a 40% reduction in extracellular dopamine by in vivo microdialysis in conscious rats after administration of 5 mg/kg of PCP twice daily for 7 days. In contrast, Lindefors et al. (79) reported that daily administration of 25 mg/kg of ketamine for 7 days increased prefrontal dopamine concentrations without altering concentrations of dopamine metabolites. The explanation for the conflicting results obtained with subchronic ketamine versus phencyclidine administration is not clear but may reflect the shorter half-life of ketamine (19). It is interesting to note that chronic administration of NMDA receptor antagonists results in decreased expression of the dopamine D$_1$ receptor mRNA in the prefrontal cortex of rats and monkeys (19, 80, 81). The D$_1$ receptor has been shown to be critical for working memory function (82).

Revisions of the dopamine hypothesis for schizophrenia have posited diminished dopaminergic activity in the prefrontal cortex and a reciprocal dopaminergic hyperactivity in the mesolimbic pathways (83). Consistent with this model, chronic PCP administration also increases subcortical dopamine release, particularly in the nucleus accumbens (68, 84). Increased mesolimbic dopaminergic activity associated with long-term administration of PCP produces sensitization to the behavioral effects of NMDA receptor antagonists such as PCP, ketamine, and MK801 (85–87), dopamine agonists (88, 89), and stress (89). Chronic administration of PCP also leads to increased mesolimbic dopamine response to haloperidol (89). Together, these findings emphasize the reciprocal modulation of glutamate and dopamine neuronal systems and are consistent with the "sensitization model" of schizophrenia (90), which may account for the progressive course of the illness and the vulnerability to stress of individuals with the illness.

Antipsychotic Drugs and Glutamate

A characteristic feature of schizophrenia is the inability to adapt to an auditory stimulus that is preceded by a low-level warning tone, a response that is known as prepulse inhibition and is believed to reflect a defect in attentional "filtering" of nonnovel stimuli (91). The atypical antipsychotic drugs clozapine, olanzapine, remoxipride, and quetiapine have all been found to reverse ketamine-induced deficits in prepulse inhibition (92–94). Haloperidol and selective antagonists at D_1, D_2 and serotonin$_2$ (5-HT$_2$) receptors did not correct the deficit in sensory gating caused by NMDA receptor antagonists (92, 95, 96), whereas the α_1-adrenergic antagonist prazosin blocked the disruptive effects of PCP (97). Chlorpromazine also blocks the effects of ketamine on prepulse inhibition, possibly by means of mediation by its potent antagonism of α_1-adrenergic receptors (96). Both clozapine and olanzapine attenuated the ketamine-induced increase in cortical metabolic activation measured by [^{14}C]-2-deoxyglucose in rats, an effect that was not achieved with either haloperidol or risperidone and that required a higher dose of olanzapine (10 mg/kg) than would be expected to produce maximal D_2 and 5-HT$_2$ blockade (98, 99). Corbett et al. (100) reported that olanzapine (0.25 mg/kg) and clozapine (2.5 mg/kg) but not haloperidol or risperidone reversed PCP-induced social withdrawal in rats. In another model, Olney (15) performed a series of experiments comparing the efficacy of antipsychotic drugs in preventing neuronal degeneration induced by NMDA receptor antagonists in the posterior cingulate and retrosplenial cortex in rats. Olanzapine, clozapine, and fluperlapine strongly prevented the neurotoxicity, whereas haloperidol and thioridazine displayed intermediate effectiveness (101–103). Neuroprotective effects have also been observed with muscarinic receptor antagonists, benzodiazepines, σ receptor ligands, and α_2-adrenergic receptor agonists, thereby making the clinical implications of activity in this complex model unclear (104).

Antipsychotic drugs can affect glutamatergic neurotransmission by modulating release of glutamate, by interacting with glutamate receptors, or by altering the density or subunit composition of glutamate receptors. Recent research has demonstrated that antipsychotic drugs acting through the D_2 receptor promote the phosphorylation of the NR$_1$ subunit of the NMDA receptor, thereby enhancing its function and consequent gene expression (105). Thus, dopamine-glutamate interactions occur intraneuronally as well as intrasynaptically (106). Free glutamate concentrations in the striatum measured by in vivo dialysis were increased by as much as fivefold by chronic administration of haloperidol or fluphenazine but were unaffected by clozapine (107–109). The augmentation of glutamate release in the striatum by conventional antipsychotic drugs appears to be mediated by D_2 inhibitory axoaxonic synapses on glutamatergic corticostriatal terminals (109), although long-term haloperidol treatment has also been shown to decrease expression of the glial glutamate transporter GLT-1 in the rat striatum (110). The elevation of excitatory amino acid concentrations may have important clinical consequences, as indicated by significant correlations between ratings of tardive dysk-

inesia and CSF concentrations of aspartate and glutamate in neuroleptic-treated patients (111, 112). In addition, perforated synapses in the caudate, which have been associated with haloperidol-induced extrapyramidal side effects, have been shown to occur in glutamatergic synapses and to be mediated by NMDA receptors (113).

Growing evidence suggests that the effects of certain atypical antipsychotics on NMDA receptors may differentiate these agents from conventional antipsychotics. Lidsky et al. (114) measured haloperidol and clozapine displacement of [^{3}H]MK801 binding in rat striatal and cortical membranes and found that haloperidol did not significantly interact with NMDA receptors at clinically relevant concentrations but that clozapine displaced the ligand from the NMDA receptor at therapeutic levels. Using intracellular recordings and a voltage clamp, Arvanov et al. (115) found that clozapine but not haloperidol produced an enhancement of NMDA-receptor-mediated neurotransmission. Both the selective 5-HT$_{2A}$ antagonist M100907 and clozapine prevented PCP-induced blockade of NMDA receptors, as measured by depolarization of rat medial cortical pyramidal neurons (116), whereas selective D_2 blockers had no effect. Clozapine and several conventional agents have also been reported to act as partial agonists at the glycine modulatory site of the NMDA receptor, increasing neuronal depolarization at low concentrations and inhibiting depolarization at high concentrations (117, 118). Consistent with this interpretation, an increase in extracellular glycine attenuated the potentiation by haloperidol of NMDA-receptor-evoked response (119). In contrast, long-term administration of antipsychotics may result in desensitization of the glycine modulatory site of the NMDA receptor, as evidenced by a reduction in strychnine-insensitive glycine binding associated with both clozapine and conventional agents (120). These findings suggest that the glutamatergic effects of antipsychotics are importantly concentration-dependent and that, depending on their relative dose-response curves, different agents may act either as agonists or antagonists at therapeutic concentrations.

Several investigators have found that chronic antipsychotic treatment alters the expression of mRNA encoding glutamate receptor subunits, which varies depending on the drug type, the subunit, and the brain region (27, 121–123). In general, conventional antipsychotics increased the amount of mRNA encoding NMDA receptor subunits (NR$_1$ and NR$_2$) in the striatum, whereas clozapine treatment produced no change (122). This difference may reflect differential liability for extrapyramidal side effects. Conventional and atypical antipsychotics also differed in their effects on certain AMPA receptor subunits (GluR$_2$ and GluR$_4$), whereas GluR$_1$ was increased and GluR$_3$ decreased by both haloperidol and clozapine (123). Dissimilarities also were found for kainic acid receptors, with only clozapine reported to elevate expression of mRNA encoding GluR$_6$, GluR$_7$, and KA2 (123).

Pharmacologic Interventions at Glutamate Receptors

Evidence for hypoactivity of NMDA receptors in schizophrenia has led to therapeutic trials with agents that indirectly activate the receptor. Direct agonists at the NMDA receptor have not been studied because of the risk that excessive stimulation may cause excitotoxic damage to neurons (124). A more promising target is the glycine modulatory site on the NMDA receptor. Early trials of glycine administered orally at doses of 5–15 g/day produced inconsistent results, probably because glycine poorly crosses the blood-brain barrier (125–128). More recently, Javitt, Heresco-Levy, and colleagues (129–131) performed a series of placebo-controlled crossover trials with high doses of glycine (30–60 g/day) added to antipsychotic drugs and have demonstrated selective improvement in negative symptoms. In a 6-week trial, glycine also significantly improved subjects' ratings on the cognitive subscale of the Positive and Negative Syndrome Scale (131). Javitt and colleagues (23) demonstrated that glycine inhibits PCP-induced stimulation of subcortical dopamine release in a dose-related fashion in rats. Glycine transport inhibitors were also found to block PCP-induced behavioral hyperactivity (23), and they may represent a potential therapeutic approach. In another therapeutic approach with a full agonist at the glycine modulatory site, Tsai et al. (132) added D-serine to ongoing antipsychotic medication at a daily dose of 30 mg/kg for 8 weeks and reported significant improvements, compared to effects of placebo, in negative symptoms, psychosis, and cognitive function as measured by the cognitive subscale of the Positive and Negative Syndrome Scale and performance on the Wisconsin Card Sorting Test.

In a related approach, several groups have administered D-cycloserine, an antitubercular drug that acts as a relatively selective partial agonist at the glycine modulatory site over a narrow range of concentrations (133). Compared to glycine, D-cycloserine produces approximately 60% activation of the NMDA receptor, thus acting as an agonist in the presence of low concentrations of glycine (and related endogenous agonists) and as an antagonist in the presence of high concentrations of glycine. In an initial placebo-controlled, partly blinded, dose-finding study of D-cycloserine added to conventional neuroleptics, Goff et al. (134) found an inverted U-shaped dose response with significant reductions in negative symptoms and improvement in performance on a test of working memory at a D-cycloserine dose of 50 mg/day. Van Berkel et al. (135) administered D-cycloserine in a small, open trial to medication-free schizophrenia patients and observed selective improvement of negative symptoms at a D-cycloserine dose of 100 mg/day. In an 8-week, fixed-dose, placebo-controlled, parallel-group trial involving 46 patients who met criteria for the deficit syndrome of schizophrenia (126), 50 mg/day of D-cycloserine significantly improved

negative symptoms when added to conventional antipsychotics, but it did not improve performance on a cognitive battery (136). It is noteworthy that a full response was not achieved until weeks 4–6. Rosse et al. (137) found no improvement in negative symptoms when 15 mg/day or 30 mg/day of D-cycloserine was added to molindone.

Since clozapine (arguably) produces substantial therapeutic effects on negative symptoms in patients who respond poorly to typical neuroleptics and since its effects on glutamatergic systems differ from those of conventional agents, it was of interest to determine whether the addition of D-cycloserine would have further ameliorative effects in clozapine responders. Two separate trials of 50 mg/day of D-cycloserine added to clozapine resulted in worsening of negative symptoms (138, 139). In contrast, controlled trials in which the full agonists glycine and D-serine were added to clozapine produced no change in negative symptoms or cognitive function (140–142). One possible explanation for these findings is that clozapine may exert its effects on negative symptoms partly by increasing occupancy of the glycine modulatory site on the NMDA receptor, thereby transforming the partial agonist D-cycloserine into an antagonist and precluding additional therapeutic effects with the exogenous full agonists glycine and D-serine.

A final but quite preliminary area of investigation involves the study of drugs acting at the AMPA receptor that have recently become available for clinical trials. This family of drugs, known as ampakines, act as positive modulators of the AMPA receptor complex. CX516, the first drug of this class to be studied, has been shown to increase the peak and duration of glutamate-induced AMPA receptor-gated inward currents (143). In rats, ampakines increased hippocampal neuronal activity in response to stimulation of glutamatergic afferents and enhanced long-term potentiation (144, 145). These findings suggest that ampakines, by potentiating AMPA receptor-induced depolarization, indirectly enhance NMDA receptor function. In behavioral models to test learning in rats, ampakines improved acquisition and retention in the radial arm maze, water maze, and olfactory cue tasks (146). CX516 also synergistically blocked methamphetamine-induced rearing behavior in rats when it was added to clozapine and to conventional antipsychotic agents, an effect believed to predict antipsychotic efficacy (147).

CX516 was added to clozapine in a placebo-controlled, 4-week, escalating-dose trial involving six patients with schizophrenia and in a placebo-controlled, fixed-dose, parallel-group design with an additional 13 patients; the combination was well tolerated without significant adverse effects (148). Combined results from the two trials (N=19) revealed a consistent pattern of improvement in performance on tests of attention, memory, and distractibility. Comparisons between groups demonstrated moderate-to-large effect sizes favoring CX516 over placebo for most cognitive tests, but inferential tests of statistical sig-

1372

nificance were not performed due to the small number of subjects. Although the ampakines show promise as a treatment for cognitive deficits of schizophrenia, these preliminary data require replication in larger groups of patients.

Conclusions

Multiple lines of evidence have linked abnormalities in glutamatergic receptor expression, subunit composition, and function in schizophrenia. Similarities between behavioral effects of NMDA receptor antagonists and the clinical symptoms of schizophrenia have focused attention on treatment trials targeting a putative hypoactivity of a subpopulation of NMDA receptors. However, currently available antipsychotic drugs alter glutamatergic activity in multiple ways by enhancing release of glutamate in the striatum, directly interacting with NMDA receptors, altering glutamate receptor density, and changing the subunit composition of glutamate receptors. Many of these effects are regionally selective and vary among the antipsychotic drugs, with important differences emerging between atypical and conventional drugs. Clinical trials in which NMDA receptor activity was enhanced by agents acting at the glycine modulatory site have demonstrated decreases in negative symptoms and variable improvements in cognitive function. Electrophysiologic and neurochemical evidence suggests that clozapine, aside from its interactions with aminergic receptors, may also be acting through the NMDA receptor in affecting negative symptoms. Although the findings are preliminary, recent work with an ampakine indicates that positive modulation of the AMPA receptor may also provide another glutamatergic approach to treat cognitive deficits in schizophrenia. Thus, drugs that modulate glutamatergic neurotransmission hold promise for novel treatments for schizophrenia, especially for the cognitive impairments and negative symptoms associated with the disorder.

Received June 2, 2000; revisions received Nov. 29, 2000, and Feb. 27, 2001; accepted March 12, 2001. From the Schizophrenia Program, Massachusetts General Hospital, Boston; and the Consolidated Department of Psychiatry, Harvard Medical School. Address reprint requests to Dr. Coyle, Consolidated Department of Psychiatry, Harvard Medical School, 115 Mill St., Belmont, MA 02478; joseph_coyle@hms.harvard.edu (e-mail).
Supported in part by NIMH grants MH-51290 and MH-606450 (to Dr. Coyle) and MH-54245 and MH-57708 (to Dr. Goff).

References

1. Krystal JH, D'Souza DC, Petrakis IL, Belger A, Berman R, Charney DS, Abi-Saab W, Madonick S: NMDA agonists and antagonists as probes of glutamatergic dysfunction and pharmacotherapies for neuropsychiatric disorders. Harv Rev Psychiatry 1999; 7:125–133
2. Goff DC: Glutamate receptors in schizophrenia and antipsychotic drugs, in Neurotransmitter Receptors in Actions of Antipsychotic Medications. Edited by Lidow MS. New York, CRC Press, 2000, pp 121–136

3. Meador-Woodruff JH, Healy DJ: Glutamate receptor expression in schizophrenic brain. Brain Res Rev 2000; 31:288–294
4. Gao X-M, Sakai K, Roberts RC, Conley RR, Dean B, Tamminga CA: Ionotropic glutamate receptors and expression of N-methyl-D-aspartate receptor subunits in subregions of human hippocampus: effects of schizophrenia. Am J Psychiatry 2000; 157:1141–1149
5. Ibrahim HM, Hogg AJ Jr, Healy DJ, Haroutunian V, Davis KL, Meador-Woodruff JH: Ionotropic glutamate receptor binding and subunit mRNA expression in thalamic nuclei in schizophrenia. Am J Psychiatry 2000; 157:1811–1823
6. Heckers S, Goff D, Schacter D, Savage C, Fischman A, Alpert N, Rausch S: Functional imaging of memory retrieval in deficit vs nondeficit schizophrenia. Arch Gen Psychiatry 1999; 56:1117–1123
7. Heckers S, Curran T, Goff D, Rauch SL, Fischman AJ, Alpert NM, Schacter DL: Abnormalities in the thalamus and prefrontal cortex during episodic object recognition in schizophrenia. Biol Psychiatry 2000; 48:651–657
8. Akbarian S, Bunney WJ, Potkin S, Wigal S, Hagman J, Sandman C, Jones E: Altered distribution of nicotinamide-adenine dinucleotide phosphate-diaphorase cells in frontal lobe of schizophrenics implies disturbances of cortical development. Arch Gen Psychiatry 1993; 50:169–177
9. Akbarian S, Vinuela A, Kim J, Potkin S, Bunney WJ, Jones E: Distorted distribution of nicotinamide-adenine dinucleotide phosphate-diaphorase neurons in temporal lobe of schizophrenics implies anomalous cortical development. Arch Gen Psychiatry 1993; 50:178–187
10. McGlashan TH, Hoffman RE: Schizophrenia as a disorder of developmentally reduced synaptic connectivity. Arch Gen Psychiatry 2000; 57:637–648
11. McDonald JW, Johnston MV: Physiological and pathophysiological roles of excitatory amino acids during central nervous system development. Brain Res Rev 1990; 15:41–70
12. Kerwin RW: Glutamate receptor, microtubule associated proteins and developmental anomaly in schizophrenia: an hypothesis. Psychol Med 1993; 13:547–551
13. Komuro H, Rakic P: Modulation of neuronal migration by NMDA receptors. Science 1993; 260:95–97
14. Choi DW: Glutamate neurotoxicity and diseases of the nervous system. Neuron 1988; 1:623–634
15. Olney JW: New mechanisms of excitatory transmitter neurotoxicity. J Neural Transm Suppl 1994; 43:47–51
16. Carlsson M, Carlsson A: Interactions between glutamatergic and monoaminergic systems within the basal ganglia—implications for schizophrenia and Parkinson's disease. Trends Neurosci 1990; 13:272–276
17. Nakanishi S: Molecular diversity of glutamate receptors and implications for brain function. Science 1992; 258:597–603
18. Dawson TM, Zhang J, Dawson VL, Snyder SH: Nitric oxide: cellular regulation and neuronal injury. Prog Brain Res 1994; 103:365–369
19. Jentsch J, Roth R: The neuropsychopharmacology of phencyclidine: from NMDA receptor hypofunction to the dopamine hypothesis of schizophrenia. Neuropsychopharmacology 1999; 20:201–225
20. Huettner JE: Competitive antagonism of glycine at the N-methyl-D-aspartate (NMDA) receptor. Biochem Pharmacol 1991; 41:9–16
21. Bergeron R, Meyer T, Coyle J, Greene R: Modulation of N-methyl-D-aspartate receptor function by glycine transport. Proc Natl Acad Sci USA 1998; 95:15730–15734
22. Danysza W, Parsons CG: Glycine and N-methyl-D-aspartate receptors: physiological significance and possible therapeutic applications. J Neurophysiol 1998; 80:3336–3340

181

23. Javitt DC, Balla A, Sershen H, Lajtha A: Reversal of the behavioral and neurochemical effects of phencyclidine by glycine and glycine transport inhibitors. Biol Psychiatry 1999; 45:668–679

24. Bliss T, Collingridge G: A synaptic model of memory: long-term potentiation in the hippocampus. Nature 1993; 361:31–39

25. Kuner T, Schoepfer R: Multiple structural elements determine subunit specificity of Mg^{2+} block in NMDA receptor channels. J Neurosci 1996; 16:3549–3558

26. Grunze HC, Rainnie DG, Hasselmo ME, Barkai E, Hearn EF, McCarley RW, Greene RW: NMDA-dependent modulation of CA1 local circuit inhibition. J Neurosci 1996; 16:2034–2043

27. Fitzgerald LW, Deutch AY, Gasic G, Heinemann SF, Nestler EJ: Regulation of cortical and subcortical glutamate receptor subunit expression by antipsychotic drugs. J Neurosci 1995; 15: 2453–2461

28. Breese CR, Freedman R, Leonard SS: Glutamate receptor subtype expression in human postmortem brain tissue from schizophrenics and alcohol abusers. Brain Res 1995; 674:82–90

29. Kim JS, Kornhuber HH, Schmid-Burgk W, Holzmuller B: Low cerebrospinal glutamate in schizophrenic patients and a new hypothesis on schizophrenia. Neurosci Lett 1980; 20:379–382

30. Bjerkenstedt L, Edman G, Hagenfeldt L, Sedvall G, Wiesel FA: Plasma amino acids in relation to cerebrospinal fluid monoamine metabolites in schizophrenic patients and healthy controls. Br J Psychiatry 1985; 147:276–282

31. Macciardi F, Lucca A, Catalano M, Marino C, Zanardi R, Smeraldi E: Amino acid patterns in schizophrenia: some new findings. Psychiatry Res 1989; 32:63–70

32. Gattaz WF, Gattaz D, Beckmann H: Glutamate in schizophrenics and healthy controls. Arch Psychiatr Nervenkr 1982; 231:221–225

33. Perry TL: Normal cerebrospinal fluid and brain glutamate levels in schizophrenia do not support the hypothesis of glutamatergic neuronal dysfunction. Neurosci Lett 1982; 28:81–85

34. Tsai G, van Kammen D, Chen S, Kelley M, Grier A, Coyle J: Glutamatergic neurotransmission involves structural and clinical deficits of schizophrenia. Biol Psychiatry 1998; 44:667–674

35. Tsai G, Passani LA, Slusher BS, Carter R, Baer L, Kleinman JE, Coyle JT: Abnormal excitatory neurotransmitter metabolism in schizophrenic brains. Arch Gen Psychiatry 1995; 52:829–836

36. Coyle J: The nagging question of the function of N-acetylaspartylglutamate. Neurobiol Dis 1997; 4:231–238

37. Kegles L, Humaran TJ, Mann JJ: In vivo neurochemistry of brain in schizophrenia as revealed by magnetic resonance spectroscopy. Biol Psychiatry 1998; 44:382–388

38. Tsai G, Coyle JT: N-Acetylaspartate in neuropsychiatric disorders. Prog Neurobiol 1995; 46:531–540

39. Deakin JFW, Slater P, Simpson MDC, Gilchrist AC, Skan WJ, Royston MC, Reynolds GP, Cross AJ: Frontal cortical and left temporal glutamatergic dysfunction in schizophrenia. J Neurochem 1989; 52:1781–1786

40. Nishikawa T, Takashima M, Toru M: Increased [^{3}H] kainic acid binding in the prefrontal cortex in schizophrenia. Neurosci Lett 1983; 40:245–250

41. Kerwin RW, Patel S, Meldrum BS, Czudek C, Reynolds GP: Asymmetrical loss of glutamate receptor subtype in left hippocampus in schizophrenia. Lancet 1988; 1:583–584

42. Kerwin R, Patel S, Meldrum B: Quantitative autoradiographic analysis of glutamate binding sites in the hippocampal formation in normal and schizophrenic brain post mortem. Neuroscience 1990; 39:25–32

43. Ishimaru M, Kurumaji A, Toru M: NMDA-associated glycine binding site increases in schizophrenic brains (letter). Biol Psychiatry 1992; 32:379–381

44. Ishimaru M, Kurumaji A, Toro M: Increases in strychnine-insensitive glycine binding sites in cerebral cortex of chronic schizophrenics: evidence for glutamate hypothesis. Biol Psychiatry 1994; 35:84–95

45. Simpson MDC, Slater P, Royston MC, Deaking JFW: Regionally selective deficits in uptake sites for glutamate and gamma-aminobutyric acid in the basal ganglia in schizophrenia. Psychiatry Res 1992; 42:273–282

46. Harrison PJ, McLaughlin D, Kerwin RW: Decreased hippocampal expression of a glutamate receptor gene in schizophrenia. Lancet 1991; 337:450–452

47. Eastwood SL, McDonald B, Burnet PWJ, Beckwith JP, Kerwin RW, Harrison PJ: Decreased expression of mRNAs encoding non-NMDA glutamate receptors GluR1 and GluR2 in medial temporal lobe neurons in schizophrenia. Mol Brain Res 1995; 29: 211–223

48. Akbarian S, Sucher NJ, Bradley D, Tafazzoli A, Trinh D, Hetrick WP, Potkin SG, Sandman CA, Bunney WE, Jones EG: Selective alterations in gene expression for NMDA receptor subunits in prefrontal cortex of schizophrenics. J Neurosci 1996; 16:19–30

49. Mohn A, Gainetdinov R, Caron M, Koller B: Mice with reduced NMDA receptor expression display behaviors related to schizophrenia. Cell 1999; 98:427–436

50. Luby ED, Cohen BD, Rosenbaum G, Gottlieb JS, Kelley R: Study of a new schizophrenomimetic drug—sernyl. Arch Neurol Psychiatry 1959; 81:363–369

51. Javitt DC, Zukin SR: Recent advances in the phencyclidine model of schizophrenia. Am J Psychiatry 1991; 148:1301–1308

52. Itil T, Keskiner A, Kiremitci N, Holden JMC: Effect of phencyclidine in chronic schizophrenics. Can Psychiatr Assoc J 1967; 12: 209–212

53. Krystal JH, Karper LP, Seibyl JP, Freeman GK, Delaney R, Bremner JD, Heninger GR, Bowers MBJ, Charney DS: Subanesthetic effects of the noncompetitive NMDA antagonist, ketamine, in humans: psychotomimetic, perceptual, cognitive, and neuroendocrine responses. Arch Gen Psychiatry 1994; 51:199–214

54. Cohen B, Rosenbaum G, Luby E, Gottlieb J: Comparison of phencyclidine hydrochloride (sernyl) with other drugs: simulation of schizophrenic performance with phencyclidine hydrochloride (sernyl), lysergic acid diethylamide (LSD-25), and amobarbital (Amytal) sodium, II: symbolic and sequential thinking. Arch Gen Psychiatry 1962; 6:79–85

55. Moller P, Husby R: The initial prodrome in schizophrenia: searching for core dimensions of experience and behavior. Schizophr Bull 2000; 26:217–232

56. Malhotra A, Pinals D, Weingartner H, Sirocco K, Missar C, Pickar D, Breier A: NMDA receptor function and human cognition: the effects of ketamine in healthy volunteers. Neuropsychopharmacology 1996; 14:301–307

57. Newcomer J, Farber N, Jevtovic-Todorovic V, Selke G, Melson A, Hershey T, Craft S, Olney J: Ketamine-induced NMDA receptor hypofunction as a model of memory impairment and psychosis. Neuropsychopharmacology 1999; 20:106–118

58. Lahti AC, Koffel B, LaPorte D, Tamminga CA: Subanesthetic doses of ketamine stimulate psychosis in schizophrenia. Neuropsychopharmacology 1995; 13:9–19

59. Malhotra A, Pinals D, Adler C, Elman I, Clifton A, Pickar D, Breier A: Ketamine-induced exacerbation of psychotic symptoms and cognitive impairment in neuroleptic-free schizophrenics. Neuropsychopharmacology 1997; 17:141–150

60. Krystal JH, Belger A, D'Souza C, Anand A, Charney DS, Aghajanian GK, Moghaddam B: Therapeutic implications of the hyperglutamatergic effects of NMDA antagonists. Neuropsychopharmacology 1999; 22:S143–S157

61. Breier A, Malhotra A, Pinals DA, Weisenfeld NI, Pickar D: Association of ketamine-induced psychosis with focal activation of

1374

182

the prefrontal cortex in healthy volunteers. Am J Psychiatry 1997; 154:805–811

62. Lahti AC, Holcomb HH, Medoff DR, Tamminga CA: Ketamine activates psychosis and alters limbic blood flow in schizophrenia. Neuroreport 1995; 6:869–872

63. Vollenweider FX, Leenders KL, Oye I, Hell D, Angst J: Differential psychopathology and patterns of cerebral glucose utilisation produced by (S)- and (R)-ketamine in healthy volunteers using positron emission tomography (PET). Eur Neuropsychopharmacol 1997; 7:25–38

64. Vollenweider FX, Leenders KL, Scharfetter C, Antonini A, Maguire P, Missimer J, Angst J: Metabolic hyperfrontality and psychopathology in the ketamine model of psychosis using positron emission tomography (PET) and [18F] fluorodeoxyglucose (FDG). Eur Neuropsychopharmacol 1997; 7:9–24

65. Hertzmann M, Reba RC, Kotlyarove EV: Single photon emission computed tomography in phencyclidine and related drug abuse (letter). Am J Psychiatry 1990; 147:255–256

66. Wu JC, Buchsbaum MS, Bunney EW: Positron emission tomography study of phencyclidine users as a possible drug model of schizophrenia. Yakubutsu Seishin 1991; 11:47–48

67. Jentsch J, Redmond DJ, Elsworth J, Taylor J, Youngren K, Roth R: Enduring cognitive deficits and cortical dopamine dysfunction in monkeys after long-term administration of phencyclidine. Science 1997; 277:953–955

68. Deutch AY, Tam S-Y, Freeman AS, Bowers MBJ, Roth RH: Mesolimbic and mesocortical dopamine activation induced by phencyclidine: contrasting pattern to striatal response. Eur J Pharmacol 1987; 134:257–264

69. Bowers MBJ, Bannon MJ, Hoffman FJJ: Activation of forebrain dopamine systems by phencyclidine and footshock stress: evidence for distinct mechanisms. Psychopharmacology (Berl) 1987; 93:133–135

70. Verma A, Moghaddam B: NMDA receptor antagonists impair prefrontal cortex function as assessed via spatial delayed alternation performance in rats: modulation by dopamine. J Neurosci 1996; 16:373–379

71. Moghaddam B, Adams B, Verma A, Daly D: Activation of glutamatergic neurotransmission by ketamine: a novel step in the pathway from NMDA receptor blockade to dopaminergic and cognitive disruptions associated with the prefrontal cortex. J Neurosci 1997; 17:2921–2927

72. Svensson TH, Mathe JM, Andersson JL, Nomikos GG, Hildebrand BE, Marcus M: Mode of action of atypical neuroleptics in relation to the phencyclidine model of schizophrenia: role of 5-HT2 receptor and alpha1-adrenoreceptor antagonism. J Clin Psychopharmacol 1995; 15:11S–18S

73. Smith GS, Schloesser R, Brodie JD, Dewey SL, Logan J, Vitkun SA, Simkowitz P, Hurley A, Cooper T, Volkow ND, Cancro R: Glutamate modulation of dopamine measured in vivo with positron emission tomography (PET) and 11C-raclopride in normal human subjects. Neuropsychopharmacology 1998; 18:18–25

74. Breier A, Adler CM, Weisenfeld N, Su TP, Elman I, Picken L, Malhotra AK, Pickar D: Effects of NMDA antagonism on striatal dopamine release in healthy subjects: application of a novel PET approach. Synapse 1998; 29:142–147

75. Vollenweider FX, Vontobel P, Oye I, Hell D, Leenders KL: Effects of (S)-ketamine on striatal dopamine: a [11C]raclopride PET study of a model psychosis in humans. J Psychiatr Res 2000; 34:35–43

76. Tsukada H, Harada N, Nishiyama S, Ohba H, Sato K, Fukumoto D, Kakiuchi T: Ketamine decreased striatal [11C]raclopride binding with no alterations in static dopamine concentrations in the striatal extracellular fluid in the monkey brain: multiparametric PET studies combined with microdialysis analysis. Synapse 2000; 37:95–103

77. Jentsch J, Tran A, Le D, Youngren K, Roth R: Subchronic phencyclidine administration reduces mesoprefrontal dopamine utilization and impairs prefrontal cortical-dependent cognition in the rat. Neuropsychopharmacology 1997; 17:92–99

78. Jentsch JD, Dazzi L, Chhatwal JP, Verrico CD, Roth RH: Reduced prefrontal dopamine, but not acetylcholine, release in vivo after repeated, intermittent phencyclidine administration to rats. Neurosci Lett 1998; 24:175–178

79. Lindefors N, Barati S, O'Connor W: Differential effects of single and repeated ketamine administration on dopamine, serotonin, and GABA transmission in rat prefrontal cortex. Brain Res 1997; 759:202–212

80. Healy DJ, Meador-Woodruff JH: Differential regulation, by MK-801, of dopamine receptor gene expression in rat nigrostriatal and mesocorticolimbic systems. Brain Res 1996; 708:38–44

81. Healy DJ, Meador-Woodruff JH: Dopamine receptor gene expression in hippocampus is differentially regulated by the NMDA receptor antagonist MK-801. Eur J Pharmacol 1996; 306:257–264

82. Sawaguchi T, Goldman-Rakic PS: D1 dopamine receptors in prefrontal cortex: involvement in working memory. Science 1991; 251:947–950

83. Davis KL, Kahn RS, Ko G, Davidson M: Dopamine in schizophrenia: a review and reconceptualization. Am J Psychiatry 1991; 148:1474–1486

84. Jentsch J, Elsworth J, Redmond DJ, Roth R: Phencyclidine increases forebrain monoamine metabolism in rats and monkeys: modulation by the isomers of HA966. J Neurosci 1997; 17:1769–1776

85. Scalzo F, Holson R: The ontogeny of behavioral sensitization to phencyclidine. Neurotoxicol Teratol 1992; 14:7–14

86. Wolf M, Diener J, Lajeunesse C, Shriqui C: Low-dose bromocriptine in neuroleptic-resistant schizophrenia: a pilot study. Biol Psychiatry 1992; 31:1166–1168

87. Xu X, Domino E: Phencyclidine-induced behavioral sensitization. Pharmacol Biochem Behav 1994; 47:603–608

88. Lannes B, Micheletti G, Warter J, Kempf E, DiScala G: Behavioral, pharmacological, and biochemical effects of acute and chronic administration of ketamine in the rat. Neurosci Lett 1991; 128:177–181

89. Jentsch J, Taylor J, Roth R: Subchronic phencyclidine administration increases mesolimbic dopamine system responsivity and augments stress and amphetamine-induced hyperlocomotion. Neuropsychopharmacology 1998; 19:105–113

90. Lieberman J, Sheitman B, Kinon B: Neurochemical sensitization in the pathophysiology of schizophrenia: deficits and dysfunction in neuronal regulation and plasticity. Neuropsychopharmacology 1997; 17:205–229

91. Braff DL, Geyer MA: Sensorimotor gating and schizophrenia. Arch Gen Psychiatry 1990; 47:181–188

92. Bakshi VP, Swerdlow NR, Geyer MA: Clozapine antagonizes phencyclidine-induced deficits in sensorimotor gating of the startle response. J Pharmacol Exp Ther 1994; 271:787–794

93. Bakshi V, Geyer M: Antagonism of phencyclidine-induced deficits in prepulse inhibition by the putative atypical antipsychotic drug olanzapine. Psychopharmacology (Berl) 1995; 122:198–201

94. Swerdlow N, Bakshi V, Geyer M: Seroquel restores sensorimotor gating in phencyclidine-treated rats. J Pharmacol Exp Ther 1996; 279:1290–1299

95. Johansson C, Jackson D, Svensson L: The atypical antipsychotic, remoxipride, blocks phencyclidine-induced disruption of prepulse inhibition in the rat. Psychopharmacology (Berl) 1994; 116:437–442

96. Swerdlow N, Bakshi V, Waikar M, Taaid N, Geyer M: Seroquel, clozapine and chlorpromazine restore sensorimotor gating in

ketamine-treated rats. Psychopharmacology (Berl) 1998; 140: 75–80

97. Bakshi VP, Geyer MA: Reversal of phencyclidine-induced deficits in prepulse inhibition by prazosin, an alpha-1 adrenergic antagonist. J Pharmacol Exp Ther 1997; 283:666–674

98. Duncan GE, Leipzig JN, Mailman RB, Lieberman JA: Differential effects of clozapine and haloperidol on ketamine-induced brain metabolic activation. Brain Res 1998; 812:65–75

99. Duncan GE, Miyamoto S, Leipzig JN, Lieberman JA: Comparison of the effects of clozapine, risperidone, and olanzapine on ketamine-induced alterations in regional brain metabolism. J Pharmacol Exp Ther 2000; 293:8–14

100. Corbett R, Camacho F, Woods AT, Kerman LL, Fishkin RJ, Brooks K, Dunn RW: Antipsychotic agents antagonize non-competitive N-methyl-D-aspartate antagonist-induced behaviors. Psychopharmacology (Berl) 1995; 120:67–74

101. Olney JW, Farber NB: Efficacy of clozapine compared with other antipsychotics in preventing NMDA-antagonist neurotoxicity. J Clin Psychiatry 1994; 55(9, suppl B):43–46

102. Farber N, Foster J, Duhan N, Olney J: Olanzapine and fluperlapine mimic clozapine in preventing MK-801 neurotoxicity. Schizophr Res 1996; 21:33–37

103. Farber NB, Price MT, Labruyere J, Nemnich J, St Peter H, Wozniak DF, Olney JW: Antipsychotic drugs block phencyclidine receptor-mediated neurotoxicity. Biol Psychiatry 1993; 34: 119–121

104. Olney JW, Farber NB: Glutamate receptor dysfunction and schizophrenia. Arch Gen Psychiatry 1995; 52:998–1007

105. Leveque JC, Macias W, Rajadhyaksha A, Carlson RR, Barczak A, Kang S, Li X-M, Coyle JT, Huganier RL, Heckers S, Konradi C: Intracellular modulation of NMDA receptor function by antipsychotic drugs. J Neurosci 2000; 20:4011–4020

106. Snyder GI, Allen PB, Feinberg AA, Valle CG, Huganier RI, Nairn AC, Greengard P: Regulation of phosphorylation of the GluR1 AMPA receptor in the neostriatum by dopamine and stimulants in vivo. J Neurosci 2000; 20:4480–4488

107. Yamamoto BK, Cooperman MA: Differential effects of chronic antipsychotic drug treatment on extracellular glutamate and dopamine concentrations. J Neurosci 1994; 14:4159–4166

108. Yamamoto BK, Pehek EA, Meltzer HY: Brain region effects of clozapine on amino acid and monoamine transmission. J Clin Psychiatry 1994; 55(9, suppl B):8–14

109. See R, Lynch A: Duration-dependent increase in striatal glutamate following prolonged fluphenazine administration in rats. Eur J Pharmacol 1996; 308:279–282

110. Schneider J, Wade T, Lidsky T: Chronic neuroleptic treatment alters expression of glial glutamate transporter GLT-1 mRNA in the striatum. Neuroreport 1998; 9:133–136

111. Goff DC, Tsai G, Beal MF, Coyle JT: Tardive dyskinesia and substrates of energy metabolism in CSF. Am J Psychiatry 1995; 152: 1730–1736

112. Tsai G, Goff DC, Chang RW, Flood J, Baer L, Coyle JT: Markers of glutamatergic neurotransmission and oxidative stress associated with tardive dyskinesia. Am J Psychiatry 1998; 155:1207–1213

113. Meshul C, Bunker G, Mason J, Allen C, Janowsky A: Effects of subchronic clozapine and haloperidol on striatal glutamatergic synapses. J Neurochem 1996; 67:1965–1973

114. Lidsky TI, Yablonsky-Alter E, Zuck L, Banerjee SP: Antiglutamatergic effects of clozapine. Neurosci Lett 1993; 163: 155–158

115. Arvanov V, Liang X, Schwartz J, Grossman S, Wang R: Clozapine and haloperidol modulate N-methyl-D-aspartate and non-N-methyl-D-aspartate receptor-mediated neurotransmission in rat prefrontal cortical neurons in vitro. J Pharmacol Exp Ther 1997; 283:226–234

116. Wang RY, Liang X: M100907 and clozapine, but not haloperidol or raclopride, prevent phencyclidine-induced blockade of NMDA responses in pyramidal neurons of the rat medial prefrontal cortical slice. Neuropsychopharmacology 1998; 19:74–85

117. Banerjee SP, Zuck LG, Yablonsky-Alter E, Lidsky TI: Glutamate agonist activity: implications for antipsychotic drug action and schizophrenia. Neuroreport 1995; 6:2500–2504

118. Lidsky TI, Yablonsky-Alter E, Zuck LG, Banerjee SP: Antipsychotic drug effects on glutamatergic activity. Brain Res 1997; 764:46–52

119. Fletcher EJ, MacDonald JF: Haloperidol interacts with the strychnine-insensitive glycine site at the NMDA receptor in cultured mouse hippocampal neurones. Eur J Pharmacol 1993; 235:291–295

120. McCoy L, Richfield EK: Chronic antipsychotic treatment alters glycine-stimulated NMDA receptor binding in rat brain. Neurosci Lett 1996; 213:137–141

121. Healy D, Meador-Woodruff J: Clozapine and haloperidol differentially affect AMPA and kainate receptor subunit mRNA levels in rat cortex and striatum. Mol Brain Res 1997; 47:331–338

122. Riva M, Tascedda F, Lovati E, Racagni G: Regulation of NMDA receptor subunit messenger RNA levels in the rat brain following acute and chronic exposure to antipsychotic drugs. Mol Brain Res 1997; 50:136–142

123. Meador-Woodruff J, King R, Damask S, Bovenkerk K: Differential regulation of hippocampal AMPA and kainate receptor subunit expression by haloperidol and clozapine. Mol Psychiatry 1996; 1:41–53

124. Lawlor BA, Davis KL: Does modulation of glutamatergic function represent a viable therapeutic strategy in Alzheimer's disease? Biol Psychiatry 1992; 31:337–350

125. Waziri R: Glycine therapy of schizophrenia (letter). Biol Psychiatry 1988; 23:209–214

126. Rosse RB, Theut SK, Banay-Schwartz M, Leighton M, Scarcella E, Cohen CG, Deutsch SI: Glycine adjuvant therapy to conventional neuroleptic treatment in schizophrenia: an open-label, pilot study. Clin Neuropharmacol 1989; 12:416–424

127. Costa J, Khaled E, Sramek J, Bunney W, Potkin SG: An open trial of glycine as an adjunct to neuroleptics in chronic treatment-refractory schizophrenics (letter). J Clin Psychopharmacol 1990; 10:71–72

128. D'Souza DC, Charney D, Krystal J: Glycine site agonists of the NMDA receptor: a review. CNS Drug Rev 1995; 1:227–260

129. Javitt DC, Zylberman I, Zukin SR, Heresco-Levy U, Lindenmayer JP: Amelioration of negative symptoms in schizophrenia by glycine. Am J Psychiatry 1994; 151:1234–1236

130. Heresco-Levy U, Javitt D, Ermilov M, Mordel C, Horowitz A, Kelly D: Double-blind, placebo-controlled, crossover trial of glycine adjuvant therapy for treatment-resistant schizophrenia. Br J Psychiatry 1996; 169:610–617

131. Heresco-Levy U, Javitt D, Ermilov M, Mordel C, Silipo G, Lichenstein M: Efficacy of high-dose glycine in the treatment of enduring negative symptoms of schizophrenia. Arch Gen Psychiatry 1999; 56:29–36

132. Tsai G, Yang P, Chung L-C, Lange N, Coyle J: D-Serine added to antipsychotics for the treatment of schizophrenia. Biol Psychiatry 1998; 44:1081–1089

133. Watson GB, Bolanowski MA, Baganoff MP, Deppeler CL, Lanthorn TH: D-Cycloserine acts as a partial agonist at the glycine modulatory site of the NMDA receptor expressed in Xenopus oocytes. Brain Res 1990; 510:158–160

134. Goff DC, Tsai G, Manoach DS, Coyle JT: Dose-finding trial of D-cycloserine added to neuroleptics for negative symptoms in schizophrenia. Am J Psychiatry 1995; 152:1213–1215

135. van Berckel BN, Hijman R, van der Linden JA, Westenberg HG, van Ree JM, Kahn RS: Efficacy and tolerance of D-cycloserine in

184

drug-free schizophrenic patients. Biol Psychiatry 1996; 40: 1298–1300

136. Goff D, Tsai G, Levitt J, Amico E, Manoach D, Schoenfeld D, Hayden D, McCarley R, Coyle J: A placebo-controlled trial of D-cycloserine added to conventional neuroleptics in patients with schizophrenia. Arch Gen Psychiatry 1999; 56:21–27

137. Rosse R, Fay-McCarthy M, Kendrick K, Davis R, Deutsch S: D-Cycloserine adjuvant therapy to molindone in the treatment of schizophrenia. Clin Neuropharmacol 1996; 19:444–450

138. Goff DC, Tsai G, Manoach DS, Flood J, Darby DG, Coyle JT: D-Cycloserine added to clozapine for patients with schizophrenia. Am J Psychiatry 1996; 153:1628–1630

139. Goff D, Henderson D, Evins A, Amico E: A placebo-controlled crossover trial of D-cycloserine added to clozapine in patients with schizophrenia. Biol Psychiatry 1999; 45:512–514

140. Potkin SG, Jin Y, Bunney BG, Costa J, Gulasekaram B: Effect of clozapine and adjunctive high-dose glycine in treatment-resistant schizophrenia. Am J Psychiatry 1999; 156:145–147

141. Tsai GE, Yang P, Chung L-C, Tsai I-C, Tsai C-W, Coyle JT: D-Serine added to clozapine for the treatment of schizophrenia. Am J Psychiatry 1999; 156:1822–1825

142. Evins AE, Fitzgerald SM, Wine L, Roselli R, Goff DC: Placebo-controlled trial of glycine added to clozapine in schizophrenia. Am J Psychiatry 2000; 157:826–828

143. Arai A, Kessler M, Rogers G, Lynch G: Effects of a memory-enhancing drug on DL-alpha-amino-3-hydroxy-5-methyl-4-isoxazolepropionic acid receptor currents and synaptic transmission in hippocampus. J Pharmacol Exp Ther 1996; 278:1–12

144. Staubli U, Perez Y, Xu F, Rogers G, Ingvar M, Stone-Elander S, Lynch G: Centrally active modulators of glutamate receptors facilitate the induction of long-term potentiation in vivo. Proc Natl Acad Sci USA 1994; 91:11158–11162

145. Sirvio J, Larson J, Quach L, Rogers G, Lynch G: Effects of pharmacologically facilitating glutamatergic transmission in the trisynaptic intrahippocampal circuit. Neuroscience 1996; 74: 1025–1035

146. Staubli U, Rogers G, Lynch G: Facilitation of glutamate receptors enhances memory. Proc Natl Acad Sci USA 1994; 91:777–781

147. Johnson S, Luu N, Herbst T, Knapp R, Lutz D, Arai A, Rogers G, Lynch G: Synergistic interactions between ampakines and antipsychotic drugs. J Pharmacol Exp Ther 1999; 289:392–397

148. Goff D, Berman I, Posever T, Herz L, Leahy L, Lynch G: A preliminary dose escalation trial of CX516 (Ampakine) added to clozapine in schizophrenia. Schizophr Res 1999; 36:280

185

Cortical Abnormalities in Schizophrenia Identified by Structural Magnetic Resonance Imaging

Jill M. Goldstein, PhD; Julie M. Goodman, PhD; Larry J. Seidman, PhD; David N. Kennedy, PhD; Nikos Makris, MD, PhD; Hang Lee, PhD; Jason Tourville; Verne S. Caviness, Jr, MD, DPhil; Stephen V. Faraone, PhD; Ming T. Tsuang, MD, PhD

Background: Relatively few magnetic resonance imaging studies of schizophrenia have investigated the entire cerebral cortex. Most focus on only a few areas within a lobe or an entire lobe. To assess expected regional alterations in cortical volumes, we used a new method to segment the entire neocortex into 48 topographically defined brain regions. We hypothesized, based on previous empirical and theoretical work, that dorsolateral prefrontal and paralimbic cortices would be significantly volumetrically reduced in patients with schizophrenia compared with normal controls.

Methods: Twenty-nine patients with *DSM-III-R* schizophrenia were systematically sampled from 3 public outpatient service networks in the Boston, Mass, area. Healthy subjects, recruited from catchment areas from which the patients were drawn, were screened for psychopathological disorders and proportionately matched to patients by age, sex, ethnicity, parental socioeconomic status, reading ability, and handedness. Analyses of covariance of the volumes of brain regions, adjusted for age- and sex-corrected head size, were used to compare patients and controls.

Results: The greatest volumetric reductions and largest effect sizes were in the middle frontal gyrus and paralimbic brain regions, such as the frontomedial and frontoorbital cortices, anterior cingulate and paracingulate gyri, and the insula. In addition, the supramarginal gyrus, which is densely connected to prefrontal and cingulate cortices, was also significantly reduced in patients. Patients also had subtle volumetric increases in other cortical areas with strong reciprocal connections to the paralimbic areas that were volumetrically reduced.

Conclusion: Findings using our methods have implications for understanding brain abnormalities in schizophrenia and suggest the importance of the paralimbic areas and their connections with prefrontal brain regions.

Arch Gen Psychiatry. 1999;56:537-547

S EVERAL MODELS have been proposed to explain the widespread brain abnormalities in patients with schizophrenia. Early anatomical models were based largely on hypothesized focal abnormalities in particular brain regions,[1] derived mainly from adult lesion models of neuropsychiatric disorders. Schizophrenia has more recently been understood as, in part, a neurodevelopmental disorder[2,3] in which altered connectivity or multifocal abnormalities are more likely than focal disorders.[4-6] The most frequently replicated findings have been in subcortical structures, such as the hippocampal region[7-10] and thalamus.[10,11] An increasing number of studies, however, have demonstrated abnormalities in cortical brain regions,[12-21] indicative of developmental origins.[12,13,20,22-24] Neuropathologic and neural network findings have suggested that schizophrenia may involve a defect in neuronal migration,[22-24] myelination,[5] and/or corticocortical pruning.[25-27]

Despite the current emphasis on the importance of cortical abnormalities in schizophrenia, structural imaging studies of the entire cortex are relatively few. In fact, of 67 studies recently reviewed,[8] only 16 examined more than one cortical brain region in more than one lobe. Studies that have examined the entire cortex have sampled primarily men and acquired images with relatively large slices—5-mm slices with 2.5-mm gaps.[17,20,21] The relatively small number of cortical structural imaging studies may be due, in part, to the difficult and time-consuming nature of segmenting these relatively small areas of the brain. Furthermore, until recently, methods to assess in vivo the subtle volumetric reductions in small cortical regions, which require fine distinctions between brain regions, were not available for the analysis of brain images. Thus far, most of the subtle abnormalities in the cortex have been identified at the cellular level using postmortem techniques.

The affiliations of the authors appear in the acknowledgement section at the end of the article.

187

METHODS

SAMPLE

Patients were systematically sampled from the universe of outpatients at 3 public psychiatric hospitals in the Boston, Mass, area that serve primarily patients with psychotic disorders.[45-47] Inclusion criteria consisted of ages between 25 and 66 years, at least an eighth-grade education, English as the first language, and an estimated IQ of at least 70. Exclusion criteria for subjects were substance abuse within the past 6 months, history of a head injury with documented cognitive sequelae or loss of consciousness longer than 5 minutes, neurologic disease or damage, mental retardation, medical illnesses that substantially impair neurocognitive function, and a history of electroconvulsive treatment. Written informed consent was obtained after a complete description of the study was given to the subjects.

Healthy control subjects were recruited through advertisements in the catchment areas and notices posted on bulletin boards at the hospitals from which the patients were recruited. They were proportionately matched to patients by age, sex, ethnicity, parental socioeconomic status,[49] reading ability, and handedness. Control subjects were screened for current psychopathological disorders using a short form of the Minnesota Multiphasic Personality Inventory[50] and a family history of psychoses or psychiatric hospital admissions. We excluded potential controls if they had a current psychopathological disorder; a lifetime history of any psychosis; a family history of psychosis or psychiatric hospitalization; or a score on any clinical or validity scale on the Minnesota Multiphasic Personality Inventory, except the Masculinity-Femininity scale, above 70.

Patients were included if they had a DSM-III-R[31] clinical diagnosis of schizophrenia. (Patients were rediagnosed by research criteria, as described in the subsection "Diagnostic Procedures.") The sample consisted of 29 patients, 17 (59%) of them male. **Table 1** presents a summary of the sociodemographic and clinical characteristics of the patients and controls.

The patients were a middle-aged sample, primarily non-Hispanic white (25 [86%]), with an average education of partial college, who came from a middle to lower-middle socioeconomic status. Measures of premorbid and current IQ were in the average range. They had a mean ± SD age at illness onset of 23.6 ± 5.8 years (range, 16-45 years), with 4.2 ± 3.1 hospital admissions, reflecting 22.0 ± 9.9 months of hospitalization and 20.9 ± 10.2 years of illness. The daily chlorpromazine-equivalent dose was 689.9 ± 591.6 mg of typical neuroleptic medications. In general, the patients were clinically stable, being treated long term as outpatients, although they were rated as having mild to moderate negative and positive symptoms.[52,53]

The healthy controls were a proportionately matched comparison group. There were no significant differences in sex distribution, age, ethnicity, parental socioeconomic status, education, Wide Range Achievement Reading[54] score, Wechsler Adult Intelligence Scale–Revised[55,56] vocabulary score, and handedness. There was a significant ($P = .01$) difference in IQ, which is typical for schizophrenia.

DIAGNOSTIC PROCEDURES

Research DSM-III-R diagnoses were based on the Schedule for Affective Disorders and Schizophrenia[57] and a systematic review of the medical record. Patients primarily had undifferentiated or paranoid subtypes (Table 1). Interviews were obtained by master's level interviewers with extensive diagnostic interviewing experience. Senior investigators (Drs Goldstein and Seidman) reviewed the transcripts from the interview and the medical records to determine the consensus, best-estimate, lifetime diagnosis. Blindness of assessments among psychiatric and MRI data was maintained.

IMAGING PROCEDURES

Image Acquisition

Magnetic resonance imaging scans were acquired at the Nuclear Magnetic Resonance Center of the Massachusetts General Hospital, Boston, with a 1.5-T MRI scanner (General Electric Signa scanner; General Electric Corporation, Waukesha, Wis). Contiguous 3.1-mm coronal spoiled-gradient echo images of the entire brain were obtained using the following parameters: repetition time, 40 milliseconds; echo time, 8 milliseconds; flip angle, 50°; field of view, 30 cm; matrix, 256×256; and averages, 1. The MRI scans were processed and analyzed at the Massachusetts General Hospital Center for Morphometric Analysis for further processing and analysis.

Data were analyzed using image analysis workstations (Sun Microsystems Inc, Mountain View, Calif). Images were positionally normalized by imposing a standard 3-dimensional coordinate system on each 3-dimensional MRI scan, using the midpoints of the decussations of the anterior and posterior commissures and the midsagittal plane at the level of the posterior commissure as points of reference for rotation and (nondeformation) transformation. Scans were then resliced into normalized 3.1-mm coronal, 1.0-mm axial, and 1.0-mm sagittal scans and were analyzed. Positional normalization overcomes potential problems caused by variation in head position of subjects during scanning.

Gray Matter–White Matter Image Segmentation

Each slice of the T_1-weighted, positionally normalized, 3-dimensional coronal scans was segmented into gray and white

---

Neuropathologic studies of schizophrenia have identified abnormalities of cell size, orientation, and receptor density in the anterior cingulate gyrus[22] and prefrontal areas.[12,13,28] Structural magnetic resonance imaging (MRI) studies have shown volumetric abnormalities in schizophrenia in the frontal lobe and prefrontal subregions (eg, orbital[14] and dorsolateral[15,29]); the prefrontal areas in general[21]; and the temporal lobe, including the parahippocampal gyrus[7,16] and auditory cortex (eg, the superior temporal gyrus,[7,18,29-31] planum temporale,[19,32] and related sylvian fissure region[33]). A few studies—eg, Schlaepfer et al[29]—have implicated the parietal cortex and occipital lobe (reviewed in Shenton et al[8]), but findings in these areas have been equivocal. Cortical volume reductions have been estimated[34,35] to range from only 4% to 6%. In general, previous cortical studies suggested that prefrontal, paralimbic, and left frontotemporal lobe areas are subtly but significantly reduced in patients with schizophrenia.

188

matter and ventricular structures using a semiautomated intensity contour–mapping algorithm[38] and signal-intensity histogram distributions. This technique, described in detail elsewhere[38,58,59] and illustrated in **Figure 1**, yields separate compartments of neocortex, subcortical gray nuclei, white matter, and ventricular system subdivisions that generally correspond to the natural tissue boundaries distinguished by signal intensities in the T_1-weighted images.

The focus of the present study was the subdivision of the neocortex into parcellation units (PUs).

Parcellation of the Neocortex

The neocortex, defined by the gray-white matter segmentation procedure, was subdivided or "parcellated" into 48 bilateral PUs based on the system originally described by Rademacher,[36] modified in Caviness et al,[37] and shown in Figure 1. This is a comprehensive system of neocortical subdivision designed to approximate architectonic and functional subdivisions and based on specific anatomical landmarks present in all brains.[37]

Two types of landmarks specify the boundaries of the PUs: major fissures of the hemisphere (Figure 1) and anatomically specified single nodal points along the longitudinal axis of the brain. The fissures and nodal points are easily identifiable and normally present in all brains. Nodal points are specified by diverse anatomical structures, most of which lie in the cortex itself (eg, the intersection of 2 sulci or a sulcus within the hemispheric margin). Four nodal points are specified by subcortical landmarks—the splenium and genu of the corpus callosum, the decussation of the anterior commissure, and the lateral geniculate bodies. The PUs are mainly bounded by the major fissures of the brain (Figure 1). Where the anterior or posterior border of a PU is not completely specified by major fissures, this boundary is closed by a coronal plane through a nodal point. Following parcellation, volumes were calculated for each PU by multiplying the area measurement of the PU on each slice by the slice thickness and then summing all slices on which the PU appeared.

RELIABILITY

Our collaborators at the Massachusetts General Hospital Center for Morphometric Analysis (Drs Kennedy, Makris, and Caviness), who developed these procedures, trained and maintained quality control of the segmentation of the data. In previous studies[37] using these procedures, reliability was good. For our study, the brains of 10 subjects were completely parcellated into 48 PUs in the right and left hemispheres by 2 well-trained image analysts who had a background in neuroanatomy. **Table 2** presents the intraclass correlation coefficients (ICCs) for the 48 PUs, which were generally good.

Forty percent of the PUs had excellent reliabilities ($ICC \geq 0.80$), and about 69% were very good ($ICC \geq 0.70$). There were several PUs with ICCs of 0.55 or less. The brains of 10 additional subjects were analyzed, after a discussion of areas in which raters disagreed, and ICCs of these areas were presented in the third column of Table 2. The ICCs remained low for only 3 areas: frontal operculum, basal forebrain, and occipital pole. Finally, intrarater reliability was conducted using images from 6 subjects (Table 2, last column) and was generally excellent. Only the fusiform gyrus, lingual gyrus, and superior parietal lobule had fair reliabilities ($ICC = 0.50$, $ICC = 0.57$, and $ICC = 0.62$, respectively).

DATA ANALYSES

Three approaches were used to test for volumetric differences between patients and controls, given disagreement among the investigators in the field as to the ideal statistical model. Adjusted PU volumes were expressed as a percentage of the total cerebral volume—PU volume divided by total cerebral volume—to control for individual variations in brain size. The total cerebral volume was also used as a covariate in an analysis of covariance (ANCOVA). Finally, the z-score method[60] was used to adjust for a normal variation in age- and sex-corrected head size, as measured by the total cerebral volume. Thus, z scores reflected volumetric estimates for the patients relative to volumes expected from normal subjects of a particular head size, age, and sex.[17,21,34,60]

Adjusted brain volumes and the z scores of the PUs were analyzed using ANCOVA to assess the effect of the group (ie, subjects with schizophrenia vs controls), controlled for age, sex, and sex-by-group interaction. An ANCOVA was appropriate because tests of normality showed that the PU volumes were, in general, normally distributed. A multivariate ANCOVA using all PUs would not be statistically powerful with our sample size and, thus, would not provide accurate covariance structure estimates. However, we had some specific hypotheses about particular PUs. Thus, as suggested by Rothman,[61] a multivariate ANCOVA was used that included PUs hypothesized to be different between groups (the middle frontal gyrus, frontomedial cortex, fronto-orbital cortex, divisions of the cingulate and parahippocampal gyri, and insula), to control for a type I error. We were also interested in whether other areas, which were reflected in exploratory analyses, distinguished patients from healthy controls. In addition, relative volume differences and effect sizes[62] between patients and controls were estimated (**Table 3**). Effect sizes are unaffected by the sample size and, thus, can be compared across studies.

We introduce the application of a new brain segmentation technique to study patients with schizophrenia, with the goal of the better identification of subtly altered cortical tissue. The method, based on conceptual models of the cortex, was developed to divide the entire neocortex into 48 topographically defined brain areas[36,37] and has been applied successfully to healthy subjects.[37-39] The unique advantage of this technique is that it allows an estimation of the relative differences in volume in specific areas of the entire cortex between patients with schizophrenia and normal controls.

Neuropsychological studies,[40-44] including our own, some[45-47] using the same patients as in this study, have demonstrated impairments in working memory and other executive functions, verbal and visual short-term memory, attention, olfaction, and motivation. These functions rely heavily on circuitry that primarily includes the frontal lobes (ie, working memory, executive functions, and ol-

189

Table 1. Demographic, Cognitive, and Clinical Measures in Patients With Schizophrenia Compared With Normal Controls*

Variable	Controls (n = 26)	Patients (n = 29)
Male sex, No. (%)	12 (46)	17 (59)
Ethnicity white, No. (%)	24 (92)	25 (86)
Right-handed, No. (%)	22 (85)	23 (79)
Age, y	39.8 ± 11.5	44.8 ± 10.5
Parental SES	2.8 ± 1.0	2.7 ± 1.4
Education, y	14.4 ± 2.3	13.5 ± 2.5
WAIS-R Vocabulary score	11.3 ± 2.7	10.1 ± 2.6
WAIS-R Block Design score	10.7 ± 2.5	9.1 ± 3.2†
IQ estimate	106.9 ± 12.2	97.8 ± 14.0†
WRAT-R reading score	104.5 ± 10.6	106.1 ± 12.1
DSM-III-R schizophrenia, No. (%)		
Undifferentiated	...	12 (41)
Paranoid	...	11 (38)
Disorganized	...	5 (17)
Schizoaffective, depressed	...	1 (3)
Age at onset, y	...	23.6 ± 5.8
Duration, y	...	22.0 ± 9.9
No. of hospitalizations	...	4.24 ± 3.10
Global negative and positive symptom rating‡		
Affective flattening	...	1.9 ± 1.2
Alogia	...	1.4 ± 1.3
Avolition	...	1.7 ± 1.3
Anhedonia	...	2.4 ± 1.4
Attention	...	1.1 ± 1.2
Hallucinations	...	2.1 ± 1.8
Delusions	...	1.9 ± 2.0
Bizarre behavior	...	0.5 ± 0.7
Formal thought disorder	...	1.3 ± 1.3

*Data are given as mean ± SD unless otherwise indicated. SES indicates socioeconomic status; WAIS-R, Wechsler Adult Intelligence Scale–Revised; WRAT-R, Wide Range Achievement Test–Revised; and ellipses, not applicable. IQ estimate was derived from Vocabulary and Block Design age-scaled scores (from Brooker and Cyr[56]).
†P<.05.
‡Negative symptoms rated using Scale for the Assessment of Negative Symptoms (from Andreasen[52]), and positive symptoms rated using Scale for the Assessment of Positive Symptoms (from Andreasen[53]).

faction) and frontolimbic (verbal and visual short-term memory) or paralimbic (attention and motivation) regions. Based on previous reports, we hypothesize that the primary cortical abnormalities in schizophrenia will be in the prefrontal, especially dorsolateral prefrontal cortex, and paralimbic[48] regions (eg, cingulate and parahippocampal gyri and the frontal orbital cortex)—ie, areas involved in communication between the prefrontal and limbic brain regions. Although these hypothesized areas are not unique, this study is the first to examine all cortical areas in one study in a substantial number of subjects with schizophrenia.

RESULTS

The unadjusted (mean ± SD) total cerebral volume was significantly different between groups (patients, 1140.9 ± 116.9 cm³; and controls, 1077.3 ± 97.4 cm³) (t_{53} = 2.2, unpaired, 2-tailed test of significance; P = .03) but was not significant when adjusted for the total brain volume (patients, 87.1 ± 0.9 cm³; and controls, 88.7 ± 0.9

cm³). The total neocortex was 591.4 ± 60.2 cm³ for patients and 575.2 ± 65.8 cm³ for controls. Adjusted for the total cerebral volume, the cortex was 51.9% ± 2.3% for patients and 53.4% ± 2.7% for controls (t_{53} = −2.2; P = .03).

Table 3 presents the unadjusted mean volumes in cubic centimeters for the PUs and total volumes by lobe. Tests of differences between the groups were based on the adjusted values and z scores, and these did not differ across statistical methods, with significant differences illustrated in **Figure 2**. First, the overall F test (Wilks λ) from the multivariate ANCOVA for our hypothesized regions was significant ($F_{9,45}$ = 3.17; P≤.005), suggesting that patients and controls significantly differed in volumes of these areas. Table 3 shows that, within the frontal lobe, the middle frontal gyrus ($F_{1,52}$ = 4.87; P = .03) and the frontomedial cortex ($F_{1,52}$ = 8.41; P = .005) were significantly reduced in patients with schizophrenia. The relative volumetric reductions for patients compared with controls were 8.80% and 14.89%, respectively. When we examined the right and left hemispheres separately for hypothesized areas, only the right fronto-orbital cortex was significantly reduced in patients and not the left ($F_{1,52}$ = 3.94; P = .05) (relative volumetric reduction of the right fronto-orbital cortex among the patients was 8.5% compared with controls; effect size, 0.56). The middle frontal gyrus and frontomedial cortex were bilaterally reduced, although the middle frontal gyrus showed greater reduction on the left. Patients also exhibited significant volumetric reductions in PUs approximating the medial paralimbic cortex, in particular, the anterior cingulate gyrus ($F_{1,52}$ = 3.79; P = .05) and paracingulate gyrus ($F_{1,52}$ = 9.46; P = .003), with reductions of 11.14% and 7.99%, respectively, compared with controls. In addition, there was a large and significant volumetric reduction of the insula in patients ($F_{1,52}$ = 11.90; P = .001) by almost 1 SD below that of controls (effect size, 0.88). Exploratory analyses of other cortical temporal areas showed no significant volumetric reductions in patients.

The parietal and occipital cortices also showed few significant differences in individual PUs. The posterior supramarginal gyrus, however, was significantly and bilaterally reduced in patients compared with controls ($F_{1,52}$ = 3.95; P = .05). When combined to encompass the inferior parietal cortex as a whole—ie, anterior and posterior supramarginal gyri, angular gyrus, and parietal operculum—the volume was not significantly reduced among the patients. All analyses were rerun after omitting 8 subjects aged 60 years or older, equally distributed across the groups, and results were unchanged. In addition, in patients, cortical volumes of the significant PUs were uncorrelated with the neuroleptic medication dose.

COMMENT

This study provides new evidence that there are cortical abnormalities in schizophrenia, detectable using structural MRI. The brain areas that showed a significant reduction in patients with schizophrenia compared with well-matched healthy controls were primarily in PUs that approximated regions of the prefrontal and medial paralimbic cortices. Significant frontal lobe reductions

190

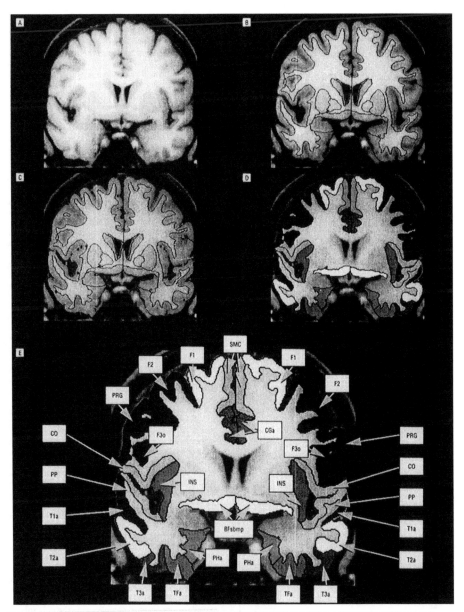

Figure 1. Cortical parcellation method. A, Normalized midbrain coronal slice at the level of the anterior commissure. B, Gray and white matter segmented; subcortical areas are shown. C, Cortical parcellation begins with the identification of cortical sulci using axial, sagittal, and coronal views. Shown here are several sulci (multicolored) that indicate where the final sulcal lines (shown in yellow) are drawn. These yellow lines delineate the cortical parcellation units. D, Nodal points based on anatomical criteria define anterior and posterior boundaries of the cortical parcellation units after sulci are identified (from Caviness et al[37]). The resulting parcellation units are shown. E, Cortical brain regions are identified by parcellation units. The labels for the regions are as shown in the first 2 columns of Tables 2 and 3. BFsbmp indicates basal forebrain subcomponent.

191

Table 2. Intraclass Correlation Coefficients (ICCs) for the Cortical Parcellation Units*

Parcellation Units	Label	2 Raters ICCs (n = 10)	ICCs (n = 10)	ICCs, Intrarater (n = 6)
Frontal Lobe				
Superior frontal gyrus	F1	0.89	...	0.99
Middle frontal gyrus	F2	0.77	...	0.83
Frontal pole	FP	0.86	...	0.97
Inferior frontal gyrus	F3o	0.85	...	0.83
Inferior frontal gyrus	F3t	0.60	...	0.94
Frontomedial cortex	FMC	0.11	0.64	0.94
Frontoorbital cortex	FOC	0.59	...	0.94
Precentral gyrus	PRG	0.93	...	0.73
Supplementary motor cortex	SMC	0.55	0.86	0.98
Frontal operculum	FO	0.25	0.34	0.92
Central operculum	CO	0.73	...	0.90
Basal forebrain	BF	0.41	0.03	0.88
Parietal Lobe				
Postcentral gyrus	POG	0.21	0.71	0.73
Superior parietal lobule	SPL	0.27	0.84	0.62
Supramarginal gyrus, ant	SGa	0.41	0.84	0.94
Supramarginal gyrus, post	SGp	0.35	0.87	0.89
Angular gyrus	AG	0.52	0.68	0.77
Precuneus	PCN	0.75	...	0.77
Parietal operculum	PO	0.72	...	0.94
Occipital Lobe				
Occipital lateral gyri, sup	OLs	0.62	0.78	0.72
Occipital lateral gyri, inf	OLi	0.007	0.71	0.74
Occipital pole	OP	0.11	0.31	0.91
Cuneus	CN	0.77	...	0.76
Lingual gyrus	LG	0.55	0.74	0.57
Fusiform gyrus	OF	0.05	0.76	0.50
Calcarine sulcus	calc	0.64	0.93	0.92
Temporal Lobe				
Temporal pole	TP	0.96	...	1.00
Superior temporal gyrus, ant	T1a	0.60	0.85	0.99
Superior temporal gyrus, post	T1p	0.92	...	0.88
Middle temporal gyrus, ant	T2a	0.59	...	0.99
Middle temporal gyrus, post	T2p	0.76	...	0.91
Middle temporal gyrus	TO2	0.86	...	0.84
Inferior temporal gyrus, ant	T3a	0.78	...	0.93
Inferior temporal gyrus, post	T3p	0.46	0.62	0.85
Inferior temporal gyrus	TO3	0.35	0.79	0.75
Fusiform gyrus, ant	TFa	0.68	...	0.93
Fusiform gyrus, post	TFp	0.77	...	0.87
Fusiform gyrus	TOF	0.52	0.73	0.89
Planum polare	PP	0.81	...	0.95
Insula	INS	0.80	...	0.98
Heschl gyrus	H1	0.76	...	0.84
Planum temporal	PT	0.12	0.81	0.78
Medial Paralimbic Cortices				
Subcallosal cortex	SC	0.50	0.69	0.92
Paracingulate cortex	PAC	0.88	...	0.94
Cingulate gyrus, ant	CGa	0.84	...	0.99
Cingulate gyrus, post	CGp	0.83	...	0.75
Parahippocampal gyrus, ant	PHa	0.92	...	0.88
Parahippocampal gyrus, post	PHp	0.11	0.81	0.93

*ant indicates anterior; post, posterior; sup, superior; inf, inferior; and ellipses, not applicable.

were in the middle, medial, and right-sided fronto-orbital cortices, the last 2 of which are considered part of the paralimbic cortices.[48] The anterior cingulate and paracingulate gyri and insula were also significantly reduced in patients compared with controls, the last 2 by almost 1 SD. The relative differences in volumes between patients and controls were primarily in the range of 7% to 15%. The largest effect sizes were in the middle frontal gyrus and right fronto-orbital cortex, the insula, and the anterior cingulate and paracingulate gyri.

In general, our findings are consistent with those of several previous MRI and neuropathological studies. Previous MRI studies that segmented specific prefrontal areas reported significant reductions in dorsolateral prefrontal (ie, middle frontal gyrus)[15,29,63] and orbital[14] cortices. A recent study[64] using sophisticated segmentation procedures did not find significant prefrontal volumetric reductions. The investigators' sample size of 15, however, would have only 26% to 38% statistical power to detect a medium effect size of 0.50, and effect sizes of the frontal gyri in our study ranged from 0.10 to 0.62. Their findings also suggested that connectivity with prefrontal areas was abnormal in schizophrenia, which may be consistent with our findings.

The largest effect sizes in our study were demonstrated in paralimbic cortices, eg, anterior cingulate and paracingulate gyri and the insula. This is consistent with previous postmortem studies that reported cytoarchitectonic and structural abnormalities in the cingulate[22,65] and imaging studies that showed anterior cingulate gyral volumetric reductions[66,67] and hypofunction[68] in patients. Lesion and functional neuroimaging studies of the anterior cingulate gyrus have shown a variety of neurobehavioral deficits[69,70] and associations with internally initiated thought and behavior,[71,72] attention to action,[73] divided attention,[74,75] and learning.[76] Thus, it has been suggested that abnormalities of the cingulate gyrus may be central in understanding schizophrenia.[22]

We would argue that our findings are not due to sample bias because patients were representative of a large outpatient network serving 3 major hospitals in the Boston area. Furthermore, the healthy controls were similar in sociodemographic background, including education, a variable typically affected by the illness. Finally, as in Pearlson et al,[16] we used 3 different statistically analytic approaches to test our hypotheses, and these demonstrated consistent findings across methods, suggesting their validity.

What is most striking about our results is that, although we included 48 cortical PUs, the significant reductions were in paralimbic cortices (ie, cingulate gyrus, insula, and frontomedial and fronto-orbital cortices) and the prefrontal area—the middle frontal gyrus—which has strong reciprocal connections to paralimbic and limbic brain regions.[48,77] Furthermore, in a previous presentation of these patients,[10] it was shown that among 10 subcortical regions tested, the thalamus and amygdala-hippocampal complex were the only subcortical areas significantly volumetrically reduced—areas with reciprocal connections[48,77,78] to the cortical areas that we found reduced in patients. (The pallidum and ventricles were significantly increased.[10])

192

Table 3. Mean ± SD Differences in Volumes (in Cubic Centimeters) of Cortical Areas for Schizophrenic Patients vs Normal Controls*

Region	Label	Schizophrenics (n = 29)	Controls (n = 26)	Effect Size	Relative Difference, %
		Frontal Lobe			
Frontal pole	FP	62.99 ± 9.64	56.65 ± 10.36	−0.41	−5.49
Superior frontal gyrus	F1	29.50 ± 3.81	28.84 ± 4.13	0.26	3.07
Middle frontal gyrus	F2	27.09 ± 5.25	27.98 ± 3.98	0.62	8.80†
Inferior frontal gyrus	F3o	9.67 ± 2.51	9.30 ± 3.26	0.10	2.98
Inferior frontal gyrus	F3t	6.40 ± 1.82	6.83 ± 1.99	0.42	11.17
Precentral gyrus	PRG	39.06 ± 6.64	39.07 ± 5.80	0.34	5.00
Supplementary motor cortex	SMC	6.29 ± 2.11	6.10 ± 1.73	0.03	2.59
Frontomedial cortex	FMC	4.04 ± 0.76	4.52 ± 1.13	0.16	14.89‡
Frontoorbital cortex	FOC	15.17 ± 2.60	15.20 ± 2.11	0.56§	8.45§
Frontal operculum	FO	4.29 ± 1.37	3.94 ± 1.31	−0.05	−1.61
Central operculum	CO	10.17 ± 2.22	9.37 ± 1.92	−0.16	−2.91
Basal forebrain	BF	3.58 ± 1.69	3.66 ± 1.56	−0.17	−7.26
Total frontal lobe		218.26 ± 21.26	211.45 ± 23.00	0.02	2.32
		Medial Paralimbic Cortex			
Cingulate gyrus, ant	CGa	12.38 ± 3.74	13.06 ± 2.74	0.50	11.14‖
Cingulate gyrus, post	CGp	12.94 ± 2.69	12.09 ± 2.36	0.01	0.19
Paracingulate cortex	PAC	14.11 ± 2.06	14.55 ± 2.41	0.78	7.99‡
Subcallosal cortex	SC	5.43 ± 1.06	5.02 ± 0.98	−0.14	−2.22
Parahippocampal gyrus, ant	PHa	6.00 ± 1.48	5.31 ± 0.93	−0.29	−5.92
Parahippocampal gyrus, post	PHp	5.49 ± 1.32	5.42 ± 0.78	0.21	4.59
Total medial paralimbic cortex		56.35 ± 8.30	55.46 ± 5.73	0.03	4.43
		Temporal Lobe			
Superior temporal gyrus	T1	13.06 ± 2.14	11.81 ± 2.04	−0.32	−4.53
Heschl gyrus	H1	2.90 ± 0.87	3.01 ± 0.76	0.37	8.81
Planum temporal	PT	6.34 ± 1.49	5.99 ± 1.25	0.004	0.08
Temporal pole	TP	21.68 ± 4.77	21.97 ± 3.82	0.41	6.79
Middle temporal gyrus, ant	T2	16.35 ± 2.65	15.75 ± 2.27	0.15	1.91
Middle temporal gyrus, post	TO2	8.77 ± 2.34	8.25 ± 2.13	−0.01	−0.32
Inferior temporal gyrus, ant	T3	13.27 ± 2.23	12.35 ± 2.03	−0.11	−1.49
Inferior temporal gyrus, post	TO3	7.47 ± 2.63	6.84 ± 1.98	−0.07	−2.03
Fusiform gyrus, ant	TF	13.16 ± 2.50	12.53 ± 2.04	0.08	1.23
Fusiform gyrus, post	TOF	6.06 ± 2.01	6.01 ± 1.69	0.18	4.74
Planum polare	PP	3.64 ± 0.74	3.44 ± 0.84	−0.01	−0.33
Insula	INS	15.88 ± 1.73	16.28 ± 1.89	0.88	7.62¶
Total temporal lobe		196.45 ± 24.15	186.88 ± 23.10	0.004	0.58
		Parietal Lobe			
Precuneus	PCN	25.76 ± 3.59	24.63 ± 4.67	0.06	0.67
Postcentral gyrus	POG	32.09 ± 4.98	30.27 ± 4.79	−0.006	−0.07
Superior parietal lobule	SPL	9.22 ± 3.31	10.10 ± 4.83	0.31	11.74
Supramarginal gyrus, ant	SGa	8.57 ± 2.48	7.83 ± 3.25	−0.14	−4.50
Supramarginal gyrus, post	SGp	10.36 ± 3.59	11.72 ± 4.85	0.44	15.13†
Angular gyrus	AG	12.50 ± 5.58	10.50 ± 2.95	−0.30	−11.60
Parietal operculum	PO	5.41 ± 1.40	4.73 ± 1.01	−0.29	−6.74
Total parietal lobe		103.91 ± 13.32	99.79 ± 15.49	0.007	1.16
		Occipital Lobe			
Occipital pole	OP	15.09 ± 10.15	14.41 ± 7.66	0.009	0.57
Cuneus	CN	5.22 ± 1.89	5.57 ± 2.23	0.34	11.60
Occipital lateral gyrus, sup	OLs	42.12 ± 9.90	42.42 ± 6.97	0.40	6.66
Occipital lateral gyrus, inf	OLi	23.41 ± 5.93	22.90 ± 4.21	0.22	3.82
Lingual gyrus	LG	15.39 ± 2.90	14.66 ± 2.95	0.05	0.68
Fusiform gyrus	OF	8.07 ± 1.94	8.02 ± 1.72	0.23	4.59
Total occipital lobe		117.39 ± 19.12	115.87 ± 14.36	0.03	4.46

*Unadjusted mean volumes are presented. Tests of differences, however, are based on analyses of brain volumes, adjusted for total cerebral volume and controlled for sex effects, using the z-score method (Mathalon et al[60]) to adjust for normal variations in age- and sex-corrected head size. Effect size (ES) between normal controls (nc) and schizophrenic patients (sz) is calculated as follows: $ES = (mean_{nc} - mean_{sz})/(pooled\ SD)$—ie, the difference in SD units (Cohen[62] for adjusted volumes. Relative difference (RD) is calculated as follows: $RD = [(mean_{nc} - mean_{sz})/mean_{nc}] \times 100\%$—ie, the percentage difference between adjusted volumes of controls and patients. ant indicates anterior; post, posterior; sup, superior; and inf, inferior.
†Left side is significant (P<.05).
‡P<.01.
§Right side is significant (P<.05).
‖Total is significant (P<.05).
¶P<.001.

193

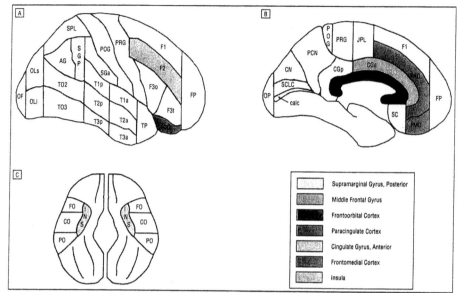

Figure 2. Cortical brain regions significantly reduced in patients compared with normal controls. Topography is based on methods described by Caviness et al[37]; A, lateral surface; B, medial surface; and C, inferior surface. Areas of significant cortical volume reduction in schizophrenic patients vs normal controls are in color. All reductions were bilateral, except in the fronto-orbital cortex, in which only the right side was significantly reduced (P = .05). The labels for the regions are as shown in the first 2 columns of Tables 2 and 3.

The functional consequences of the reduced size of the insula in patients is as yet unclear. The insular cortex, however, is highly interconnected with somatosensory and other cortical areas and limbic structures (perirhinal and entorhinal cortex and amygdala). It plays a role in sensory, motor, and language functions and has been described[79] as a limbic-integration area. In addition, the insula has connections to several brain areas that were found to be volumetrically reduced in this sample of patients, including the orbital and medial frontal cortices, the cingulate gyrus, and the amygdala. Insular abnormalities in schizophrenia may be related to an impairment in integrating sensory stimuli with internal motivational states, a hypothesis that warrants further investigation in patients with schizophrenia.

The importance of the paralimbic areas is also suggested by 2 of our previous analyses[44,46] of neuropsychological deficits of patients, including those in the present study. Olfactory and executive function deficits appeared to separate patients into 2 groups with distinct cognitive profiles, suggesting some heterogeneity among patients with cognitive deficits that may be associated with the fronto-orbital and hippocampal divisions[48,77] of the paralimbic cortices. Furthermore, these patients have exhibited other significant cognitive deficits that are dependent on limbic and paralimbic cortices, ie, executive function, attention, olfaction, and memory functions. [45,46]

We also found a significant volumetric reduction in the posterior supramarginal gyrus, which is densely connected to prefrontal and cingulate cortices. This is a potentially important finding, given the area's role in attention and memory identified in lesion and functional imaging studies.[75,80,81] Although most studies[8,82] have shown that the parietal cortex as a whole is not significantly reduced in patients with schizophrenia, previous work[29] reported significant reductions in specific areas, such as the inferior parietal cortex—ie, the supramarginal and angular gyri. We have further suggested that volumetric reductions in this cortex may be in area 40, rather than the angular gyrus (area 39). Structural deficits in area 40 are consistent with functional studies[71,72,75,81] of attention in patients with schizophrenia and healthy subjects. These studies showed abnormalities in perfusion or activation in this area during sustained attention tasks.

We also found that several cortical PUs—the basal forebrain, subcallosal cortex, operculum, and the frontal pole—were larger, although not significantly, in patients than in controls. These subtle volumetric increases were in cortical areas that have strong reciprocal connections to the areas we found significantly reduced. This may reflect an orchestrated developmental mechanism representing brain plasticity. There is some precedent for posing this hypothesis because it is consistent with animal models and functional studies[5,25,42,83] of schizophrenia that showed hypofunction in particular cortical areas (eg, dorsolateral prefrontal cortex) and hyperfunction in subcortical (eg, hippocampus) or other cortical areas. It is also consistent with a

ARCH GEN PSYCHIATRY/VOL 56, JUNE 1999
544

194

recent study of schizophrenia[84] that suggested disruptions in the dopaminergic regulation of intracortical and corticostriatal connectivity associated with the orbitofrontal cortex. Thus, there may not be a focally acting pathological process producing volumetric reductions in specific brain regions in patients with schizophrenia. Rather, there may be cortical systems, ie, limbic-paralimbic, that exhibit subtle abnormalities in their connections that result in reductions in some cortical areas and increases in others. Although this study did not test this hypothesis, it warrants further investigation.

There were no significant volumetric reductions in other cortical regions, and the effect sizes of volumetric reductions in other cortical areas were negligible, except for visual primary and association cortices, ie, 0.34 and 0.40, respectively, in the cuneus and superior lateral occipital gyrus. This is consistent with a recent study[13] that reported cytoarchitectonic abnormalities in neuronal density in patients with schizophrenia in the primary visual cortex, area 17.

Schizophrenia, however, is a heterogeneous disorder. Other brain areas—in particular, the superior temporal, Heschl and parahippocampal gyri, and planum temporale—have been found[7,16,18,29,30-32,85,86] to be volumetrically reduced in patients. In all studies, of the superior temporal gyrus, however, the samples were men only or a 2:1,[16] 3:1,[31] or approximately 5:1[30] ratio of men to women. Furthermore, some of these samples were patients with primarily positive symptoms,[7] and positive symptoms, such as hallucinations and thought disorder, have been associated with superior temporal gyral abnormalities.[7,18]

Our sample was a mix of male and female patients with mixed symptomatology. In fact, DeLisi et al[19] had a similar sex distribution to ours and found no significant reduction in the superior temporal gyrus. Reite et al[87] found that only men had reduced superior temporal and Heschl gyri,[85] whereas Vogeley et al,[88] in a postmortem study, found that men had increased volumes in anterior and posterior superior temporal gyri, but women had a reduced superior temporal gyrus in the middle compartment. A reduction in women only was also found by Schlaepfer et al,[29] whereas men showed atypical laterality in the planum temporale.[33] These studies raise the possibility that only subgroups of patients exhibit particular volumetric abnormalities (eg, one sex, patients with primarily positive or negative symptoms, or those with asymmetry abnormalities rather than volumetric reductions[18,19,85,87]). Given that our method allows for the assessment of topographically identified cortical and subcortical areas of the entire brain, we are in an advantageous position to ask questions about abnormalities in anatomical and functional neural systems as they relate to the heterogeneity of the expression of schizophrenia.

In this study, we demonstrated cortical volumetric abnormalities in the paralimbic system that have important implications for understanding the development of and functional consequences for schizophrenia. In future studies, we will investigate the effect of these anatomical abnormalities on symptoms and cognitive function in subgroups of patients with schizophrenia.

Accepted for publication February 10, 1999.

From the Department of Psychiatry (Drs Goldstein, Goodman, Seidman, Lee, Faraone, and Tsuang) and the Institute of Psychiatric Epidemiology and Genetics (Drs Goldstein, Seidman, Lee, Faraone, and Tsuang), Massachusetts Mental Health Center; the Departments of Neurology and Radiology Services, Center for Morphometric Analysis, Massachusetts General Hospital (Drs Goodman, Kennedy, Makris, and Caviness and Mr Tourville), Harvard Medical School; and the Department of Epidemiology, Harvard School of Public Health (Dr Tsuang), Boston; and the Department of Psychiatry, Harvard Medical School and Brockton–West Roxbury Veterans Affairs Medical Center (Drs Goldstein, Seidman, Faraone, and Tsuang), Brockton, Mass. Dr Lee is now at the Center for Vaccine Research, University of California–Los Angeles Medical Center.

This work was supported by grants K21 MH00976 (1992-1994) and RO1 MH56956 (1997-2000) (Dr Goldstein) and Merit Award MH 43518 (Dr Tsuang) from the National Institute of Mental Health, Bethesda, Md; a grant from the Fairway Trust (Dr Kennedy); and a Dissertation Award from the Scottish Rite Foundation, Lexington, Mass (Dr Goodman).

Reprints: Jill M. Goldstein, PhD, Harvard Institute of Psychiatric Epidemiology and Genetics, Massachusetts Mental Health Center, 74 Fenwood Rd, Boston, MA 02115 (e-mail: jill_goldstein@hms.harvard.edu).

REFERENCES

1. Andreasen NC, ed. Can Schizophrenia Be Localized in the Brain? Washington, DC: American Psychiatric Press; 1986.
2. Murray RM. Neurodevelopmental schizophrenia: the rediscovery of dementia praecox. Br J Psychiatry. 1994;165(suppl 25):6-12.
3. Weinberger DR. Implications of normal brain development for the pathogenesis of schizophrenia. Arch Gen Psychiatry. 1987;44:660-669.
4. Seidman LJ. Schizophrenia and brain dysfunction: an integration of recent neurodiagnostic findings. Psychol Bull. 1983;94:195-238.
5. Weinberger DR, Lipska BK. Cortical maldevelopment, anti-psychotic drugs, and schizophrenia: a search for common ground. Schizophr Res. 1995;16:87-110.
6. Swerdlow NR, Koob GF. Dopamine, schizophrenia, mania, and depression: towards a unified hypothesis of cortico-striato-pallido-thalamic function. Behav Brain Sci. 1987;10:197-245.
7. Shenton ME, Kikinis R, Jolesz FA, Pollak SD, LeMay M, Wible CG, Hokama H, Martin J, Metcalf D, Coleman M, McCarley RW. Abnormalities of the left temporal lobe and thought disorder in schizophrenia: a quantitative magnetic resonance imaging study. N Engl J Med. 1992;327:604-612.
8. Shenton ME, Wible CG, McCarley RW. A review of magnetic resonance imaging studies of brain abnormalities in schizophrenia. In: Krishman KRR, Doraiswamy PM, eds. Brain Imaging in Clinical Psychiatry. New York, NY: Marcel Dekker Inc; 1997:297-380.
9. Heckers S. Neuropathology of schizophrenia: cortex, thalamus, basal ganglia, and neurotransmitter-specific projection systems. Schizophr Bull. 1997;23:403-421.
10. Seidman LJ, Faraone SV, Goldstein JM, Goodman JM, Kremen WS, Matsuda G, Hoge E, Kennedy DN, Makris N, Caviness VS, Tsuang MT. Reduced subcortical brain volumes in nonpsychotic siblings of schizophrenic patients: a pilot magnetic resonance imaging study. Am J Med Genet. 1997;74:507-514.
11. Andreasen NC, Arndt S, Swayze V II, Cizadlo T, Flaum M, O'Leary D, Ehrhardt JC, Yuh WTC. Thalamic abnormalities in schizophrenia visualized through magnetic resonance image averaging. Science. 1994;266:294-298.
12. Akbarian S, Bunney WE Jr, Potkin SG, Wigal SB, Hagman JO, Sandman CA, Jones EG. Altered distribution of nicotinamide-adenine dinucleotide phosphate-diaphorase cells in frontal lobe of schizophrenics implies disturbances of cortical development. Arch Gen Psychiatry. 1993;50:169-177.
13. Selemon LD, Rajkowska G, Goldman-Rakic PS. Abnormally high neuronal density in the schizophrenic cortex: a morphometric analysis of prefrontal area 9 and occipital area 17. Arch Gen Psychiatry. 1995;52:805-818.

195

14. Jernigan TL, Zisook S, Heaton RK, Moranville JT, Hesselink JR, Braff DL. Magnetic resonance imaging abnormalities in lenticular nuclei and cerebral cortex in schizophrenia. *Arch Gen Psychiatry.* 1991;48:881-890.
15. Seidman LJ, Yurgelun-Todd D, Kremen WS, Woods BT, Goldstein JM, Faraone SV, Tsuang MT. Relationship of prefrontal and temporal lobe MRI measures to neuropsychological performance in chronic schizophrenia. *Biol Psychiatry.* 1994; 35:235-246.
16. Pearlson GD, Barta PE, Powers RE, Menon RR, Richards SS, Aylward EH, Federman EB, Chase GA, Petty RG, Tien AY. Ziskind-Somerfield Research Award 1996: medial and superior temporal gyral volumes and cerebral asymmetry in schizophrenia versus bipolar disorder. *Biol Psychiatry.* 1997;41:1-14.
17. Zipursky RB, Lim KO, Sullivan EV, Brown BW, Pfefferbaum A. Widespread cerebral gray matter volume deficits in schizophrenia. *Arch Gen Psychiatry.* 1992; 49:195-205.
18. Barta PE, Pearlson GD, Powers RE, Richards SS, Tune LE. Auditory hallucinations and smaller superior temporal gyral volume in schizophrenia. *Am J Psychiatry.* 1990;147:1457-1462.
19. DeLisi LE, Hoff AL, Neale C, Kushner M. Asymmetries in the superior temporal lobe in male and female first-episode schizophrenic patients: measures of the planum temporale and superior temporal gyrus by MRI. *Schizophr Res.* 1994; 12:19-28.
20. Lim KO, Tew W, Kushner M, Chow K, Matsumoto B, DeLisi LE. Cortical gray matter volume deficit in patients with first-episode schizophrenia. *Am J Psychiatry.* 1996;153:1548-1553.
21. Sullivan EV, Lim KO, Mathalon D, Marsh L, Beal DM, Harris D, Hoff AL, Faustman WO, Pfefferbaum A. A profile of cortical gray matter volume deficits characteristic of schizophrenia. *Cereb Cortex.* 1998;8:117-124.
22. Benes F. Neurobiological investigations in cingulate cortex of schizophrenic brain. *Schizophr Bull.* 1993;19:537-549.
23. Jakob H, Beckman H. Prenatal development disturbances in the limbic allocortex in schizophrenia. *J Neural Transm.* 1986;65:303-326.
24. Arnold SE, Hyman BT, Van Hoesen GW, Damasio AR. Some cytoarchitectural abnormalities of the entorhinal cortex in schizophrenia. *Arch Gen Psychiatry.*1991; 48:625-632.
25. Friston KJ. The disconnection hypothesis. *Schizophr Res.* 1998;30:115-125.
26. Feinberg I. Schizophrenia: caused by a fault in programmed synaptic elimination during adolescence? *J Psychiatr Res.* 1982;17:319-334.
27. Keshavan MS, Anderson S, Pettegrew JW. Is schizophrenia due to excessive synaptic pruning in the prefrontal cortex? the Feinberg hypothesis revisited. *J Psychiat Res.* 1994;28:239-265.
28. Akbarian S, Kim JJ, Potkin SG, Hagman JO, Tafazzoli A, Bunney WE Jr, Jones EG. Gene expression for glutamic acid decarboxylase is reduced without loss of neurons in prefrontal cortex of schizophrenics. *Arch Gen Psychiatry.* 1995;52: 258-266.
29. Schlaepfer TE, Harris GJ, Tien AY, Peng LW, Lee S, Federman EB, Chase GA, Barta PE, Pearlson GD. Decreased regional cortical gray matter volume in schizophrenia. *Am J Psychiatry.* 1994;151:842-848.
30. Hirayasu Y, Shenton ME, Salisbury DF, Dickey CC, Fischer IA, Mazzoni P, Kisler T, Arakaki H, Kwon JS, Anderson JE, Yurgelun-Todd D, Tohen M, McCarley RW. Lower left temporal lobe MRI volumes in patients with first-episode schizophrenia compared with psychotic patients with first-episode affective disorder and normal subjects. *Am J Psychiatry.* 1998;155:1384-1391.
31. DeLisi LE, Tew W, Xie S, Hoff AL, Sakuma M, Kushner M, Lee G, Shediack K, Smith AM, Grimson R. A prospective follow-up study of brain morphology and cognition in first-episode schizophrenic patients: preliminary findings. *Biol Psychiatry.* 1995;38:349-360.
32. Rossi A, Stratta P, Mattei P, Cupillari M, Bozzao A, Gallucci M, Casacchia M. Planum temporale in schizophrenia: a magnetic resonance study. *Schizophr Res.* 1992;7:19-22.
33. Falkai P, Bogerts B, Greve B, Pfeiffer U, Machus B, Folsch-Reetz B, Majtenyi C, Ovary I. Loss of sylvian fissure asymmetry in schizophrenia: a quantitative postmortem study. *Schizophr Res.* 1992;7:23-32.
34. Lim KO, Harris D, Beal M, Hoff AL, Minn K, Csernansky JG, Faustman WO, Marsh L, Sullivan EV, Pfefferbaum A. Gray matter deficits in young onset schizophrenia are independent of age of onset. *Biol Psychiatry.* 1996;40:4-13.
35. Bogerts B. The temporolimbic system theory of positive schizophrenic symptoms. *Schizophr Bull.* 1997;23:423-435.
36. Rademacher J. Human cerebral cortex: localization, parcellation and morphometry with magnetic resonance imaging. *J Cogn Neurosci.* 1992;4:352-373.
37. Caviness VS Jr, Meyer J, Makris N, Kennedy DN. MRI-based anatomically defined parcellation of human neocortex: an efficient method with estimate of reliability. *J Cogn Neurosci.* 1996;8:566-587.
38. Kennedy DN, Filipek P, Caviness VS. Anatomic segmentation and volumetric calculation in nuclear magnetic resonance imaging. *IEEE Trans Med Imaging.* 1989; 8:1-7.

39. Makris N, Worth AJ, Sorensen AG, Papadimitriou GM, Wu O, Reese TG, Wedeer VJ, Davis TL, Stakes JW, Caviness VS, Kaplan E, Rosen BR, Pandya DN, Kennedy DN. Morphometry of in vivo human white matter association pathways with diffusion-weighted magnetic resonance imaging. *Ann Neurol.* 1997;42:951-962.
40. Goldberg E, Seidman LJ. Higher cortical functions in normals and in schizophrenia: a selective review. In: Zubin J, Steinhauer S, Gruzelier J, eds. *Handbook of Schizophrenia, Vol 5: Neuropsychology, Psychophysiology, and Information Processing.* New York, NY: Elsevier Science Inc; 1991:553-597.
41. Gold JM, Weinberger DR. Frontal lobe structure, function, and connectivity in schizophrenia. In: Kerwin R, ed. *Neurobiology and Psychiatry.* Vol 1. Cambridge, Mass: Cambridge University Press; 1995:39-59.
42. Bilder RM, Bogerts B, Ashtari M, Wu H, Alvir JM, Jody D, Reiter G, Bell L, Lieberman JA. Anterior hippocampal volume reductions predict frontal lobe dysfunction in first episode schizophrenia. *Schizophr Res.* 1995;17:47-58.
43. Berman KF, Illowsky BP, Weinberger DR. Physiological dysfunction of dorsolateral prefrontal cortex in schizophrenia, IV: further evidence for regional and behavioral specificity. *Arch Gen Psychiatry.* 1988;45:616-622.
44. Seidman LJ, Oscar-Berman M, Kalinowski AG, Ajilor O, Kremen WS, Faraone SV, Tsuang MT. Experimental and clinical neuropsychological measures of prefrontal dysfunction in schizophrenia. *Neuropsychology.* 1995;9:481-490.
45. Goldstein JM, Seidman LJ, Goodman JM, Koren D, Lee H, Weintraub S, Tsuang MT. Are there sex differences in neuropsychological functions among patients with schizophrenia? *Am J Psychiatry.* 1998;155:1358-1364.
46. Seidman LJ, Goldstein JM, Goodman JM, Koren D, Turner WM, Faraone SV, Tsuang MT. Sex differences in olfactory identification and Wisconsin Card Sorting performance in schizophrenia: relationship to attention and verbal ability. *Biol Psychiatry.* 1997;42:104-115.
47. Kremen WS, Seidman LJ, Faraone SV, Pepple JR, Lyons MJ, Tsuang MT. The "3Rs" and neuropsychological function in schizophrenia: an empirical test of the matching fallacy. *Neuropsychology.* 1996;10:22-31.
48. Mesulam MM. Large-scale neurocognitive networks and distributed processing for attention, language, and memory. *Ann Neurol.* 1990;28:597-613.
49. Hollingshead AB. *Four Factor Index of Social Status.* New Haven, Conn: Dept of Sociology, Yale University Press; 1975.
50. Vincent KR, Castillo IM, Hauser RI, Zapata JA, Stuart HJ, Cohn CK, O'Shanick GJ. *MMPI-168 Codebook.* Norwood, NJ: Ablex Publishing Corp; 1984.
51. American Psychiatric Association. *Diagnostic and Statistical Manual of Mental Disorders, Revised Third Edition.* Washington, DC: American Psychiatric Association; 1987.
52. Andreasen NC. *Scale for the Assessment of Negative Symptoms (SANS).* Iowa City: University of Iowa; 1981.
53. Andreasen NC. *Scale for the Assessment of Positive Symptoms (SAPS).* Iowa City: University of Iowa; 1983.
54. Jastak S, Wilkinson GS. *Wide Range Achievement Test–Revised.* Wilmington, Del: Jastak Assoc; 1984.
55. Wechsler D. *Wechsler Adult Intelligence Scale–Revised.* New York, NY: Psychological Corp; 1981.
56. Brooker BH, Cyr JJ. Tables for clinicians to use to convert WAIS-R short forms. *J Clin Psychol.* 1986;42:983-986.
57. Spitzer RL, Endicott J. *Schedule for Affective Disorders and Schizophrenia.* New York: Biometrics Research Dept, New York State Psychiatric Institute; 1978.
58. Filipek PA, Kennedy DN, Caviness VS Jr. Volumetric analyses of central nervous system neoplasm based on MRI. *Pediatr Neurol.* 1991;7:347-351.
59. Seidman LJ, Faraone SV, Goldstein JM, Goodman JM, Kremen WS, Matsuda G, Hoge EA, Kennedy DN, Makris N, Caviness VS, Tsuang MT. Reduced subcortical brain volumes in nonpsychotic siblings of schizophrenic patients: a pilot magnetic resonance imaging study. *Am J Med Genet.* 1997;74:507-514.
60. Mathalon DH, Sullivan EV, Rawles JM, Pfefferbaum A. Correction for head size in brain-imaging measurements [published correction appears in *Psychiatry Res.* 1994;55:179]. *Psychiatry Res.* 1993;50:121-139.
61. Rothman KJ. No adjustments are needed for multiple comparisons. *Epidemiology.* 1990;1:43-46.
62. Cohen J. *Statistical Power Analysis for the Behavioral Sciences.* Rev ed. New York, NY: Academic Press Inc; 1977.
63. Breier A, Buchanan RW, Elkashef A, Munson RC, Kirkpatrick B, Gellad F. Brain morphology and schizophrenia: a magnetic resonance imaging study of limbic, prefrontal cortex, and caudate structures. *Arch Gen Psychiatry.* 1992;49: 921-926.
64. Wible CG, Shenton ME, Hokama H, Kikinis R, Jolesz FA, Metcalf D, McCarley RW. Prefrontal cortex and schizophrenia: a quantitative magnetic resonance imaging study. *Arch Gen Psychiatry.* 1995;52:279-288.
65. Albanese AM, Merlo AB, Mascitti TA, Tornese EB, Gomez EE, Konopka V, Albanese EF. Inversion of the hemispheric laterality of the anterior cingulate gyrus in schizophrenics. *Biol Psychiatry.* 1995;38:13-21.
66. Noga JT, Aylward E, Barta PE, Pearlson GD. Cingulate gyrus in schizophrenic

196

patients and normal volunteers. *Psychiatry Res.* 1995;61:201-208.

67. Ohnuma T, Kimura M, Takahashi T, Iwamoto N, Arai H. A magnetic resonance imaging study in first-episode disorganized-type patients with schizophrenia. *Psychiatry Clin Neurosci.* 1997;51:9-15.

68. Haznedar MM, Buchsbaum MS, Luu C, Hazlett EA, Siegel BV Jr, Lohr J, Wu J, Haier RJ, Bunney WE Jr. Decreased anterior cingulate gyrus metabolic rate in schizophrenia. *Am J Psychiatry.* 1997;154:682-684.

69. Devinsky O, Morrell M, Vogt B. Contributions of anterior cingulate cortex to behaviour. *Brain.* 1995;118:279-306.

70. Smith WK. The results of ablation of the cingular region of the cerebral cortex. *Fed Proc.* 1994;3:42-43.

71. Frith CD, Friston K, Liddle PF, Frackowiak RS. Willed action and the prefrontal cortex in man: a study with PET. *Proc R Soc Lond B Biol Sci.* 1991;244: 241-246.

72. Petrides M, Alivisatos B, Evans AC. Functional activation of the human ventrolateral frontal cortex during mnemonic retrieval of verbal information. *Proc Natl Acad Sci U S A.* 1995;92:5803-5807.

73. Pardo JV, Pardo PJ, Janer KW, Raichle ME. The anterior cingulate cortex mediates processing selection in the Stroop attentional conflict paradigm. *Proc Natl Acad Sci U S A.* 1990;87:256-259.

74. Corbetta M, Miezin FM, Dobmeyer S, Shulman GL, Petersen SE. Selective and divided attention during visual discriminations of shape, color, and speed: functional anatomy by positron emission tomography. *J Neurosci.* 1991;11: 2383-2402.

75. Seidman LJ, Breiter HC, Goodman JM, Goldstein JM, Woodruff PWR, O'Craven K, Savoy R, Tsuang MT, Rosen BR. A functional magnetic resonance imaging study of auditory vigilance with low and high information processing demands. *Neuropsychology.* 1998;12:505-518.

76. Raichle ME, Fiez JA, Videen TO, MacLeod AM, Pardo JV, Fox PT, Petersen SE. Practice-related changes in human brain functional anatomy during nonmotor learning. *Cereb Cortex.* 1994;4:8-26.

77. Mega MS, Cummings JL, Salloway S, Malloy P. The limbic system: an anatomic, phylogenetic, and clinical perspective. *J Neuropsychiatry Clin Neurosci.* 1997;9:315-330.

78. Mufson EJ, Mesulam MM. Thalamic connections of the insula in the rhesus monkey and comments on the paralimbic connectivity of the medial pulvinar nucleus. *J Comp Neurol.* 1984;227:109-120.

79. Augustine JR. Circuitry and functional aspects of the insular lobe in primates including humans. *Brain Res Brain Res Rev.* 1996;22:229-244.

80. Posner M, Petersen SE. The attention system of the human brain. *Annu Rev Neurosci.* 1990;13:25-42.

81. Fletcher PC, McKenna PJ, Frith CD, Grasby PM, Friston KJ, Dolan RJ. Brain activations in schizophrenia during a graded memory task studied with functional neuroimaging. *Arch Gen Psychiatry.* 1998;55:1001-1008.

82. Nopoulos P, Torres I, Flaum M, Andreasen NC, Ehrhardt JC, Yuh WT. Brain morphology in first-episode schizophrenia. *Am J Psychiatry.* 1995;152:1721-1723.

83. Liddle PF. Brain imaging. In: Hirsch SR, Weinberger DR, eds. *Schizophrenia.* Cambridge, Mass: Blackwell Science; 1995:425-439.

84. Meador-Woodruff JH, Haroutunian V, Powchik P, Davidson M, Davis KL, Watson SJ. Dopamine receptor transcript expression in striatum and prefrontal and occipital cortex: focal abnormalities in orbitofrontal cortex in schizophrenia. *Arch Gen Psychiatry.* 1997;54:1089-1095.

85. Rojas DC, Teale P, Sheeder J, Simon J, Reite M. Sex-specific expression of Heschl's gyrus functional and structural abnormalities in paranoid schizophrenia. *Am J Psychiatry.* 1997;154:1655-1662.

86. Menon RR, Barta PE, Aylward EH, Richards SS, Vaughn DD, Tien AY, Harris GJ, Pearlson GD. Posterior superior temporal gyrus in schizophrenia: grey matter changes and clinical correlates. *Schizophr Res.* 1995;16:127-135.

87. Reite M, Sheeder J, Teale P, Adams M, Richardson D, Simon J, Jones RH, Rojas DC. Magnetic source imaging evidence of sex differences in cerebral lateralization in schizophrenia. *Arch Gen Psychiatry.* 1997;54:433-440.

88. Vogeley K, Hobson T, Schneider-Axmann T, Honer WG, Bogerts B, Falkai P. Compartmental volumetry of the superior temporal gyrus reveals sex differences in schizophrenia: a post-mortem study. *Schizophr Res.* 1998;31:83-87.

197

Brain (1999), 122, 593–624

INVITED REVIEW

The neuropathology of schizophrenia
A critical review of the data and their interpretation

Paul J. Harrison

University Department of Psychiatry, Warneford Hospital, Oxford, UK

Correspondence to: Dr P. J. Harrison, Neurosciences Building, University Department of Psychiatry, Warneford Hospital, Oxford OX3 7JX, UK E-mail: paul.harrison@psychiatry.ox.ac.uk

Summary
Despite a hundred years' research, the neuropathology of schizophrenia remains obscure. However, neither can the null hypothesis be sustained—that it is a 'functional' psychosis, a disorder with no structural basis. A number of abnormalities have been identified and confirmed by meta-analysis, including ventricular enlargement and decreased cerebral (cortical and hippocampal) volume. These are characteristic of schizophrenia as a whole, rather than being restricted to a subtype, and are present in first-episode, unmedicated patients. There is considerable evidence for preferential involvement of the temporal lobe and moderate evidence for an alteration in normal cerebral asymmetries. There are several candidates for the histological and molecular correlates of the macroscopic features. The probable proximal explanation for decreased cortical volume is reduced neuropil and neuronal size, rather than a loss of neurons. These morphometric changes are in turn suggestive of alterations in synaptic, dendritic and axonal organization, a view supported by immunocytochemical and ultra-structural findings. Pathology in subcortical structures is not well established, apart from dorsal thalamic nuclei, which are smaller and contain fewer neurons. Other cytoarchitectural features of schizophrenia which are often discussed, notably entorhinal cortex heterotopias and hippocampal neuronal disarray, remain to be

confirmed. The phenotype of the affected neuronal and synaptic populations is uncertain. A case can be made for impairment of hippocampal and corticocortical excitatory pathways, but in general the relationship between neurochemical findings (which centre upon dopamine, 5-hydroxytryptamine, glutamate and GABA systems) and the neuropathology of schizophrenia is unclear. Gliosis is not an intrinsic feature; its absence supports, but does not prove, the prevailing hypothesis that schizophrenia is a disorder of prenatal neurodevelopment. The cognitive impairment which frequently accompanies schizophrenia is not due to Alzheimer's disease or any other recognized neurodegenerative disorder. Its basis is unknown. Functional imaging data indicate that the pathophysiology of schizophrenia reflects aberrant activity in, and integration of, the components of distributed circuits involving the prefrontal cortex, hippocampus and certain subcortical structures. It is hypothesized that the neuropathological features represent the anatomical substrate of these functional abnormalities in neural connectivity. Investigation of this proposal is a goal of current neuropathological studies, which must also seek (i) to establish which of the recent histological findings are robust and cardinal, and (ii) to define the relationship of the pathological phenotype with the clinical syndrome, its neurochemistry and its pathogenesis.

Keywords: Alzheimer's disease; cytoarchitecture; morphometry; synapse; psychosis

Abbreviations: DLPFC = dorsolateral prefrontal cortex; 5-HT = 5-hydroxytryptamine; VBR = ventricle : brain ratio

Introduction
A hundred years ago, Kraeplin described the syndrome now called schizophrenia. He was convinced that it was an organic brain disease, and it was his colleague Alzheimer who began the neuropathological investigation before moving to a more

fruitful research area. Subsequently the subject has continued to fascinate and exasperate researchers in equal measure, generating more heat than light and being notable for memorable quotes rather than durable data. The most

594 *P. J. Harrison*

infamous, that schizophrenia is the 'graveyard of neuropathologists' (Plum, 1972), was a statement which, together with critical reviews of the work up to that time (Corsellis, 1976), marked the nadir of the field.

Over the past 20 years, signs of life have appeared in the graveyard, reflected in the return of schizophrenia to the latest edition of *Greenfield's Neuropathology* (Roberts *et al.*, 1997), having been omitted from the previous two. The significant progress which has been made began with CT findings, followed by MRI and by post-mortem studies using improved methodologies and new techniques. The progress allowed Ron and Harvey (1990) to charge that '[to] have forgotten that schizophrenia is a brain disease will go down as one of the great aberrations of twentieth century medicine'. In a similar vein, Weinberger (1995) stated '20 years ago, the principal challenge for schizophrenia research was to gather objective scientific evidence that would implicate the brain. That challenge no longer exists.' On the other hand, it is undoubtedly an overstatement to claim that there is 'an avalanche of consistent . . . evidence of microscopic pathology' (Bloom, 1993); the current challenge is to establish the characteristics of the pathological changes (Shapiro, 1993; Chua and McKenna, 1995). This review summarizes the present state of knowledge, including the issues of hemispheric asymmetry, dementia in schizophrenia, neurodevelopment and neurochemistry. An integration of structure with function is attempted, with elaboration of the proposal that the neuropathology of schizophrenia represents the anatomical substrate of aberrant functional connectivity.

Review coverage and methodology

The review focuses on the key points of agreement and of controversy affecting the robustness of the data and their interpretation. It comprises a comprehensive survey of contemporary (post-1980) neurohistopathological research, with restricted coverage of earlier work and of related fields such as neuroimaging and neurochemistry.

The sources for the review consisted of: (i) papers identified using a range of keywords for on-line searches of Medline, PsycLIT and *Biological Abstracts* (last search, October 1998), (ii) weekly scanning of *Reference Update* (deluxe edition, customized to 350 journals) from 1989 to October 1998 using a similar range of keywords, and (iii) an extensive reprint collection and perusal of each article's reference list. Only data published in full papers in peer-reviewed English-language journals were considered for inclusion.

Clinical features of schizophrenia

Schizophrenia remains a clinical diagnosis, based upon the presence of certain types of delusions, hallucinations and thought disorder (McKenna, 1994; Andreasen, 1995). These 'positive' symptoms are often complemented by the 'negative' symptoms of avolition, alogia and affective flattening. The criteria of the Diagnostic and Statistical

Manual of Mental Disorders (American Psychiatric Association, 1994), used for most research studies, require symptoms to have been present for at least 6 months; there must also be impaired personal functioning, and the symptoms must not be secondary to another disorder (e.g. depression, substance abuse). The peak age of onset is in the third decade, occurring a few years earlier in males than in females (Hafner *et al.*, 1998). The course and outcome are remarkably variable, but better than sometimes believed; only a minority of patients have a chronic, deteriorating course, though many others have enduring symptoms or functional deficits (Davidson and McGlashan, 1997; Huber, 1997). There is a significant excess of mortality from suicide and natural causes (Brown, 1997). The lifetime risk of schizophrenia is just under 1% (Cannon and Jones, 1996). It has a predominantly genetic aetiology, but no chromosomal loci or genes have been unequivocally demonstrated (McGuffin *et al.*, 1995).

The diagnosis of schizophrenia is reliable, but as with any other syndromal diagnosis there are problems establishing its validity and debate as to where its external and internal boundaries should be drawn (Jablensky, 1995). These issues have implications for research into its pathological basis just as they do for the search for the causative genes (Kennedy, 1996). For example, is schizophrenia a categorical or dimensional construct? What is the relationship of schizoaffective and schizotypal disorders to schizophrenia? Are there separate pathological counterparts of schizophrenic subsyndromes or specific symptoms, given that each has its own pathophysiological correlates (Liddle *et al.*, 1992; Silbersweig *et al.*, 1995; Sabri *et al.*, 1997)? The delineation of type I and type II schizophrenia was an important, if now rather outmoded, attempt to address this issue (Crow, 1980). As an analogy, is schizophrenia—neuropathologically speaking—comparable to dementia, to a specific dementing disorder or to a domain of memory impairment? Comparisons with epilepsy are also pertinent (Bruton *et al.*, 1994; Stevens, 1997). Clearly, the prospects for success in finding the neuropathology of schizophrenia depend on which of these parallels proves closest. These issues are touched upon later in the review but for the most part, predicated on the design of the studies being discussed, schizophrenia is considered as a single entity.

Structural imaging in schizophrenia
The cardinal findings

Contemporary research into the structural basis of schizophrenia can be traced to the landmark report of Johnstone *et al.* (1976) describing dilatation of the lateral ventricles in a small group of patients with chronic schizophrenia. This CT finding, which was consistent with earlier pneumoencephalographic data (Haug, 1982), has been followed by a large number of CT and MRI studies with ever-improving resolution and sophistication of analysis. The key findings are as follows.

There is enlargement of the lateral and third ventricles in schizophrenia. The magnitude has been estimated in several ways. Comprehensive reviews of lateral ventricle : brain ratio (VBR) indicate an increase of 20–75% (Daniel *et al.*, 1991; van Horn and McManus, 1992), whilst a meta-analysis of CT studies up to 1989 showed a VBR effect size (*d*) of 70, corresponding to a 43% non-overlap between cases and controls (Raz and Raz, 1990). A median 40% increase in ventricular size was reported in a recent systematic review of volumetric MRI studies (Lawrie and Abukmeil, 1998). Of note, VBR in schizophrenia follows a single normal distribution, indicating that structural pathology, at least in terms of this parameter, is not restricted to an 'organic' subgroup but is present to a degree in all cases (Daniel *et al.*, 1991). Conversely, despite the group differences, there is a significant overlap between subjects with schizophrenia and controls for every imaging (and neuropathological) parameter to be discussed. For this reason, as well as the fact that changes such as increased VBR and decreased brain size lack diagnostic specificity, it is worth emphasizing that schizophrenia cannot be diagnosed using either a brain scan or a microscope. It remains a moot point whether this situation will change.

The ventricular enlargement is accompanied by a loss of brain tissue averaging 3% (Lawrie and Abukmeil, 1998) with = −0.26 (Ward *et al.*, 1996). However, no consistent correlation has been observed between the degree of ventricular enlargement and that of the decreased brain volume. This may reflect the relative sizes of the ventricles and cerebral cortex, such that a given percentage change in ventricular volumes corresponds to a much smaller percentage change in cortical substance (and hence one which is difficult to measure accurately). Or it may suggest that the ventricular enlargement is due to disproportionate reductions in unidentified, localized periventricular structures, or even that independent pathological processes are at work.

Evidence for regional pathology has emerged from volumetric MRI studies which indicate larger reductions in the temporal lobe overall (~8%) and in medial temporal structures (hippocampus, parahippocampal gyrus and amygdala, 4–12%; Lawrie and Abukmeil, 1998) present after correction for total brain volume (Nelson *et al.*, 1998). In support of this conclusion, the brain size reduction is significantly greater in the axial (*d* = −0.60) than the sagittal (= −0.09) plane (Ward *et al.*, 1996), suggesting a relative decrease in mediolateral breadth and a greater involvement of regions typically included in axial slices, such as the temporal lobes. Grey matter appears to be reduced more than white matter (Lawrie and Abukmeil, 1998; Zipursky *et al.*, 1998).

Valuable information has come from imaging studies of monozygotic twins discordant for schizophrenia. In virtually all pairs the affected twin has the larger ventricles (Reveley *et al.*, 1982; Suddath *et al.*, 1990) and smaller cortical and hippocampal size (Noga *et al.*, 1996). In the MRI study of Suddath *et al.* (1990), the affected twin was distinguishable even more clearly by the smaller size of his or her temporal lobes and hippocampi. The discordant monozygotic twin study design allows two conclusions to be drawn. First, that structural abnormalities are a consistent finding in schizophrenia, their identification being aided by controlling for genetic influences on neuroanatomy (Bartley *et al.*, 1997) and, to a large degree, for variation due to environmental factors. Secondly, that the alterations are associated with expression of the schizophrenia phenotype rather than merely with the underlying, shared genotype. Family studies support this interpretation, in that schizophrenics have bigger ventricles and smaller brains than do their unaffected relatives (Honer *et al.*, 1994; Sharma *et al.*, 1998; Silverman *et al.*, 1998). However, the relatives who are obligate carriers [i.e. unaffected by schizophrenia but transmitting the gene(s)] have larger ventricles than relatives who are not; moreover, both groups of relatives have larger ventricles and smaller brain structures than equivalent control subjects from families without schizophrenia (Lawrie *et al.*, 1999; Sharma *et al.*, 1998). These data indicate that a proportion of the structural pathology of schizophrenia may be a marker of genetic liability to the disorder. (By inference, the same applies to the accompanying histological features, though there have been no post-mortem studies of relatives.)

Imaging of subcortical structures in schizophrenia has produced few clear findings. One firm conclusion is that the striatal enlargement reported in some studies is, unlike other changes, due to antipsychotic medication (Chakos *et al.*, 1994; Keshavan *et al.*, 1994*b*). Indeed, in unmedicated and first-episode patients, caudate volumes are probably reduced (Keshavan *et al.*, 1998; Shihabuddin *et al.*, 1998). Two MRI studies suggest that the thalamus is smaller in schizophrenia (Andreasen *et al.*, 1994; Buchsbaum *et al.*, 1996); though this evidence is weak (Portas *et al.*, 1998), it is complemented by relatively strong neuropathological data (see below). Finally, reports of structural abnormalities in the cerebellum in schizophrenia (Katsetos *et al.*, 1997) merit further investigation, given accumulating evidence for its patho-physiological involvement in the disorder (Andreasen *et al.*, 1996).

Progression, heterogeneity and clinicopathological correlations

Knowledge of the timing of the brain changes is essential for understanding their aetiological significance. Ventricular enlargement and cortical volume reduction are both present in first-episode cases (Degreef *et al.*, 1992; Lim *et al.*, 1996; Gur *et al.*, 1998; Whitworth *et al.*, 1998; Zipursky *et al.*, 1998), excluding the possibility that they are a consequence of chronic illness or its treatment. Moreover, adolescents and young adults who are at high risk of developing schizophrenia by virtue of their family history show enlarged ventricles (Cannon *et al.*, 1993) and smaller medial temporal lobes (Lawrie *et al.*, 1999), suggesting that the brain pathology precedes the onset of symptoms (Harrison, 1999a) and supporting a neurodevelopmental model of schizophrenia (discussed below).

It is less clear what happens to the structural pathology after symptoms emerge. Neither VBR nor cortical volume reduction, nor the smaller size of the medial temporal lobe (Marsh *et al.*, 1994), correlate with disease duration, suggesting that the alterations are largely static. However, longitudinal studies, which now span 4–8 years, are equivocal. Some support the view that there is no progression (Jaskiw *et al.*, 1994; Vita *et al.*, 1997) whilst others find continuing divergence from controls (DeLisi *et al.*, 1997a; Nair *et al.*, 1997; Gur *et al.*, 1998). This may reflect a subgroup of subjects with a deteriorating course (Davis *et al.*, 1998) or who receive high doses of antipsychotics (Madsen *et al.*, 1998), but other studies have not shown such correlations. Overall, the question whether brain pathology in schizophrenia is progressive or static, or even fluctuating, remains controversial, and has an uncertain relationship with the clinical heterogeneity of the syndrome.

It is uncertain whether sex is a confounder. Greater structural abnormalities in men than women with schizophrenia have been reported (Flaum *et al.*, 1990; Nopoulos *et al.*, 1997), perhaps related to sex differences in clinical and aetiological factors (Tamminga, 1997). However, sex differences have not been found consistently (Lauriello *et al.*, 1997) and they were not apparent in the meta-analysis of Lawrie and Abukmeil (1998).

Numerous correlations have been reported between brain structure and the individual subtypes and symptoms of schizophrenia, but they are less well established than those involving cerebral metabolism (e.g. Buchanan *et al.*, 1993; Gur *et al.*, 1994). One of the few reasonably robust correlations is that between decreased superior temporal gyrus size and the severity of thought disorder and auditory hallucinations (Barta *et al.*, 1990; Shenton *et al.*, 1992; Marsh *et al.*, 1997).

In the rare childhood-onset schizophrenia, similar brain and ventricular abnormalities are observed as in adults (Frazier *et al.*, 1996), with progression of the changes during the early phase of the illness (Rapaport *et al.*, 1997; Jacobsen *et al.*, 1998).

Neuropathological findings in schizophrenia

By 1980, the growing evidence for structural brain changes in schizophrenia provided by CT studies had spurred a return to post-mortem investigations. These have focused on three overlapping areas, which I consider in turn. First, attempts have been made to confirm whether the alterations were replicable in direct measurements of the brain. Secondly, research has sought to clarify the frequency and nature of neurodegenerative abnormalities in schizophrenia, especially to ascertain whether gliosis is present and whether Alzheimer's disease occurs at an increased frequency, as earlier authors had suggested. As will be seen, the results

indicate strongly that neurodegenerative processes do ■ represent the neuropathology of schizophrenia and th cannot explain the smaller brain volume. In the context these negative findings, the third, and largest, area of resear has been to investigate the cytoarchitecture of the cereb cortex.

Contemporary neuropathological investigations schizophrenia have, unlike their predecessors, been by a large well designed and appropriately analysed. Th renaissance has coincided with the advent of molecu techniques and computerized image analysis, allowing m powerful and quantitative experimental approaches (Harris 1996). Nevertheless, it is worth mentioning three limitatic which continue to apply, to varying degrees, to most studi First, few have been carried out according to stereologi principles (Howard and Reed, 1998) and hence are subj to errors and biases which may be particularly important this instance, given the subtlety of the alterations bei sought. Secondly, research groups have tended to use differi methods, measuring different parameters, and have stud different regions of the brain. It is therefore difficult to kn whether inconsistent results reflect genuine pathological anatomical heterogeneity or methodological factors, or a simply contradictory. Thirdly, sample sizes have continu to be small, leading inevitably to both false-positive a false-negative results and meaning that potential complexiti such as diagnosis × gender interactions and discr clinicopathological correlations, have barely been address

Macroscopic features

The CT and MRI findings in schizophrenia are partly b not unequivocally corroborated by measurements of the br post-mortem. The key positive autopsy studies report decrease in brain weight (Brown *et al.*, 1986; Pakkenbe 1987; Bruton *et al.*, 1990), brain length (Bruton *et al.*, 199 and volume of the cerebral hemispheres (Pakkenberg, 198° Concerning regional alterations, there are several post-morte replications of the imaging findings, especially enlargeme of the lateral ventricles (Brown *et al.*, 1986; Pakkenbe 1987; Crow *et al.*, 1989), reduced size of temporal lo structures (Bogerts *et al.*, 1985, 1990b; Brown *et al.*, 198 Falkai and Bogerts, 1986; Falkai *et al.*, 1988; Jeste and Lo 1989; Altshuler *et al.*, 1990; Vogeley *et al.*, 1998), decreas thalamic volume (Pakkenberg, 1990, 1992; Danos *et c* 1998) and enlarged basal ganglia (Heckers *et al.*, 1991« Whilst this convergence of autopsy and *in vivo* results encouraging, there are negative post-mortem reports for ea parameter (Rosenthal and Bigelow, 1972; Bogerts *et c* 1990b; Heckers *et al.*, 1990; Pakkenberg, 1990; Arnold *et a* 1995a; for further details, see Arnold and Trojanowski, 199 Dwork, 1997).

As a meta-analysis of the post-mortem studies is n feasible, the robustness of the positive findings and the sour of the discrepancies remain unclear. In any event, the relian upon such measurements has been diminished by MRI, whi allows most of the indices to be measured accurately in life. The real value of neuropathological studies, and hence the primary focus here, is now in elucidating the microscopic and molecular features of schizophrenia which remain beyond the reach of neuroimaging.

Coincidental pathological abnormalities

A high proportion (~50%) of brains from patients with schizophrenia contain non-specific focal degenerative abnormalities, such as small infarcts and white matter changes (Stevens, 1982; Jellinger, 1985; Bruton *et al.*, 1990; Riederer *et al.*, 1995). These are presumably coincidental, in that they are variable in distribution and nature, do not affect the clinical picture (Johnstone *et al.*, 1994) and in some instances are documented as having occurred long after the onset of symptoms. The issue is whether the frequency of lesions is a sign that the brain in schizophrenia is vulnerable to neurodegenerative and vascular impairment, perhaps in conjunction with chronic antipsychotic treatment, or whether the finding is merely a collection artefact (see below). A related point is that ~3-5% of cases diagnosed as schizophrenia turn out to be due to an atypical presentation of a neurological disorder, such as temporal lobe epilepsy, syphilis, Wilson's disease and metachromatic leucodystrophy (Davison, 1983; Johnstone *et al.*, 1987). One school of thought argues that cases in both these categories should be included in neuropathological studies of schizophrenia since there are no grounds a priori for exclusion, and these 'outliers' may provide crucial and unexpected clues—and if not will at least help establish the pathological heterogeneity of the syndrome (Heckers, 1997; Stevens, 1997). On the other hand, the omission of subjects with coincidental pathologies and those with a neurological schizophrenia-like disorder allows 'true' schizophrenia to be examined (Bruton *et al.*, 1990; Dwork, 1997); an argument in favour of the latter strategy is that the excess of miscellaneous lesions in schizophrenia may be an artefact of how tissue is acquired: researchers can afford to pick and choose control brains, but cases with schizophrenia are scarce and hence more likely to be included even if there is a complex or incomplete medical history. Note that the cytoarchitectural findings to be discussed later all come from brain series which were 'purified' to varying extents.

Gliosis

Stevens (1982), in keeping with observations going back as far as Alzheimer (Nieto and Escobar, 1972; Fisman, 1975), found fibrillary gliosis (reactive astrocytosis) in ~70% of her cases of schizophrenia. The gliosis was usually located in periventricular and subependymal regions of the diencephalon or in adjacent basal forebrain structures. As gliosis is a sign of past inflammation (Kreutzberg *et al.*, 1997), this finding supported a number of aetiopathogenic scenarios for

schizophrenia involving infective, ischaemic, autoimmune or neurodegenerative processes.

Because of these implications for the nature of the disease and its position as the first major neuropathological study of schizophrenia in the modern era, Stevens' paper has been important and influential. However, many subsequent investigations of schizophrenia have not found gliosis (Roberts *et al.*, 1986, 1987; Stevens *et al.*, 1988*b*; Casanova *et al.*, 1990; Arnold *et al.*, 1996). The illuminating study of Bruton *et al.* (1990) found that, when gliosis was present, it was in the cases exhibiting separate neuropathological abnormalities mentioned above. These findings together suggest strongly that gliosis is not a feature of the disease but is a sign of coincidental or superimposed pathological changes (Harrison, 1997*b*). Though this view is now widely accepted, it is subject to several caveats. First, the recognition and definition of gliosis is not straightforward (Miyake *et al.*, 1988; da Cunha, 1993; Halliday *et al.*, 1996). Secondly, several of the key studies have determined gliosis by GFAP (glial fibrillary acidic protein) immunoreactivity (Roberts *et al.*, 1986, 1987; Arnold *et al.*, 1996), but the sensitivity of this method for detection of chronic gliosis relative to the traditional Holzer technique has been questioned (Stevens *et al.*, 1988*a*, 1992). An alternative method sometimes used, that of counting or sizing glia in Nissl-stained material (Benes *et al.*, 1986; Pakkenberg, 1990; Rajkowska *et al.*, 1998), though reassuringly reaching the same negative conclusion in schizophrenia, has the problem of distinguishing astrocytes from small neurons and other cell types. Thirdly, recent studies have focused on the cerebral cortex rather than on the diencephalic regions where the gliosis of Stevens (1982) were concentrated. Since lesions do not always produce gliosis in distant areas, even those heavily interconnected, it cannot be assumed that a lack of gliosis in the cortex precludes it in other structures (Anezaki *et al.*, 1992; Jones, 1997*a*). Finally, the subgroup of schizophrenics who are demented (see below) do have an increased number of GFAP-positive astrocytes (Arnold *et al.*, 1996). Inclusion of such cases in post-mortem studies, where the cognitive status of individuals is usually unknown, may therefore contribute to the uncertainty concerning gliosis in schizophrenia.

The gliosis debate has been fuelled by the implications it has for the nature of schizophrenia. The gliotic response is said not to occur until the end of the second trimester *in utero* (Friede, 1989). Hence an absence of gliosis is taken as prima facie evidence for an early neurodevelopmental origin of schizophrenia (discussed below), whereas the presence of gliosis would imply that the disease process occurred after that time and raise the possibility that it is a progressive and degenerative disorder. In this respect the lack of gliosis is an important issue. Unfortunately, there are problems with this dichotomous view of the meaning of gliosis. Despite the widely cited time point at which the glial response is said to begin, it has not been well investigated (Roessmann and Gambetti, 1986; Aquino *et al.*, 1996) and may be regionally variable (Ajtai *et al.*, 1997). Hence it is prudent not to time

Table 1 *Neuronal morphometric findings in schizophrenia*

	Cases/ controls	Methods and parameters	Main findings in schizophrenia
(A) Temporal lobe			
Kovelman and Scheibel, 1984	10/8	Nissl stain; HC neuron orientation and density	More variability of orientation (disarray) at CA2/CA1 and CA1/subiculum borders. Density unchanged
Jakob and Beckmann, 1986	64/0*	Nissl stain; qualitative neuron organization in ERC and ventral insula	Cytoarchitectonic abnormalities (e.g. abnormal lamina II islands; displaced neurons) in a third of cases[†]
Falkai and Bogerts, 1986	13/11	Nissl stain; HC neuron number and density	Decreased neuron number. Neuron density unchanged
Altshuler et al., 1987	7/6	Nissl stain; HC neuron orientation	No differences
Falkai et al., 1988	13/11	Nissl stain; ERC neuron number	Decreased (−37%)
Christison et al., 1989	17/32	Nissl stain; neuron orientation; shape and size at CA1/subiculum border	No differences
Jeste and Lohr, 1989	13/16*	Nissl stain; HC neuron density	Decreased (~30%) in CA3 and CA4
Pakkenberg, 1990	12/12	Nissl stain, physical disector, neuron number in basolateral amygdala	No differences
Arnold et al., 1991a	6/16	Nissl stain; qualitative ERC neuron organization	Neuron disorganization and displacement
Benes et al., 1991b	14/9	Nissl stain; HC neuron size, density and orientation	Decreased size (~15%). Density and variability of orientation unchanged
Conrad et al., 1991	11/7	Nissl stain; HC neuron orientation	More disarray at CA1/CA2 and CA2/CA3 borders
Heckers et al., 1991b	13/13	Nissl stain, optical disector; HC neuron number and density	No differences
Akbarian et al., 1993b	7/7	ICC; NADPHd neurons in MTL and BA 21	Decreased (−40%) in MTL and GM of BA 21; increased (>40%) in deep WM of BA 21
Pakkenberg, 1993b	8/16	Giemsa stain, optical disector; neuron number and neuron density in temporal lobe	Density increased (29%), number unchanged (as lobar volume reduced)
Arnold et al., 1995a	14/10	Nissl stain; neuron size, density and orientation in HC and ERC	Decreased size (−10%). Density and variability of orientation unchanged
Akil and Lewis, 1997	10/10	Nissl stain; neuron organization in ERC	No differences
Arnold et al., 1997a	8/8	Nissl stain, spatial point pattern analyses of ERC neuron organization	Abnormal clustering and higher 'density' in lamina III; lower density in lamina II
Cotter et al., 1997	8/11	ICC; number, staining intensity and orientation of MAP-2 HC neurons	Increased staining of non-phosphorylated MAP-2 in subiculum and CA1. Neuron number and orientation unchanged
Jønsson et al., 1997	4/8	Nissl stain; neuron density and orientation in HC	Density decreased and correlated with more variable orientation in CA1–CA3
Krimer et al., 1997b	14/14	Nissl stain, optical disector; neuron number, density and laminar volumes of ERC	No differences. No evidence for cytoarchitectural abnormalities. Trend for decreased neuron number and density
Zaidel et al., 1997a	14/17	Nissl stain; HC neuron size, shape and orientation	Decreased size (−7%) and altered shape (less pyramidal) in some subfields. Orientation variability unchanged
Zaidel et al., 1997b	14/18	Nissl stain; HC neuron density	Increased in right CA3 (22%) and CA1 (25%). Altered correlations between subfields
Benes et al., 1998	11/10*	Nissl stain; HC neuron number, density and size	Decreased number and density of CA2 interneurons
(B) Frontal lobe			
Benes et al., 1986	10/9	Nissl stain; neuron density and size in BA 4, 10 and 24	Decreased density (~−25%) in lamina III of BA 4, lamina V of BA 24, deep laminae of BA 10. Size unchanged (laminae III and VI measured)
Benes and Bird, 1987	10/10	Nissl stain, spatial arrangement of neurons in BA 4, 10 and 24	Smaller and more dispersed neuron clusters in lamina II of BA 24
Benes et al., 1991a	18/12	Nissl stain; neuron density in BA 10 and 24	Small interneurons decreased, mainly lamina II (−30%); pyramidal neurons increased (33%) in lamina V of BA 24

Table 1 *continued*

	Cases/ controls	Methods and parameters	Main findings in schizophrenia
Akbarian *et al.*, 1993*a*	5/5	ICC; NADPHd neuron density in BA 9	Decreased in superficial WM, increased in deep WM
Pakkenberg, 1993*b*	8/16	Giemsa stain, optical disector; neuron number in frontal lobe	No differences
Akbarian *et al.*, 1995	10/10	Nissl stain; neuron density in BA 9	No differences
Arnold *et al.*, 1995*a*	14/10	Nissl stain; neuron density and size in lamina III of BA 4 and lamina V of BA 17	No differences
Daviss and Lewis, 1995	5/5	ICC; CB and CR interneuron density in BA 9/46	Increased (50%) CB neurons
Selemon *et al.*, 1995	16/19*	Nissl stain, 3D-counting box; neuron density in BA 9 and 17	Pyramidal and non-pyramidal neuron density increased by 17% in BA 9 and 10% in BA 17
Akbarian *et al.*, 1996	20/20	ICC; MAP-2, NADPHd and NPNF neurons in WM of BA 46	All decreased in superficial WM; MAP-2 and NPNF neurons increased in deep WM
Anderson *et al.*, 1996	5/5	ICC; MAP-2 neuron density and size in WM of BA 9/46	Increased (44%) density overall; no change in deep WM
Beasley and Reynolds, 1997	18/22	ICC; PV neuron density in BA 10	Decreased, mainly in laminae III and IV (−35%)
Kalus *et al.*, 1997	5/5	Nissl stain and PV ICC; neuron density in BA 24	Increased (40%) in lamina V. No change in total neuron density
Rajowska *et al.*, 1998	9/10*	Methods as Selemon *et al.*, 1995; neuron size, and density × size, in BA 9 and 17	Decreased neuron size (4–9%) in BA 9; large lamina IIIc neurons most affected, and fewer of them. Density of small neurons increased (70–140%). No changes in BA 17
Selemon *et al.*, 1998	10/9*	As Selemon *et al.*, 1995, in BA 46	Increased (21%). Lamina II thinner (−13%)
(C) Subcortical areas			
Thalamus			
Pakkenberg, 1990	12/12	Nissl stain, physical disector; neuron number in mediodorsal nucleus	Fewer (−40%) neurons
Danos *et al.*, 1998	12/14	Nissl stain and PV ICC; neuron density in anteroventral nucleus	Decreased (−35%) PV neuron density
Other regions			
Averback, 1981	14/29*	Various stains; neurons in substantia nigra	Swollen, degenerating, lipid-laden neurons
Reyes and Gordon, 1981	12/8	Nissl stain; Purkinje cell density	Decreased (−39%) per unit length; increased (+39%) surface density
Arendt *et al.*, 1983	3/14	Nissl stain; neuron density in nucleus basalis and globus pallidus	No differences
Bogerts *et al.*, 1983	6/6*	Nissl stain; neuron density in substantia nigra	Decreased in medial part
Lohr and Jeste, 1988	15/13	Nissl stain; neuron density and size in locus coeruleus	No differences
Pakkenberg, 1990	12/12	Nissl stain; physical disector; neuron number in nucleus accumbens and ventral pallidum	Fewer (−48%) neurons in nucleus accumbens. No change in ventral pallidum
Garcia-Rill *et al.*, 1995	9/5*	NADPH ICC for cholinergic mesopontine neurons; TH ICC for noradrenergic locus coeruleus neurons	Increased mesopontine neuron number (60%). No change in locus coeruleus
Beckmann and Lauer, 1997	9/9	Nissl stain, optical disector; striatal neuron number	Increased (18%), caudate > putamen
Bernstein *et al.*, 1998	10/13*	NOS ICC; optical disector; neuron number and density in hypothalamus	Decreased number (−25%) and density (−31%) in paraventricular nucleus
Briess *et al.*, 1998	9/6*	Nissl stain; optical disector; mammillary body size, neuron number and neuron density	Enlarged (+34%); neuron density decreased (−34%); unchanged neuron number
Tran *et al.*, 1998	14/13	Nissl stain; Purkinje cell size and density in vermis	Cells smaller (−8%). Unchanged density

BA = Brodmann area; CB = calbindin; CR = calretinin; ERC = entorhinal cortex; GM = grey matter; HC = hippocampus; ICC = immunocytochemistry; MAP = microtubule-associated protein; NADPHd = nicotinamide-adenine dinucleotide phosphate-diaphorase; NOS = nitric oxide synthase; NPNF = non-phosphorylated epitope of 160 and 200 kDa neurofilament; PV = parvalbumin; TH = tyrosine hydroxylase; WM = white matter. *Psychiatric control group(s) also used. †Additional data in Jakob and Beckmann (1989).

Table 2 *Synaptic, axonal and dendritic findings in schizophrenia*[†]

	Cases/controls	Methods and parameters	Main findings in schizophrenia
(A) Hippocampal formation			
Arnold *et al.*, 1991*b*	6/5*	MAP-2 and MAP-5 ICC.	Decreased staining, mainly dendritic, in subiculum and ERC
Browning *et al.*, 1993	7/7	IB for synaptophysin and synapsin I and IIb	Decreased synapsin I (–40%)
Eastwood *et al.*, 1995*a*	7/13	ISH and ICC for synaptophysin	Decreased synaptophysin mRNA (–30%) except in CA1
Eastwood and Harrison, 1995	11/14	IAR for synaptophysin	Decreased (–25%)
Goldsmith and Joyce, 1995	11/8*	Modified Timm's stain for mossy fibres	Decreased intensity of staining
Adams *et al.*, 1995	10/11*	Modified Timm's stain for mossy fibres	No differences
Harrison and Eastwood, 1998	11/11	ISH and IAR for complexin I and II	Both decreased, complexin II > I
Young *et al.*, 1998	13/13	ELISA, IB and ICC for SNAP-25 and synaptophysin	Decreased SNAP-25
(B) Frontal and temporal lobe			
Benes *et al.*, 1987	7/7	ICC; NF-labelled axons in BA 24	Increased density (25%) of vertically orientated axons
Aganova and Uranova, 1992	5/7	EM; synaptic density in BA 24	Increased axospinous (225%), decreased axodendritic (–40%) synapses
Perrone-Bizzozero *et al.*, 1996	6/6	IB for synaptophysin in BA 9, 10, 17 and 20	Decreased (30–50%) in BA 9, 10 and 20
Benes *et al.*, 1997	10/15	ICC; TH fibres in BA 10 and 24	Shift of terminals from large to small neurons in lamina II of BA 24
Gabriel *et al.*, 1997	19/16*	IB for synaptophysin, SNAP-25 and syntaxin in BA 7, 8, 20 and 24	All increased in BA 24 (~25%). Unchanged in BA 7, 8 and 20
Honer *et al.*, 1997	18/24	As Gabriel *et al.* (1997) in BA 24	Increased syntaxin (30%)
Glantz and Lewis, 1997	10/10*	ICC for synaptophysin in BA 9, 46 and 17	Decreased (15%) in BA 9, 46. Unchanged in BA 17
Tcherepanov and Sokolov, 1997	22/10	RT-PCR for synaptophysin and synapsin Ia and Ib mRNAs in BA 21 and 22	Unchanged. (Increased, if comparison limited to the nine cases < 75 years old)
Garey *et al.*, 1998	13/9	Golgi stain; dendritic spines on lamina III pyramidal neurons in BA 38	Decreased density (–60%). Similar finding in BA 11
Thompson *et al.*, 1998	5/7*	IB for SNAP-25 in BA 9, 10, 17 and 20	Decreased in BA 10 (–56%) and BA 20 (–33%); increased in BA 9 (32%); unchanged in BA 17
Woo *et al.*, 1998	15/15*	ICC; density of GABAergic axon terminals in BA 9 and 46	Selective decrease (–40%) of chandelier neuron terminals
(C) Other regions			
Striatum			
Roberts *et al.*, 1996	6/6	EM; area of dendritic spines	Smaller (–30%)
Uranova *et al.*, 1996	7/7	EM; synaptic size in left caudate	Larger postsynaptic densities in axospinous synapses
Kung *et al.*, 1998	6/7*	EM; proportions, densities and sizes of different synaptic types	Fewer symmetrical, axodendritic and perforated synapses; more axospinous synapses. No size changes
Corpus callosum			
Nasrallah *et al.*, 1983	18/11*	Silver stain; density of myelinated fibres	No differences
Casanova *et al.*, 1989	11/13	Silver stains; fibre counts	No differences
Highley *et al.*, 1999	26/29	Silver stain; fibre number and density	Decreased number and density in female schizophrenics
Thalamus			
Blennow *et al.*, 1996	19/27	IB for rab-3a	Decreased

ELISA = enzyme-linked immunosorbent assay; EM = electron microscopy; IAR = immunoautoradiography; IB = immunoblotting; ISH = *in situ* hybridization; NF = neurofilament (200 kDa subunit); RT-PCR = reverse transcriptase–polymerase chain reaction; SNAP-25 = 25 kDa synaptosome-associated protein. Other abbreviations as in Table 1. *Psychiatric control group(s) also used. [†]Studies using markers of plasticity rather than structure (e.g. GAP-43, N-CAM) omitted.

the pathology of schizophrenia with spurious accuracy or certainty based upon the available data. Additionally, gliosis is not always demonstrable or permanent after (postnatal) neural injury (Kalman *et al.*, 1993; Dell'Anna *et al.*, 1995; Berman *et al.*, 1998), nor does it accompany apoptosis, another process which hypothetically might be involved in hizophrenia. Furthermore, it is a moot point whether the btle kinds of morphometric disturbance to be described in hizophrenia, whenever and however they occurred, would sufficient to trigger gliosis or other signs of ongoing urodegeneration (Horton *et al.*, 1993). Thus the lack of iosis does not mean, in isolation, that schizophrenia must a neurodevelopmental disorder of prenatal origin; it is erely one argument in favour of that conclusion.

chizophrenia, its dementia and Alzheimer's *sease*

ognitive impairment has been a neglected feature of hizophrenia. Its importance is now being appreciated inically as a major factor contributing to the failure to habilitate some patients despite relief of their psychotic mptoms (Green, 1996), and as being a putative therapeutic rget (Davidson and Keefe, 1995). Neuropsychological normalities are demonstrable in first-episode patients (Hoff al., 1992; Saykin *et al.*, 1994; Kenny *et al.*, 1997) and emorbidly (Jones, 1997b; Russell *et al.*, 1997), and though eir progression remains unclear (Bilder *et al.*, 1992; oldberg *et al.*, 1993; Waddington and Youssef, 1996), in a zeable minority of chronic schizophrenics their severity arrants the label of dementia (Davidson *et al.*, 1996). here is particular involvement of memory and executive nctioning (McKenna *et al.*, 1990; Saykin *et al.*, 1991) ainst a background of a generalized deficit (Blanchard and eale, 1994; for review, see David and Cutting, 1994). (As ith the neuropathological abnormalities, it is worth pointing at that the mean size of these differences is small. Many dividuals with schizophrenia score within the normal range, d some are well above average. On the other hand, there no evidence that cognitive impairment is limited to a bgroup, and it may be that even in high-functioning subjects ere has been a decline from, or failure to attain, their ll neuropsychological potential.) The final controversies garding neurodegenerative processes in schizophrenia ncern the neuropathological explanation for the cognitive eficits, and the alleged increased prevalence of Alzheimer's sease in schizophrenia (e.g. Plum, 1972).

The belief that Alzheimer's disease is commoner in hizophrenia, regardless of cognitive status, seems to have iginated from two German papers in the 1930s (Corsellis,)62). It was supported by three retrospective, uncontrolled udies (Buhl and Bojsen-Møller, 1988; Soustek, 1989; ohovnik *et al.*, 1993) and the suggestion that antipsychotic ugs promote Alzheimer-type changes (Wisniewski *et al.*,)94). However, corroborating Corsellis' opinion (Corsellis,)62), a meta-analysis (Baldessarini *et al.*, 1997) and additional ethodologically sound studies show conclusively that lzheimer's disease is not commoner than expected in hizophrenia (Arnold *et al.*, 1998; Murphy *et al.*, 1998; Niizato al., 1998; Purohit *et al.*, 1998). Even amongst elderly hizophrenics with unequivocal, prospectively assessed

dementia (mean Mini-Mental State score = 12), detailed immunocytochemical analyses find no evidence for Alzheimer's disease or any other neurodegenerative disorder (Arnold *et al.*, 1996, 1998). In keeping with this negative conclusion, apolipoprotein E4 allele frequencies are unchanged (Arnold *et al.*, 1997b; Powchik *et al.*, 1997; Thibaut *et al.*, 1998) and cholinergic markers are preserved (Arendt *et al.*, 1983; Haroutunian *et al.*, 1994) in schizophrenia. Moreover, the evidence as a whole does not support the view that antipsychotic drugs predispose to neurofibrillary pathology (Baldessarini *et al.*, 1997; Harrison *et al.*, 1997b).

How, therefore, is the cognitive impairment of schizophrenia explained? One possibility is that it is a more severe manifestation of whatever substrate underlies schizophrenia itself rather than resulting from the superimposition of a separate process. Or it may be that the brain in schizophrenia is rendered more vulnerable to cognitive impairment in response to a normal age-related amount of neurodegeneration, or even that the pathological findings so far discovered actually relate to the cognitive impairment rather than to the psychotic features by which the disorder is defined. A final, speculative suggestion is that the gliosis observed in demented schizophrenics (Arnold *et al.*, 1996) is a sign of an as yet unrecognized novel neurodegenerative disorder. These possibilities cannot be distinguished at present since few neuropsychologically evaluated patients have been studied neuropathologically; inclusion of subjects with comorbid schizophrenia and mental retardation may be valuable when addressing the issue (Doody *et al.*, 1998).

The cytoarchitecture of schizophrenia

Since neurodegenerative abnormalities are uncommon in, and probably epiphenomenal to, schizophrenia, the question is raised as to what the pathology of the disorder is, and how the macroscopic findings are explained at the microscopic level. This brings us to the heart of recent schizophrenia neuropathology research, which has been the increasingly sophisticated measurement of the cortical cytoarchitecture. The focus has been mainly on the extended limbic system [hippocampus, dorsolateral prefrontal cortex (DLPFC) and cingulate gyrus], encouraged by suggestions that psychotic symptoms originate in these regions (Stevens, 1973; Torrey and Peterson, 1974).

Table 1 summarizes the morphometric investigations in which neuronal parameters such as density, number, size, shape, orientation, location and clustering have been determined. Table 2 summarizes the studies of synapses, dendrites and axons, evaluated either ultrastructurally or indirectly using immunological and molecular markers. Both tables are subdivided by brain region. Only the major findings are listed; details such as laterality effects are omitted. In the following sections the main themes of this literature are discussed, although even the choice of what to highlight is problematic given that controversy surrounds nearly every point.

Studies of neurons

Cytoarchitectural abnormalities in entorhinal cortex.

An influential paper reported the presence of various abnormalities in the cytoarchitecture and lamination of the entorhinal cortex (anterior parahippocampal gyrus) in schizophrenia (Jakob and Beckmann, 1986). The changes were prominent in lamina II, with a loss of the normal clustering of the constituent pre-α cells, which appeared shrunken, misshapen and heterotopic. Despite extensions (Jakob and Beckmann, 1989) and partial replications (Arnold et al., 1991a), the findings remain questionable for several reasons, which are elaborated because of the importance attributed to them in the neurodevelopmental model of schizophrenia. First, no normal control group was used; the comparisons were made with brains from 10 patients with other psychiatric or neurological disorders. Whilst this criticism does not apply to the study of Arnold et al. (1991a), both are limited by the lack of objective criteria for the cytoarchitectural disturbance. The later work of Arnold et al. (1995a, 1997a) overcomes this deficiency in different ways and provides some further evidence for a disturbance in the location, clustering and/or size of entorhinal cortex neurons, though of much lesser magnitude and frequency than reported by Jakob and Beckmann. The most serious problem is that none of these studies have fully allowed for the heterogeneous cytoarchitecture of the entorhinal cortex (Beall and Lewis, 1992; Insausti et al., 1995) and its variation between individuals (Heinsen et al., 1996; Krimer et al., 1997a; West and Slomianka, 1998). For example, as Akil and Lewis (1997) point out, Jakob and Beckmann (1986) sampled their material based on external landmarks which may shift relative to the entorhinal cortex in schizophrenia, resulting in differences in the rostrocaudal location of the sections, which could account for their findings. Notably, the two studies that most closely attend to the issue of anatomical complexity within the entorhinal cortex found no differences in its cytoarchitecture in schizophrenia (Akil and Lewis, 1997; Krimer et al., 1997a).

Disarray of hippocampal pyramidal neurons.

A second parameter of cytoarchitectural disturbance in schizophrenia, a disarray of hippocampal pyramidal neurons, has also been given prominence disproportionate to the strength of the data. Normally, pyramidal neurons in Ammon's horn are aligned, as in a palisade, with the apical dendrite orientated towards the stratum radiatum. Kovelman and Scheibel (1984) reported that this orientation was more variable and even reversed in schizophrenia, hence the term 'neuronal disarray'. The disarray was present at the boundaries of CA1 with CA2 and subiculum. The basic finding of greater variability of hippocampal neuronal orientation was extended in subsequent studies from the same group (Altshuler et al., 1987; Conrad et al., 1991) and independently (Jønsson et al., 1997; Zaidel et al., 1997a). However, none of these studies constitutes true replication.

Conrad et al. (1991) came closest, but located the disarray at the boundaries of CA2 rather than CA1; Altshuler et al. (1987) found no differences between cases and controls merely a correlation between the degree of disarray and severity of psychosis within the schizophrenic group; disarray in the small study of Jønsson et al. (1997) was the central part of each CA field, and Zaidel et al. (199? found no overall difference in orientation but, in a post h analysis, found an asymmetrical variability limited to a p of CA3. Furthermore, there are three entirely negative stud (Christison et al., 1989; Benes et al., 1991b; Arnold et a 1995a). Thus, even a charitable overview of the data wo accept that the site and frequency of hippocampal neuro disarray in schizophrenia remains uncertain, while a scepti view would be that the phenomenon has not be unequivocally demonstrated. Certainly, as with the entorhi cortex abnormalities, it seems inappropriate to place too mu interpretative weight on such insecure empirical foundatio

Location of cortical subplate neurons.

The subpl is a key structure in the formation of the cortex and i orderly ingrowth of thalamic axons (Allendoerfer and Sha 1994). Some of the subplate neurons persist as interstit neurons in the subcortical white matter and contribute cortical and corticothalamic circuits. Stimulated by t entorhinal and hippocampal cytoarchitectural findin suggestive of aberrant neuronal migration, subplate neurc have been studied in schizophrenia, since changes in t density and distribution of these neurons would probably a correlate of such a disturbance. Using nicotinamide-adeni dinucleotide phosphate-diaphorase histochemistry as marker, these neurons were found to be distributed mc deeply in the frontal and temporal cortex white matter schizophrenics than in controls (Akbarian et al., 1993a, A subsequent survey using additional markers and a larg sample confirmed the observation of fewer interstitial neurc in superficial white matter compartments of DLPFC schizophrenia (Akbarian et al., 1996).

These data are more convincing than the reports entorhinal cortex dysplasias and hippocampal neuron disarr and the studies are noteworthy for being embedded in known cellular biology of cortical development. Neverthele it would be premature to consider maldistribution of surviv subplate neurons, and by inference aberrant neuro migration, to be an established feature of schizophrenia. Fir Dwork (1997) has drawn attention to the doubtful statistic significance of the original results (Akbarian et al., 1993a, Secondly, in the follow-up study (Akbarian et al., 1996) abnormalities were milder and less prevalent, and th statistical significance was enhanced by the apparent retenti of the original cases. Thirdly, considerable variation in abundance of interstitial neurons has been found betwe individuals and between frontal and temporal white mat (Rojiani et al., 1996), suggesting that sample sizes larg than those employed to date may be necessary to ident clearly any alterations associated with schizophrenia. Fina as shown in Table 1B, Anderson *et al.* (1996) found essentially the opposite result from that of Akbarian *et al.* (1996). Further investigations are therefore essential to corroborate the potentially key observations of Akbarian and colleagues.

Hippocampal and cortical neuron density and number. A loss of hippocampal neurons is another oft-stated feature of schizophrenia. In fact only two studies have found reductions in neuron density (Jeste and Lohr, 1989; Jønsson *et al.*, 1997) and one reported a lower number of pyramidal neurons (Falkai and Bogerts, 1986). In contrast, several have found no change in density (Kovelman and Scheibel, 1984; Falkai and Bogerts, 1986; Benes *et al.*, 1991*b*; Arnold *et al.*, 1995*a*) and one found a localized increase (Zaidel *et al.*, 1997*b*). Since none of these studies were stereological, their value is limited by the inherent weaknesses of neuron counts when measured in this way (Mayhew and Gundersen, 1996)—although not to the extent that they should be discounted (Guillery and Herrup, 1997). Nevertheless, the fact that the single stereological study that has been carried out found no difference in neuronal number or density in any subfield (Heckers *et al.*, 1991*a*) supports the view that there is no overall change in the neuron content of the hippocampus in schizophrenia. In this context, single reports of altered neuronal density restricted to a specific neuronal type or subfield (Zaidel *et al.*, 1997*a*; Benes *et al.*, 1998) must be replicated before discussion is warranted.

The prefrontal cortex has also been examined. A careful stereologically based study found an increased neuronal density in DLPFC (Selemon *et al.*, 1995, 1998), and a similar trend was seen for the whole frontal lobe by Pakkenberg (1993*b*). The higher packing density identified by Selemon and colleagues affected small and medium-sized neurons more than large pyramidal ones. Other neuronal density studies in the prefrontal cortex have not produced consistent findings (Table 1B). For example, Benes *et al.* (1986, 1991*a*) identified a variety of lamina-, area- and cell type-specific differences, whilst unaltered neuronal density has been reported in the motor cortex (Arnold *et al.*, 1995*a*) and DLPFC (Akbarian *et al.*, 1995). These discrepancies may be due to anatomical heterogeneity or may be the consequence of differences in the stereological purity of the studies. The total number of neurons in the frontal cortex is not altered in schizophrenia (Pakkenberg, 1993*b*), which probably reflects the net effect of anatomical variation in the neuronal density changes within the frontal lobe and/or the trend for cortical grey matter to be thinner in schizophrenia, which compensates for the increased packing density of neurons therein (Pakkenberg, 1987; Selemon *et al.*, 1998; Woo *et al.*, 1998).

Hippocampal and cortical neuronal size. With the advent of user-friendly image analysis it has become relatively straightforward to measure the size of the cell body of neurons, either by tracing around the perikaryal outline or by measuring the smallest circle within which the soma fits.

Three studies, each counting large numbers of neurons, have now identified a smaller mean size of hippocampal pyramidal neurons in schizophrenia (Benes *et al.*, 1991*a*; Arnold *et al.*, 1995*a*; Zaidel *et al.*, 1997*a*). Although different individual subfields reached significance in the latter two studies, the same downward trend was present in all CA fields and in the subiculum. The non-replications comprise Christison *et al.* (1989) and Benes *et al.* (1998), perhaps because measurements were limited to a restricted subset of neurons. Smaller neuronal size has also been reported in DLPFC, especially affecting large lamina IIIc neurons (Rajkowska *et al.*, 1998). A degree of anatomical specificity to the size reductions is apparent, since this study found no differences in the visual cortex of the same cases, in agreement with the unchanged cell size found in that region as well as in the motor cortex by Arnold *et al.* (1995*a*) and Benes *et al.* (1986).

Neuronal morphometric changes in other regions. Outside the cerebral cortex, consistent cytoarchitectural data are limited to the thalamus (Table 1C). Pakkenberg (1990) found markedly lower numbers of neurons in the dorsomedial nucleus, which projects mainly to the prefrontal cortex. A similar finding was observed in the anteroventral nucleus, which also has primarily prefrontal connections, the significant deficit affecting parvalbumin-immunoreactive cells, a marker for thalamocortical neurons (Danos *et al.*, 1998). Whether similar changes occur in thalamic nuclei not intimately related to cortical regions implicated in schizophrenia remains to be determined.

In summary, a range of differences in neuronal parameters have been reported to occur in schizophrenia. The abnormalities most often taken to be characteristic of the disorder—disarray, displacement and paucity of hippocampal and cortical neurons—are in fact features which have not been clearly demonstrated. This undermines attempts to date the pathology of schizophrenia to the second trimester *in utero* based on their presence (see below). In contrast, decreased neuron size, especially affecting neurons in the hippocampus and DLPFC, has been shown fairly convincingly; some studies suggest that the size reduction is accompanied by increased neuron density. The other relatively robust cytoarchitectural abnormality in schizophrenia is in the dorsal thalamus, which is smaller and contains fewer neurons.

Studies of synapses and dendrites. Synaptic abnormalities represent a potential site for significant pathology in schizophrenia which would be undetectable using standard histological approaches. The term 'synaptic pathology' is used here to denote abnormalities in axons and dendrites in addition to those affecting the synaptic terminals themselves.

Practical issues. Qualitative studies identified a range of ultrastructural abnormalities of neuronal and synaptic elements in schizophrenia (Tatetsu *et al.*, 1964; Miyakawa *et al.*, 1972; Averback, 1981; Soustek, 1989; Ong and Garey,

1993). However, because of the difficulties and limitations of electron microscopy in post-mortem human brain tissue, especially for quantitative analysis, much contemporary research into synaptic pathology in schizophrenia has adopted a complementary approach whereby the expression and abundance of proteins concentrated in presynaptic terminals, such as synaptophysin, are used as proxies for synapses. This approach has been validated in several experimental and disease states (Masliah and Terry, 1993; Eastwood et al., 1994a). For example, in Alzheimer's disease, synaptophysin mRNA and protein levels correlate inversely with the clinical and pathological severity of dementia (Terry et al., 1991; Heffernan et al., 1998). Note, however, that although synaptic protein measurements are widely interpreted as reflecting synaptic density, an assumption almost certainly true in neurodegenerative disorders, in principle changes in synaptic protein expression could instead be due to alterations in synaptic size or number of vesicles per terminal, or to a structural abnormality of the presynaptic region. Such possibilities should not be ignored in schizophrenia, given that ultrastructural features of this kind were suggested by some of the electron microscopy studies mentioned above.

Hippocampal formation. Synaptic protein determinations in the hippocampal formation (hippocampus and parahippocampal gyrus) in schizophrenia have fairly consistently found levels to be reduced (Table 2A), although not all reach statistical significance for reasons other than just inadequate sample size. First, subfields may be differentially affected (Eastwood and Harrison, 1995; Eastwood et al., 1995a), and localized changes may be masked if homogenized tissue is used. Secondly, the synaptic proteins studied change to varying degrees, probably reflecting their concentration in differentially affected synaptic populations. For example, synaptophysin, which is present in all synapses, shows only slight reductions (Browning et al., 1993; Eastwood and Harrison, 1995; Eastwood et al., 1995a), whereas SNAP-25 (Young et al., 1998) and complexin II (Harrison and Eastwood, 1998), which are both concentrated in subsets of synapses, show greater decrements. Furthermore, complexin II is primarily expressed by excitatory neurons, unlike complexin I, which is mainly present in inhibitory neurons and is less affected in schizophrenia (Harrison and Eastwood, 1998). Thus, these data suggest a particular involvement of excitatory pathways in this region, a conclusion in keeping with neurochemical studies of the glutamatergic system (see below). A final example of current attempts to dissect out the nature of hippocampal synaptic involvement in schizophrenia is provided by a study of the expression of the neuronal growth-associated protein-43 (GAP-43), a marker of synaptic plasticity (Benowitz and Routtenberg, 1997). A loss of hippocampal GAP-43 mRNA was found, suggesting that hippocampal synapses may be remodelled less actively in schizophrenia (Eastwood and Harrison, 1998).

Less attention has been paid to postsynaptic elements of the hippocampal circuitry. However, dendritic abnormalities have been reported, with decreased and aberrant expression of the dendritic microtubule-associated protein MAP-2 in some subfields (Arnold et al., 1991b; Cotter et al., 1997).

Neocortex. Two studies have found synaptophysin to be reduced in DLPFC in schizophrenia (Perrone-Bizzozero et al. 1996; Glantz and Lewis, 1997). The inferred decrease of presynaptic terminals is complemented by a lower density of dendritic spines (to which many of the synapses are apposed) on layer III pyramidal neurons (Garey et al. 1998). The pattern of synaptophysin alteration is not uniform throughout the cortex, since levels are unchanged in the visual cortex (Perrone-Bizzozero et al., 1996; Glantz and Lewis, 1997) and increased in the cingulate gyrus (Gabriel et al., 1997). The suggestion that there is a discrete profile of synaptic pathology in the cingulate gyrus is noteworthy given the other cytoarchitectural and ultrastructural findings in that region (Tables 1B and 2B), such as increased glutamatergic axons (Benes et al., 1987, 1992a) and axospinous synapses (Aganova and Uranova, 1992), and deficits in inhibitory interneurons (Benes et al., 1991a) which have not been reported elsewhere. However, further direct comparisons are needed before it can be concluded that the cingulate exhibits a different pattern of pathology.

Thalamus. A marked reduction of the synaptic protein rab3a from the thalamus was found in a large group of schizophrenics compared with controls (Blennow et al. 1996). These data, in concert with the morphometric and imaging findings (Table 1C), highlight the thalamus as meriting active investigation in schizophrenia (Jones, 1997a) a somewhat belated return to the one brain region for which the earlier generation of studies had produced potentially meaningful findings (David, 1957).

Striatum. In the striatum, electron microscopy rather than immunocytochemical measurements has continued to be used to investigate synaptic pathology in schizophrenia. Altered sizes and proportions of synapses in the caudate nucleus have been found compared with controls (Table 2C). It is difficult to interpret these findings and integrate them with those in other regions because of the methodological differences and the greater concern about confounding effect of antipsychotic medication in basal ganglia (see below). Nevertheless, they broadly support the view that synaptic organization is altered in schizophrenia.

In summary, synaptic studies in the hippocampus and DLPFC in schizophrenia show decrements in presynaptic markers and, though less extensively studied, in postsynaptic markers too. The simplest interpretation is that these changes reflect a reduction in the number of synaptic contacts formed and received in these areas, bearing in mind the caveat about alternative possibilities such as abnormal synaptic vesicle composition or even dysregulation of synaptic protein gene transcription. In pathogenic terms, the direction of the synaptic alterations in the hippocampus and DLPFC supports hypotheses of excessive (Keshavan *et al.*, 1994*a*) rather than inadequate (Feinberg, 1982) synaptic pruning in schizophrenia. Since the reductions are not uniform in magnitude or location, it is likely that certain synaptic populations are more affected than others; preliminary evidence suggests glutamatergic synapses may be especially vulnerable in the hippocampus and perhaps the DLPFC, with predominantly GABAergic involvement in the cingulate gyrus. There is a need not only to extend the work (e.g. to include confocal microscopy and to measure additional synaptic proteins) but to integrate it with further Golgi staining and electron microscope investigations directly visualizing synapses and dendrites.

Integrating the neuronal and synaptic pathological findings

Despite the limitations of the neuronal (Table 1) and synaptic (Table 2) data in schizophrenia, there is an encouraging convergence between the two, at least in the hippocampus and DLPFC, from where most data have been obtained (Fig. 1). In particular, the fact that presynaptic and dendritic markers are generally decreased in schizophrenia is in keeping with the finding of smaller neuronal cell bodies, since perikaryal size is proportional to the extent of the dendritic (Hayes and Lewis, 1996; Elston and Rosa, 1998) and axonal (Ho *et al.*, 1992; Pierce and Lewin, 1994) tree. It is also consistent with the findings of increased neuron density, in that dendrites, axons and synapses are the major component of the neuropil and, if the latter is reduced, neurons will pack more closely together (Schlaug *et al.*, 1993). Moreover, there is a correspondence with the results of proton MRS (magnetic resonance spectroscopy) and MRS-imaging studies of the hippocampus and DLPFC in schizophrenia, which have shown reductions in signal for the neuronal marker NAA (*N*-acetyl-aspartate) (Maier *et al.*, 1995; Bertolino *et al.*, 1996; Deicken *et al.*, 1997, 1998), as one would predict if the constituent neurons are on average smaller and have less extensive axonal arborizations. (Given the morphometric findings in schizophrenia, this is a more plausible explanation than attributing the NAA reduction to a lower neuronal density.) Parenthetically, the lowered NAA signal is seen in unmedicated (Bertolino *et al.*, 1998) and first-episode (Renshaw *et al.*, 1995) schizophrenia, as are alterations in ^{31}P-MRS phosphoester signals suggestive of synaptic pathology (Kegeles *et al.*, 1998). These findings imply that the cytoarchitectural abnormalities seen in post-mortem studies, which inevitably are limited to chronic schizophrenia, may also be present at this early stage.

Schizophrenia and cerebral asymmetry

Neuropathological findings have been prominent in maintaining the persistent belief that there is an important

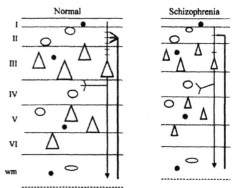

Fig. 1 Schematic cartoon exaggerating the putative cytoarchitectural features of schizophrenia. The grey matter contains an unchanged number of neurons, but the pyramidal neurons (black triangles) are smaller and more densely packed. The cortex is thinner, especially in laminae II and III. The reduced neuron size and increased neuron density are both correlates of a reduced neuropil volume, which in turn reflects abnormalities affecting the axonal (green) and dendritic (red) arborizations of some neurons. For example, there may be less extensive, or otherwise aberrant, synaptic connections formed by incoming corticocortical fibres (hollow green lines, shown as having shorter terminations on dendritic spines, denoted by thin red lines) and by axon collaterals (solid green lines, shown as being shorter and in a different position) of efferent pyramidal neurons. Glia (grey filled circles) are unaffected. Although the figure illustrates the situation in the prefrontal neocortex, a similar diagram could be drawn for the hippocampus. For clarity, possible differences in the distribution and synaptic organization of interneuron subpopulations (blue and brown) and white matter (wm) neurons (purple), as well as the pattern of changes in the cingulate gyrus and subcortical structures, are omitted.

interaction between schizophrenia and cerebral asymmetry (Crichton-Browne, 1879). Interest in this question was rekindled by the report that schizophrenia-like psychosis is commoner in temporal lobe epilepsy when the focus is in the left hemisphere (Flor-Henry, 1969), and has been reinforced by the observations in schizophrenia of decreased left parahippocampal width (Brown *et al.*, 1986) and ventricular enlargement limited to the left temporal horn (Crow *et al.*, 1989). Several other recent reports indicate that normal asymmetries are reduced or even reversed in schizophrenia, and that the pathological findings—as well as neuropsychological, neurochemical and electrophysiological abnormalities—are more pronounced in the left hemisphere (Crow, 1997).

Key studies which have been able to address the issue of lateralized pathology in schizophrenia are summarized in Table 3. Though no firm conclusion can be drawn, alterations in normal asymmetries, and a left-sided 'preference' of the pathology, are findings that seem to be more common than one would expect by chance. Insofar as there is a phenomenon

Table 3 *Cerebral asymmetry and the neuropathology of schizophrenia*

	Key positive reports*	Relevant negative reports[†]
Macroscopic features		
Decreased fronto-occipital torque	Bilder *et al.*, 1994; DeLisi *et al.*, 1997*b*	DeLisi *et al.*, 1997*b*
Decreased size of left superior temporal gyrus	Shenton *et al.*, 1992	Flaum *et al.*, 1995
Reversal of left > right planum temporale size asymmetry	Falkai *et al.*, 1995; Barta *et al.*, 1997[‡]	Kulynych *et al.*, 1996
Loss of left > right sylvian fissure length	Falkai *et al.*, 1992	
Left parahippocampal thinning	Brown *et al.*, 1986[§]	
Left temporal horn enlargement	Crow *et al.*, 1989	
Left medial temporal lobe reductions	Bogerts *et al.*, 1990*a*; Pearlson *et al.*, 1997	Altshuler *et al.*, 1990; Bogerts *et al.*, 1990*b*; Nelson *et al*, 1998
Progressive left ventricular enlargement in severe cases	Davis *et al.*, 1998	
Cytoarchitectural asymmetries		
Asymmetrical size and shape changes in hippocampal neurons	Zaidel *et al.*, 1997*a*	
Increased right hippocampal neuron density	Zaidel *et al.*, 1997*b*	
Loss of synaptic protein from left thalamus	Blennow *et al.*, 1996	

For additional references see Falkai and Bogerts (1993) and Crow (1997). *With clear evidence for lateralised change (e.g. diagnosis × side interaction on ANOVA). [†]Studies where the change was found bilaterally. [‡]Planum temporale area reduced unilaterally, but volume reduced bilaterally. [§]Relative to affective disorder controls.

to be explained, two hypotheses exist. Crow's evolving and evolutionary theory is that schizophrenia, cerebral dominance, handedness and language are inextricably and causally linked to each other and to a single gene (Crow, 1990, 1997). Alternatively, altered asymmetry in schizophrenia is viewed as an epiphenomenon of its *in utero* origins, a process which interferes with subsequent brain lateralization (Bracha, 1991; Roberts, 1991). Clarifying how the neuropathology interacts with cerebral asymmetry thus requires not only additional, appropriately designed studies of schizophrenia and other neurodevelopmental disorders, but also a better understanding of the causes and consequences of histological asymmetries *per se* (Galaburda, 1994; Hayes and Lewis, 1996; Anderson and Rutledge, 1996). Interactions between asymmetry, gender and schizophrenia introduce further complexity to the issue (Highley *et al.*, 1998, 1999; Vogeley *et al.*, 1998).

Interpretation of the neuropathology of schizophrenia

Neuropathology and the neurodevelopmental model

The concept of developmental insanity was proposed by Clouston in 1891 (Murray and Woodruff, 1995) and elaborated in neuropathological terms early this century (Southard, 1915). However, it is only in the past decade that a neurodevelopmental origin for schizophrenia has become the prevailing pathogenic hypothesis for the disorder; indeed the principle is now largely unchallenged (Murray and Lewis, 1987; Weinberger, 1987, 1995). The model receives support from various sources, the neuropathological data forming an important component of the evidence (Table 4) (Harrison, 1997*a*; Raedler *et al.*, 1998).

The most influential and specific form of the theory is that the pathology of schizophrenia originates in the middle stage of intrauterine life (Roberts, 1991; Bloom, 1993; Roberts *et al.*, 1997). An earlier timing is excluded since overt abnormalities in the structure and cellular content of the cerebral cortex would be expected if neurogenesis were affected, whilst the absence of gliosis is taken to mean that the changes must have occurred prior to the third trimester. The conclusion that, by default, the pathological process originates in the second trimester is bolstered by reference to certain of the cytoarchitectural abnormalities of schizophrenia. However, this 'strong' form of the neurodevelopmental model is weak on two grounds. First, because of the limitations of the absence-of-gliosis argument mentioned earlier. Secondly, the types of cytoarchitectural disturbance adduced in favour are those of neuronal disarray, heterotopias and malpositioning suggestive of aberrant migration (Kovelman and Scheibel, 1984; Jakob and Beckmann, 1986; Arnold *et al.*, 1991*a*; Akbarian *et al.*, 1993*a*, *b*), processes which occur at the appropriate gestational period; yet, as described above, none of these cytoarchitectural abnormalities has been unequivocally established to be a feature of schizophrenia. By comparison, the other cytoarchitectural findings, such as alterations in neuronal size and synaptic and dendritic organization, could well originate much later, being susceptible to ongoing environmental influences (Jones and Schallert, 1994; Moser *et al.*, 1994; Saito *et al.*, 1994; Andrade *et al.*, 1996; Kolb and Whishaw, 1998), ageing (Huttenlocher, 1979; Braak and Braak, 1986; Masliah *et al.*, 1993; de Brabander *et al.*, 1998) and perhaps also to genetic factors (Vaughn *et al.*, 1977; Williams *et al.*, 1998).

Other versions of the neurodevelopmental theory of

Table 4 *Key points of evidence for a neurodevelopmental origin of schizophrenia*

Neuropathological evidence
  Ventricular enlargement and decreased cortical volume present at onset of symptoms, if not earlier
  Presence and nature of cytoarchitectural abnormalities
  Absence of gliosis and other neurodegenerative features
  Increased prevalence of abnormal septum pellucidum (Shioiri *et al.*, 1996; Kwon *et al.*, 1998)

Other evidence
  The environmental risk factors are mostly obstetric complications (Geddes and Lawrie, 1995)
  Children destined to develop schizophrenia in adulthood show neuromotor, behavioural and intellectual impairment (Jones, 1997*b*)
  Increased prevalence of abnormal dermatoglyphics and minor physical anomalies (Buckley, 1998)
  Experimental neonatal lesions have delayed effects on relevant behavioural and neurochemical indices

For additional references see text.

schizophrenia postulate additional or alternative abnormalities in processes such as cell adhesion, myelination and synaptic pruning (e.g. Keshavan *et al.*, 1994*a*; Benes *et al.*, 1994; Akbarian *et al.*, 1996; Arnold and Trojanowski, 1996; Lewis, 1997) or allow for a mixture of maturational and degenerative processes (e.g. Murray *et al.*, 1992; Garver, 1997). Overall, a parsimonious view is that the extant cytoarchitectural abnormalities and lack of gliosis are indicative merely of an essentially neurodevelopmental as opposed to neurodegenerative disease process, rather than as pointing directly to a particular mechanism or timing. It is only by consideration of the pathological features in conjunction with the other evidence (Table 4) that a strong case for a significant early childhood, including foetal, component to schizophrenia can be made. Even then, it is unknown whether neurodevelopmental deviance is either necessary or sufficient. Moreover, any such model has a problem explaining the onset and outcome of the disorder: how is an abnormality in the cortical cytoarchitecture, present since early in life and presumably persistent, reconciled with the onset of symptoms in adulthood and a typically relapsing and remitting course thereafter? Regarding the explanation for the timing of psychosis, one can take refuge in the similar difficulties in explaining some epilepsies, and point to the fact that pathological and behavioural effects can clearly be long delayed after relevant neonatal lesions (Beauregard *et al.*, 1995; Lipska and Weinberger, 1995; Saunders *et al.*, 1998). It can also be argued that the expression of psychotic symptoms requires a brain which has reached a certain stage of biochemical and anatomical maturation. Explaining the course of the disorder is more difficult and entirely speculative. It may be hypothesized that the aberrant circuitry is rendered 'unstable' (e.g. is more susceptible to neurochemical fluctuations which precipitate recurrence) or is unable to undergo normal plasticity in response to age-related and environmental factors (Stevens, 1992; DeLisi, 1997; Lieberman *et al.*, 1997).

Neuropathology and neurochemistry

The neurochemical pathology of schizophrenia is outside the scope of this review, but it is pertinent to summarize some key recent findings (Table 5) and their relationship to the neuropathology. For more extensive coverage see Owen and Simpson (1995) and Reynolds (1995).

Dopamine

The dopamine hypothesis proposes that the symptoms of schizophrenia are due to dopaminergic overactivity. This might arise due to excess dopamine itself or to an elevated sensitivity to it, e.g. because of increased numbers of dopamine receptors. The hypothesis originated with the discovery that all effective antipsychotic drugs are dopamine (D_2) receptor antagonists, and that dopamine-releasing agents such as amphetamine can produce a paranoid psychosis. It received support from findings of increased dopamine content and higher densities of D_2 receptors in schizophrenia (summarized in Roberts *et al.*, 1997). However, despite the longevity of this hypothesis there is still no consensus as to the nature of the supposed abnormality or any evidence that dopamine has a causal role in the disorder (Davis *et al.*, 1991; Joyce and Meador-Woodruff, 1997). There are two main difficulties. First, antipsychotics have marked effects on the dopamine system, seriously confounding all studies of medicated subjects. Secondly, the molecular characterization of the dopamine receptor family has greatly increased the number of potential sites of dysfunction and the mechanisms by which it might occur in schizophrenia.

There is no doubt that D_2 receptor densities are increased in schizophrenia, but considerable doubt as to what proportion is not attributable to antipsychotic treatment (Zakzanis and Hansen, 1998), especially given that PET studies of D_2 receptors in drug-naive, first-episode cases are largely negative (Nordstrom *et al.*, 1995). There are reports of altered D_1 (Okubo *et al.*, 1997) and D_3 (Gurevich *et al.*, 1997) receptors in schizophrenia, but these are either unconfirmed or contradicted by other studies (see Harrison, 1999*b*). The D_4 receptor has proved particularly controversial following a report that its density was increased several-fold in schizophrenia, seemingly independently of medication (Seeman *et al.*, 1993). However, it appears that the result was due to a 'D_4-like site' rather than the true D_4 receptor (Reynolds, 1996; Seeman *et al.*, 1997). In summary, the status

Table 5 *Summary of recent neurochemical findings in schizophrenia*

	Strength of evidence
Dopamine	
Increased striatal D_2 receptors	++++*
Increased dopamine content or metabolism	+++*
Increased amphetamine-stimulated dopamine transmission	+++
Decreased cortical D_1 receptors	+
Increased cortical D_3 receptors	+
Increased D_4 receptors	+/–
Abnormal configuration of D_2 receptors	+/–
Altered dopamine receptor–G protein coupling	+/–
5-HT	
Decreased cortical 5-HT_{2A} receptors	+++
Increased cortical 5-HT_{1A} receptors	++
CSF 5-HIAA concentrations related to negative symptoms	+
Glutamate	
Decreased expression of hippocampal non-NMDA receptors	++
Increased cortical expression of some NMDA receptor subunits	++
Increased glutamate reuptake in frontal cortex	+
Decreased cortical glutamate release	·+
Altered concentrations of glutamate and metabolites	+/–

+/– = weak ; + = moderate; ++ = good; +++ = strong; ++++ = shown by meta-analysis. *Though much of the increase is c to antipsychotic medication (see text).

of dopamine receptors in schizophrenia is still contentious. In contrast, there is emerging evidence for a presynaptic dopaminergic abnormality in schizophrenia, with PET and single photon emission tomography displacement studies indicating an elevated dopamine release in response to amphetamine (Laruelle *et al.*, 1996; Breier *et al.*, 1997; Abi-Dargham *et al.*, 1998), implying a dysregulation and hyper-responsiveness of dopaminergic neurons. This is a potentially important finding which needs further investigation.

5-Hydroxytryptamine (5-HT; serotonin)

The idea that 5-HT is involved in schizophrenia has long been advocated because the hallucinogen LSD is a 5-HT agonist. Current interest centres on the role of the 5-HT_{2A} receptor (Harrison and Burnet, 1997) because a high affinity for the receptor may explain the different therapeutic and side-effect profile of novel antipsychotics (Meltzer, 1996), and polymorphisms of the gene are reported to be a minor risk factor for schizophrenia (Williams *et al.*, 1997) and response to the atypical antipsychotic drug clozapine (Arranz *et al.*, 1998). Neurochemically, many studies have found lowered 5-HT_{2A} receptor expression in the frontal cortex in schizophrenia (Harrison, 1999b), and there is a blunted neuroendocrine response to 5-HT_2 agonists (Abi-Dargham *et al.*, 1997). An elevated number of cortical 5-HT_{1A} receptors is also a replicated finding (Burnet *et al.*, 1997). Both the 5-HT_{1A} and 5-HT_{2A} receptor alterations are seen in unmedicated subjects post-mortem, but a preliminary PET study has not shown any change in 5-HT_{2A} receptors in younger, medication-free patients (Trichard *et al.*, 1998), suggesting

that the abnormalities may emerge during the course the illness.

Hypotheses to explain 5-HT involvement in schizophre include alterations in the trophic role of 5-HT neurodevelopment, impaired 5-HT_{2A} receptor-media activation of the prefrontal cortex, and interactions betw 5-HT and dopamine (Kapur and Remington, 1996).

Glutamate

Phencyclidine and other non-competitive antagonists of NMDA (N-methyl-D-aspartate) subtype of glutamate recep produce a psychosis closely resembling schizophrenia (Ja and Zukin, 1991). This has driven the hypothesis glutamatergic dysfunction in schizophrenia. In support, th is now considerable evidence for abnormalities in pre-postsynaptic glutamate indices (Table 5). For example, in medial temporal lobe, glutamatergic markers are decrea and there is reduced expression of non-NMDA subtypes glutamate receptor (Kerwin *et al.*, 1990; Eastwood *et* 1995b, 1997b; Porter *et al.*, 1997). However, a differ pattern is seen in other brain regions, affecting other glutam receptor subtypes (Roberts *et al.*, 1997), precluding simple conclusion regarding the nature of glutamater abnormality in schizophrenia (Tamminga, 1998).

Mechanisms proposed to explain glutamatergic invol ment in schizophrenia centre on its interactions w dopamine (Carlsson and Carlsson, 1990), subtle forms excitotoxicity (Olney and Farber, 1995) and a developme abnormality of corticocortical connections (Deakin Simpson, 1997).

Relationship between neurochemical and neuropathological findings

Even from this brief, selective review it is apparent that there is still no clear picture as to the cardinal neurochemical features of schizophrenia or their position in the pathogenesis of the disorder. The main point, *vis a vis* neuropathology, is that the presence of structural abnormalities, however slight, must be taken into account. That is, a change in the level of a neurotransmitter, receptor or any other molecule may be due to dysfunction in the cells producing it or a change in the cellular constituents of the tissue being evaluated, rather than being indicative of a molecularly specific abnormality. This applies to *in vivo* functional imaging as well to neurochemistry, and affects discussions as to the putative causes and consequences of any alteration. Whilst an obvious point to make, it has not always been appreciated in schizophrenia research, perhaps because of the belief that the brain is entirely normal, structurally speaking. As an example, consider the case of 5-HT receptors. In the prefrontal cortex in schizophrenia, we and others have found a loss of 5-HT$_{2A}$ receptors and an accompanying increase of 5-HT$_{1A}$ receptors (Burnet *et al.*, 1996, 1997). In this region, the 5-HT$_{2A}$ receptor is expressed by pyramidal neurons, interneurons and perhaps glia (Burnet *et al.*, 1995; Jakab and Goldman-Rakic, 1998), whilst the 5-HT$_{1A}$ receptor is expressed exclusively, or virtually so, by pyramidal neurons (Burnet *et al.*, 1995). Thus it is unclear whether the 5-HT receptor changes seen in schizophrenia arise from differential involvement of the cell types concerned or from opposing abnormalities in the regulation of expression of each receptor subtype. Similarly, it is difficult to interpret unambiguously the various glutamatergic and dopaminergic abnormalities reported in schizophrenia, or the deficits in GABA which are also apparent (Simpson *et al.*, 1989; Benes *et al.*, 1992*b*; Akbarian *et al.*, 1995), independently of the morphometric alterations in excitatory and inhibitory neurons and their synapses discussed above. More sophisticated analyses are needed in order to establish when a neurochemical finding in schizophrenia is really that, and when it is a reflection of neuropathology.

Neuropathology and aberrant functional connectivity

Bleuler, who coined the term schizophrenia, stated 'the thousands of associations guiding our thought are interrupted by this disease . . . The thought processes, as a result, become strange and illogical, and the associations find new paths' (Bleuler, 1950). His view that the key symptoms of schizophrenia were those of 'psychic splitting' now have their counterparts in neuropsychological models and in imaging studies which have implicated aberrant functional connectivity between different brain regions as the patho-physiological mechanism of psychosis (Friston and Frith, 1995; McGuire and Frith, 1996; Andreasen *et al.*, 1996;

Bullmore *et al.*, 1998). Although the evidence in favour of altered connectivity in schizophrenia remains circumstantial and its details poorly specified, the concept has been widely promulgated. Examples are shown in Table 6.

Here the specific hypothesis is elaborated that aberrant connectivity in schizophrenia has neuroanatomical roots: the neuropathology of the disorder is that of a miswiring of the neural circuitry within and between certain brain regions. This 'hard-wiring' theme (Mesulam, 1990), which can be traced back to Wernicke, is apparent in a number of experimental and theoretical perspectives (Table 6). However, aberrant functional connectivity does not presuppose or require an anatomical substrate, and neither is it synonymous with regional brain dysfunction (Friston, 1998). Hence the pathological evidence in schizophrenia must be considered on its own merits before attempts are made to integrate structure with function. Certainly, schizophrenia is not a disconnectivity syndrome akin to Alzheimer's disease, in which there is frank loss of connections due to neuronal and synaptic degeneration (Pearson and Powell, 1989; De Lacoste and White, 1993), but it is argued here that schizophrenia is a dysconnectivity or misconnectivity syndrome which affects the precise organization of the neural circuitry, and perhaps its plasticity characteristics (Randall, 1983; Haracz, 1985; Goodman, 1989; Walker and Diforio, 1997). It is in such terms that the cytoarchitectural abnormalities reported in schizophrenia can reasonably be interpreted as being a putative basis for at least a proportion of the aberrant connectivity. That is, the types of neuronal, synaptic and dendritic findings reviewed above are entirely consistent with aberrant functional connectivity. For example (Fig. 1), in DLPFC, lamina III pyramidal neurons are smaller (Rajkowska *et al.*, 1998), have fewer dendritic spines (Garey *et al.*, 1998) and receive fewer inhibitory inputs (Woo *et al.*, 1998); moreover there is a reduction in synaptophysin in this region (Glantz and Lewis, 1997). Since the layer III pyramidal neurons are the origin of corticocortical projections, it is reasonable to propose that this combination of abnormalities will result in dysfunction of pathways to and from the DLPFC, in keeping with the many neuropsychological and functional imaging data attesting to the involvement of this region in the pathophysiology of schizophrenia (Weinberger, 1987; Andreasen *et al.*, 1996; Pantelis *et al.*, 1997).

Much remains to be done before the hypothesized association between structure and function can be confirmed and shown to be causal. It will not be easy to falsify or to clarify its detail, and the overriding need at present is still to improve the robustness of the contributory data. Nevertheless, the goal should be kept firmly in mind when designing neuropathological investigations into schizo-phrenia.

Methodological issues

It is all too evident that schizophrenia pushes neuropathology to its technical and conceptual limit. As well as sharing the

Table 6 *Concepts of dysconnectivity in schizophrenia*

Approach	Comments and examples of findings in schizophrenia
Experimental	
Patterns of correlations	
of regional cerebral blood flow	Inverted temporal lobe activity correlation during frontal lobe tasks (Frith *et al.*, 1995)
of regional glucose metabolism	Fewer corticothalamic correlations (Katz *et al.*, 1996)
of regional brain volumes	Frontotemporal (Woodruff *et al.*, 1997) or thalamocortical (Portas *et al.*, 1998) dissociation
of volume with rCBF	Hippocampal size correlates with frontal rCBF (Weinberger *et al.*, 1992)
of volume with function	Hippocampal size correlates with frontal test performance (Bilder *et al.*, 1995)
of neuron density	Asymmetrical change in subfield correlations within and between hippocampi (Zaidel *et al.*, 1997b)
of gene expression	Increased inter-areal correlations of GAP-43 mRNA (Eastwood and Harrison, 1998)
Distribution of abnormalities	
Cytoarchitectural	Hippocampal (Arnold *et al.*, 1995a) and corticocortical (Rajkowska *et al.*, 1998) pathways
Neurochemical	Frontotemporal glutamatergic circuitry (Deakin and Simpson, 1997)
Profile of neuropsychological deficits	Frontostriatal dysfunction (Pantelis *et al.*, 1997)
Theoretical	
Comparison with other disorders affecting connectivity	Inattention syndromes (Mesulam and Geschwind, 1978); metachromatic leucodystrophy (Hyde *et al.*, 1992)
Anatomical considerations	Intrinsic DLPFC circuitry (Lewis, 1997); heteromodal association cortex (Pearlson *et al.*, 1996)
Pharmacoanatomical considerations	Corticostriatal glutamatergic dysfunction (Carlsson and Carlsson, 1990)
Evolutionary	Myelination (Randall, 1983); callosal pathways and language representation (Crow, 1998)
Modelling	Dopamine system (Cohen and Servan-Schreiber, 1992); synaptic pruning (Hoffman and Dobscha, 1989)
Other	Functional clustering (Tononi *et al.*, 1998)

Table 7 *Methodological problems in schizophrenia neuropathology*

Issues especially pertinent to neuropathological studies
  Availability of enough cases, with adequate documentation
  Duration of disease prior to death
  Dealing with other pathologies which may have produced a schizophrenia-like psychosis
  Confounding by concurrent illnesses
  Confounding by perimortem factors (e.g. mode of death, autopsy delay, tissue processing)
  Hemispheric structural asymmetries
  Is the neuropathology a result of schizophrenia? (e.g. caused by persistent symptoms, or a poor environment?)
  Selecting which brain areas to study
  Adherence to stereological principles
Issues common to all schizophrenia research
  Validity of the diagnosis
  Does the variable being measured relate to the syndrome of schizophrenia, or to a symptom? Is it categorical or dimensional?
  Is there heterogeneity?
  Is the variable affected by antipsychotic drugs or other treatments?
  Are subjects included in research representative?
  Use of a psychiatric control group

For further discussion of the methodological issues affecting neuropathological studies of schizophrenia, see Kleinman *et al.* (1995), Harrison (1996) and Hill *et al.* (1996).

difficulties inherent in schizophrenia research, neuropathological investigations are faced with additional problems, some of which have already been alluded to (Table 7). None are unique to schizophrenia, but they take on disproportionate importance given the nature of the pathology and the low signal-to-noise ratio.

Confounding by antipsychotic medication is almost unavoidable. However, it is a somewhat overemphasized problem, certainly for cortical cytoarchitectural studies, in that no correlations have been found with treatment exposure in any of the studies mentioned, and little or no effect of the drugs upon similar parameters has been found in the rat brain (Harrison, 1993). Though reassuring, these approaches cannot wholly eliminate medication as a confounder; study of brain

Table 8 *Certainty and doubt in schizophrenia neuropathology*

	Strength of evidence
Macroscopic findings	
Enlarged lateral and third ventricles	++++
Decreased cortical volume	++++
The above changes present in first-episode patients	+++
Disproportionate volume loss from temporal lobe (incl. hippocampus)	+++
Decreased thalamic volume	++
Cortical volume loss affects grey rather than white matter	++
Enlarged basal ganglia secondary to antipsychotic medication	+++
Histological findings	
Absence of gliosis as an intrinsic feature	+++
Smaller cortical and hippocampal neurons	+++
Fewer neurons in dorsal thalamus	+++
Reduced synaptic and dendritic markers in hippocampus	++
Maldistribution of white matter neurons	+
Entorhinal cortex dysplasia	+/−
Cortical or hippocampal neuron loss	+/−
Disarray of hippocampal neurons	+/−
Miscellaneous	
Alzheimer's disease is not commoner in schizophrenia	++++
Pathology interacts with cerebral asymmetries	++

+/− = weak ; + = moderate; ++ = good; +++ = strong; ++++ = shown by meta-analysis.

collected in the pre-antipsychotic era does (e.g. Altshuler *et al.*, 1987; Falkai *et al.*, 1988; Arnold *et al.*, 1991*b*), but has its own limitations such as the age of the material, changes in diagnostic practice, and the frequent occurrence of leucotomy, insulin coma and other potentially neurotoxic therapies (e.g. Lohr and Jeste, 1988; Pakkenberg, 1993*a*). In the striatum and substantia nigra there is greater evidence for antipsychotic drug-induced neuronal and synaptic changes, both in animals (Harrison, 1993; Eastwood *et al.*, 1994*b*, 1997*a*; Kelley *et al.*, 1997) and in post-mortem series (Christensen *et al.*, 1970; Jellinger, 1977). Investigations in these regions must therefore continue to take particular care to distinguish the effects of disease from those of medication.

Of all the factors listed in Table 7, the main one affecting the design and execution of neuropathological studies of schizophrenia is simply the collection of brains. This problem has worsened with the fall in autopsy rates, and is exaggerated by community care, which means that most deaths occur outside hospital and are frequently referred to the coroner, making acquisition of tissue for research practically and legally difficult. The decreased supply is compounded by exclusion of some potentially suitable subjects because of a lack of sufficient information about the clinical history or other confounders. A significant effort is needed to overcome these problems and allow continuing collection of brain tissue of adequate quality and quantity from subjects with schizophrenia and suitable controls, both healthy and those with other psychiatric disorders. This is not an undertaking to be embarked on lightly, nor is it easily funded, but it has been productively implemented in several centres (Arnold *et al.*, 1995*b*; Johnston *et al.*, 1997; Garey *et al.*, 1998).

A final issue to consider is how the types of neuropathological abnormality described in schizophrenia relate to the clinical phenotype, whether defined in terms of psychotic symptoms or neuropsychological profile (Elliott and Sahakian, 1995). Features such as decreased cortical volume and cytoarchitectural abnormalities are diagnostically non-specific, overlapping with those observed in other psychiatric and neurological conditions. There could be a diagnostic lesion characteristic of schizophrenia still going unrecognized, though this is increasingly implausible. Or it could be the precise combination of alterations and their location and timing which produces schizophrenia. Some clarification will emerge as other idiopathic, putatively neurodevelopmental conditions such as bipolar disorder (Benes *et al.*, 1998; Drevets *et al.*, 1998), autism (Raymond *et al.*, 1996; Bailey *et al.*, 1998) and Rett's syndrome (Belichenko *et al.*, 1997) begin to be investigated in the same fashion. A complete answer, however, will also probably require identification of the causative genes and a better understanding of the pathogenesis, not just the pathology, of schizophrenia. At this point, one re-encounters the circular problem: the goal of the research is to find a valid endophenotype, yet without one the goal may be unattainable.

Conclusions

Despite the many controversies and contradictions, there are now established facts about the neuropathology of schizophrenia (Table 8). The disorder is associated with ventricular enlargement and decreased cortical volume. The pathology is neither focal nor uniform, being most convincingly demonstrated in the hippocampus, prefrontal cortex and dorsal thalamus. The pattern of abnormalities is suggestive of a disturbance of connectivity within and between these regions, most likely originating during brain development. At the cellular level, the changes are manifested as abnormalities, mainly decrements, in perikaryal, presynaptic and dendritic parameters (Tables 1 and 2; Fig. 1). The phenotype of the affected neurons and synapses is unclear, though there is some evidence for preferential glutamatergic involvement in the hippocampus. The sorts of cytoarchitectural changes being proposed, whilst still speculative and perhaps better viewed as aberrant neuroanatomy rather than neuropathology *per se*, are in keeping with the clinical complexity of the syndrome which they are being invoked to explain, as well as with the results of various functional imaging, neurochemical and neuropsychological findings. Progress is now constrained more by the subtlety of the target pathology than by methodological limitations of the work; indeed, the best contemporary studies are prime examples of innovative, quantitative neuropathology research.

In 1915 the neuropathologist Southard boldly stated that 'structural (visible or invisible) changes of a maldevelopmental nature lie at the bottom of the [schizophrenia] disease process . . . Aside from the left-sidedness of the lesions and internal hydrocephalus, very striking is the preference of these changes to occupy the association centres of Fleschig'. A positive view of the field today is that empirical data are belatedly proving the correctness of these assertions. Conversely, a cynic might suggest that it is the invisibility which has proved the most robustly demonstrable, or that the current histological findings remain sufficiently vague and numerous to cover all possibilities, ensuring that one will turn out, with hindsight, to be similarly prescient. Certainly it is time to implement still better research, driven by specific hypotheses (e.g. Benes, 1998; Weickert and Weinberger, 1998). In this way the small but increasingly steady steps which are finally being taken can proceed to a clear identification of the pathological substrate(s) of schizophrenia.

Acknowledgements

I am grateful to the Wellcome Trust and the Stanley Foundation for research support. I wish to thank Tim Crow, Sharon Eastwood, Margaret Esiri, Gareth Roberts and the many other colleagues upon whose findings and ideas the review is based. Margaret Cousin kindly provided secretarial support.

References

Abi-Dargham A, Laruelle M, Aghajanian GK, Charney D, Krystal J. The role of serotonin in the pathophysiology and treatment of schizophrenia. [Review]. J Neuropsychiatry Clin Neurosci 1997; 9: 1–17.

Abi-Dargham A, Gil R, Krystal J, Baldwin RM, Seibyl JP, Bowers M, et al. Increased striatal dopamine transmission in schizophrenia: confirmation in a second cohort. Am J Psychiatry 1998; 155: 761–7.

Adams CE, DeMasters BK, Freedman R. Regional zinc staining in postmortem hippocampus from schizophrenic patients. Schizophr Res 1995; 18: 71–7.

Aganova EA, Uranova NA. Morphometric analysis of synaptic contacts in the anterior limbic cortex in the endogenous psychoses. Neurosci Behav Physiol 1992; 22: 59–65.

Ajtai BM, Kallai L, Kalman M. Capability for reactive gliosis develops prenatally in the diencephalon but not in the cortex of rats. Exp Neurol 1997; 146: 151–8.

Akbarian S, Bunney WE Jr, Potkin SG, Wigal SB, Hagman JO, Sandman CA, et al. Altered distribution of nicotinamide-adenine dinucleotide phosphate-diaphorase cells in frontal lobe of schizophrenics implies disturbances of cortical development. Arch Gen Psychiatry 1993a; 50: 169–77.

Akbarian S, Vinuela A, Kim JJ, Potkin SG, Bunney WE Jr, Jones EG. Distorted distribution of nicotinamide-adenine dinucleotide phosphate-diaphorase neurons in temporal lobe of schizophrenics implies anomalous cortical development. Arch Gen Psychiatry 1993b; 50: 178–87.

Akbarian S, Kim JJ, Potkin SG, Hagman JO, Tafazzoli A, Bunney WE Jr, et al. Gene expression for glutamic acid decarboxylase is reduced without loss of neurons in prefrontal cortex of schizophrenics [see comments]. Arch Gen Psychiatry 1995; 52: 258–66.

Akbarian S, Kim JJ, Potkin SG, Hetrick WP, Bunney WE Jr, Jones EG. Maldistribution of interstitial neurons in prefrontal white matter of the brains of schizophrenic patients. Arch Gen Psychiatry 1996; 53: 425–36.

Akil M, Lewis DA. Cytoarchitecture of the entorhinal cortex in schizophrenia. Am J Psychiatry 1997; 154: 1010–2.

Allendoerfer KL, Shatz CJ. The subplate, a transient neocortical structure: its role in the development of connections between thalamus and cortex. [Review]. Annu Rev Neurosci 1994; 17: 185–218.

Altshuler LL, Conrad A, Kovelman JA, Scheibel A. Hippocampal pyramidal cell orientation in schizophrenia. A controlled neurohistologic study of the Yakovlev collection. Arch Gen Psychiatry 1987; 44: 1094–8.

Altshuler LL, Casanova MF, Goldberg TE, Kleinman JE. The hippocampus and parahippocampus in schizophrenia, suicide, and control brains [published erratum appears in Arch Gen Psychiatry 1991; 48; 442]. Arch Gen Psychiatry 1990; 47: 1029–34.

American Psychiatric Association. Diagnostic and statistical manual of mental disorders. DSM-IV. 4th ed. Washington (DC): American Psychiatric Association; 1994.

Anderson B, Rutledge V. Age and hemisphere effects on dendritic structure. Brain 1996; 119: 1983–90.

Anderson SA, Volk DW, Lewis DA. Increased density of microtubule associated protein 2-immunoreactive neurons in the prefrontal white matter of schizophrenic subjects. Schizophr Res 1996; 19: 111–9.

ndrade JP, Castanheira-Vale AJ, Paz-Dias PG, Madeira MD, Paula-arbosa MM. The dendritic trees of neurons from the hippocampal rmation of protein-deprived adult rats. A quantitative Golgi study. xp Brain Res 1996; 109: 419–33.

ndreasen NC. Symptoms, signs, and diagnosis of schizophrenia. Review]. Lancet 1995; 346: 477–81.

ndreasen NC, Arndt S, Swayze V 2nd, Cizadlo T, Flaum M, *Leary D, et al. Thalamic abnormalities in schizophrenia visualized rough magnetic resonance image averaging [see comments]. cience 1994; 266: 294–8. Comment in: Science 1994; 266: 221.

ndreasen NC, O'Leary DS, Cizadlo T, Arndt S, Rezai K, Ponto L, et al. Schizophrenia and cognitive dysmetria: a positron-nission tomography study of dysfunctional prefrontal-thalamic-rebellar circuitry. Proc Natl Acad Sci USA 1996; 93: 9985–90.

nezaki T, Yanagisawa K, Takahashi H, Nakajima T, Miyashita K, hikawa A, et al. Remote astrocytic response of prefrontal cortex caused by the lesions in the nucleus basalis of Meynert, but not the ventral tegmental area. Brain Res 1992; 574: 63–9.

quino DA, Padin C, Perez JM, Peng D, Lyman WD, Chiu FC. nalysis of glial fibrillary acidic protein, neurofilament protein, tin and heat shock proteins in human fetal brain during the second mester. Brain Res Dev Brain Res 1996; 91: 1–10.

rendt T, Bigl V, Arendt A, Tennstedt A. Loss of neurons in the cleus basalis of Meynert in Alzheimer's disease, paralysis agitans d Korsakoff's disease. Acta Neuropathol (Berl) 1983; 61: 101–8.

rnold SE, Trojanowski JQ. Recent advances in defining the uropathology of schizophrenia. [Review]. Acta Neuropathol (Berl) 96; 92: 217–31.

rnold SE, Hyman BT, Van Hoesen GW, Damasio AR. Some toarchitectural abnormalities of the entorhinal cortex in hizophrenia. Arch Gen Psychiatry 1991a; 48: 625–32.

rnold SE, Lee VM-Y, Gur RE, Trojanowski JQ. Abnormal pression of two microtubule-associated proteins (MAP2 and AP5) in specific subfields of the hippocampal formation in hizophrenia. Proc Natl Acad Sci USA 1991b; 88: 10850–4.

rnold SE, Franz BR, Gur RC, Gur RE, Shapiro RM, Moberg PJ, al. Smaller neuron size in schizophrenia in hippocampal subfields at mediate cortical-hippocampal interactions. Am J Psychiatry 95a; 152: 738–48.

rnold SE, Gur RE, Shapiro RM, Fisher KR, Moberg PJ, Gibney R, et al. Prospective clinicopathologic studies of schizophrenia: crual and assessment of patients. Am J Psychiatry 1995b; 152: 1–7.

rnold SE, Franz BR, Trojanowski JQ, Moberg PJ, Gur RE. ial fibrillary acidic protein-immunoreactive astrocytosis in elderly tients with schizophrenia and dementia. Acta Neuropathol (Berl) 96; 91: 269–77.

rnold SE, Ruscheinsky DD, Han LY. Further evidence of abnormal toarchitecture of the entorhinal cortex in schizophrenia using atial point pattern analyses. Biol Psychiatry 1997a; 42: 639–47.

rnold SE, Joo E, Martinoli MG, Roy N, Trojanowski JQ, Gur RE, al. Apolipoprotein E genotype in schizophrenia: frequency, age onset, and neuropathologic features [see comments]. Neuroreport 97b; 8: 1523–6. Comment in: Neuroreport 1997; 8: i–ii.

Arnold SE, Trojanowski JQ, Gur RE, Blackwell P, Han LY, Choi C. Absence of neurodegeneration and neural injury in the cerebral cortex in a sample of elderly patients with schizophrenia. Arch Gen Psychiatry 1998; 55: 225–32.

Arranz MJ, Munro J, Sham P, Kirov G, Murray RM, Collier DA, et al. Meta-analysis of studies on genetic variation in 5-HT$_{2A}$ receptors and clozapine response. Schizophr Res 1998; 32: 93–9.

Averback P. Lesions of the nucleus ansae peduncularis in neuropsychiatric disease. Arch Neurol 1981; 38: 230–5.

Bailey A, Luthert P, Dean A, Harding B, Janota I, Montgomery M, et al. A clinicopathological study of autism. Brain 1998; 121: 889–905.

Baldessarini RJ, Hegarty JD, Bird ED, Benes FM. Meta-analysis of postmortem studies of Alzheimer's disease-like neuropathology in schizophrenia [published erratum appears in Neuroreport 1997; 154: 1180]. Neuroreport 1997; 154: 861–3.

Barta PE, Pearlson GD, Powers RE, Richards SS, Tune LE. Auditory hallucinations and smaller superior temporal gyral volume in schizophrenia. Am J Psychiatry 1990; 147: 1457–62.

Barta PE, Pearlson GD, Brill LB 2nd, Royall R, McGilchrist IK, Pulver AE, et al. Planum temporale asymmetry reversal in schizophrenia: replication and relationship to gray matter abnormalities. Am J Psychiatry 1997; 154: 661–7.

Bartley AJ, Jones DW, Weinberger DR. Genetic variability of human brain size and cortical gyral patterns. Brain 1997; 120: 257–69.

Beall MJ, Lewis DA. Heterogeneity of layer II neurons in human entorhinal cortex. J Comp Neurol 1992; 321: 241–66.

Beasley CL, Reynolds GP. Parvalbumin-immunoreactive neurons are reduced in the prefrontal cortex of schizophrenics. Schizophr Res 1997; 24: 349–55.

Beauregard M, Malkova L, Bachevalier J. Stereotypies and loss of social affiliation after early hippocampectomy in primates. Neuroreport 1995; 6: 2521–6.

Beckmann H, Lauer M. The human striatum in schizophrenia. II. Increased number of striatal neurons in schizophrenics. Psychiatry Res 1997; 68: 99–109.

Belichenko PV, Hagberg B, Dahlstrom A. Morphological study of neocortical areas in Rett syndrome. Acta Neuropathol (Berl) 1997; 93: 50–61.

Benes FM. Model generation and testing to probe neural circuitry in the cingulate cortex of postmortem schizophrenic brain. [Review]. Schizophr Bull 1998; 24: 219–30.

Benes FM, Bird ED. An analysis of the arrangement of neurons in the cingulate cortex of schizophrenic patients. Arch Gen Psychiatry 1987; 44: 608–16.

Benes FM, Davidson J, Bird ED. Quantitative cytoarchitectural studies of the cerebral cortex of schizophrenics. Arch Gen Psychiatry 1986; 43: 31–5.

Benes FM, Majocha RE, Bird ED, Marotta CA. Increased vertical axon numbers in cingulate cortex of schizophrenics. Arch Gen Psychiatry 1987; 44: 1017–21.

Benes FM, McSparren J, Bird ED, SanGiovanni JP, Vincent SL. Deficits in small interneurons in prefrontal and cingulate cortices of schizophrenic and schizoaffective patients. Arch Gen Psychiatry 1991a; 48: 996–1001.

Benes FM, Sorensen I, Bird ED. Reduced neuronal size in posterior hippocampus of schizophrenic patients. Schizophr Bull 1991b; 17: 597–608.

Benes FM, Sorensen I, Vincent SL, Bird ED, Sathi M. Increased density of glutamate-immunoreactive vertical processes in superficial laminae in cingulate cortex of schizophrenic brain. Cereb Cortex 1992a; 2: 503–12.

Benes FM, Vincent SL, Alsterberg G, Bird ED, SanGiovanni JP. Increased GABA$_A$ receptor binding in superficial layers of cingulate cortex in schizophrenics. J Neurosci 1992b; 12: 924–9.

Benes FM, Turtle M, Khan Y, Farol P. Myelination of a key relay zone in the hippocampal formation occurs in the human brain during childhood, adolescence, and adulthood. Arch Gen Psychiatry 1994; 51: 477–84.

Benes FM, Todtenkopf MS, Taylor JB. Differential distribution of tyrosine hydroxylase fibers on small and large neurons in layer II of anterior cingulate cortex of schizophrenic brain. Synapse 1997; 25: 80–92.

Benes FM, Kwok EW, Vincent SL, Todtenkopf MS. A reduction of nonpyramidal cells in sector CA2 of schizophrenics and manic depressives. Biol Psychiatry 1998; 44: 88–97.

Benowitz LI, Routtenberg A. GAP-43: an intrinsic determinant of neuronal development and plasticity. [Review]. Trends Neurosci 1997; 20: 84–91.

Berman NE, Raymond LA, Warren KA, Raghavan R, Joag SV, Narayan O, et al. Fractionator analysis shows loss of neurons in the lateral geniculate nucleus of macaques infected with neurovirulent simian immunodeficiency virus. Neuropathol Appl Neurobiol 1998; 24: 44–52.

Bernstein HG, Stanarius A, Baumann B, Henning H, Krell D, Danos P, et al. Nitric oxide synthase-containing neurons in the human hypothalamus: reduced number of immunoreactive cells in the paraventricular nucleus of depressive patients and schizophrenics. Neuroscience 1998; 83: 867–75.

Bertolino A, Nawroz S, Mattay VS, Barnett AS, Duyn JH, Moonen CT, et al. Regionally specific pattern of neurochemical pathology in schizophrenia as assessed by multislice proton magnetic resonance spectroscopic imaging. Am J Psychiatry 1996; 153: 1554–63.

Bertolino A, Callicott JH, Elman I, Mattay VS, Tedeschi G, Frank JA, et al. Regionally specific neuronal pathology in untreated patients with schizophrenia: a proton magnetic resonance spectroscopic imaging study. Biol Psychiatry 1998; 43: 641–8.

Bilder RM, Lipschutz-Broch L, Reiter G, Geisler SH, Mayerhoff DI, Lieberman JA. Intellectual deficits in first-episode schizophrenia: evidence for progressive deterioration. Schizophr Bull 1992; 18: 437–48.

Bilder RM, Wu H, Bogerts B, Degreef G, Ashtari M, Alvir JM, et al. Absence of regional hemispheric volume asymmetries in first-episode schizophrenia. Am J Psychiatry 1994; 151: 1437–47.

Bilder RM, Bogerts B, Ashtari M, Wu H, Alvir JM, Jody et al. Anterior hippocampal volume reductions predict frontal dysfunction in first episode schizophrenia. Schizophr Res 1995; 47–58.

Blanchard JJ, Neale JM. The neuropsychological signature schizophrenia: generalized or differential deficit? Am J Psych 1994; 151: 40–8.

Blennow K, Davidsson P, Gottfries C-G, Ekman R, Heilig Synaptic degeneration in thalamus in schizophrenia [letter]. La 1996; 348: 692–3.

Bleuler E. Dementia praecox or the group of schizophrenias I Transl. J. Zinkin. New York: International Universities Press; I

Bloom FE. Advancing a neurodevelopmental origin schizophrenia. [Review]. Arch Gen Psychiatry 1993; 50: 224–

Bogerts B, Hantsch J, Herzer M. A morphometric study of dopamine-containing cell groups in the mesencephalon of norm Parkinson patients, and schizophrenics. Biol Psychiatry 1983; 951–69.

Bogerts B, Meertz E, Schonfeldt-Bausch R. Basal ganglia limbic system pathology in schizophrenia. Arch Gen Psych 1985; 42: 784–91.

Bogerts B, Ashtari M, Degreef G, Alvir JM, Bilder RM, Lieber JA. Reduced temporal limbic structure volumes on magn resonance images in first episode schizophrenia. Psychiatry 1990a; 35: 1–13.

Bogerts B, Falkai P, Haupts M, Greve B, Ernst S, Tapernon-F U, et al. Post-mortem volume measurements of limbic system basal ganglia structures in chronic schizophrenics. Initial re from a new brain collection. Schizophr Res 1990b; 3: 295–30

Braak H, Braak E. Ratio of pyramidal cells versus non-pyram cells in the human frontal isocortex and changes in ratio with ag and Alzheimer's disease. Prog Brain Res 1986; 70: 185–212.

Bracha HS. Etiology of structural asymmetry in schizophrenia alternative hypothesis [letter]. Schizophr Bull 1991; 17: 551–3

Breier A, Su TP, Saunders R, Carson RE, Kolachana BS, Bartolomeis A, et al. Schizophrenia is associated with elev amphetamine-induced synaptic dopamine concentrations: evide from a novel positron emission tomography method. Proc . Acad Sci USA 1997; 94: 2569–74.

Briess D, Cotter D, Doshi R, Everall I. Mammillary b abnormalities in schizophrenia [letter]. Lancet 1998; 352: 789–

Brown S. Excess mortality of schizophrenia. A meta-analysis. . Psychiatry 1997; 171: 502–8.

Brown R, Colter N, Corsellis JA, Crow TJ, Frith CD, Ja R, et al. Postmortem evidence of structural brain changes schizophrenia. Differences in brain weight, temporal horn area, parahippocampal gyrus compared with affective disorder. Arch Psychiatry 1986; 43: 36–42.

Browning MD, Dudek EM, Rapier JL, Leonard S, Freedmar Significant reductions in synapsin but not synaptophysin spe activity in the brains of some schizophrenics. Biol Psychiatry 1 34: 529–35.

Bruton CJ, Crow TJ, Frith CD, Johnstone EC, Owens DG, Roberts GW. Schizophrenia and the brain: a prospective clinico-neuropathological study. Psychol Med 1990; 20: 285–304.

Bruton CJ, Stevens JR, Frith CD. Epilepsy, psychosis, and schizophrenia: clinical and neuropathologic correlations. Neurology 1994; 44: 34–42.

Buchanan RW, Breier A, Kirkpatrick B, Elkashef A, Munson RC, Gellad F, et al. Structural abnormalities in deficit and nondeficit schizophrenia. Am J Psychiatry 1993; 150: 59–65.

Buchsbaum MS, Someya T, Teng CY, Abel L, Chin S, Najafi A, et al. PET and MRI of the thalamus in never-medicated patients with schizophrenia. Am J Psychiatry 1996; 153: 191–9.

Buckley PF. The clinical stigmata of aberrant neurodevelopment in schizophrenia. [Review]. J Nerv Ment Dis 1998; 186: 79–86.

Buhl L, Bojsen-Møller M. Frequency of Alzheimer's disease in a postmortem study of psychiatric patients. Dan Med Bull 1988; 35: 288–90.

Bullmore ET, Woodruff PW, Wright IC, Rabe-Hesketh S, Howard RJ, Shuriquie N, et al. Does dysplasia cause anatomical dysconnectivity in schizophrenia? Schizophr Res 1998; 30: 127–35.

Burnet PW, Eastwood SL, Lacey K, Harrison PJ. The distribution of 5-HT$_{1A}$ and 5-HT$_{2A}$ receptor mRNA in human brain. Brain Res 1995; 676: 157–68.

Burnet PW, Eastwood SL, Harrison PJ. 5-HT$_{1A}$ and 5-HT$_{2A}$ receptor mRNAs and binding site densities are differentially altered in schizophrenia. Neuropsychopharmacology 1996; 15: 442–55.

Burnet PW, Eastwood SL, Harrison PJ. [^{3}H]WAY-100635 for 5-HT$_{1A}$ receptor autoradiography in human brain: a comparison with [^{3}H]8-OH-DPAT and demonstration of increased binding in the frontal cortex in schizophrenia. Neurochem Int 1997; 30: 565–74.

Cannon M, Jones P. Schizophrenia. [Review]. J Neurol Neurosurg Psychiatry 1996; 60: 604–13.

Cannon TD, Mednick SA, Parnas J, Schulsinger F, Praestholm J, Vestergaard A. Developmental brain abnormalities in the offspring of schizophrenic mothers. I. Contributions of genetic and perinatal factors [see comments]. Arch Gen Psychiatry 1993; 50: 551–64. Comment in: Arch Gen Psychiatry 1995; 52: 157–9.

Carlsson M, Carlsson A. Schizophrenia: a subcortical neurotransmitter imbalance syndrome? [Review]. Schizophr Bull 1990; 16: 425–32.

Casanova MF, Zito M, Bigelow LB, Berthot B, Sanders RD, Kleinman JE. Axonal counts of the corpus callosum of schizophrenic patients. J Neuropsychiatry Clin Neurosci 1989; 1: 391–3.

Casanova MF, Stevens JR, Kleinman JE. Astrocytosis in the molecular layer of the dentate gyrus: a study in Alzheimer's disease and schizophrenia. Psychiatry Res 1990; 35: 149–66.

Chakos MH, Lieberman JA, Bilder RM, Borenstein M, Lerner G, Bogerts B, et al. Increase in caudate nuclei volumes of first-episode schizophrenic patients taking antipsychotic drugs. Am J Psychiatry 1994; 151: 1430–6.

Crichton-Browne J. On the weight of the brain and its component parts in the insane. Brain 1879; 2: 42–67.

Christensen E, Moller JE, Faurbye A. Neuropathological investigation of 28 brains from patients with dyskinesia. Acta Psychiatr Scand 1970; 46: 14–23.

Christison GW, Casanova MF, Weinberger DR, Rawlings R, Kleinman JE. A quantitative investigation of hippocampal pyramidal cell size, shape, and variability of orientation in schizophrenia. Arch Gen Psychiatry 1989; 46: 1027–32.

Chua SE, McKenna PJ. Schizophrenia—a brain disease? A critical review of structural and functional cerebral abnormality in the disorder. [Review]. Br J Psychiatry 1995; 166: 563–82.

Cohen JD, Servan-Schreiber D. Context, cortex, and dopamine: a connectionist approach to behavior and biology in schizophrenia. [Review]. Psychol Rev 1992; 99: 45–77.

Conrad AJ, Abebe T, Austin R, Forsythe S, Scheibel AB. Hippocampal pyramidal cell disarray in schizophrenia as a bilateral phenomenon. Arch Gen Psychiatry 1991; 48: 413–7.

Corsellis JAN. Mental illness and the ageing brain. Institute of Psychiatry Maudsley Monographs No. 9. London: Oxford University Press; 1962.

Corsellis JAN. Psychoses of obscure pathology. In: Blackwood W, Corsellis JAN, editors. Greenfield's neuropathology. 3rd ed. London: Edward Arnold; 1976. p. 903–15.

Cotter D, Kerwin R, Doshi B, Martin CS, Everall IP. Alterations in hippocampal non-phosphorylated MAP2 protein expression in schizophrenia. Brain Res 1997; 765: 238–46.

Crow TJ. Molecular pathology of schizophrenia: more than one disease process? [Review]. Br Med J 1980; 280: 66–8.

Crow TJ. Temporal lobe asymmetries as the key to the etiology of schizophrenia. [Review]. Schizophr Bull 1990; 16: 433–43.

Crow TJ. Schizophrenia as failure of hemispheric dominance for language [see comments]. [Review]. Trends Neurosci 1997; 20: 339–43. Comment in: Trends Neurosci 1998; 21: 145–7.

Crow TJ. Schizophrenia as a transcallosal misconnection syndrome. Schizophr Res 1998; 30: 111–4.

Crow TJ, Ball J, Bloom SR, Brown R, Bruton CJ, Colter N, et al. Schizophrenia as an anomaly of development of cerebral asymmetry. Arch Gen Psychiatry 1989; 46: 1145–50.

da Cunha A, Jefferson JJ, Tyor WR, Glass JD, Jannotta FS, Vitkovic L. Gliosis in human brain: relationship to size but not other properties of astrocytes. Brain Res 1993; 600: 161–5.

Daniel DG, Goldberg TE, Gibbons RD, Weinberger DR. Lack of a bimodal distribution of ventricular size in schizophrenia: a Gaussian mixture analysis of 1056 cases and controls. Biol Psychiatry 1991; 30: 887–903.

Danos P, Baumann B, Bernstein H-G, Franz M, Stauch R, Northoff G, et al. Schizophrenia and anteroventral thalamic nucleus: selective decrease of parvalbumin-immunoreactive thalamocortical projection neurons. Psychiatry Res 1998; 82: 1–10.

David GB. The pathological anatomy of the schizophrenias. In: Richter D, editor. Schizophrenia: somatic aspects. London: Pergamon Press; 1957. p. 93–130.

David AS, Cutting JC. The neuropsychology of schizophrenia. Hove (UK): Lawrence Erlbaum; 1994.

Davidson M, Keefe RS. Cognitive impairment as a target for pharmacological treatment in schizophrenia. [Review]. Schizophr Res 1995; 17: 123–9.

Davidson L, McGlashan TH. The varied outcomes of schizophrenia [review]. Can J Psychiatry 1997; 42: 34–43.

Davidson M, Harvey P, Welsh KA, Powchik P, Putnam KM, Mohs RC. Cognitive functioning in late-life schizophrenia: a comparison of elderly schizophrenic patients and patients with Alzheimer's disease. Am J Psychiatry 1996; 153: 1274–9.

Davis KL, Kahn RS, Ko G, Davidson M. Dopamine in schizophrenia: a review and reconceptualization [see comments]. Am J Psychiatry 1991; 148: 1474–86. Comment in: Am J Psychiatry 1992; 149: 1284–5. Comment in: Am J Psychiatry 1992; 149: 1620–1.

Davis KL, Buchsbaum MS, Shihabuddin L, Spiegel-Cohen J, Metzger M, Frecska E, et al. Ventricular enlargement in poor-outcome schizophrenia [see comments]. Biol Psychiatry 1998; 43: 783–93. Comment in: Biol Psychiatry 1998; 43: 781–2.

Davison K. Schizophrenia-like psychoses associated with organic cerebral disorders: a review. [Review]. Psychiatr Dev 1983; 1: 1–33.

Daviss SR, Lewis DA. Local circuit neurons of the prefrontal cortex in schizophrenia: selective increase in the density of calbindin-immunoreactive neurons. Psychiatry Res 1995; 59: 81–96.

de Brabander JM, Kramers RJK, Uylings HBM. Layer-specific dendritic regression of pyramidal cells with ageing in the human prefrontal cortex. Eur J Neurosci 1998; 10: 1261–9.

De Lacoste M-C, White CL, 3d. The role of cortical connectivity in Alzheimer's disease pathogenesis: a review and model system [see comments]. [Review]. Neurobiol Aging 1993; 14: 1–16. Comment in: Neurobiol Aging 1993; 14: 49–50, Comment in: Neurobiol Aging 1993; 14: 51–4; disc 55–6.

Deakin JF, Simpson MD. A two-process theory of schizophrenia: evidence from studies in post-mortem brain. [Review]. J Psychiat Res 1997; 31: 277–95.

Degreef G, Ashtari M, Bogerts B, Bilder RM, Jody DN, Alvir JM, et al. Volumes of ventricular system subdivisions measured from magnetic resonance images in first-episode schizophrenic patients. Arch Gen Psychiatry 1992; 49: 531–7.

Deicken RF, Zhou L, Corwin F, Vinograd S, Weiner MW. Decreased left frontal lobe N-acetylaspartate in schizophrenia. Am J Psychiatry 1997; 154: 688–90.

Deicken RF, Zhou L, Schuff N, Fein G, Weiner MW. Hippocampal neuronal dysfunction in schizophrenia as measured by proton magnetic resonance spectroscopy. Biol Psychiatry 1998; 43: 483–8.

DeLisi LE. Is schizophrenia a lifetime disorder of brain plasticity, growth and aging? [Review]. Schizophr Res 1997; 23: 119–29.

DeLisi LE, Sakuma M, Tew W, Kushner M, Hoff AL, Grimson R. Schizophrenia as a chronic active brain process: a study of progressive brain structural change subsequent to the onset of schizophrenia. Psychiatry Res 1997a; 74: 129–40.

DeLisi LE, Sakuma M, Kushner M, Finer DL, Hoff AL, Crow TJ. Anomalous cerebral asymmetry and language processing in schizophrenia [published erratum appears in Schizophr Bull 1997; 23: 536]. Schizophr Bull 1997b; 23: 255–71.

Dell'Anna ME, Geloso MC, Draisci G, Luthman J. Transient changes in fos and GFAP immunoreactivity precede neuronal loss in the rat hippocampus following neonatal anoxia. Exp Neurol 1995; 131: 144–56.

Doody GA, Johnstone EC, Sanderson TL, Owens DGC, Muir WJ. 'Pfropfschizophrenie' revisited: schizophrenia in people with mild learning disability. Br J Psychiatry 1998; 173: 145–53.

Drevets WC, Ongur D, Price JL. Neuroimaging abnormalities in the subgenual prefrontal cortex: implications for the pathophysiology of familial mood disorders. Mol Psychiatry 1998; 3: 220–6.

Dwork AJ. Postmortem studies of the hippocampal formation in schizophrenia. [Review]. Schizophr Bull 1997; 23: 385–402.

Eastwood SL, Harrison PJ. Decreased synaptophysin in the medial temporal lobe in schizophrenia demonstrated using immuno-autoradiography. Neuroscience 1995; 69: 339–43.

Eastwood SL, Harrison PJ. Hippocampal and cortical growth-associated protein-43 messenger RNA in schizophrenia. Neuroscience 1998; 86: 437–48.

Eastwood SL, Burnet PWJ, McDonald B, Clinton J, Harrison PJ. Synaptophysin gene expression in human brain: a quantitative in situ hybridization and immunocytochemical study. Neuroscience 1994a; 59: 881–92.

Eastwood SL, Burnet PW, Harrison PJ. Striatal synaptophysin expression and haloperidol-induced synaptic plasticity. Neuroreport 1994b; 5: 677–80.

Eastwood SL, Burnet PW, Harrison PJ. Altered synaptophysin expression as a marker of synaptic pathology in schizophrenia. Neuroscience 1995a; 66: 309–19.

Eastwood SL, McDonald B, Burnet PW, Beckwith JP, Kerwin RW, Harrison PJ. Decreased expression of mRNAs encoding non-NMDA glutamate receptors GluR1 and GluR2 in medial temporal lobe neurons in schizophrenia. Brain Res Mol Brain Res 1995b; 29: 211–23.

Eastwood SL, Heffernan J, Harrison PJ. Chronic haloperidol treatment differentially affects the expression of synaptic and neuronal plasticity-associated genes. Mol Psychiatry 1997a; 2: 322–9.

Eastwood SL, Kerwin RW, Harrison PJ. Immunoautoradiographic evidence for a loss of alpha-amino-3-hydroxy-5-methyl-4-isoxazole propionic-acid-preferring non-N-methyl-D-aspartate glutamate receptors within the medial temporal lobe in schizophrenia. Biol Psychiatry 1997b; 41: 636–43.

Elliott R, Sahakian, BJ. The neuropsychology of schizo-phrenia: relations with clinical and neurobiological dimen-sions. [Review]. Psychol Med 1995; 25: 581–94.

Elston GN, Rosa MG. Morphological variation of layer III pyramidal neurones in the occipitotemporal pathway of the macaque monkey visual cortex. Cereb Cortex 1998; 8: 278–94.

Falkai P, Bogerts B. Cell loss in the hippocampus of schizophrenics. Eur Arch Psychiatry Neurol Sci 1986; 236: 154–61.

Falkai P, Bogerts B. Cytoarchitectonic and developmental studies in schizophrenia. In: Kerwin RW, editor. Neurobiology and psychiatry, Vol. 2. Cambridge: Cambridge University Press; 1993. p. 43–70.

Falkai P, Bogerts B, Rozumek M. Limbic pathology in schizophrenia: the entorhinal region—a morphometric study. Biol Psychiatry 1988; 24: 515–21.

Falkai P, Bogerts B, Greve B, Pfeiffer U, Machus B, Folsch-Reetz B, et al. Loss of sylvian fissure asymmetry in schizophrenia. A quantitative post-mortem study. Schizophr Res 1992; 7: 23–32.

Falkai P, Bogerts B, Schneider T, Greve B, Pfeiffer U, Pilz K, et al. Disturbed planum temporale asymmetry in schizophrenia. A quantitative post-mortem study. Schizophr Res 1995; 14: 161–76.

Feinberg I. Schizophrenia: caused by a fault in programmed synaptic elimination during adolescence? J Psychiatr Res 1982; 17: 319–34.

Fisman M. The brain stem in psychosis. Br J Psychiatry 1975; 126: 414–22.

Flaum M, Arndt S, Andreasen NC. The role of gender in studies of ventricle enlargement in schizophrenia: a predominantly male effect [see comments]. Am J Psychiatry 1990; 147: 1327–32. Comment in: Am J Psychiatry 1991; 148: 1754–6.

Flaum M, Swayze VW 2nd, O'Leary DS, Yuh WT, Ehrhardt JC, Arndt SV, et al. Effects of diagnosis, laterality, and gender on brain morphology in schizophrenia. Am J Psychiatry 1995; 152: 704–14.

Flor-Henry P. Psychosis and temporal lobe epilepsy. A controlled investigation. Epilepsia 1969; 10: 363–95.

Frazier JA, Giedd JN, Hamburger SD, Albus KE, Kaysen D, Vaituzis AC, et al. Brain anatomic magnetic resonance imaging in childhood-onset schizophrenia. Arch Gen Psychiatry 1996; 53: 617–24.

Friede RL. Developmental neuropathology. Berlin: Springer Verlag; 1989.

Friston KJ. The disconnection hypothesis. Schizophr Res 1998; 30: 115–25.

Friston KJ, Frith CD. Schizophrenia: a disconnection syndrome? [Review]. Clin Neurosci 1995; 3: 89–97.

Frith CD, Friston KJ, Herold S, Silbersweig D, Fletcher P, Cahill C, et al. Regional brain activity in chronic schizophrenic patients during the performance of a verbal fluency task. Br J Psychiatry 1995; 167: 343–9.

Gabriel SM, Haroutunian V, Powchik P, Honer WG, Davidson M, Davies P, et al. Increased concentrations of presynaptic proteins in the cingulate cortex of subjects with schizophrenia [published erratum appears in Arch Gen Psychiatry 1997; 54: 912]. 559–66.

Galaburda AM. Anatomic basis for cerebral dominance. In: Richardson RE, Hugdahl K, editors. Cerebral asymmetry. Boston: MIT Press; 1994. p. 51–73.

Garcia-Rill E, Biedermann JA, Chambers T, Skinner RD, Mrak RE, Husain M, et al. Mesopontine neurons in schizophrenia. Neuroscience 1995; 66: 321–35.

Garey LJ, Ong WY, Patel TS, Kanani M, Davis A, Mortimer AM, et al. Reduced dendritic spine density on cerebral cortical pyramidal neurons in schizophrenia. J Neurol Neurosurg Psychiatry 1998; 65: 446–53.

Garver DL. The etiologic heterogeneity of schizophrenia. Harvard Rev Psychiatry 1997; 4: 317–27.

Geddes JR, Lawrie SM. Obstetric complications and schizophrenia: a meta-analysis. Br J Psychiatry 1995; 167: 786–93.

Glantz LA, Lewis DA. Reduction of synaptophysin immunoreactivity in the prefrontal cortex of subjects with schizophrenia. Regional and diagnostic specificity [corrected and republished article originally appeared in Arch Gen Psychiatry 1997; 54: 660–9]. Arch Gen Psychiatry 1997; 54: 943–52.

Goldberg TE, Hyde TM, Kleinman JE, Weinberger DR. Course of schizophrenia: neuropsychological evidence for a static encephalopathy. [Review]. Schizophr Bull 1993; 19: 797–804.

Goldsmith SK, Joyce JN. Alterations in hippocampal mossy fiber pathway in schizophrenia and Alzheimer's disease. Biol Psychiatry 1995; 37: 122–6.

Goodman R. Neuronal misconnections and psychiatric disorder. Is there a link? [see comments]. [Review]. Br J Psychiatry 1989; 154: 292–9. Comment in: Br J Psychiatry 1989; 155: 129–30.

Green MF. What are the functional consequences of neurocognitive deficits in schizophrenia? [see comments]. [Review]. Am J Psychiatry 1996; 153: 321–30. Comment in: Am J Psychiatry 1997; 154: 443–4.

Guillery RW, Herrup K. Quantification without pontification: choosing a method for counting objects in sectioned tissues [comment]. J Comp Neurol 1997; 386: 2–7. Comment on: J Comp Neurol 1996; 364: 6–15.

Gur RE, Mozley PD, Shtasel DL, Cannon TD, Gallacher F, Turetsky B, et al. Clinical subtypes of schizophrenia: differences in brain and CSF volume [see comments]. Am J Psychiatry 1994; 151: 343–50. Comment in: Am J Psychiatry 1995; 152: 817–8.

Gur RE, Cowell P, Turetsky BI, Gallacher F, Cannon T, Bilker W, et al. A follow-up magnetic resonance imaging study of schizophrenia. Arch Gen Psychiatry 1998; 55: 145–52.

Gurevich EV, Bordelon Y, Shapiro RM, Arnold SE, Gur RE, Joyce JN. Mesolimbic dopamine D_3 receptors and use of antipsychotics in patients with schizophrenia. A postmortem study. Arch Gen Psychiatry 1997; 54: 225–32.

Hafner H, an der Heiden W, Behrens S, Gattaz WF, Hambrecht M, Loffler W, et al. Causes and consequences of the gender difference in age at onset of schizophrenia. [Review]. Schizophr Bull 1998; 24: 99–113.

Halliday GM, Cullen KM, Kril JJ, Harding AJ, Harasty J. Glial fibrillary acidic protein (GFAP) immunohistochemistry in human cortex: a quantitative study using different antisera. Neurosci Lett 1996; 209: 29–32.

Haracz JL. Neural plasticity in schizophrenia. Schizophr Bull 1985; 11: 191–229.

Haroutunian V, Davidson M, Kanof PD, Perl DP, Powchik P, Losonczy M, et al. Cortical cholinergic markers in schizophrenia. Schizophr Res 1994; 12: 137–44.

Harrison PJ. Effects of neuroleptics on neuronal and synaptic structure. In: Barnes TRE, editor. Antipsychotic drugs and their side-effects. London: Academic Press; 1993. p. 99–110.

Harrison PJ. Advances in post-mortem molecular neurochemistry and neuropathology: examples from schizophrenia research. [Review]. Br Med Bull 1996; 52: 527–38.

Harrison PJ. Schizophrenia: a disorder of neurodevelopment? [Review]. Curr Opin Neurobiol 1997a; 7: 285–9.

Harrison PJ. Schizophrenia and its dementia. In: Esiri MM, Morris JH, editors. The neuropathology of dementia. Cambridge: Cambridge University Press; 1997b. p. 385–97.

Harrison PJ. Brains at risk of schizophrenia [Editorial]. Lancet 1999a; 353: 3–4.

Harrison PJ. Neurochemical alterations in schizophrenia affecting the putative targets of atypical antipsychotics: focus on dopamine (D_1, D_3, D_4) and 5-HT_{2A} receptors. Br J Psychiatry 1999b; 174 Suppl 38: 41–51.

Harrison PJ, Burnet PW. The 5-HT_{2A} (serotonin$_{2A}$) receptor gene in the aetiology, pathophysiology and pharmacotherapy of schizophrenia. J Psychopharmacol (Oxf) 1997; 11: 18–20.

Harrison PJ, Eastwood SL. Preferential involvement of excitatory neurons in the medial temporal lobe in schizophrenia. Lancet 1998; 352: 1669–73.

Haug JO. Pneumoencephalographic evidence of brain atrophy in acute and chronic schizophrenic patients. Acta Psychiatr Scand 1982; 66: 374–83.

Hayes TL, Lewis DA. Magnopyramidal neurons in the anterior motor speech region. Dendritic features and interhemispheric comparisons. Arch Neurol 1996; 53: 1277–83.

Heckers S. Neuropathology of schizophrenia: cortex, thalamus, basal ganglia, and neurotransmitter-specific projection systems. [Review]. Schizophr Bull 1997; 23: 403–21.

Heckers S, Heinsen H, Heinsen YC, Beckmann H. Limbic structures and lateral ventricle in schizophrenia: a quantitative postmortem study [see comments]. Arch Gen Psychiatry 1990; 47: 1016–22. Comment in: Arch Gen Psychiatry 1991; 48: 956–8.

Heckers S, Heinsen H, Heinsen Y, Beckmann H. Cortex, white matter, and basal ganglia in schizophrenia: a volumetric postmortem study. Biol Psychiatry 1991a; 29: 556–66.

Heckers S, Heinsen H, Geiger B, Beckmann H. Hippocampal neuron number in schizophrenia: a stereological study. Arch Gen Psychiatry 1991b; 48: 1002–8.

Heffernan JM, Eastwood SL, Nagy Z, Sanders MW, McDonald B, Harrison PJ. Temporal cortex synaptophysin mRNA is reduced in Alzheimer's disease and is negatively correlated with the severity of dementia. Exp Neurol 1998; 150: 235–9.

Heinsen H, Gossmann E, Rub U, Eisenmenger W, Bauer M, Ulmar G, et al. Variability in the human entorhinal region may confound neuropsychiatric diagnoses. Acta Anat (Basel) 1996; 157: 226–37.

Highley JR, Esiri MM, McDonald B, Cortina-Borja M, Cooper SJ, Herron BM et al. Anomalies of cerebral asymmetry in schizophrenia interact with gender and age of onset: a post-mortem study. Schizophr Res 1998; 34: 13–25.

Highley JR, Esiri MM, McDonald B, Cortina-Borja M, Herron BM, Crow TJ. The size and fibre composition of the corpus callosum with respect to gender and schizophrenia: a post-mortem study. Brain 1999; 122: 99–110.

Hill C, Keks N, Roberts S, Opeskin K, Dean B, MacKinnon A, et al. Problem of diagnosis in postmortem brain studies of schizophrenia. Am J Psychiatry 1996; 153: 533–7.

Ho K-C, Gwozdz JT, Hause LL, Antuono PG. Correlation of neuronal cell body size in motor cortex and hippocampus with body height, body weight, and axonal length. Int J Neurosci 1992; 65: 147–53.

Hoff AL, Riordan H, O'Donnell DW, Morris L, DeLisi LE. Neuropsychological functioning of first-episode schizophreniform patients. Am J Psychiatry 1992; 149: 898–903.

Hoffman RE, Dobscha SK. Cortical pruning and the development of schizophrenia: a computer model [see comments]. Schizophr Bull 1989; 15: 477–90. Comment in: Schizophr Bull 1990; 16: 567–70.

Honer WG, Bassett AS, Smith GN, Lapointe JS, Falkai P. Temporal lobe abnormalities in multigenerational families with schizophrenia. Biol Psychiatry 1994; 36: 737–43.

Honer WG, Falkai P, Young C, Wang T, Xie J, Bonner J, et al. Cingulate cortex synaptic terminal proteins and neural cell adhesion molecule in schizophrenia. Neuroscience 1997; 78: 99–110.

Horton K, Forsyth CS, Sibtain N, Ball S, Bruton CJ, Royston MC, et al. Ubiquitination as a probe for neurodegeneration in the brain in schizophrenia: the prefrontal cortex. Psychiatry Res 1993; 48: 145–52.

Howard CV, Reed MG. Unbiased stereology. Oxford: Bios; 1998.

Huber G. The heterogeneous course of schizophrenia. Schizophr Res 1997; 28: 177–85.

Huttenlocher PR. Synaptic density in human frontal cortex: developmental changes and effects of aging. Brain Res 1979; 163: 195–205.

Hyde TM, Ziegler JC, Weinberger DR. Psychiatric disturbances in metachromatic leukodystrophy: insights into the neurobiology of psychosis [see comments]. Arch Neurol 1992; 49: 401–6. Comment in: Arch Neurol 1993; 50: 131.

Insausti R, Tunon T, Sobreviela T, Insausti AM, Gonzalo LM. The human entorhinal cortex: a cytoarchitectonic analysis. J Comp Neurol 1995; 355: 171–98.

Jablensky A. Schizophrenia: recent epidemiologic issues. [Review]. Epidemiol Rev 1995; 17: 10–20.

Jacobsen LK, Giedd JN, Castellanos FX, Vaituzis AC, Hamburger SD, Kumra S, et al. Progressive reduction of temporal lobe structures in childhood-onset schizophrenia. Am J Psychiatry 1998; 155: 678–85.

Jakab RL, Goldman-Rakic PS. 5-Hydroxytryptamine$_{2A}$ serotonin receptors in the primate cerebral cortex: possible site of action of hallucinogenic and antipsychotic drugs in pyramidal cell apical dendrites. Proc Natl Acad Sci USA 1998; 95: 735–40.

kob H, Beckmann H. Prenatal developmental disturbances in the
nbic allocortex in schizophrenics. J Neural Transm 1986; 65:
03–26.

kob H, Beckmann H. Gross and histological criteria for
evelopmental disorders in brains of schizophrenics. [Review]. J R
oc Med 1989; 82: 466–9.

skiw GE, Juliano DM, Goldberg TE, Hertzman M, Urow-Hamell
, Weinberger DR. Cerebral ventricular enlargement in
hizophreniform disorder does not progress. A seven year follow-
p study. Schizophr Res 1994; 14: 23–8.

vitt DC, Zukin SR. Recent advances in the phencyclidine model
' schizophrenia [see comments]. [Review]. Am J Psychiatry 1991;
48: 1301–8. Comment in: Am J Psychiatry 1992; 149: 848-9.

llinger K. Neuropathologic findings after neuroleptic long-term
erapy. In: Roizin L, Shiraki H, Grcevic N, editors.
eurotoxicology. New York: Raven Press; 1977. p. 25–42.

llinger K. Neuromorphological background of pathochemical
dies in major psychoses. In: Beckmann H, Riederer P, editors.
thochemical markers in major psychoses. Berlin: Springer; 1985.
1–23.

ste DV, Lohr JB. Hippocampal pathologic findings in
hizophrenia. A morphometric study. Arch Gen Psychiatry 1989;
: 1019–24.

hnston NL, Cervenak J, Shore AD, Torrey EF, Yolken RH.
ultivariate analysis of RNA levels from postmortem human brains
measured by three different methods of RT-PCR [published
ratum appears in J Neurosci Methods 1998; 79: 233]. J Neurosci
ethods 1997; 77: 83–92.

hnstone EC, Crow TJ, Frith CD, Husband J, Kreel L. Cerebral
entricular size and cognitive impairment in chronic schizophrenia.
ancet 1976; 2: 924–6.

hnstone EC, McMillan JF, Crow TJ. The occurrence of organic
sease of possible or probable aetiological significance in a
pulation of 268 cases of first episode schizophrenia. Psychol Med
87; 17: 371–9.

hnstone EC, Bruton CJ, Crow TJ, Frith CD, Owens DG. Clinical
rrelates of postmortem brain changes in schizophrenia: decreased
ain weight and length correlate with indices of early impairment.
Neurol Neurosurg Psychiatry 1994; 57: 474–9.

nes EG. Cortical development and thalamic pathology in
hizophrenia [see comments]. [Review]. Schizophr Bull 1997a;
' 483–501. Comment in: Schizophr Bull 1997; 23: 509–12,
mment in: Schizophr Bull 1997; 537-40.

nes P. The early origins of schizophrenia. [Review]. Br Med Bull
97b; 53: 135–55.

nes TA, Schallert T. Use-dependent growth of pyramidal neurons
er neocortical damage. J Neurosci 1994; 14: 2140–52.

nsson SA, Luts A, Guldberg-Kjaer N, Brun A. Hippocampal
ramidal cell disarray correlates negatively to cell number:
plications for the pathogenesis of schizophrenia. Eur Arch
ychiatry Clin Neurosci 1997; 247: 120–7.

Joyce JN, Meador-Woodruff JH. Linking the family of D$_2$ receptors
to neuronal circuits in human brain: insights into schizophrenia.
[Review]. Neuropsychopharmacology 1997; 16: 375–84.

Kalman M, Csillag A, Schleicher A, Rind C, Hajos F, Zilles K.
Long-term effects of anterograde degeneration on astroglial reaction
in the rat geniculo-cortical system as revealed by computerized
image analysis. Anat Embryol (Berl) 1993; 187: 1–7.

Kalus P, Senitz D, Beckmann H. Altered distribution of parvalbumin-
immunoreactive local circuit neurons in the anterior cingulate cortex
of schizophrenic patients. Psychiatry Res 1997; 75: 49–59.

Kapur S, Remington G. Serotonin-dopamine interaction and its
relevance to schizophrenia. [Review]. Am J Psychiatry 1996; 153:
466–76.

Katsetos CD, Hyde TM, Herman MM. Neuropathology of the
cerebellum in schizophrenia—an update: 1996 and future directions.
[Review]. Biol Psychiatry 1997; 42: 213–24.

Katz M, Buchsbaum MS, Siagel BV Jr, Wu J, Haier RJ, Bunney
WE Jr Correlational patterns of cerebral glucose metabolism in
never-medicated schizophrenics. Neuropsychobiology 1996; 33:
1–11.

Kegeles LS, Humaran J, Mann JJ. In vivo neurochemistry of
the brain in schizophrenia as revealed by magnetic resonance
spectroscopy. Biol Psychiatry 1998; 44: 382–98.

Kelley JJ, Gao XM, Tamminga CA, Roberts RC. The effect of
chronic haloperidol treatment on dendritic spines in the rat striatum.
Exp Neurol 1997; 146: 471–8.

Kennedy JL. Schizophrenia genetics: the quest for an anchor
[editorial]. Am J Psychiatry 1996; 153: 1513–4.

Kenny JT, Friedman L, Findling RL, Swales TP, Strauss ME,
Jesberger JA, et al. Cognitive impairment in adolescents with
schizophrenia. Am J Psychiatry 1997; 154: 1613–5.

Kerwin R, Patel S, Meldrum B. Quantitative autoradiographic
analysis of glutamate binding sites in the hippocampal formation
in normal and schizophrenic brain post-mortem. Neuroscience 1990;
39: 25–32.

Keshavan MS, Anderson S, Pettegrew JW. Is schizophrenia due to
excessive synaptic pruning in the prefrontal cortex? The Feinberg
hypothesis revisited. [Review]. J Psychiatr Res 1994a; 28: 239–65.

Keshavan MS, Bagwell WW, Haas GL, Sweeney JA, Schooler NR,
Pettegrew JW. Changes in caudate volume with neuroleptic treatment
[letter]. Lancet 1994b; 344: 1434.

Keshavan MS, Rosenberg D, Sweeney JA, Pettegrew JW. Decreased
caudate volume in neuroleptic-naive psychotic patients. Am J
Psychiatry 1998; 155: 774–8.

Kleinman JE, Hyde TM, Herman MM. Methodological issues in
the neuropathology of mental illness. In: Bloom FE, Kupfer DJ,
editors. Psychopharmacology. The fourth generation of progress.
New York: Raven Press; 1995. p. 859–64.

Kolb B, Whishaw IQ. Brain plasticity and behavior. [Review]. Annu
Rev Psychol 1998; 49: 43–64.

Kovelman JA, Scheibel AB. A neurohistological correlate of
schizophrenia. Biol Psychiatry 1984; 19: 1601–21.

Kreutzberg GW, Blakemore WF, Graeber MB. Cellular pathology of the central nervous system. In: Graham DI, Lantos PL, editors. Greenfield's neuropathology. 6th ed. London: Edward Arnold; 1997. p. 85–156.

Krimer LS, Herman MM, Saunders RC, Boyd JC, Hyde TM, Carter JM, et al. A qualitative and quantitative analysis of the entorhinal cortex in schizophrenia. Cereb Cortex 1997a; 7: 732–9.

Krimer LS, Hyde TM, Herman MM, Saunders RC. The entorhinal cortex: an examination of cyto- and myeloarchitectonic organization in humans. Cereb Cortex 1997b; 7: 722–31.

Kulynych JJ, Vladar K, Jones DW, Weinberger DR. Superior temporal gyrus volume in schizophrenia: a study using MRI morphometry assisted by surface rendering. Am J Psychiatry 1996; 153: 50–6.

Kung L, Conley R, Chute DJ, Smialek J, Roberts RC. Synaptic changes in the striatum of schizophrenic cases: a controlled postmortem ultrastructural study. Synapse 1998; 28: 125–39.

Kwon JS, Shenton ME, Hirayasu Y, Salisbury DF, Fischer IA, Dickey CC, et al. MRI study of cavum septi pellucidi in schizophrenia, affective disorder, and schizotypal personality disorder. Am J Psychiatry 1998; 155: 509–15.

Laruelle M, Abi-Dargham A, van Dyck CH, Gil R, D'Souza CD, Erdos J, et al. Single photon emission computerized tomography imaging of amphetamine-induced dopamine release in drug-free schizophrenic subjects. Proc Natl Acad Sci USA 1996; 93: 9235–40.

Lauriello J, Hoff A, Wieneke MH, Blankfeld H, Faustman WO, Rosenbloom M, et al. Similar extent of brain dysmorphology in severely ill women and men with schizophrenia. Am J Psychiatry 1997; 154: 819–25.

Lawrie SM, Abukmeil SS. Brain abnormality in schizophrenia. A systematic and quantitative review of volumetric magnetic resonance imaging studies. [Review]. Br J Psychiatry 1998; 172: 110–20.

Lawrie SM, Whalley H, Kestelman JN, Abukmeil SS, Byrne M, Hodges A, et al. Magnetic resonance imaging of the brain in subjects at high risk of developing schizophrenia. Lancet 1999; 353: 30–3.

Lewis DA. Development of the prefrontal cortex during adolescence: insights into vulnerable neural circuits in schizophrenia. [Review]. Neuropsychopharmacology 1997; 16: 385–98.

Liddle PF, Friston KJ, Frith CD, Hirsch SR, Jones T, Frackowiak RS. Patterns of cerebral blood flow in schizophrenia. Br J Psychiatry 1992; 160: 179–86.

Lieberman JA, Sheitman BB, Kinon BJ. Neurochemical sensitization in the pathophysiology of schizophrenia: deficits and dysfunction in neuronal regulation and plasticity. [Review]. Neuropsychopharmacology 1997; 17: 205–29.

Lim KO, Tew W, Kushner M, Chow K, Matsumoto B, DeLisi LE. Cortical gray matter volume deficit in patients with first-episode schizophrenia. Am J Psychiatry 1996; 153: 1548–53.

Lipska BK, Weinberger DR. Genetic variation in vulnerability to the behavioral effects of neonatal hippocampal damage in rats. Proc Natl Acad Sci USA 1995; 92: 8906–10.

Lohr JB, Jeste DV. Locus ceruleus morphometry in aging and schizophrenia. Acta Psychiatr Scand 1988; 77: 689–97.

Madsen AL, Keiding N, Karle A, Esbjerg S, Hemmingsen. Neuroleptics in progressive structural brain abnormalities psychiatric illness [letter]. Lancet 1998; 352: 784–5.

Maier M, Ron MA, Barker GJ, Tofts PS. Proton magnetic resonan spectroscopy: an in vivo method of estimating hippocampal neuro depletion in schizophrenia [published erratum appears in Psyc. Med 1996; 26: 877]. Psychol Med 1995; 25: 1201–9.

Marsh L, Suddath RL, Higgins N, Weinberger DR. Medial tempo lobe structures in schizophrenia: relationship of size to duration illness. Schizophr Res 1994; 11: 225–38.

Marsh L, Harris D, Lim KO, Beal M, Hoff AL, Minn K, et Structural magnetic resonance imaging abnormalities in men w severe chronic schizophrenia and an early age at clinical ons Arch Gen Psychiatry 1997; 54: 1104–12.

Masliah E, Terry R. The role of synaptic proteins in the pathogene of disorders of the central nervous system. [Review]. Brain Pat 1993; 3: 77–85.

Masliah E, Mallory M, Hansen L, DeTeresa R, Terry R Quantitative synaptic alterations in the human neocortex dur normal aging. Neurology 1993; 43: 192–7.

Mayhew TM, Gundersen HJ. 'If you assume, you can make an out of u and me': a decade of the disector for stereological count of particles in 3D space. [Review]. J Anat 1996; 188: 1–15.

McGuffin P, Owen MJ, Farmer AE. Genetic basis of schizophren Lancet 1995; 346: 678–82.

McGuire PK, Frith CD. Disordered functional connectivity schizophrenia [editorial]. Psychol Med 1996; 26: 663–7.

McKenna PJ. Schizophrenia and related syndromes. Oxford: Oxf University Press; 1994.

McKenna PJ, Tamlyn D, Lund CE, Mortimer AM, Hammond Baddeley AD. Amnesic syndrome in schizophrenia. Psychol M 1990; 20: 967–72.

Meltzer HY. Pre-clinical pharmacology of atypical antipsychc drugs: a selective review. [Review]. Br J Psychiatry 1996; Suppl 29: 23–31.

Mesulam M-M. Schizophrenia and the brain [editorial; commen N Engl J Med 1990; 322: 842–5. Comment on: N Engl J M 1990; 322: 789-94.

Mesulam M-M, Geschwind N. On the possible role of neocortex a its limbic connections in the process of attention and schizophren clinical cases of inattention in man and experimental anatomy monkey. J Psychiatr Res 1978; 14: 249–59.

Miyakawa T, Sumiyoshi S, Deshimaru M, Suzuki T, Tomon H. Electron microscopic study on schizophrenia. Mechanism pathological changes. Acta Neuropathol (Berl) 1972; 20: 67–77.

Miyake T, Kitamura T, Takamatsu T, Fujita S. A quantitat analysis of human astrocytosis. Acta Neuropathol (Berl) 1988; 535–7.

Moser M-B, Trommald M, Andersen P. An increase in dendr spine density on hippocampal CA1 pyramidal cells following spa learning in adult rats suggests the formation of new synapses. P Natl Acad Sci USA 1994; 91: 12673–5.

Murphy GM Jr, Lim KO, Wieneke M, Ellis WG, Forno LS, Hoff AL, et al. No neuropathologic evidence for an increased frequency of Alzheimer's disease among elderly schizophrenics. Biol Psychiatry 1998; 43: 205–9.

Murray RM, Lewis SW. Is schizophrenia a neurodevelopmental disorder? [editorial] Br Med J 1987; 295: 681–2.

Murray RM, Woodruff PWR. Developmental insanity or dementia praecox: a new perspective on an old debate. Neurol Psychiatry Brain Res 1995; 3: 167–76.

Murray RM, O'Callaghan E, Castle DJ, Lewis SW. A neurodevelopmental approach to the classification of schizophrenia. [Review]. Schizophr Bull 1992; 18: 319–32.

Nair TR, Christensen JD, Kingsbury SJ, Kumar NG, Terry WM, Garver DL. Progression of cerebroventricular enlargement and the subtyping of schizophrenia. Psychiatry Res 1997; 74: 141–50.

Nasrallah HA, McCalley-Whitters M, Bigelow LB, Rauscher FP. A histological study of the corpus callosum in chronic schizophrenia. Psychiatry Res 1983; 8: 251–60.

Nelson MD, Saykin AJ, Flashman LA, Riordan HJ. Hippocampal volume reduction in schizophrenia as assessed by magnetic resonance imaging: a meta-analytic study. Arch Gen Psychiatry 1998; 55: 433–40.

Nieto D, Escobar A. Major psychoses. In: Minckler J, editor. Pathology of the nervous system. New York: McGraw-Hill; 1972. p. 2655–65.

Niizato K, Arai T, Kuroki N, Kase K, Iritani S, Ikeda K. Autopsy study of Alzheimer's disease brain pathology in schizophrenia. Schizophr Res 1998; 31: 177–84.

Noga JT, Bartley AJ, Jones DW, Torrey EF, Weinberger DR. Cortical gyral anatomy and gross brain dimensions in monozygotic twins discordant for schizophrenia. Schizophr Res 1996; 22: 27–40.

Nopoulos P, Flaum M, Andreasen NC. Sex differences in brain morphology in schizophrenia [see comments]. 48–54. Comment in: Am J Psychiatry 1997; 154: 1637–9.

Nordstrom AL, Farde L, Eriksson L, Halldin C. No elevated D_2 dopamine receptors in neuroleptic-naive schizophrenic patients revealed by positron emission tomography and [^{11}C]N-methylspiperone [see comments]. Psychiatry Res 1995; 61: 67–83. Comment in: Psychiatry Res 1996; 67: 159-62.

Okubo Y, Suhara T, Suzuki K, Kobayashi K, Inoue O, Terasaki O, et al. Decreased prefrontal dopamine D1 receptors in schizophrenia revealed by PET [see comments]. Nature 1997; 385: 634–6. Comment in: Nature 1997; 385: 578-9.

Olney JW, Farber NB. Glutamate receptor dysfunction and schizophrenia [see comments]. Arch Gen Psychiatry 1995; 52: 998–1007. Comment in: Arch Gen Psychiatry 1997; 54: 578-80.

Ong WY, Garey LJ. Ultrastructural features of biopsied temporopolar cortex (area 38) in a case of schizophrenia. Schizophr Res 1993; 10: 15–27.

Owen F, Simpson MDC. The neurochemistry of schizophrenia. In: Hirsch SR, Weinberger DR, editors. Schizophrenia. Oxford: Blackwell Science; 1995. p. 358–78.

Pakkenberg B. Post-mortem study of chronic schizophrenic brains. Br J Psychiatry 1987; 151: 744–52.

Pakkenberg B. Pronounced reduction of total neuron number in mediodorsal thalamic nucleus and nucleus accumbens in schizophrenics. Arch Gen Psychiatry 1990; 47: 1023–8.

Pakkenberg B. The volume of the mediodorsal thalamic nucleus in treated and untreated schizophrenics. Schizophr Res 1992; 7: 95–100.

Pakkenberg B. Leucotomized schizophrenics lose neurons in the mediodorsal thalamic nucleus. Neuropathol Appl Neurobiol 1993a; 19: 373–80.

Pakkenberg B. Total nerve cell number in neocortex in chronic schizophrenics and controls estimated using optical disectors. Biol Psychiatry 1993b; 34: 768–72.

Pantelis C, Barnes TR, Nelson HE, Tanner S, Weatherley L, Owen AM, et al. Frontal–striatal cognitive deficits in patients with chronic schizophrenia. Brain 1997; 120: 1823–43.

Pearlson GD, Petty RG, Ross CA, Tien AY. Schizophrenia: a disease of heteromodal association cortex. [Review]. Neuropsychopharmacology 1996; 14: 1–17.

Pearlson GD, Barta PE, Powers RE, Menon RR, Richards SS, Aylward EH, et al. Medial and superior temporal gyral volumes and cerebral asymmetry in schizophrenia versus bipolar disorder. Biol Psychiatry 1997; 41: 1–14.

Pearson RCA, Powell TPS. The neuroanatomy of Alzheimer's disease. Rev Neurosci 1989; 2: 101–22.

Perrone-Bizzozero NI, Sower AC, Bird ED, Benowitz LI, Ivins KJ, Neve RL. Levels of the growth-associated protein GAP-43 are selectively increased in association cortices in schizophrenia. Proc Natl Acad Sci USA 1996; 93: 14182–7.

Pierce JP, Lewin GR. An ultrastructural size principle. [Review]. Neuroscience 1994; 58: 441–6.

Plum F. Prospects for research on schizophrenia. 3. Neurophysiology. Neuropathological findings. Neurosci Res Program Bull 1972; 10: 384–8.

Portas CM, Goldstein JM, Shenton ME, Hokama HH, Wible CG, Fischer I, et al. Volumetric evaluation of the thalamus in schizophrenic male patients using magnetic resonance imaging. Biol Psychiatry 1998; 43: 649–59.

Porter RH, Eastwood SL, Harrison PJ. Distribution of kainate receptor subunit mRNAs in human hippocampus, neocortex and cerebellum, and bilateral reduction of hippocampal GluR6 and KA2 transcripts in schizophrenia. Brain Res 1997; 751: 217–31.

Powchik P, Friedman J, Haroutunian V, Greenberg D, Altsteil L, Purohit D, et al. Apolipoprotein E4 in schizophrenia: a study of one hundred sixteen cases with concomitant neuropathological examination. Biol Psychiatry 1997; 42: 296–8.

Prohovnik I, Dwork AJ, Kaufman MA, Willson N. Alzheimer-type neuropathology in elderly schizophrenia patients. Schizophr Bull 1993; 19: 805–16.

Purohit DP, Perl DP, Haroutunian V, Powchik P, Davidson M, Davies KL. Alzheimer disease and related neurodegenerative diseases in elderly patients with schizophrenia: a postmortem neuropathologic study of 100 cases. Arch Gen Psychiatry 1998; 55: 205–11.

Raedler TJ, Knable MB, Weinberger DR. Schizophrenia as a developmental disorder of the cerebral cortex. [Review]. Curr Opin Neurobiol 1998; 8: 157–61.

Rajkowska G, Selemon LD, Goldman-Rakic PS. Neuronal and glial somal size in the prefrontal cortex: a postmortem morphometric study of schizophrenia and Huntington disease. Arch Gen Psychiatry 1998; 55: 215–24.

Randall PL. Schizophrenia, abnormal connection, and brain evolution. Med Hypotheses 1983; 10: 247–80.

Rapoport JL, Giedd J, Kumra S, Jacobsen L, Smith A, Lee P, et al. Childhood-onset schizophrenia. Progressive ventricular change during adolescence [see comments]. Arch Gen Psychiatry 1997; 54: 897–903. Comment in: Arch Gen Psychiatry 1997; 54: 913-4.

Raymond GV, Bauman ML, Kemper TL. Hippocampus in autism: a Golgi analysis. Acta Neuropathol (Berl) 1996; 91: 117–9.

Raz S, Raz N. Structural brain abnormalities in the major psychoses: a quantitative review of the evidence from computerized imaging. Psychol Bull 1990; 108: 93–108.

Renshaw PF, Yurgelun-Todd DA, Tohen M, Gruber S, Cohen BM. Temporal lobe proton magnetic resonance spectroscopy of patients with first-episode psychosis. Am J Psychiatry 1995; 152: 444–6.

Reveley AM, Reveley MA, Clifford CA, Murray RM. Cerebral ventricular size in twins discordant for schizophrenia. Lancet 1982; 1: 540–1.

Reyes MG, Gordon A. Cerebellar vermis in schizophrenia [letter]. Lancet 1981; 2, 700–1.

Reynolds GP. Neurotransmitter systems in schizophrenia. [Review]. Int Rev Neurobiol 1995; 38: 305–39.

Reynolds GP. Dopamine D4 receptors in schizophrenia [letter; comment]. J Neurochem 1996; 66: 881–3. Comment on: J Neurochem 1995; 64: 1413-5.

Riederer P, Gsell W, Calza L, Franzek E, Jungkunz G, Jellinger K, et al. Consensus on minimal criteria of clinical and neuropathological diagnosis of schizophrenia and affective disorders for post-mortem research. [Review]. J Neural Transm Gen Sect 1995; 102: 255–64.

Roberts GW. Schizophrenia: a neuropathological perspective. [Review]. Br J Psychiatry 1991; 158: 8–17.

Roberts GW, Colter N, Lofthouse R, Bogerts B, Zech M, Crow TJ. Gliosis in schizophrenia: a survey. Biol Psychiatry 1986; 21: 1043–50.

Roberts GW, Colter N, Lofthouse R, Johnstone EC, Crow TJ. Is there gliosis in schizophrenia? Investigation of the temporal lobe. Biol Psychiatry 1987; 22: 1459–68.

Roberts RC, Conley R, Kung L, Peretti FJ, Chute DJ. Reduced striatal spine size in schizophrenia: a postmortem ultrastructural study. Neuroreport 1996; 7: 1214–8.

Roberts GW, Royston MC, Weinberger DR. Schizophrenia. In: Graham DI, Lantos PL, editors. Greenfield's neuropathology. 6th ed. London: Edward Arnold; 1997. p. 897–929.

Roessmann U, Gambetti P. Pathological reaction of astrocytes perinatal brain injury. Immunohistochemical study. Ac Neuropathol (Berl) 1986; 70: 302–7.

Rojiani AM, Emery JA, Anderson KJ, Massey JK. Distributic of heterotopic neurons in normal hemispheric white matter morphometric analysis. J Neuropathol Exp Neurol 1996; 55: 178–8

Ron MA, Harvey I. The brain in schizophrenia [see comments [Review]. J Neurol Neurosurg Psychiatry 1990; 53: 725–6. Comme in: J Neurol Neurosurg Psychiatry 1992; 55: 522, Comment in: Neurol Neurosurg Psychiatry 1992; 55: 981.

Rosenthal R, Bigelow LB. Quantitative brain measurements : chronic schizophrenia. Br J Psychiatry 1972; 121: 259–64.

Russell AJ, Munro JC, Jones PB, Hemsley DR, Murray RN Schizophrenia and the myth of intellectual decline. Am J Psychiatr 1997; 154: 635–9.

Sabri O, Erkwoh R, Schreckenberger M, Owega A, Sass H, Bue U. Correlation of positive symptoms exclusively to hyperperfusic or hypoperfusion of cerebral cortex in never-treated schizophrenic Lancet 1997; 349: 1735–9.

Saito S, Kobayashi S, Ohashi Y, Igarashi M, Komiya Y, Ando S Decreased synaptic density in aged brains and its prevention b rearing under enriched environment as revealed by synaptophysi contents. J Neurosci Res 1994; 39: 57–62.

Saunders RC, Kolachana BS, Bachevalier J, Weinberger DF Neonatal lesions of the medial temporal lobe disrupt prefronta cortical regulation of striatal dopamine. Nature 1998; 393: 169–7

Saykin AJ, Gur RC, Gur RE, Mozley PD, Mozley LH, Resnic SM, et al. Neuropsychological function in schizophrenia. Selectiv impairment in memory and learning. Arch Gen Psychiatry 199 48: 618–24.

Saykin AJ, Shtasel DL, Gur RE, Kester DB, Mozley LH, Stafiniak I et al. Neuropsychological deficits in neuroleptic naive patients wit first-episode schizophrenia. Arch Gen Psychiatry 1994; 51: 124–3

Schlaug G, Armstrong E, Schleicher A, Zilles K. Layer V pyramid cells in the adult human cingulate cortex. A quantitative Golg study. Anat Embryol (Berl) 1993; 187: 515–22.

Sedvall G, Farde L. Chemical brain anatomy in schizophrenia [se comments]. [Review]. Lancet 1995; 346: 743–9. Comment ir Lancet 1995; 346: 1302-3.

Seeman P, Guan H-C, Van Tol HH. Dopamine D4 receptor elevated in schizophrenia [see comments]. Nature 1993; 365: 441- 5. Comment in: Nature 1993; 365: 393.

Seeman P, Corbett R, Van Tol HH. Atypical neuroleptics have lov affinity for dopamine D2 receptors or are selective for D4 receptors [Review]. Neuropsychopharmacology 1997; 16: 93–110.

Selemon LD, Rajkowska G, Goldman-Rakic PS. Abnormally higl neuronal density in the schizophrenic cortex. A morphometri analysis of prefrontal area 9 and occipital area 17. Arch Ge Psychiatry 1995; 52: 805–18.

Selemon LD, Rajkowska G, Goldman-Rakic PS. Elevated neurona density in prefrontal area 46 in brains from schizophrenic patients application of a three-dimensional, stereologic counting method. Comp Neurol 1998; 392: 402–12.

Shapiro RM. Regional neuropathology in schizophrenia: where are we? Where are we going? [Review]. Schizophr Res 1993; 10: 187–239.

Sharma T, Lancaster E, Lee D, Lewis S, Sigmundsson T, Takei N, et al. Brain changes in schizophrenia. Br J Psychiatry 1998; 173: 132–8.

Shenton ME, Kikinis R, Jolesz FA, Pollak SD, LeMay M, Wible CG, et al. Abnormalities of the left temporal lobe and thought disorder in schizophrenia. A quantitative magnetic resonance imaging study. N Engl J Med 1992; 327: 604–12.

Shihabuddin L, Buchsbaum MS, Hazlett EA, Haznedar MM, Harvey PD, Newman A, et al. Dorsal striatal size, shape, and metabolic rate in never-medicated and previously medicated schizophrenics performing a verbal learning task. Arch Gen Psychiatry 1998; 55: 235–43.

Shioiri T, Oshitani Y, Kato T, Murashita J, Hamakawa H, Inubushi T, et al. Prevalence of cavum septum pellucidum detected by MRI in patients with bipolar disorder, major depression and schizophrenia. Psychol Med 1996; 26: 431–4.

Silbersweig DA, Stern E, Frith C, Cahill C, Holmes A, Grootoonk S, et al. A functional neuroanatomy of hallucinations in schizophrenia. Nature 1995; 378: 176–9.

Silverman JM, Smith CJ, Guo SL, Mohs RC, Siever LJ, Davis KL. Lateral ventricular enlargement in schizophrenic probands and their siblings with schizophrenia-related disorders. Biol Psychiatry 1998; 43: 97–106.

Simpson MD, Slater P, Deakin JF, Royston MC, Skan WJ. Reduced GABA uptake sites in the temporal lobe in schizophrenia. Neurosci Lett 1989; 107: 211–5.

Soustek Z. Ultrastructure of cortical synapses in the brain of schizophrenics. Zentralbl Allg Pathol 1989; 135: 25–32.

Southard EE. On the topographical distribution of cortex lesions and anomalies in dementia praecox, with some account of their functional significance. Am J Insan 1915; 71: 603–71.

Stevens JR. An anatomy of schizophrenia? Arch Gen Psychiatry 1973; 29: 177–89.

Stevens JR. Neuropathology of schizophrenia. Arch Gen Psychiatry 1982; 39: 1131–9.

Stevens JR. Abnormal reinnervation as a basis for schizophrenia: a hypothesis [published erratum appears in Arch Gen Psychiatry 1992; 49: 708]. [Review]. Arch Gen Psychiatry 1992; 49: 238–43.

Stevens JR. Anatomy of schizophrenia revisited. [Review]. Schizophr Bull 1997; 23: 373–83.

Stevens J, Casanova M, Bigelow L. Gliosis in schizophrenia [published erratum appears in Biol Psychiatry 1988; 25: 121]. Biol Psychiatry 1988a; 24: 727–9.

Stevens CD, Altshuler LL, Bogerts B, Falkai P. Quantitative study of gliosis in schizophrenia and Huntington's chorea. Biol Psychiatry 1988b; 24: 697–700.

Stevens JR, Casanova M, Poltorak M, Germain L, Buchan GC. Comparison of immunocytochemical and Holzer's methods for detection of acute and chronic gliosis in human postmortem material

[see comments]. J Neuropsychiatry Clin Neurosci 1992; 4: 168–73. Comment in: J Neuropsychiatry Clin Neurosci 1993; 5: 225-7.

Suddath RL, Christison GW, Torrey EF, Casanova MF, Weinberger DR. Anatomical abnormalities in the brains of monozygotic twins discordant for schizophrenia [published erratum appears in N Engl J Med 1990; 322: 1616] [see comments]. N Engl J Med 1990; 322: 789–94. Comment in: N Engl J Med 1990; 322: 842-5, Comment in: N Engl J Med 1990; 323: 545-8.

Tamminga CA. Gender and schizophrenia. [Review]. J Clin Psychiatry 1997; 58 Suppl 15: 33–7.

Tamminga CA. Schizophrenia and glutamatergic transmission. [Review]. Crit Rev Neurobiol 1998; 12: 21–36.

Tatetsu S. A contribution to the morphological background of schizophrenia: with special reference to the findings in the telencephalon. Acta Neuropathol (Berl) 1964; 3: 558–71.

Tcherepanov AA, Sokolov BP. Age-related abnormalities in expression of mRNAs encoding synapsin 1A, synapsin 1B, and synaptophysin in the temporal cortex of schizophrenics. J Neurosci Res 1997; 49: 639–44.

Terry RD, Masliah E, Salmon DP, Butters N, DeTeresa R, Hill R, et al. Physical basis of cognitive alterations in Alzheimer's disease: synapse loss is the major correlate of cognitive impairment. Ann Neurol 1991; 30: 572–80.

Thibaut F, Coron B, Hannequin D, Segard L, Martin C, Dollfus S, et al. No association of apolipoprotein epsilon 4 allele with schizophrenia even in cognitively impaired patients. Schizophr Res 1998; 30: 149–53.

Thompson PM, Sower AC, Perrone-Bizzozero NI. Altered levels of the synaptosomal associated protein SNAP-25 in schizophrenia. Biol Psychiatry 1998; 43: 239–43.

Tononi G, McIntosh AR, Russell DP, Edelman GM. Functional clustering: identifying strongly interactive brain regions in neuroimaging data. Neuroimage 1998; 7: 133–49.

Torrey EF, Peterson MR. Schizophrenia and the limbic system. [Review]. Lancet 1974; 2: 942–6.

Tran KD, Smutzer GS, Doty RL, Arnold SE. Reduced Purkinje cell size in the cerebellar vermis of elderly patients with schizophrenia. Am J Psychiatry 1998; 155: 1288–90.

Trichard C, Paillere-Martinot ML, Attar-Levy D, Blin J, Feline A, Martinot JL. No serotonin 5-HT$_{2A}$ receptor density abnormality in the cortex of schizophrenic patients studied with PET. Schizophr Res 1998; 31: 13–7.

Uranova NA, Casanova MF, DeVaughn NM, Orlovskaya DD, Denisov DV. Ultrastructural alterations of synaptic contacts and astrocytes in postmortem caudate nucleus of schizophrenic patients [letter]. Schizophr Res 1996; 22: 81–3.

Van Horn JD, McManus IC. Ventricular enlargement in schizophrenia. A meta-analysis of studies of the ventricle: brain ratio (VBR) [see comments]. Br J Psychiatry 1992; 160: 687–97. Comment in: Br J Psychiatry 1992; 161: 278, Comment in: Br J Psychiatry 1992; 161: 714-5.

Vaughn JE, Matthews DA, Barber RP, Wimer CC, Wimer RE. Genetically-associated variations in the development of hippocampal pyramidal neurons may produce differences in mossy fiber connectivity. J Comp Neurol 1977; 173: 41–52.

Vita A, Dieci M, Giobbio GM, Tenconi F, Invernizzi G. Time course of cerebral ventricular enlargement in schizophrenia supports the hypothesis of its neurodevelopmental nature. [Review]. Schizophr Res 1997; 23: 25–30.

Vogeley K, Hobson T, Schneider-Axmann T, Honer WG, Bogerts B, Falkai P. Compartmental volumetry of the superior temporal gyrus reveals sex differences in schizophrenia—a post-mortem study. Schizophr Res 1998; 31: 83–7.

Waddington JL, Youssef HA. Cognitive dysfunction in chronic schizophrenia followed prospectively over 10 years and its longitudinal relationship to the emergence of tardive dyskinesia. Psychol Med 1996; 26: 681–8.

Walker EF, Diforio D. Schizophrenia: a neural diathesis-stress model. Psychol Rev 1997; 104: 667–85.

Ward KE, Friedman L, Wise A, Schulz SC. Meta-analysis of brain and cranial size in schizophrenia. Schizophr Res 1996; 22: 197–213.

Weickert CS, Weinberger DR. A candidate molecule approach to defining developmental pathology in schizophrenia. [Review]. Schizophr Bull 1998; 24: 303–16.

Weinberger DR. Implications of normal brain development for the pathogenesis of schizophrenia. Arch Gen Psychiatry 1987; 44: 660–9.

Weinberger DR. From neuropathology to neurodevelopment. [Review]. Lancet 1995; 346: 552–7.

Weinberger DR, Berman KF, Suddath R, Torrey EF. Evidence of dysfunction of a prefrontal-limbic network in schizophrenia: a magnetic resonance imaging and regional cerebral blood flow study of discordant monozygotic twins. Am J Psychiatry 1992; 149: 890–7.

West MJ, Slomianka L. Total number of neurons in the layers of the human entorhinal cortex. Hippocampus 1998; 8: 69–82.

Whitworth AB, Honeder M, Kremser C, Kemmler G, Felber S, Hausmann A, et al. Hippocampal volume reduction in male schizophrenic patients. Schizophr Res 1998; 31: 73–81.

Williams J, McGuffin P, Nothen MM, Owen MJ. Meta-analysis of the association between the 5-HT$_{2A}$ receptor T102C polymorphism and schizophrenia [letter]. Lancet 1997; 349: 1221.

Williams RW, Strom RC, Goldowitz D. Natural variation in neuron number in mice is linked to a major quantitative trait locus on Chr 11. J Neurosci 1998; 18: 138–46.

Wisniewski HM, Constantinidis J, Wegiel J, Bobinski M, Tarnawski M. Neurofibrillary pathology in brains of elderly schizophrenics treated with neuroleptics. Alzheimer Dis Assoc Disord 1994; 8: 211–27.

Woo TU, Whitehead RE, Melchitzky DS, Lewis DA. A subclass of prefrontal gamma-aminobutyric acid axon terminals are selectively altered in schizophrenia. Proc Natl Acad Sci USA 1998; 95: 5341–6.

Woodruff PW, Wright IC, Shuriquie N, Russouw H, Rushe T, Howard RJ, et al. Structural brain abnormalities in male schizophrenics reflect fronto-temporal dissociation. Psychol Med 1997; 27: 1257–66.

Young CE, Arima K, Xie J, Hu L, Beach TG, Falkai P, et al. SNAP-25 deficit and hippocampal connectivity in schizophrenia. Cereb Cortex 1998; 8: 261–8.

Zaidel DW, Esiri MM, Harrison PJ. Size, shape, and orientation of neurons in the left and right hippocampus: investigation of normal asymmetries and alterations in schizophrenia. Am J Psychiatry 1997a; 154: 812–8.

Zaidel DW, Esiri MM, Harrison PJ. The hippocampus in schizophrenia: lateralized increase in neuronal density and altered cytoarchitectural asymmetry. Psychol Med 1997b; 27: 703–13.

Zakzanis KK, Hansen KT. Dopamine D$_2$ receptor densities and the schizophrenic brain. Schizophr Res 1998; 32: 201–6.

Zipursky RB, Lambe EK, Kapur S, Mikulis DJ. Cerebral gray matter volume deficits in first episode psychosis. Arch Gen Psychiatry 1998; 55: 540–6.

Received 18 September, 1998. Revised November 11, 1998. Accepted 3 December, 1998

Proc. Natl. Acad. Sci. USA
Vol. 93, pp. 9235–9240, August 1996
Neurobiology

Single photon emission computerized tomography imaging of amphetamine-induced dopamine release in drug-free schizophrenic subjects

MARC LARUELLE*†‡, ANISSA ABI-DARGHAM*†, CHRISTOPHER H. VAN DYCK*, ROBERTO GIL*†,
CYRIL D. D'SOUZA*†, JOSEPH ERDOS*†, ELINORE MCCANCE*, WILLIAM ROSENBLATT§, CHRISTINE FINGADO*†,
SAMI S. ZOGHBI¶, RONALD M. BALDWIN*†, JOHN P. SEIBYL¶, JOHN H. KRYSTAL*†, DENNIS S. CHARNEY*†,
AND ROBERT B. INNIS*†

Departments of *Psychiatry, ¶Diagnostic Radiology, and §Anesthesiology, Yale University School of Medicine, New Haven, CT 06520; and †Veterans Affairs Medical Center, West Haven, CT 06516

Communicated by Patricia S. Goldman-Rakic, Yale University, New Haven, CT, May 24, 1996 (received for review March 12, 1996)

ABSTRACT   The dopamine hypothesis of schizophrenia proposes that hyperactivity of dopaminergic transmission is associated with this illness. However, direct observation of abnormalities of dopamine function in schizophrenia has remained elusive. We used a newly developed single photon emission computerized tomography method to measure amphetamine-induced dopamine release in the striatum of fifteen patients with schizophrenia and fifteen healthy controls. Amphetamine-induced dopamine release was estimated by the amphetamine-induced reduction in dopamine D_2 receptor availability, measured as the binding potential of the specific D_2 receptor radiotracer $[^{123}I](S)$-$(-)$-3-iodo-2-hydroxy-6-methoxy-N-[(1-ethyl-2-pyrrolidinyl)methyl]benzamide ($[^{123}I]$IBZM). The amphetamine-induced decrease in $[^{123}I]$IBZM binding potential was significantly greater in the schizophrenic group ($-19.5 \pm 4.1\%$) compared with the control group ($-7.6 \pm 2.1\%$). In the schizophrenic group, elevated amphetamine effect on $[^{123}I]$IBZM binding potential was associated with emergence or worsening of positive psychotic symptoms. This result suggests that psychotic symptoms elicited in this experimental setting in schizophrenic patients are associated with exaggerated stimulation of dopaminergic transmission. Such an observation would be compatible with an abnormal responsiveness of dopaminergic neurons in schizophrenia.

The dopamine hypothesis of schizophrenia, formulated about 30 years ago, proposes that hyperactivity of dopaminergic transmission is associated with this illness (1). This hypothesis is based on the observation that dopamine D_2 receptor antagonists alleviate symptoms of the illness (mostly positive symptoms), while dopamine agonists can induce psychotic states characterized by some salient features of schizophrenia (2). These pharmacological effects suggest, but do not establish, a dysregulation of dopamine systems in schizophrenia. Despite decades of effort to validate this hypothesis, documentation of abnormalities of dopamine function in schizophrenia has remained elusive. Postmortem studies measuring dopamine and its metabolites in the brain of schizophrenic patients have yielded inconsistent results (for review, see ref. 3). Increased density of striatal dopamine D_2 and D_2-like receptors has been reported in postmortem studies, but this observation is difficult to interpret, given that neuroleptic drugs upregulate these receptors (4, 5). Positron emission tomography and single photon emission computerized tomography (SPECT) studies of striatal D_2 and D_2-like receptors density in neuroleptic-naive schizophrenic patients have been inconclusive. While

one group reported increased striatal D_2-like receptors density in schizophrenia (6, 7), other groups reported negative results (8–12). The lack of clear evidence for increased dopaminergic indices in schizophrenia might indicate that dopaminergic transmission is enhanced only relative to other systems, such as serotonergic or glutamatergic systems (13, 14). On the other hand, the absence of data supporting the dopamine hypothesis of schizophrenia might be due to the difficulty of obtaining direct measurement of dopamine transmission in the living human brain.

Over the past few years, several groups have provided evidence that competition between neurotransmitters and radioligands for neuroreceptor binding allows measuring changes in synaptic neurotransmitter levels with in vivo binding techniques. In rodents, decreased uptake of D_2 radioligands has been measured following amphetamine and other dopamine enhancing drugs, whereas the opposite effect (i.e., increased tracer accumulation) has been induced by drugs that decrease dopamine concentration (15–17). In baboons, decreased specific uptake of positron emission tomography or SPECT D_2 radiotracers has been reported following amphetamine challenge (18–20). In humans, decreased accumulation of the D_2 antagonist $[^{11}C]$raclopride has been observed following challenges with amphetamine (21) or methylphenidate (22).

We recently developed and validated a protocol to measure amphetamine-induced dopamine release with SPECT and $[^{123}I](S)$-$(-)$-3-iodo-2-hydroxy-6-methoxy-N-[(1-ethyl-2-pyrrolidinyl)methyl]benzamide ($[^{123}I]$IBZM). This radiotracer, an iodinated analog of raclopride, is a selective antagonist at the D_2 and D_3 receptors (23). We initially observed that amphetamine challenge reduced the $[^{123}I]$IBZM binding potential in baboons (the binding potential is the product of the density and affinity of free receptors; ref. 24). Since amphetamine is devoid of significant affinity for D_2 receptors (amphetamine IC_{50} for $[^{123}I]$IBZM in vitro is >100 μM; unpublished results), we postulated that this effect was mediated by increased dopamine release and displacement of $[^{123}I]$IBZM specific binding by dopamine. This mechanism was confirmed by the observation that pretreatment with the dopamine depleter α-methyl-p-tyrosine prevented the effect of amphetamine on $[^{123}I]$IBZM binding potential (24). In addition, we established the existence of a good correlation between amphetamine-induced dopamine release measured with microdialysis and amphetamine-induced decrease in $[^{123}I]$IBZM binding potential measured with SPECT (24).

Abbreviations: SPECT, single photon emission computerized tomography; $[^{123}I]$IBZM, $[^{123}I](S)$-$(-)$-3-iodo-2-hydroxy-6-methoxy-N-[(1-ethyl-2-pyrrolidinyl)methyl]benzamide.
‡To whom reprint requests should be sent at the present address: New York State Psychiatric Institute, 722 West 168th Street, Unit 28, New York, NY 10032.

Therefore, measuring the reduction in [^{123}I]IBZM binding potential following amphetamine provides a noninvasive method to estimate the magnitude of amphetamine-induced dopamine release in the vicinity of the receptors (which includes, but is not restricted to, the synaptic space). Preliminary experiments in healthy volunteers demonstrated the feasibility of this method in humans (25).

Acute exposure to amphetamine induces emergence or worsening of positive symptoms in schizophrenic patients at doses that do not produce psychotic symptoms in healthy subjects (for review, see ref. 26). The neuronal mechanisms underlying this sensitivity of schizophrenic patients to the psychotogenic effect of amphetamine are not known. Preclinical data suggest that this exaggerated response might be associated with enhanced dopamine release (27). To test this hypothesis, we measured the amphetamine-induced reduction in [^{123}I]IBZM binding potential in fifteen drug free patients with schizophrenia and fifteen healthy controls matched for age, gender, race, and parental socioeconomic status.

METHODS

The study was performed according to protocols approved by Yale School of Medicine and West Haven Veterans Affairs Internal Review Boards. Inclusion criteria for patients were as follows: (*i*) diagnosis of schizophrenia according to Diagnostic and Statistical Manual (DSM-IV); (*ii*) no other DSM-IV axis I diagnosis; (*iii*) no history of alcohol or substance abuse or dependence; (*iv*) absence of any psychotropic medication for at least 21 days before the study (with the exception of lorazepam, which was allowed at a maximal dose of 3 mg per day up to 24 h before the study); (*v*) no concomitant or past severe medical conditions; (*vi*) no pregnancy; (*vii*) no current suicidal or homicidal ideation; and (*viii*) ability to provide informed consent. After explanation of the nature and risks of the study, the ability of the patient to provide informed consent was formally evaluated by asking the patient to complete a multiple-choice questionnaire (available on request). According to the recommendation of the National Alliance for the Mentally Ill (Arlington, VA), consent from involved family members was also obtained. All patients were admitted to a research ward for the duration of the study (including the washout period).

Inclusion criteria for healthy controls were as follows: (*i*) absence of past or present neurological or psychiatric illnesses; (*ii*) no concomitant or past severe medical conditions; (*iii*) no pregnancy; and (*iv*) informed consent. Healthy controls were individually matched to patients for age (±5 years), gender, race, and parental socioeconomic level. Socioeconomic level was assessed by education and employment using the Hollingstead scale (A. Hollingstead, Four-Factor Index of Social Status; work published by the author, 1975).

SPECT experiments were carried out as described (25). [^{123}I]IBZM with specific activity >5000 Ci/mmol and radiochemical purity >95% was prepared by direct electrophilic radioiodination of the desiodoprecursor BZM. An i.v. catheter was inserted in each arm of the subject, for drug administration and blood sampling, respectively. A total [^{123}I]IBZM dose of 10.5 ± 0.5 mCi (with this and subsequent values expressed as mean ± SEM) was given as a bolus (4.0 ± 0.2 mCi) followed by a continuous infusion at a rate of 1.1 ± 0.1 mCi/h for the duration of the experiment (375 min, with this and all subsequent times given in reference to the beginning of the radiotracer administration). This protocol of administration (bolus plus constant infusion) was shown, in preliminary experiments, to induce a state of sustained binding equilibrium: in the absence of amphetamine injection, both the specific and nonspecific activity remained at a constant level from 150 min to the end of the experiment (25).

SPECT data were acquired on the PRISM 3000 (Picker, Cleveland, OH) with high-resolution fan beam collimators (resolution at full-width half-maximum, 11 mm; ^{123}I point source sensitivity, 16.5 counts/s per μCi). Two scanning sessions were obtained for each subject (before and after amphetamine injection). Each scanning session consisted of eight consecutive acquisitions of 8 min each. The first scanning session was obtained from 180 min to 244 min. After completion of the first scanning session, amphetamine (dextroamphetamine sulfate) was injected i.v. at a dose of 0.3 mg/kg over 30 s. Experiments in baboons established that it takes ≈60 min for [^{123}I]IBZM displacement to be achieved after amphetamine challenge. Therefore, subjects were not scanned during the 60 min following the amphetamine injection and were available for evaluation of the psychiatric response to amphetamine. The second scanning session (post-amphetamine session) was obtained from 310 min to 374 min.

Plasma metabolite-corrected [^{123}I]IBZM steady-state concentration (C_{SS}) was measured by extraction followed by high-pressure liquid chromatography on nine venous samples collected at 20-min intervals from 180 to 300 min (25). Determination of the plasma [^{123}I]IBZM free fraction (f_1) was performed by ultrafiltration (Centrifree; Amicon) (28). Plasma [^{123}I]IBZM clearance was calculated as the ratio of C_{SS} to infusion rate. Amphetamine plasma concentration was measured by gas chromatography (National Medical Services, Willow Grove, PA) on three venous samples obtained at 10, 20, and 40 min post-amphetamine injection. Because no statistically significant differences were observed between these three amphetamine measurements (repeated measures ANOVA, $P = 0.17$), the average values were used in subsequent analyses.

The clinical response to the amphetamine challenge was evaluated with the Positive and Negative Symptom Scales (29). Baseline ratings were obtained 60 min before the first scanning session. Post-amphetamine ratings were obtained 30 min after the injection of amphetamine (i.e., during the interval between the first and second scanning session). For positive and negative subscales, a change of at least four points relative to baseline was considered clinically significant. Behavioral response was also rated by the subjects using a simplified version of the Amphetamine Interview Rating Scale (30). Self ratings for euphoria, restlessness, alertness, and anxiety were obtained at various intervals, using a ten-point analog scale (25). Responses were calculated as peak minus baseline scores.

SPECT data were analyzed blind to the diagnosis. Count projections were prefiltered using a Wiener 0.5 filter and backprojected using a ramp filter. SPECT images were reoriented to the cantho-meatal line as visualized by four external fiducial markers glued to the subject's head. The four slices with highest striatal uptake were summed and attenuation corrected assuming uniform attenuation. Standard region of interest profiles (striatum 556 mm^2; occipital 2204 mm^2) were positioned on the summed images. The camera resolution did not allow differentiating counts originating from the dorsal (sensorimotor) or ventral (limbic) striatum. Thus, the striatal region included both components. Right and left striatal regions were averaged. Striatal specific binding was calculated as striatal minus occipital activity. The occipital region was selected as the background region because (*i*) the density of dopamine D$_2$ receptors is negligible in this region compared with the striatum (31); (*ii*) this region can be identified with greater reliability than the cerebellum; and (*iii*) in humans, [^{123}I]IBZM activity in the occipital region is equal to the nonspecific activity in the striatum (32).

The baseline [^{123}I]IBZM binding potential (ml·g^{-1}), corresponding to the product of the free receptor density (B_{max}, nM, or pmol per g of brain tissue) and affinity (1/K_D, nM^{-1}, or ml of plasma per pmol), was calculated as the ratio of striatal specific binding (μCi per g of brain tissue) to the steady-state free unmetabolized plasma tracer concentration (f_1C_{SS}, μCi per ml of plasma) measured during scanning session 1 (25). For each scanning session, the specific to nonspecific equilibrium partition coefficient was calculated as the ratio of striatal minus occipital to occipital activity. Under steady-state conditions, the decrease in specific to nonspecific partition coefficient is equivalent to the decrease in binding potential (see equations in ref. 25). Amphetamine-induced decrease in [^{123}I]IBZM binding potential was expressed in percentage of pre-amphetamine value.

Unless otherwise specified, between-groups comparisons were performed with two-tailed unpaired t tests. Relationships between continuous variables were analyzed with the Pearson product moment correlation coefficient. A probability value of 0.05 was selected as significance level. Because of lack or loss of the second i.v. line, plasma samples for [^{123}I]IBZM measurement could not be obtained in one patient and one control. In these subjects, the relative decrease in [^{123}I]IBZM binding potential could be calculated, but not the absolute value of the baseline binding potential. For similar reasons, plasma samples for amphetamine measurement could not be obtained in three patients and one control.

RESULTS

Eighteen patients with schizophrenia were recruited for this study. One patient was neuroleptic-naive, eight patients were neuroleptic-free at the time of recruitment for reasons unrelated to the study (such as noncompliance or intolerance), and nine patients were taking neuroleptics and/or other psychotropic drugs at the time of recruitment. Because of clinical deterioration, medication was initiated or resumed before the end of the washout period in three patients. Thus, a total of 15 patients completed the protocol with a mean time off neuroleptic medication of 192 ± 141 days (range 21 days to 5 years). Five patients received lorazepam during the washout period. Mean duration of illness was 14 ± 2 years. Brief Psychiatric Rating Scale (33) scores were 37 ± 3 points, and Positive and Negative Symptom Scales scores at baseline were 16.6 ± 1.7 points for positive symptoms subscale and 14.9 ± 1.5 points for negative symptoms subscale. One patient presented mild tardive dyskinesia at baseline. Other patients were free of motor symptoms. Controls were matched with patients for age, gender, race, and parental socioeconomic status (Table 1).

The two groups did not differ in experimental parameters such as [^{123}I]IBZM total injected dose (schizophrenics, 11.0 ± 0.6 mCi; controls, 10.4 + 0.7 mCi; $P = 0.51$), effective bolus to hourly infusion ratio (schizophrenics, 3.88 ± 0.02 h; controls 3.87 ± 0.02 h; $P = 0.59$), scanning time (start of session 1: schizophrenics, 179 ± 7 min; controls, 180 ± 8 min; $P = 0.74$; start of session 2: schizophrenics, 319 ± 7 min; controls, 316 ± 8 min; $P = 0.75$). No between-group differences were observed in [^{123}I]IBZM plasma clearance (schizophrenics, 70.3 ± 6.1 liter/h; controls, 71.6 ± 5.2 liter/h; $P = 0.87$) or in the [^{123}I]IBZM plasma free fraction (schizophrenics, 3.1 ± 0.3%; controls, 3.5 ± 0.1%; $P = 0.87$). The steady-state quality of the plasma input function was evaluated by the slope of the

metabolite-corrected plasma [^{123}I]IBZM concentration from 180 to 300 min. This slope was small and not different between groups (schizophrenics, +2.1 ± 2.5% per h; controls, +2.1 ± 1.7% per h; $P = 0.98$). Similarly, the slope of the occipital activity from the beginning of scanning session 1 to the end of scanning session 2 was negligible and did not differ between the groups (schizophrenics, +1.0 ± 0.7% per h, controls, +1.1 ± 1.2% per h; $P = 0.94$). None of these slope distributions had a mean value significantly different from zero (one-sample t test, plasma [^{123}I]IBZM, $P = 0.18$; occipital [^{123}I]IBZM, $P = 0.13$), indicating that an adequate steady-state input function was achieved in both groups.

In agreement with previous data obtained with [^{123}I]IBZM and [^{11}C]raclopride in neuroleptic-naive schizophrenic patients (8, 10, 11), the density of D$_2$ receptors at baseline was not statistically different between schizophrenics and controls ($t = 1.35$, df = 26, $P = 0.18$; Table 2). Thus, potential D$_2$ receptor upregulation induced by previous neuroleptic treatment was not observed at the time of the study. The variance of baseline [^{123}I]IBZM binding potential was not statistically different between the groups (F-test for variance ratio: $F = 1.61, P = 0.40$).

The amphetamine-induced decrease in [^{123}I]IBZM binding potential was significantly larger in schizophrenic patients ($-19.5 ± 4.1\%$) than in controls ($-7.6 ± 2.1\%$; $t = 2.62$, df = 28, $P = 0.014$, Fig. 1 and Fig. 2 and Table 2). Schizophrenic patients exhibited larger displacement than control subjects in 12 of 15 pairs (paired t test: $t = 2.73$, df = 14, $P = 0.016$). The variance of the amphetamine effect on [^{123}I]IBZM binding potential was larger in the schizophrenic than in the control groups (variance ratio 3.85, $F = 3.85$, $P = 0.0167$). Therefore,

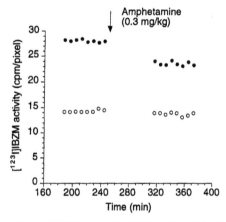

FIG. 1. [^{123}I]IBZM activity (in μCi/ml) in striatum (●) and occipital (○) before and after amphetamine challenge in a patient with schizophrenia. [^{123}I]IBZM was given as a bolus (4.6 mCi), followed by infusion at a constant rate of 1.2 mCi/h for the duration of the experiment (375 min). After establishment of steady state, a first scanning session was obtained from 180 to 244 min. Amphetamine (0.3 mg/kg i.v. bolus) was injected just after completion of the first scanning session (250 min, arrow). A second scanning session was obtained from 310 min to 374 min. Occipital activity was used to estimate the nonspecific binding in the striatum. Striatal specific binding to D$_2$ receptors was calculated by the difference between striatal and occipital activities. The reduction in [^{123}I]IBZM binding potential induced by amphetamine was calculated as the difference between the specific to nonspecific ratio measured during the first (0.99 ± 0.02) and second (0.77 ± 0.02) session and expressed in percentage of the baseline value (-22%).

Table 1. Demographic characteristics

Measure	Control subjects	Patients with schizophrenia
n	15	15
Age	41 ± 2	42 ± 2
Sex	14 M, 1 F	14 M, 1 F
Race	9 C, 5 AA, 1 H	9 C, 5 AA, 1 H
Parental SES	31 ± 3	37 ± 4
Subject SES	37 ± 4	24 ± 3*

Values are mean ± SEM. M, male; F, female; C, Caucasians; AA, African-Americans; H, Hispanics; and SES, socioeconomic status. *Unpaired two-tailed t test; $P = 0.011$.

Table 2. Measurement of D$_2$ receptor availability at baseline and after amphetamine

Measure	Control subjects	Patients with schizophrenia
Baseline [^{123}I]IBZM binding potential, ml/g	178 ± 12 (14)	204 ± 15 (14)
Amphetamine effect on [^{123}I]IBZM binding potential, % decrease	−7.6 ± 2.1% (15)	−19.5 ± 4.1% (15)*
Amphetamine plasma level, ng/ml	32 ± 3 (14)	35 ± 9 (12)

Values are mean ± SEM. Number of subjects (*n*) are in parentheses.
*Unpaired two-tailed *t* test; *P* = 0.014.

we also performed nonparametric analyses on this variable with similar results (unpaired analysis: Mann-Whitney *U*, *P* = 0.034; paired analysis: Wilcoxon Signed Rank, *P* = 0.014). No significant between-groups difference was observed in amphetamine plasma levels (*P* = 0.41; Table 2). No correlation was observed between amphetamine plasma levels and amphetamine-induced decreases in [^{123}I]IBZM binding potential, either in the entire sample (*r* = 0.08, *P* = 0.68) or in each group considered separately (schizophrenics, *r* = 0.24, *P* = 0.45; controls, *r* = 0.14, *P* = 0.63). Consequently, the group difference in amphetamine-induced [^{123}I]IBZM binding potential decrease could not be attributed to differences in amphetamine disposition. Amphetamine induced a transient (60–90 min) increase in systolic and diastolic blood pressure. The blood pressure response did not differ between the groups (peak systolic blood pressure above baseline: schizophrenics, 43 ± 5 mm Hg; controls, 49 ± 4 mm Hg, *P* = 0.31; peak diastolic above baseline: schizophrenics, 18 ± 2 mm Hg; controls, 22 ± 2 mm Hg, *P* = 0.11).

No psychotic symptoms were observed after the amphetamine injection in controls. In patients, the clinical response was heterogeneous. Amphetamine induced clinically significant worsening in positive psychotic symptoms in six patients, improvement in three patients, and no significant change in six patients. This distribution was consistent with the previously reported prevalence of psychotic reactions to acute challenge with dopamine agonists in schizophrenia (26). Negative symptoms improved significantly in four patients and did not change in 11 patients. All observable clinical changes were transient and, by the end of the experiment, patients had recovered their pre-amphetamine clinical status.

Schizophrenic patients who experienced worsening in positive symptoms showed larger reductions in [^{123}I]IBZM binding potential (−27.6 ± 6.4%, *n* = 6) than schizophrenic patients whose positive symptoms did not worsen (−14.1 ± 4.6%, *n* = 9) and healthy controls (−7.6 ± 2.1%, *n* = 15, ANOVA: *F* = 6.31, *P* = 0.0056, Kruskal–Wallis: *P* = 0.031). In the schizophrenic group, the magnitude of the amphetamine effect on [^{123}I]IBZM binding potential was positively correlated with changes in positive symptoms (*r* = 0.53, *P* = 0.038; Fig. 3). Such a correlation was not observed with changes in negative symptoms (*r* = 0.40, *P* = 0.14). Schizophrenic and controls did not differ in general behavioral activation scores measured with the Amphetamine Interview Rating Scale: euphoria (schizophrenics, +2.0 ± 0.5; controls, +2.7 ± 0.5, *P* = 0.35), restlessness (schizophrenics, +2.6 ± 0.6; controls, +1.8 ± 0.5, *P* = 0.34), alertness (schizophrenics, +2.5 ± 0.4; controls, +2.5 ± 0.7, *P* = 1), and anxiety (schizophrenics, +2.7 ± 0.5; controls, +2.6 ± 0.6, *P* = 0.87). In the schizophrenic group, the amphetamine effect on [^{123}I]IBZM binding potential was not correlated with severity of positive symptoms at baseline (*r* = 0.03, *P* = 0.92), duration of illness (*r* = 0.09, *P* = 0.75), duration of neuroleptic-free interval before the scan (*r* = 0.30, *P* = 0.30), or lifetime neuroleptic exposure (*r* = 0.33, *P* = 0.22). No difference was observed in the amphetamine effect on [^{123}I]IBZM binding potential between the schizophrenic patients who received lorazepam during the 21 days before the study (−16.6 ± 6.5%, *n* = 5) and the ones who did not (−21.0 + 5.3%, *n* = 10, *P* = 0.63). The effect of age on amphetamine-induced decrease in [^{123}I]IBZM binding potential could not be studied in these samples, because of the narrow age range of the subjects.

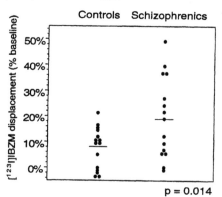

FIG. 2. Amphetamine-induced relative decrease in [^{123}I]IBZM binding potential in 15 healthy controls and 15 patients with schizophrenia, matched for age, sex, race, and parental socioeconomic level.

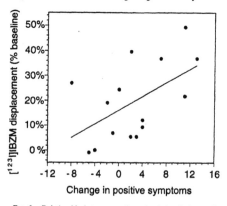

FIG. 3. Relationship between amphetamine-induced changes in positive symptoms and amphetamine-induced relative decrease in [^{123}I]IBZM binding potential in the schizophrenic group (*n* = 15, *r* = 0.53, *P* = 0.038).

DISCUSSION

This study represents the first attempt to measure directly *in vivo* striatal dopamine transmission in patients with schizophrenia. The data indicate that more D_2 receptors are occupied by dopamine following amphetamine challenge in schizophrenic patients than in matched healthy controls. This increased response to amphetamine could not be attributed to differences in peripheral amphetamine disposition, since amphetamine plasma levels were similar in both groups and not related to the amphetamine effect on [^{123}I]IBZM binding potential. Furthermore, blood pressure response to amphetamine was similar between the groups. The increased effect of amphetamine on [^{123}I]IBZM binding potential in the schizophrenic group did not appear to be related to prior neuroleptic exposure, as the effect was not associated with lifetime neuroleptic exposure or duration of the neuroleptic-free period prior to the scan. Furthermore, chronic treatment with typical neuroleptic does not affect amphetamine-induced dopamine release as measured with microdialysis in rodents (34). Similarly, the exaggerated response observed in the schizophrenic group did not appear to be due to lorazepam administration. Patients who did not receive lorazepam during the drug-free period displayed the same level of response as the five patients who did receive lorazepam. Therefore, it is plausible that the increased effect of amphetamine on [^{123}I]IBZM binding potential reflects an abnormal response of the dopaminergic system associated with the disease process *per se*.

The increased displacement of [^{123}I]IBZM binding following dopamine release observed in the schizophrenic group could reflect either an increased affinity of D_2 receptors for dopamine or an increased concentration of dopamine in the vicinity of the receptors, or some combination of both factors. Available data do not support the existence of an increased affinity of D_2 receptors for agonists in schizophrenia: the sequence of the D_2 receptor gene is not altered (35) and the binding of dopamine agonists in postmortem striata is not increased in schizophrenia (36, 37). Nevertheless, a decreased dopamine concentration at baseline would result in an effective increased affinity of the unoccupied D_2 receptors (for both agonists and antagonists). Again, available data do not support the existence of a marked reduction in baseline dopamine in schizophrenia, since the *in vivo* affinity of [^{11}C]raclopride is not elevated in patients with this condition (8, 10). Therefore, while a contribution of the affinity factor cannot be definitively excluded, an increased concentration of dopamine in the vicinity of the receptors is likely to be the predominant mechanism underlying the observed effect.

Amphetamine increases extracellular dopamine concentration by various mechanisms: facilitation of transporter-mediated release of cytoplasmic dopamine (38), redistribution of dopamine from vesicular to cytoplasmic pool (39), inhibition of uptake (40), inhibition of monoamine oxidase activity (41), and calcium-dependent stimulation of dopamine synthesis (42). Any of these factors could be implicated in the exaggerated response observed in the patients. Interestingly, a recent positron emission tomography study has reported increased accumulation of the dopamine precursor 6-[^{18}F]fluoro-L-dopa in the striatum of patients with schizophrenia (43). An increase in enzymatic activity associated with dopamine synthesis might lead to the constitution of larger cytoplasmic and/or vesicular pool and to a larger amphetamine-induced dopamine release.

The mechanism of this putative increased dopaminergic neuronal reactivity remains to be elucidated. Corticofugal glutamatergic projections that increase the responsiveness of dopaminergic subcortical systems are inhibited by dopaminergic prefrontal projections, both directly and indirectly via GABAergic interneurons (44, 45). This glutamatergic cortical control occurs primarily through projections to the dopamine

cell body area rather than the terminal region (46). In nonhuman primates, selective destruction of dopamine terminals in dorsolateral, medial, and orbital regions of the prefrontal cortex does not affect striatal baseline dopamine concentration but induces a long-lasting increase in striatal potassium-induced dopamine release (47). Since potassium, like amphetamine, stimulates both dopamine synthesis and release (48), this observation is potentially relevant to the present finding. Thus, the increased responsiveness of subcortical dopamine neurons observed in this study might be secondary to prefrontal dopaminergic or GABAergic deficits as both deficits have been proposed as constituents of the "cortical pathology" in schizophrenia (49, 50).

A large variability in the amphetamine effect was evident in the schizophrenic group, and three patients showed lower amphetamine-induced [^{123}I]IBZM displacement than their matched controls. This heterogeneity in the biochemical response to amphetamine matched the heterogeneity of the clinical response well and indicated that the abnormality revealed by this study is not present in all patients with schizophrenia. The correlation between [^{123}I]IBZM displacement and the emergence or exacerbation of positive symptoms supports the role of increased dopamine transmission in the genesis of these symptoms. Yet, this correlation was relatively weak, and two schizophrenic subjects experienced a psychotic reaction despite [^{123}I]IBZM displacement values overlapping with control values. Therefore, increased dopamine transmission at the D_2 receptors is not the only factor contributing to a psychotic response to amphetamine in schizophrenic subjects.

Several limitations of this study should be mentioned. (*i*) Because of the lack of placebo control, we could not assess the respective contribution of amphetamine and of the stress associated with the experimental setting to the induction of psychotic reactions. However, this limitation does not affect the observation that a psychotic response (whether due to amphetamine or stress or both) was associated with increased dopamine release. (*ii*) Patients included in this study were able to provide informed consent and to comply with this demanding protocol. Thus, patients devoid of insight about their illness or with major psychotic symptoms were excluded. The impact of this selection bias on the results is not known. (*iii*) While we failed to document that increased amphetamine-induced dopamine release was associated with previous neuroleptic exposure, potential impact of prior medication on the observed effect could not be definitively ruled out. Studies in neuroleptic-naive patients are needed to address this issue. (*iv*) Considerable preclinical evidence supports the hypothesis that antipsychotic drug action is associated with dopamine antagonism in the mesolimbic rather than the nigrostriatal dopaminergic projections (for review, see ref. 45). The limited resolution of the camera precluded evaluation in humans of the respective contributions of limbic versus sensorimotor striatal dopamine release in the production of psychotic symptoms. However, the results of this study might support the contention that dopamine hyperactivity in schizophrenia is not limited to the mesolimbic system (51). (*v*) This study measured only the relative increase in dopamine release following amphetamine challenge and did not provide information about dopamine release at baseline. We are currently developing a dopamine depletion paradigm which, coupled with SPECT imaging, might provide absolute measurement of baseline dopamine concentration in the vicinity of D_2 receptors.

In conclusion, this study used a newly developed noninvasive method to measure amphetamine-induced dopamine release in patients with schizophrenia and suggested the existence of a dysregulation of dopamine neurons in schizophrenia, leading to an increased dopamine transmission in response to amphetamine. If independently replicated, this observation would support the time-honored dopaminergic hypothesis of schizophrenia.

We thank the subjects who participated in this study. We also thank Danielle Abi-Saab, Donna M. Damon, Louise Brenner, Melyssa K. Madrak, Morgan Stratton, Quinn Ramsby, Richard Weiss, and Lynn Pantages-Torok for excellent technical assistance; Paul B. Hoffer, M.D., and Nallakkandra Rajeevan, Ph.D., for Nuclear Medicine expertise; the technologist staff of the NeuroSpect laboratory at Yale–New Haven Hospital; and the clinical staff of G8W at West Haven Veterans Affairs Medical Center and WS2 at Yale Psychiatric Institute. This work was supported by a young investigator award (M.L.) from the National Alliance for Research on Schizophrenia and Depression, the Department of Veterans Affairs (Schizophrenia Research Center), and the U.S. Public Health Service (Grants M01RR00125 and MH54192).

1. Rossum, V. (1966) *Arch. Int. Pharmacodyn. Ther.* 160, 492–494.
2. Angrist, B. M. & Gershon, S. (1970) *Biol. Psychiatry* 2, 95–107.
3. Davis, K. L., Kahn, R. S., Ko, G. & Davidson, M. (1991) *Am. J. Psychiatry* 148, 1474–1486.
4. Burt, D. R., Creese, I. & Snyder, S. S. (1977) *Science* 196, 326–328.
5. Seeman, P. (1987) *Synapse* 1, 133–152.
6. Wong, D. F., Wagner, H. N., Tune, L. E., Dannals, R. F., Pearlson, G. D., Links, J. M., Tamminga, C. A., Broussolle, E. P., Ravert, H. T., Wilson, A. A., Toung, J. K., Malat, J., Williams, J. A., O'Tuama, L. A., Snyder, S. H., Kuhar, M. J. & Gjedde, A. (1986) *Science* 234, 1558–1563.
7. Tune, L. E., Wong, D. F., Pearlson, G., Strauss, M., Young, T., Shaya, E. K., Dannals, R. F., Wilson, A. A., Ravert, H. T., Sapp, J., Cooper, T., Chase, G. A. & Wagner, H. N. (1994) *Psychiatry Res.* 49, 219–237.
8. Farde, L., Wiesel, F., Stone-Elander, S., Halldin, C., Nordström, A. L., Hall, H. & Sedvall, G. (1990) *Arch. Gen. Psychiatry* 47, 213–219.
9. Martinot, J. I., Paillère-Martinot, M. L., Loc'h, C., Hardy, P., Poirier, M. F., Mazoyer, B., Beaufils, B., Mazièfre, B., Alliaire, J. F. & Syrota, A. (1991) *Br. J. Psychiatry* 158, 346–350.
10. Hietala, J., Syvälahti, E., Vuorio, K., Nagren, K., Lehikoinen, P., Ruotsalainen, U., Räkköläinen, V., Lehtinen, V. & Wegelius, U. (1994) *Arch. Gen. Psychiatry* 51, 116–123.
11. Pilowsky, L. S., Costa, D. C., Ell, P. J., Verhoeff, N. P. L. G., Murray, R. M. & Kerwin, R. W. (1994) *Br. J. Psychiatry* 164, 16–26.
12. Nordström, A. L., Farde, L., Erikson, L. & Halldin, C. (1995) *Psychiatry Res.* 61, 67–83.
13. Carlsson, A. (1988) *Neuropsychopharmacology* 1, 179–186.
14. Meltzer, H. (1989) *Psychopharmacology* 99, S18–S27.
15. Köhler, C., Fuxe, K. & Ross, S. B. (1981) *Eur. J. Pharmacol.* 72, 397–402.
16. Van der Werf, J. F., Sebens, J. B., Vaalburg, W. & Korf, J. (1986) *Eur. J. Pharmacol.* 87, 259–270.
17. Ross, S. B. & Jackson, D. M. (1989) *Naunyn–Schmiedebergs Arch. Pharmakol.* 340, 6–12.
18. Logan, J., Dewey, S. L., Wolf, A. P., Fowler, J. S., Brodie, J. D., Angrist, B., Volkow, N. D. & Gatley, S. J. (1991) *Synapse* 9, 195–207.
19. Innis, R. B., Malison, R. T., Al-Tikriti, M., Hoffer, P. B., Sybirska, E. H., Seibyl, J. P., Zoghbi, S. S., Baldwin, R. M., Laruelle, M. A., Smith, E., Charney, D. S., Heninger, G., Elsworth, J. D. & Roth, R. H. (1992) *Synapse* 10, 177–184.
20. Dewey, S. L., Smith, G. S., Logan, J. & Brodie, J. D. (1993) *Neuropsychopharmacology* 8, 371–376.
21. Farde, L., Nordström, A. L., Wiesel, F. A., Pauli, S., Halldin, C. & Sedvall, G. (1992) *Arch. Gen. Psychiatry* 49, 538–544.
22. Volkow, N. D., Wang, G.-J., Fowler, J. S., Logan, J., Schlyer, D., Hitzemann, R., Lieberman, J., Angrist, B., Pappas, N., MacGregor, R., Burr, G., Cooper, T. & Wolf, A. P. (1994) *Synapse* 16, 255–262.

23. Kung, H. F., Kasliwal, R., Pan, S., Kung, M.-P., Mach, R. H. & Guo, Y.-Z. (1988) *J. Med. Chem.* 31, 1039–1043.
24. Laruelle, M., Iyer, R. N., Al-Tikriti, M. S., Zea-Ponce, Y., Malison, R., Zoghbi, S. S., Baldwin, R. M., Kung, H. F., Charney, D. S., Hoffer, P. B., Innis, R. B. & Bradberry, C. W. (1996) *Synapse*, in press.
25. Laruelle, M., Abi-Dargham, A., van Dyck, C. H., Rosenblatt, W., Zea-Ponce, Y., Zoghbi, S. S., Baldwin, R. M., Charney, D. S., Hoffer, P. B., Kung, H. F. & Innis, R. B. (1995) *J. Nucl. Med.* 36, 1182–1190.
26. Lieberman, J. A., Kane, J. M. & Alvir, J. (1987) *Psychopharmacology* 91, 415–433.
27. Gandelman, M. S., Baldwin, R. M., Zoghbi, S. S., Zea-Ponce, Y. & Innis, R. B. (1994) *J. Pharm. Sci.* 83, 1014–1019.
28. Gandelman, M. S., Baldwin, R. M., Zoghbi, S. S., Zea-Ponce, Y. & Innis, R. B. (1994) *J. Pharm. Sci.* 83, 1014–1019.
29. Kay, S. R., Fiszbein, A. & Opler, L. A. (1987) *Schizophr. Bull.* 13, 261–276.
30. van Kammen, D. P. & Murphy, D. L. (1975) *Psychopharmacologia* 44, 215–224.
31. Lidow, M. S., Goldman-Rakic, P. S., Rakic, P. & Innis, R. B. (1989) *Proc. Natl. Acad. Sci. USA* 86, 6412–6416.
32. Seibyl, J., Woods, S., Zoghbi, S., Baldwin, R., Dey, H., Goddard, A., Zea-Ponce, Y., Zubal, G., Germinne, M., Smith, E., Heninger, G. R., Charney, D. S., Kung, H., Alavi, A., Hoffer, P. & Innis, R. (1992) *J. Nucl. Med.* 33, 1964–1971.
33. Overall, J. E. & Gorham, D. R. (1962) *Psychol. Rep.* 10, 799–812.
34. Ichikawa, J. & Meltzer, H. Y. (1992) *Brain Res.* 574, 98–104.
35. Gejman, P. V., Ram, A., Gelernter, J., Friedman, E., Cao, Q., Pickar, D., Blum, K., Noble, E. P., Kranzler, H. R., O'Malley, S., Hamer, D. h., Whitsitt, F., Rao, P., DeLisi, L. E., Virkkunen, M., Linoila, M., Goldman, D. & Gershon, E. S. (1994) *J. Am. Med. Assoc.* 271, 204–208.
36. Lee, T., Seeman, P., Tourtelotte, W. W., Farley, I. J. & Hornykiewicz, O. (1978) *Nature (London)* 274, 897–900.
37. Cross, A. J., Crow, T. J., Ferrier, I. N., Johnstone, E. C., McCreadie, R. M., Owen, F., Owens, D. G. C. & Poulter, M. (1983) *J. Neural Transm. Suppl.* 18, 265–272.
38. Azzuro, A. J. & Rutledge, C. O. (1973) *Biochem. Pharmacol.* 22, 2801–2813.
39. Sulzer, D., Chen, T. K., Lau, Y. Y., Kristensen, H., Rayport, S. & Ewing, A. (1995) *J. Neurosci.* 15, 4102–4108.
40. Horn, A. S., Coyle, J. T. & Snyder, S. H. (1970) *Mol. Pharmacol.* 7, 66–90.
41. Green, A. L. & El Haut, M. J. (1978) *J. Pharm. Pharmacol.* 30, 262–263.
42. Uretsky, N. J. & Snodgrass, S. R. (1977) *J. Pharmacol. Exp. Ther.* 202, 565–580.
43. Reith, J., Benkelfat, C., Sherwin, A., Yasuhara, Y., Kuwabara, H., Andermann, F., Bachneff, S., Cumming, P., Diksic, M., Dyve, S. E., Etienne, P., Evans, A. C., Lal, S., Shevell, M., Savard, G., Wong, D. F., Chouinard, G. & Gjedde, A. (1994) *Proc. Natl. Acad. Sci. USA* 91, 11651–11654.
44. Retaux, S., Besson, M. J. & Penit-Soria, J. (1991) *Neuroscience* 43, 323–329.
45. Deutch, A. Y. (1993) *J. Neural Transm.* 91, 197–221.
46. Karreman, M. & Moghaddam, B. (1996) *J. Neurochem.* 66, 589–598.
47. Roberts, A. C., Desalvia, M. A., Wilkinson, L. S., Collins, P., Muir, J. L., Everitt, B. J. & Robbins, T. W. (1994) *J. Neurosci.* 14, 2531–2544.
48. Schwarz, R. D., Uretsky, N. J. & Bianchine, J. R. (1980) *J. Neurochem.* 35, 1120–1127.
49. Weinberger, D. R. (1987) *Arch. Gen. Psychiatry* 44, 660–669.
50. Benes, F. M., McSparren, J., Bird, E. D., Vincent, S. L. & SanGiovani, J. P. (1991) *Arch. Gen. Psychiatry* 48, 996–1001.
51. Lidsky, T. I. (1995) *Schizophr. Bull.* 21, 67–74.

Compromised White Matter Tract Integrity in Schizophrenia Inferred From Diffusion Tensor Imaging

Kelvin O. Lim, MD; Maj Hedehus, PhD; Michael Moseley, PhD; Alexander de Crespigny, PhD; Edith V. Sullivan, PhD; Adolf Pfefferbaum, MD

Background: Current investigations suggest that brain white matter may be qualitatively altered in schizophrenia even in the face of normal white matter volume. Diffusion tensor imaging provides a new approach for quantifying the directional coherence and possibly connectivity of white matter fibers in vivo.

Methods: Ten men who were veterans of the US Armed Forces and met the *DSM-IV* criteria for schizophrenia and 10 healthy, age-matched control men were scanned using magnetic resonance diffusion tensor imaging and magnetic resonance structural imaging.

Results: Relative to controls, the patients with schizophrenia exhibited lower anisotropy in white matter, despite ab-

sence of a white matter volume deficit. In contrast to the white matter pattern, gray matter anisotropy did not distinguish the groups, even though the patients with schizophrenia had a significant gray matter volume deficit. The abnormal white matter anisotropy in patients with schizophrenia was present in both hemispheres and was widespread, extending from the frontal to occipital brain regions.

Conclusions: Despite the small sample size, diffusion tensor imaging was powerful enough to yield significant group differences, indicating widespread alteration in brain white matter integrity but not necessarily white matter volume in schizophrenia.

Arch Gen Psychiatry. 1999;56:367-374

From the Nathan Kline Institute for Psychiatric Research and Long Island Jewish Medical Center, Orangeburg, NY (Dr Lim); the Departments of Radiology (Drs Hedehus, Moseley, and de Crespigny) and Psychiatry and Behavioral Sciences (Drs Sullivan and Pfefferbaum), Stanford University School of Medicine, Stanford, Calif; and the Neuropsychiatry Program, SRI International, Menlo Park, Calif (Dr Pfefferbaum).

HERE IS now little controversy regarding the claim that the brains of patients with schizophrenia are structurally and functionally compromised. Abnormalities occur in both gray matter and white matter. In vivo magnetic resonance imaging studies report volume deficits more often in cortical gray than white matter[1-4] and are consistent with neuropathologic observations of increased neuronal density and decreased neuropil[5] presence of smaller neurons in layer III of the prefrontal cortex and absence of glial cell enlargement.[6] There have also been reports of reduced prefrontal lobe white matter volume in patients with schizophrenia[7,8] and of patchy signal intensity differences between patients with schizophrenia and controls that affect white matter tracts.[9] Proton magnetic resonance spectroscopic imaging, which provides in vivo indices of some brain metabolites, has shown abnormally low white but normal gray matter signals of N-acetyl (NAc) compounds, primarily N-acetylaspartate, a putative marker for living mature neurons, in patients with schizophrenia who had abnormally small gray but not white matter volumes.[10] The low white

matter NAc signal was interpreted as potentially reflecting compromised neuronal connectivity.[11-14] Evidence from postmortem studies supports the in vivo findings of anomalous white matter in schizophrenia, including selective displacement of interstitial white matter neurons in the prefrontal and temporal[15] cortex and delayed myelination in frontal white matter.[16,17] These neuropathologic signs may be reflected in measurements sensitive to directional coherence or connectivity of fiber tracts.

Findings of abnormal white matter integrity, together with the possibility that cortical gray matter volume deficit has a neurodevelopmental genesis, have led to the hypothesis that a cortical dysconnection syndrome plays a role in the pathophysiology of schizophrenia.[18-20] Perhaps the most current support for this speculation comes from diffusion tensor imaging (DTI), a relatively new magnetic resonance imaging method[21,22] that can be used to quantitate the magnitude and directionality of tissue water mobility (ie, self-diffusion) in 3 dimensions.

Self-diffusion (hereafter called diffusion) is caused by random Brownian move-

237

SUBJECTS AND METHODS

All subjects gave written informed consent for study participation and underwent physical and psychiatric examinations. The patients were 10 men, veterans of the US Armed Forces, who met the DSM-IV criteria for schizophrenia (**Table**). They were 47.7±7.8 (mean ±SD) years old (range, 32-64 years) and had 13.9±1.9 years of education. Exclusion factors were DSM-IV criteria for Alcohol or Substance Abuse or Dependence within 3 months prior to scanning; posttraumatic stress disorder; significant medical illness; or head injury resulting in loss of consciousness exceeding 30 minutes. DSM-IV diagnoses were determined by consensus between a psychiatrist or clinical psychologist, who conducted a clinical interview, and a trained research assistant, who administered the Structured Clinical Interview for Diagnosis. All patients were receiving antipsychotic medications. Clinical condition was evaluated using an average of the 18-item Brief Psychiatric Rating Scale score[32] (mean±SD, 33.6±6.2) obtained by 2 raters with established reliability. Premorbid intelligence was assessed using the National Adult Reading Test[33] (108.1±9.9), and parental socio-occupational status was determined using the Hollingshead 2-Factor Scale[34] (2.8±1.2).

The healthy control subjects were 10 men (41.9±8.3 years; range, 30-57 years), recruited from the local community.[35,36] Seven subjects were given the Structured Clinical Interview for Diagnosis and a physical examination; 3 completed a detailed questionnaire inquiring about current and past medical and psychiatric conditions, medications, and substance use.

IMAGE ACQUISITION AND PROCESSING

Anatomical Magnetic Resonance Imaging

An initial spin-echo sagittal scout image was collected (3-mm skip, 0 mm; repetition time [TR], 600 milliseconds; echo

time [TE], 20 milliseconds; 256×256 pixel matrix; field of view, 24 cm). Using the midsagittal image, the line connecting the anterior and posterior commissures (AC-PC line) was identified. For tissue segmentation, a fast spin-echo (FSE) sequence was collected (TR, 2500 milliseconds; TE, 20/80 milliseconds; echo train length, 8; 5-mm skip, 0 mm; field of view, 24 cm; 256×256 pixel matrix; 18 slices beginning 2 cm below and aligned on the AC-PC line (**Figure 2**, A and B).

All analyses were performed blind to subject identity. Nonbrain tissue (dura, skull, and scalp) was stripped and the remaining tissue was segmented into gray matter, white matter, or cerebrospinal fluid (Figure 2, D) with a semiautomated procedure.[37,38] White-matter hyperintensities segmenting as gray matter were hand-edited for inclusion in the white matter compartment.

For regional analyses, 8 images were used for volumetric quantification and manually midlined along the interhemispheric fissure to separate the hemispheres and divided according to anatomical landmarks and a priori rules into 3 lobar regions: prefrontal, temporal-parietal, and parietal-occipital (**Figure 3**). A prefrontal region began at the anterior margin of the slice, with the posterior extent determined by the point where the anterior cingulate and adjacent white matter met at the interhemispheric fissure. Sulcal landmarks were also considered, such that on the inferior slices the inferior border fell at the juncture between the anterior-temporal pole and the frontal cortex. On superior slices, the prefrontal region included the 3 frontal-lateral gyri. A temporal-parietal region was formed by the posterior border of the prefrontal region and the anterior border of the parietal-occipital region. Included were the temporal lobes from the level of the insula and basal ganglia to the superior extents of the lateral ventricles. A parietal-occipital region had its anterior border determined by several landmarks, including the juncture at which the cortex joins white matter along the interhemispheric fissure, posterior to lateral ventricles, and the point at which the parietal sulci are horizontal (ie, perpendicular to the

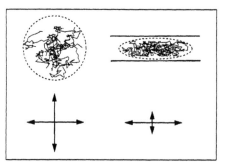

Figure 1. *A computer simulation of 2-dimensional Brownian motion. Left, Paths of 10 particles starting at the same position in a condition of no spatial constraint. The particles move randomly, with a chance of moving horizontally and vertically equally in all directions (arrows), resulting in a circular displacement profile (broken circle). This movement is termed* isotropic. *Right, Paths of 10 particles with a physical constraint in the vertical direction (solid lines). The particles move randomly, with a greater chance of moving horizontally than vertically (arrows), resulting in an ellipsoidal displacement profile. This movement is termed* anisotropic.

ment of molecules. Isotropic diffusion is characterized by identical diffusion properties in all directions, such that, after a period, a number of molecules originating at the same location would be spatially distributed over a circle in 2 dimensions (**Figure 1**, left) or a sphere in 3 dimensions. In brain tissue, the diffusion of water is impeded by structures such as cell membranes, myelin sheaths, and white matter tracts. When trapped, water molecules tend to move farther along paths that are parallel to fibers than ones that are perpendicular to fibers (Figure 1, right). The resulting distribution of water molecules becomes ellipsoid rather than circular, and the diffusion is termed *anisotropic*. The direction and shape of the ellipsoid is determined by the restricting fibers, and the degree of anisotropy can be thought of as the ratio of the long axis to the short axis of the diffusion ellipsoid.

Diffusion (expressed as the apparent diffusion coefficient) measured parallel to fiber tracts yields larger values than when measured perpendicular to tracts.[23] In heterogeneous tissue, such as the brain, it is not possible to choose diffusion directions perfectly aligned with the orientation of the fibers for all imaged voxels;

238

interhemispheric fissures). Region of interest determination was made by consensus of the 2 scorers (A.P. and E.V.S.).

Diffusion Tensor Imaging

A diffusion tensor data set was collected using a pulsed gradient spin-echo echo-planar imaging technique. The field of view was 24 cm; pixel matrix size, 128×128; 0 filled to 256×256 pixel matrix as required by scanner specifications; TE/TR, 106 milliseconds/6 seconds; and 18 oblique slices (5-mm skip, 0 mm) aligned with FSE slices. The duration of the diffusion gradient was 32 milliseconds, the maximum gradient strength was 1.4 G/cm, and the separation of the diffusion gradient pulses was maximized within the echo time (approximately 34 milliseconds). Gradients were always applied on 2 axes simultaneously, resulting in a total value of 860 s/mm². Diffusion was measured along 6 noncollinear directions: $(Gx, Gy, Gz) = [(1,1,0), (0,1,1), (1,0,1), (-1,1,0), (0,-1,1), (1,0,-1)]$. For each gradient direction, 4 diffusion-weighted images were acquired and averaged. Two additional images with no diffusion weighting were acquired and averaged. Averaging was performed after Fourier transformation. A set of cerebrospinal fluid–nulled inversion recovery images (TI $\approx$ 2100 milliseconds) was acquired with no diffusion weighting as a reference for unwarping eddy current effects in diffusion-weighted images, using the method of de Crespigny and Moseley.[39]

Using the averaged images with and without diffusion weighting, 6 maps of the apparent diffusion coefficient were calculated from which the 6 independent elements of the diffusion tensor were determined. Based on the eigenvalues, the degree of anisotropy can be calculated on a voxel-by-voxel basis. From the diffusion tensor, eigenvalues and eigenvectors were determined. Many scalar measures of anisotropy are derived from the tensor.[27] Fractional anisotropy (FA)[28] is a robust intravoxel measure that yields values between 0 (perfectly isotropic

diffusion) and 1 (the hypothetical case of a cylinder infinitely long and infinitely thin). These values were plotted to produce an image (Figure 2, C) approximating the inverse of the anatomical FSE early-echo image (Figure 2, A).

According to simulation studies,[29] rotationally invariant measures of anisotropy are "reasonably accurate and precise for signal-to-noise ratio levels greater than 20."[29(p903)] Our current signal-to-noise ratio of about 30 in the non–diffusion-weighted image is thus well within the range of acceptable accuracy in fractional anisotropy measurement.

STRUCTURE/DIFFUSION ANALYSIS

This analysis used 8 contiguous slices of the FSE and corresponding FA images that began at the anterior commissure and proceeded superiorly 40 mm. This volume encompassed the largest extent of cerebral white matter across all subjects and included the corpus callosum and centrum semiovale. Segmented FSE images (Figure 2, D) were registered with FA images (Figure 2, C). Fractional anisotropy voxels were characterized according to their tissue type (white matter, gray matter, and cerebrospinal fluid) and allocated to the 3 cortical regions of interest. Echoplanar warping, present in DTI, has the potential to hamper registration between DTI and FSE images; however, such effects were apparent only in the most anterior regions (Figure 2, E) and were minimized by use of tissue segmentation contours.

STATISTICAL ANALYSIS

The unit of DTI analysis was median FA. Group differences in FA were examined with repeated-measures analysis of variance (ANOVA) and unpaired t tests. Group differences in total FA were further tested with 3 separate analyses of covariance that used gray matter volume, white matter volume, and age as covariates. The α level for all tests was .05 (2 tailed).

Characteristics of Patients With Schizophrenia*

Subject No./ Age at Scan, y	Education, y	Secondary Diagnosis	Past Substance Abuse/Dependence†	Age When Patient Last Met Diagnosis for Substance Abuse/Dependence, y‡	Global Assessment of Functioning Scale Score	Brief Psychiatric Rating Scale Score	Medication at Scan
1/32	14	Undifferentiated	Cannabis abuse	20 (12)	57	32.0	Risperidone, Prolixin
2/44	11	Disorganized	...	...	32	45.0	Clozapine
3/46	13	Undifferentiated	Cannabis dependence, hallucinogen abuse	26 (20)	37	39.0	Risperidone, Olanzapine
4/47	13	Undifferentiated	Cannabis dependence	20 (27)	52	32.6	Clozapine
5/47	12	Undifferentiated	Cocaine dependence	41 (6)	42	35.0	Risperidone
6/48	16	Residual	Cannabis abuse	43 (5)	60	23.0	Clozapine
7/49	15	Residual	Alcohol dependence, cannabis abuse, opiod abuse	38 (11)	60	29.6	Clozapine
8/50	14	Undifferentiated	...	...	45	38.6	Clozapine
9/50	11	Undifferentiated	Alcohol abuse	22 (32)	32	32.6	Olanzapine
10/64	16	Residual	...	...	57	28.0	Risperidone

*Schizophrenia was the DSM-IV diagnosis for all subjects.
†Ellipses indicate no substance use.
‡Numbers in parentheses indicate years since patient last met this diagnosis.

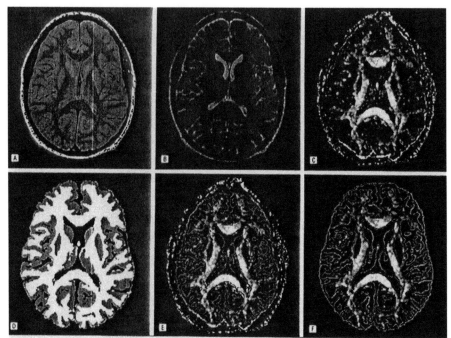

Figure 2. *Axial images from slice 3, 1.5 cm superior to the AC-PC line, from a single subject. A, Early echo. B, Late echo. C, Fractional anisotropy image. D, Fully processed image segmented into 3 tissue compartments (white matter=light gray, gray matter=dark gray, and cerebrospinal fluid=black). E, Fractional anisotropy image with segmentation contours overlaid to localize alignment and misalignment between anatomical and diffusion images. F, Fractional anisotropy voxels only for white matter, with segmentation contours overlaid. Note that the spatial distortion common to echo-planar imaging, especially at the frontal air-tissue boundaries (E), is confined primarily to cerebrospinal fluid and gray matter, with little distortion of white matter (F).*

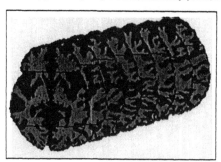

Figure 3. *Region-of-interest boundaries, marked in black lines, are superimposed on each of the 8 fast-spin echo segmented slices used in data analysis.*

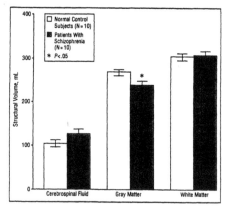

Figure 4. *Mean (SEM) cerebrospinal fluid, gray matter, and white matter volumes for the 10 normal control subjects and the 10 patients with schizophrenia.*

however, the so-called "diffusion tensor," first described by Basser et al,[24-26] contains information about the 3-dimensional geometry, orientation, and shape of the diffusion ellipsoid and thus fully characterizes the diffusion system. A tensor is a mathematical construct useful for describing multidimensional vector systems, and the diffusion tensor provides the apparent diffusion co-efficient of a certain direction, degree of anisotropy, and primary fiber tract orientation.

240

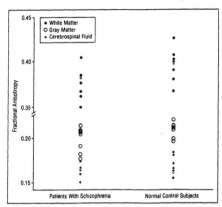

Figure 5. *Fractional anisotropy measures of cerebrospinal fluid, gray matter, and white matter for normal control subjects and patients with schizophrenia over all 8 slices analyzed.*

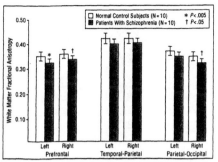

Figure 6. *White matter fractional anisotropy (mean and SEM) in the 3 regions of interest, in the left and right hemispheres, for 10 normal control subjects and 10 patients with schizophrenia.*

The degree of anisotropy in a voxel is determined by microstructural features of the tissue in that particular voxel, such as fiber diameter and density, as well as the degree of myelination,[27,28] and also by macrostructural features, such as intravoxel fiber-tract coherence.[29,30] At first glance, high anisotropy may seem to be evidence of a high degree of coherence and hence highly connected tissue (such as normal white matter), whereas low anisotropy would imply tissue with low connectivity (such as abnormal white matter); however, a high degree of connectivity with low anisotropy can be found at the junction of merging tracts,[29] where fibers with different orientations are found within the same voxel. Another example occurs in pons, where both descending and perpendicular fibers are found within a voxel. Wallerian degeneration of only the descending pathways reduces the amount of crossing fibers and increases the coherence of fibers within that particular voxel, such that the observed anisotropy increases.[30] Thus, the meaning of low anisotropy must always be interpreted in the context of the anisotropy in a corresponding normal region.

Using DTI, Buchsbaum et al[31] reported evidence of lower diffusion anisotropy in some inferior portions of prefrontal white matter in patients with schizophrenia (n=5) than in controls (n=6). Together with lower metabolic rates in the frontal cortex and striatum observed with positron emission tomographic scans in these same patients, these results were interpreted as diminished frontostriatal connectivity in schizophrenia.

Our controlled study of schizophrenia used DTI to quantify anisotropy determined from magnetic resonance images divided on the basis of tissue composition, hemisphere, and anatomically determined lobar regions. Our previous observations revealed gray but not white matter volume deficits, yet NAc concentration deficits occurred in white but not gray matter, suggesting compromised tissue composition in white matter.[10] Therefore, we hypothesized that patients with schizophrenia would exhibit gray but not white matter volume deficits

in conjunction with decreased white but not necessarily gray matter anisotropy relative to age- and sex-matched controls. Given the results of Buchsbaum et al, we anticipated that the most notable deficits would be in inferior frontal white matter in the right hemisphere.

RESULTS

Based on the segmented FSE data, a repeated-measures ANOVA for total volume revealed a group × tissue-type interaction ($F_{1,18}$=13.125, $P<.002$), indicating a volume deficit in gray but not white matter in the patients with schizophrenia relative to the controls (**Figure 4**). The FA data for gray and white matter also yielded a significant interaction ($F_{1,18}$=10.521, $P<.005$), indicating lower FA in white but not gray matter in the patients with schizophrenia than in the controls (**Figure 5**). The effect size for the white matter FA group difference was 1.5 SD. The lower white matter FA persisted with 3 separate, 2-group analyses of covariance, controlling for gray matter volume, white matter volume, and age.

Regional effects between groups in white matter FA were tested with a repeated-measures ANOVA across the 3 lobar regions and across hemispheres (**Figure 6**), with the objective of testing for a group effect (patients vs controls) and interactions involving group. This 3-way ANOVA yielded a significant effect only for group ($F_{1,18}$=9.070, $P<.008$); none of the interactions involving group was significant.

The hypothesis that FA would be especially low in inferior frontal white matter in the right hemisphere of the schizophrenic group was tested by employing separate repeated-measures ANOVAs (2 groups × 3 regions) for slice 2 (**Figure 7**; 0.5 cm superior to the AC-PC line, with inferior tips of the lateral ventricles, internal capsule, and some genu of the corpus callosum visible) and slice 3 (Figure 7; 1 cm superior to the AC-PC line, with genu and some splenium of the corpus callosum visible). For the frontal region of interest, these 2 slices appeared to correspond to those showing the greatest effects in the Buchsbaum et al[31] study. The ANOVAs yielded the same results for each slice, with significant effects only for group [slice 2: $F_{1,18}$ =9.843,

ARCH GEN PSYCHIATRY/VOL 56, APR 1999
371

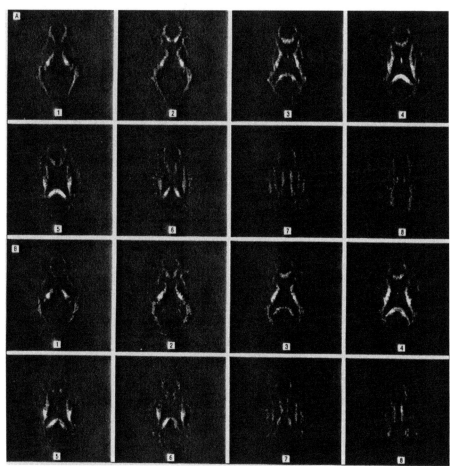

Figure 7. *Grand average images (each slice was warped to a standard size and rotation) of fractional anisotropy for 8 slices for the 10 normal control subjects (A) and the 10 patients with schizophrenia (B).*

$P<.006$; slice 3: $F_{1,18}=11.824$, $P<.003$], region [slice 2: $F_{2,36}=27.418$, $P<.001$; slice 3: $F_{2,36}=98.559$, $P<.001$], and region $\times$ hemisphere [slice 2: $F_{2,36}=5.168$, $P<.02$; slice 3: $F_{2,36}=7.155$, $P<.003$]. **Figure 8** plots the FA for each slice within each region of interest.

COMMENT

We compared anisotropy and volumes of equivalent regions of white and gray matter in patients with schizophrenia and controls and observed the following double dissociation. Although patients with schizophrenia and controls had an equivalent volume of white matter, this white matter exhibited lower anisotropy among patients with schizophrenia. By contrast, gray matter anisotropy did not distinguish the groups even though the schizophrenic group had a significant gray matter volume deficit. Furthermore, the abnormal white matter anisotropy in the patients with schizophrenia was present in both hemispheres and was widespread, extending from the frontal to occipital brain regions. A similar double dissociation was observed in our previous comparison[10] of tissue volume and tissue composition of the brain metabolite NAc; patients with schizophrenia had decreased gray matter but not white matter volume and decreased white matter but not gray matter NAc concentration.

There is no convention for a DTI outcome, and the appropriateness of traditional statistical tests in the analysis of DTI data has yet to be decided. The information

242

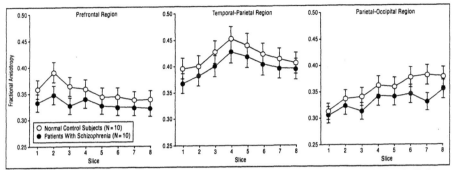

Figure 8. White matter fractional anisotropy (mean and SEM) in the 3 regions of interest (frontal, temporal-parietal, and parietal-occipital) for each of the 8 analyzed slices from the 10 normal control subjects and the 10 patients with schizophrenia.

contained in the tensor comprises complex 3-dimensional directionality, which by its very nature is difficult to condense into a scalar measure. The most quoted measure, however, is the degree of diffusion anisotropy, the simplest being the ratios between diffusivities along different directions. Such ratios are highly sensitive to noise and have small deviations in the eigenvalues.[29] Fractional anisotropy, used in our study, and relative anisotropy (RA),[27] used in the Buchsbaum study, are more robust measures that are normalized and thus appropriate for between-group comparisons. The physiologically relevant range of anisotropy is FA of 0.2 to 0.8, corresponding to a ratio of about 1:4 between the largest and smallest diffusivities in a symmetrical cylinder. In this anisotropy range, RA and FA are comparable; however, RA is the ratio of the anisotropic component of the tensor to the isotropic component; as one goes up, the other goes down, rendering RA more sensitive to variations for large degrees of anisotropy but not as sensitive in the midrange. Fractional anisotropy, on the other hand, is the ratio of the anisotropic component to the entire tensor, which is independent of the degree of anisotropy; the anisotropy that we observed in white matter (approximately 0.3 to 0.4) is in the range where FA is more sensitive than RA.

Buchsbaum et al[31] reported lower RA in frontal white matter, including the anterior limb of the external capsule only in the right hemisphere. Our study observed abnormalities in these frontal regions in both hemispheres as well as in nonfrontal regions. These 2 studies differed in the analysis approach and the anisotropy measure: Buchsbaum et al used RA, whereas we used FA. They also employed a spatial normalization method to standardized coordinates,[40] which involved stretching each slice of each subject to a common size, followed by pixel-by-pixel *t* tests corrected for multiple observations. We analyzed large regions of interest that were inherently less anatomically specific but more robust to noise and statistically more conservative. Nonetheless, the results of both studies converge on the possibility of compromised frontostriatal connectivity or directional coherence of white matter fibers in schizophrenia, although our study also points to abnormalities in other regions.

The possibility of compromised white matter connectivity suggested by our study must be considered within the context of cortical gray matter pathology noted in schizophrenia. The gray matter volume deficit is especially prominent in the heteromodal cortex,[1,4,41] which has extensive corticocortical and subcorticocortical interconnections.[42] Disruption of these interconnections could arise from several sources: abnormally small size or number of neurons producing commensurately fewer than normal arbors, disturbances in the white matter structure arising from displaced interstitial neurons, or aberrant myelination. These white matter anomalies could disrupt fiber coherence or might even result in compromised connections. Considering neuropathologic reports, either or both of these possibilities could occur in schizophrenia. White matter growth and restructuring occur from late prenatal development through late adolescence. The cortical targets—prefrontal, superior temporal, and parietal—in the heteromodal system putatively disrupted in schizophrenia are critical to higher-order cognitive functions of problem solving, working memory, sequencing, language, and spatial orientation, many of which are commonly impaired in patients with schizophrenia.[43,44] Our results note a potential substrate for functional disconnection[18,20] or for a less dramatic disruption in brain structural organization in the form of decreased fiber coherence. Decreased anisotropy could, therefore, arise from underdevelopment of these otherwise highly integrated neural networks, possibly from incomplete organization of target sites during development, and could result in decreased directional coherence of white matter fibers or vulnerability from neurotoxic sources, including neuroleptic exposure or symptom exacerbation.[45]

Limitations of our study arise from the fact that the echo-planar acquisition used in DTI introduces warping in the images due to magnetic field inhomogeneity, particularly at borders between tissue and air and especially prominent at the most inferior frontal margins of the brain. The structural images used for defining anatomical structures and tissue types for regions of FA measurement were acquired with an FSE protocol. This echo-planar warping is not present in FSE images, therefore

243

precluding perfect registration of the 2 image types. In our study, however, the misregistration appeared to be minimal except for the most anterior regions (Figure 2, E). Consequently, we used tissue segmentation as a basis for defining anatomical borders for regional FA measurements (Figure 2, F). A preferred approach may involve unwarping the DTI images,[46] which requires the acquisition of a magnetic field map at the time of data acquisition; however, such data were not available for our analysis. Despite the limitations of our study, including its restrictions in sample size and sex, the method was powerful enough to yield group differences with a 1.5-SD effect size, indicating widespread alteration in brain white matter integrity but not necessarily white matter volume in schizophrenia.

Accepted for publication December 28, 1998.

This study was supported by grants MH53313 (Dr Lim), MH30854, MH58007, and AA05965 (Dr Pfefferbaum), and NS35959 and RR09784 (Dr Moseley) from the National Institutes of Mental Health, Bethesda, Md, and the clinical resources of the Department of Veterans Affairs, Palo Alto Health Care System, Palo Alto, Calif.

Corresponding author: Kelvin O. Lim, MD, Nathan Kline Institute for Psychiatric Research, Division of Medical Physics, Center for Advanced Brain Imaging, 140 Old Orangeburg Rd, Orangeburg, NY 10962 (e-mail: lim@nki.rfmh.org).

REFERENCES

1. Schlaepfer TE, Harris GJ, Tien AY, Peng LW, Lee S, Federman EB, Chase GA, Barta PE, Pearlson GD. Decreased regional cortical gray matter volume in schizophrenia. Am J Psychiatry. 1994;151:842-848.
2. Harvey I, Persaud R, Ron MA, Baker G, Murray RM. Volumetric MRI measurements in bipolars compared with schizophrenics and healthy controls. Psychol Med. 1994;24:689-699.
3. Zipursky RB, Lim KO, Sullivan EV, Brown BW, Pfefferbaum A. Widespread cerebral gray matter volume deficits in schizophrenia. Arch Gen Psychiatry. 1992; 49:195-205.
4. Sullivan E, Lim K, Mathalon D, Marsh L, Beal D, Harris D, Hoff A, Faustman W, Pfefferbaum A. A profile of cortical gray matter volume characteristic of schizophrenia. Cereb Cortex. 1998;8:117-124.
5. Selemon LD, Rajkowska G, Goldman-Rakic PS. Abnormally high neuronal density in the schizophrenic cortex: a morphometric analysis of prefrontal area 9 and occipital area 17. Arch Gen Psychiatry. 1995;52:805-818.
6. Rajkowska G, Selemon LD, Goldman-Rakic PS. Neuronal and glial somal size in the prefrontal cortex: a postmortem morphometric study of schizophrenia and Huntington disease. Arch Gen Psychiatry. 1998;55:215-224.
7. Breier A, Buchanan RW, Elkashef A, Munson RC, Kirkpatrick B, Gellad F. Brain morphology and schizophrenia: a magnetic resonance imaging study of limbic, prefrontal cortex, and caudate structures. Arch Gen Psychiatry. 1992;49: 921-926.
8. Buchanan R, Vladar K, Barta P, Pearlson G. Structural evaluation of the prefrontal cortex in schizophrenia. Am J Psychiatry. 1998;155:1049-1055.
9. Wolkin A, Rusinek H, Vaid G, Arena L, Lafargue T, Sanfilipo M, Loneragan C, Lautin A, Rotrosen J. Structural magnetic resonance image averaging in schizophrenia. Am J Psychiatry. 1998;155:1064-1073.
10. Lim KO, Adalsteinson A, Spielman D, Rosenbloom MJ, Sullivan EV, Pfefferbaum A. Proton magnetic resonance spectroscopic imaging of cortical gray and white matter in schizophrenia. Arch Gen Psychiatry. 1998;55:346-352.
11. Pearlson GD, Petty RG, Ross CA, Tien AY. Schizophrenia: a disease of heteromodal association cortex? Neuropsychopharmacology. 1996;14:1-17.
12. McGuire PK, Frith CD. Disordered functional connectivity in schizophrenia. Psychol Med. 1996;26:663-667.
13. Friston KJ. Theoretical neurobiology and schizophrenia. Br Med Bull. 1996;52: 644-655.
14. Andreasen NC, Arndt S, Swayze V, Cizadlo T, Flaum M, O'Leary D, Ehrhardt JC, Yuh WTC. Thalamic abnormalities in schizophrenia visualized through magnetic resonance image averaging. Science. 1994;266:294-298.
15. Akbarian S, Kim JJ, Potkin SG, Hetrick WP, Bunney WE Jr, Jones EG. Maldis-

16. tribution of interstitial neurons in prefrontal white matter of the brains of schizophrenic patients. Arch Gen Psychiatry. 1996;53:425-436.
16. Benes FM. Myelination of cortical-hippocampal relays during late adolescence. Schizophr Bull. 1989;15:585-593.
17. Benes FM, Turtle M, Khan Y, Farol P. Myelination of a key relay zone in the hippocampal formation occurs in the human brain during childhood, adolescence, and adulthood. Arch Gen Psychiatry. 1994;51:477-484.
18. Weinberger DR, Lipska BK. Cortical maldevelopment, anti-psychotic drugs, and schizophrenia: a search for common ground. Schizophr Res. 1995;16:87-110.
19. Weinberger DR. On the plausibility of "The neurodevelopmental hypothesis" of schizophrenia. Neuropsychopharmacology. 1996;14:S1-S11.
20. Friston KJ, Frith CD. Schizophrenia: a disconnection syndrome? Clin Neurosci 1995;3:89-97.
21. Moseley ME, Wendland MF, Kucharczyk J. Magnetic resonance imaging of diffusion and perfusion. Top Magn Reson Imaging. 1991;3:50-67.
22. Basser PJ, Mattiello J, LeBihan D. MR diffusion tensor spectroscopy and imaging. Biophys J. 1994;66:259-267.
23. Moseley ME, Mintorovitch J, Cohen Y, Asgari HS, Derugin N, Norman D, Kucharczyk J. Early detection of ischemic injury: comparison of spectroscopy, diffusion-, T2-, and magnetic susceptibility-weighted MRI in cats. Acta Neurochir Suppl (Wien). 1990;51:207-209.
24. Basser P, Le Bihan D. Fiber orientation mapping in an anisotropic medium with NMR diffusion spectroscopy. In: Abstracts of the Society of Magnetic Resonance Annual Meeting; August 8-14, 1992:1221; Berlin, Germany.
25. Basser P, Mattiello J, Le Bihan D. Diagonal and off-diagonal components of the self-diffusion tensor: their relation to and estimation from the NMR spin-echo signal. In: Abstracts of the Society of Magnetic Resonance Annual Meeting; August 8-14, 1992; Berlin, Germany. Abstract 1222.
26. Basser P, Mattiello J, Le Bihan D. Estimation of the effective self-diffusion tensor from the NMR spin echo. J Magn Reson B. 1994;103:247-254.
27. Basser PJ. Inferring microstructural features and the physiological state of tissues from diffusion-weighted images. NMR Biomed. 1995;8:333-344.
28. Basser J, Pierpaoli C. Microstructural and physiological features of tissues elucidated by quantitative diffusion tensor MRI. J Magn Reson. 1996;111 209-219.
29. Pierpaoli C, Basser J. Toward a quantitative assessment of diffusion anisotropy Magn Reson Med. 1996;36:893-906.
30. Pierpaoli C, Barnett A, Virta A, Penix L, Chen R. Diffusion MRI of Wallerian degeneration: a new tool to investigate neural connectivity in vivo? In: Abstracts of the International Society of Magnetic Resonance in Medicine Annual Meeting April 18-24, 1998; Sydney, Australia. Abstract 1247.
31. Buchsbaum MS, Tang CY, Peled S, Gudbjartsson H, Lu D, Hazlett EA, Downhill J, Haznedar M, Fallon JH, Atlas SW. MRI white matter diffusion anisotropy and PET metabolic rate in schizophrenia. Neuroreport. 1998;9:425-430.
32. Overall JE, Gorham DR. The Brief Psychiatric Rating Scale (BPRS): recen developments in ascertainment and scaling. Psychopharmacol Bull. 1988;24 97-99.
33. Nelson HE. The National Adult Reading Test (NART). Windsor, Ontario: Nelson Publishing Co; 1982.
34. Hollingshead A, Redlich F. Social Class and Mental Illness. New York, NY: John Wiley & Sons Inc; 1958.
35. Pfefferbaum A, Mathalon DH, Sullivan EV, Rawles JM, Zipursky RB, Lim KO. A quantitative magnetic resonance imaging study of changes in brain morphology from infancy to late adulthood. Arch Neurol. 1994;51:874-887.
36. Pfefferbaum A, Sullivan EV, Rosenbloom MJ, Mathalon DH, Lim KO. A controlled study of cortical gray matter and ventricular changes in alcoholic men over a 5-year interval. Arch Gen Psychiatry. 1998;55:905-912.
37. Lim KO, Pfefferbaum A. Segmentation of MR brain images into cerebrospinal fluid spaces, white and gray matter. J Comput Assist Tomogr. 1989;13:588-593.
38. Pfefferbaum A, Sullivan E, Adalsteinsson A, Spielman D, Lim KO. In vivo spectroscopic quantification of the N-acetyl moiety, creatine and choline from large volumes of gray and white matter: effects of normal aging. J Magn Reson Imaging. 1998;41:276-284.
39. de Crespigny A, Moseley M. Eddy current induced image warping in diffusion weighted EPI. In: Abstracts of the International Society of Magnetic Resonance in Medicine; April 18-24, 1998; Sydney, Australia. Abstract 2661.
40. Bookstein FL. Morphometric Tools for Landmark Data. New York, NY: Cambridge University Press; 1991.
41. Ross CA, Pearlson GD. Schizophrenia, the heteromodal association neocortex and development: potential for a neurogenetic approach. Trends Neurosci. 1996; 19:171-176.
42. Selemon LD, Goldman-Rakic PS. Common cortical and subcortical targets of the dorsolateral prefrontal and posterior parietal cortices in the rhesus monkey: evidence for a distributed neural network subserving spatially guided behavior. J Neurosci. 1988;8:4049-4068.
43. Green MF. What are the functional consequences of neurocognitive deficits in schizophrenia? Am J Psychiatry. 1996;153:321-330.
44. Hoff AL. Neuropsychological function in schizophrenia. In: Shrique CL, Nasrallah HA, eds. Contemporary Issues in the Treatment of Schizophrenia. Washington, DC: American Psychiatric Press; 1995:187-208.
45. Wyatt RJ. Risks of withdrawing antipsychotic medications. Arch Gen Psychiatry. 1995;52:205-208.
46. Jezzard P, Balaban R. Correction for geometric distortion in echo-planar images from B0 field variations. Magn Reson Med. 1995;34:65-73.

Decreased prefrontal dopamine D1 receptors in schizophrenia revealed by PET

Yoshiro Okubo*†, Tetsuya Suhara†, Kazutoshi Suzuki†,
Kaoru Kobayashi†, Osamu Inoue†, Omi Terasaki*†,
Yasuhiro Someya*†, Takeshi Sassa*†, Yasuhiko Sudo†,
Eisuke Matsushima*, Masaomi Iyo†, Yukio Tateno†
& Michio Toru*

* Department of Neuropsychiatry, Tokyo Medical and Dental University School of
Medicine, 1-5-45 Yushima, Bunkyo-ku, Tokyo 113, Japan
† Division of Advanced Technology for Medical Imaging, National Institute of
Radiological Sciences, 4-9-1, Anagawa, Inage-ku, Chiba 263, Japan

Schizophrenia is believed to involve altered activation of dopamine receptors, and support for this hypothesis comes from the
antipsychotic effect of antagonists of the dopamine D2 receptor
(D2R)[1]. D2R is expressed most highly in the striatum, but most of
the recent positron emission tomography (PET) studies have
failed to show any change in D2R densities in the striatum of
schizophrenics[2-5], raising the possibility that other receptors may
also be involved. In particular, the dopamine D1 receptor (D1R),
which is highly expressed in the prefrontal cortex[6], has been
implicated in the control of working memory[7,8], and working
memory dysfunction is a prominent feature of schizophrenia[9]. We
have therefore used PET to examine the distribution of D1R and
D2R in brains of drug-naive or drug-free schizophrenic patients.
Although no differences were observed in the striatum relative to
control subjects, binding of radioligand to D1R was reduced in the
prefrontal cortex of schizophrenics. This reduction was related to
the severity of the negative symptoms (for instance, emotional
withdrawal) and to poor performance in the Wisconsin Card
Sorting Test[10]. We propose that dysfunction of D1R signalling in
the prefrontal cortex may contribute to the negative symptoms
and cognitive deficits seen in schizophrenia.

We examined D1R and D2R in 17 male schizophrenics and 18
healthy male volunteers. Ten of the patients were completely naive
for neuroleptics and seven were drug-free for a minimum of two
weeks before PET examination. Two PET runs were done in each
subject on the same day using [¹¹C]SCH23390 and [¹¹C]N-methyl-

Figure 1 PET visualization of D1R (left image) and D2R (right image) in a control
subject. The radioactivity distribution was obtained at the level of striatum, 14 to
40 min after injection of [¹¹C]SCH23390 and 34–60 min after [¹¹C]NMSP injection.
Images were normalized with respect to cerebellar radioactivity. The in vivo
labelling of the striatum and cortex by [¹¹C]SCH23390 (left) represents D1R, and
[¹¹C]NMSP (right) binds predominantly to D2R in the striatum but to 5-HR₂ in the
cortex.

Table 1 Mean values of D1R and D2R binding

	Controls (n = 18, 12*)	Schizophrenics Drug-naive (n = 10)	Drug-free (n = 7)	ANOVA F(P)	ANCOVA F(P)
D2 dopamine receptor (k_3); [11C]NMSP					
Striatum	0.033 ± 0.007	0.036 ± 0.006	0.032 ± 0.004	1.02(0.38)	0.43(0.65)
D1 dopamine receptor (k_3/k_4); [11C]SCH23390					
Striatum	1.29 ± 0.17	1.28 ± 0.15	1.20 ± 0.18	0.67(0.52)	0.47(0.63)
Prefrontal cortex	0.41 ± 0.06	0.35 ± 0.06†	0.33 ± 0.05†	6.15(0.005)	9.11(0.0008)
Anterior cingulate cortex	0.48 ± 0.08	0.42 ± 0.08	0.41 ± 0.07	3.40(0.046)	5.68(0.008)
Temporal cortex	0.46 ± 0.08	0.42 ± 0.06	0.38 ± 0.05	3.32(0.049)	4.35(0.022)
Occipital cortex	0.33 ± 0.05	0.33 ± 0.06	0.30 ± 0.05	1.04(0.37)	0.82(0.45)

k_3, Association rate constant; k_4, dissociation rate constant; k_3/k_4, binding potential assumed to be equal to B_{max}/K_D^{18}. According to the one-way analysis of variance (ANOVA), a significant difference ($P < 0.0083 = 0.05/6$) was considered as significant to avoid type I errors in the multiplicity of statistical analyses) among the groups was found only in the D1R of the PFC. Because we found an age effect on D1R and D2R binding, in agreement with earlier[13,23], an analysis of covariance (ANCOVA) with age as covariate was performed to test for group differences; significant differences in the PFC and anterior cingulate cortex were found.
* Twelve of the 18 control subjects underwent PET scans with [11C]SCH23390 and [11C]NMSP; 6 controls underwent PET scan with [11C]SCH23390 only.
† Duncans post hoc analysis after ANOVA showed that the mean values of D1R binding in the PFC for both patient groups were significantly smaller than for the control group (P < 0.05).

spiperone([11C]NMSP), respectively, as the PET tracers (Fig. 1 and Methods). In vivo labelling of the striatum and cortex by [11C]SCH23390 is thought to be due to binding to dopamine D1 receptors[11,12]; [11C]NMSP binds predominantly to dopamine D2 receptors in the striatum[13].

We found no difference in striatal D2R among the three groups (Table 1 and Fig. 2a). This observation is in agreement with PET findings using different radioligands[2–5] and fails to support the hypothesis that schizophrenia is related to an increased density of D2 receptors.

As for D1R, a post-mortem study showed an increased ratio of D2R/D1R in the striatum of schizophrenics[14], and a preliminary PET study has reported that D1R binding in the putamen is lower in schizophrenics, suggesting that a low D1R binding in the putamen is lower in schizophrenics, suggesting that a low D1R density may result in a reduced activity of D1R to D2R regulated feedback systems in schizophrenia[15]. However, we failed to detect this difference either in the striatal D1R (Table 1 and Fig. 2b) or in the ratio of striatal D1R to striatal D2R (data not shown).

In contrast to the lack of difference in the striatal D1R and D2R, the mean values of D1R binding potential in the prefrontal cortex (PFC) for both patient groups were significantly lower than for the control group. (Table 1 and Fig. 2c). Because the binding potential is not critically dependent on cerebral blood flow[16], such difference cannot be accounted for by its reduction. To exclude the effect of difference in the size of the regions of interest (ROIs), the number of pixels for each ROI was calculated and no significant difference was

found in any region (data not shown). Our magnetic resonance imaging (MRI) measurements (see Methods) revealed no difference in the PFC volume of schizophrenics and controls (data not shown). Reduction in D1R binding is therefore not associated with gross alterations in brain anatomy. Furthermore, the decreased D1R binding in patients who have never been treated with neuroleptics indicates that the D1R system in PFC may be involved in the disease process of schizophrenia itself.

Reduction of prefrontal D1R was related to the clinical ratings for negative symptoms (Fig. 3a) and poor performance in the Wisconsin Card Sorting Test (WCST; Fig. 3b) but was not correlated with age at onset or duration of illness.

Several lines of evidence have suggested that the PFC of schizophrenic patients may be hypodopaminergic and that this decreased mesocortical dopaminergic activity may induce poor performance in frontally mediated cognitive tasks and negative symptoms[17]: (1) local depletion of dopamine in the PFC of monkeys produced an impairment in spatial delayed alternation performance which was almost as severe as that caused by surgical ablation of the same area, and this behavioural deficit could be reversed by a dopamine agonist[18]; (2) a study of human plasma using homovanillic acid indicated that the negative symptoms of schizophrenic patients are associated with decreased dopaminergic function[19]; (3) administration of dopamine stimulant ameliorates cognitive performance on frontally mediated tasks and task-dependent activation of regional blood flow in the PFC[20] in schizophrenics; and (4) a PET study has revealed that an impaired cognitive-task-induced activation of the

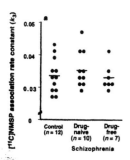
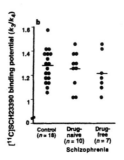
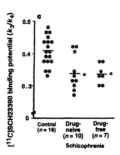

Figure 2 Distribution of D1R and D2R binding indices. Values were adjusted for age. **a**, Association rate constant (k_3) of striatal D2R: adjusted $k_3 = k_3 + 0.0006$ (age, 28.5 yr). **b**, Binding potential (k_3/k_4) of striatal D1R: adjusted $k_3/k_4 = k_3/k_4 + 0.16$ (age, 28.5 yr). **c**, Binding potential (k_3/k_4) of PFC D1R: adjusted $k_3/k_4 = k_3/k_4 + 0.06$ (age, 28.5 yr). Asterisks, Duncan's post hoc analysis after ANOVA revealed that both patient groups had reduced D1R binding in the PFC compared with the control group (P < 0.05).

247

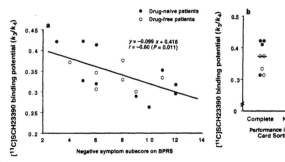

● Drug-naive patients
○ Drug-free patients

$y = -0.099 x + 0.416$
$r = -0.60 (P = 0.011)$

Negative symptom subscore on BPRS

Complete   Not complete

Performance in Wisconsin Card Sorting Test

Figure 3 a, Prefrontal D1R binding potential adjusted for age negatively correlates with the negative symptom subscore (blunted affect, emotional withdrawal, motor retardation) on the Brief Psychiatric Rating Scale (BPRS). When restricted to drug-naive patients only, the correlation was the same. Prefrontal D1R binding was not correlated with the BPRS total score or the positive-symptom subscore. **b,** Modified WCST[10] was performed in 8 drug-naive patients (filled circles) and 5 drug-treated patients (circles). Eight patients completed the required categories within two steps ('complete' group) but the other 5 patients performed poorly and could not complete the categories ('not complete' group). Two-way ANCOVA (performance on WCST × history of medication) with age as covariate revealed that patients with poor performance showed decreased D1R binding in the PFC ($*F = 9.65, P = 0.014$). There was no significant interaction between performance and history of medication.

anterior cingulate cortex in schizophrenics can be significantly modulated by dopaminergic manipulation[21].

Several findings indicate that the proposed hypodopaminergic activity in the PFC of schizophrenics may be due to hypofunction in the D1R system: (1) the human cortex contains 4 to 7 times more D1R than D2R (ref. 6); (2) administration of the D1 antagonist SCH23390 produced deficits in performance that were dose-dependent during a delayed-response task in monkeys[7]; (3) by combining iontophoretic analysis of dopamine receptors with single-cell recording delayed-response performance, the specific role of D1R in regulating neuronal activity associated with working memory in monkeys has been revealed[8].

Here we have shown that D1R binding decreases in the PFC of schizophrenic patients and that this reduction is related to negative symptoms and poor performance in the WCST. Our findings indicate that this dysfunction in the D1R modulation mechanism in the PFC may contribute to negative symptoms and cognitive deficits in schizophrenia and suggest that selective D1 agonists may be helpful in treating the negative symptoms of schizophrenia. □

Methods

Subjects. This study was approved by the Ethics and Radiation Safety Committee of the National Institute of Radiological Sciences and the Ethics Committee of Tokyo Medical and Dental university. We examined 17 patients aged 27.4 ± 5.9 yr (mean $\pm$ s.d.) and 18 controls aged 27.7 ± 5.6 yr. Ten of the patients (aged 26.1 ± 3.8 yr) were neuroleptic-naive and 7 (aged 29.2 ± 8.1 yr) had been previously treated with neuroleptics but had been drug-free for at least two weeks (median 5 weeks, maximum 4 years) before the PET study. Written informed consent was obtained from all subjects. The patients all met the ICD-10 criteria for schizophrenia. The duration of illness ranged from 4 months to 18 years (average 5.5 yr).

PET experiments. Two PET experiments were performed on the same day with a four-ring, 7-slices PET system (PCT3600W40; Hitachi). Spatial resolution of the system is 8 mm on the plane and axial resolution is 12 mm. The subject were carefully positioned with the aid of a vertical laser line so that the lowest slice included the cerebellar hemispheres and was parallel to the orbitomeatal plane. The head was immobilized during scanning with a specially designed headholder and a plastic face mask. In the first PET run, a dose of $291.2-412.2$ MBq of [11C]SCH23390 was injected to study D1R in the striatum and cortex. The radioactivity was followed for 40 min immediately following injection. Two hours after the first examination, a dose of $226.4-563.1$ MBq of [11C]NMSP was injected to study D2R in the striatum and radioactivity monitored for 60 min.

Quantification of D1R and D2R binding. Regions of interest (ROIs) were defined blindly by Y.O. on the basis of a previously used[22] semiautomatic method, which consists of two steps. First, areas in the brain were divided into several regions manually, with surrounding cerebrospinal fluid space and white matter on the PET image being referend to the brain atlas. Then the ROIs were defined by computer-controlled delineation of the percentage isocounter. The ROI for cerebellum was obtained in the lowest slice; ROIs for the striatum, PFC, anterior cingulate, temporal and occipital cortices in [11C]SCH23390 images and the ROIs for the striatum in [11C]NMSP were obtained in the slice in which the striatum was most visible (Fig. 1). Based on a two-compartment model[23], the binding potentials of D1R, which are defined as the association rate constant (k_3) divided by the dissociation rate constant (k_4) and are assumed to be equal to B_{max} (maximum receptor density)/K_D (dissociation constant) (ref. 16), were quantified in the striatum and PFC. Because the dissociation of [11C]NMSP in the striatum is negligible, the association rate constant (k_3) was used for the D2R in the striatum[24]. To compare the volume of the brain, the MRI scan was performed with 2-mm contiguous coronal sections. The measured values were summed and then divided by the cranium volume.

Received 15 August; accepted 4 December 1996.

1. Seeman, P., Lee, T., Chau-Wong, M. & Wong, K. *Nature* **261**, 717–719 (1976).
2. Hietala, J. *et al. Arch. Gen. Psychiat.* **51**, 116–123 (1994).
3. Martinot, J. L., Person-Magnan, P., Huret, J. D. & Mazoyer, B. *Am. J. Psychiat.* **147**, 44–50 (1990).
4. Nordström, A. L., Farde, L., Eriksson, L. & Halldin, C. *Psychiat. Res. Neuroimag.* **61**, 67–83 (1995).
5. Farde, L. *et al. Arch. Gen. Psychiat.* **47**, 213–219 (1990).
6. Hall, H. *et al. Neuropsychopharmacology,* **11**, 245–256 (1994).
7. Sawaguchi, T. & Goldman-Rakic, P. S. *Science* **251**, 947–950 (1991).
8. Williams, G. V. & Goldman-Rakic, P. S. *Nature* **376**, 572–575 (1995).
9. Goldman-Rakic, P. S. *J. Neuropsychiat. Clin. Neurosci.* **6**, 348–357 (1994).
10. Kashima, H. *J. Psychopharmacol.* **11**, 83–88 (1991).
11. Farde, L., Halldin, C., Stone, E. S. & Sedvall, G. *Psychopharmacology* **92**, 278–284 (1987).
12. Anderson, P. & Gronvald, F. *Life Sci.* **38**, 1507–1514 (1986).
13. Wong, D. F. *et al. Science* **226**, 1393–1396 (1984).
14. Hess, E. J., Bracha, H. S., Kleinman, J. E. & Creese, I. *Life Sci.* **40**, 1487–1497 (1987).
15. Sedvall, G. & Farde, L. *Lancet* **346**, 743–749 (1995).
16. Mintun, M. A., Raichle, M. E., Kilbourn, M. R., Wooten, G. F. & Welch, M. J. *Ann. Neurol.* **15**, 217–227 (1984).
17. Weinberger, D. R., Berman, K. F. & Zec, R. F. *Arch. Gen. Psychiat.* **43**, 114–124 (1986).
18. Brozoski, T., Brown, R., Rosvold, H. & Goldman-Rakic, P. S. *Science* **205**, 929–931 (1979).
19. Davidson, M. & Davis, K. *Arch. Gen. Psychiat.* **45**, 561–563 (1988).
20. Daniel, D., Weinberger, D. & Jones, D. *J. Neurosci.* **11**, 1907–1917 (1991).
21. Dolan, R. J. *et al. Nature* **378**, 180–182 (1995).
22. Asahina, M. *et al. Acta Neurol. Scand.* **91**, 437–443 (1995).
23. Suhara, T. *et al. Psychopharmacology* **103**, 41–45 (1991).
24. Patlak, C. & Blasberg, R. *J. Cereb. Blood Flow Metab.* **5**, 584–590 (1985).

Acknowledgements. We thank F. Shishido, H. Mori, S. Tsung and J. Ji for their help. Supported by the PET project of the National Institute of Radiological Sciences of Japan and by a grant-in-aid for Scientific Research from the Ministry of Education of Japan.

Correspondence should be addressed to Y.O. (e-mail: okubo.psyc@med.tmd.ac.jp).

Neuronal and Glial Somal Size in the Prefrontal Cortex

A Postmortem Morphometric Study of Schizophrenia and Huntington Disease

Grazyna Rajkowska, PhD; Lynn D. Selemon, PhD; Patricia S. Goldman-Rakic, PhD

Background: The cortex of patients with schizophrenia exhibits a deficit in neuropil, but the nature and extent of cellular abnormalities remain unclear. To gain further insight into this abnormality, neuronal and glial somal size were analyzed in postmortem brains from 9 patients with schizophrenia, 10 normal (control) patients, and 7 patients with Huntington disease, the latter representing a known neurodegenerative disorder.

Methods: A 3-dimensional image analyzer was used to measure the perimeters of 10 722 neuronal and 19 913 glial profiles in Brodmann areas 9 and 17. Neurons and glia classified by size and layer to assess specific vulnerabilities with respect to cortical architecture and circuitry.

Results: The schizophrenic prefrontal cortex was characterized by a downward shift in neuronal sizes accompanied by 70% to 140% per layer increases in the density of small neurons. In layer III only, a significant reduction in mean neuronal size was associated with a significant decrease in the density of very large neurons in sublayer IIIc. Neither neuronal size in occipital area 17 nor glial size in prefrontal or occipital cortexes were reduced. In cortex with Huntington disease, neuronal degeneration was evidenced by concurrence of reduced neuronal size, decreased density of large neurons, and dramatic elevation in density of large glia.

Conclusions: Distinct cytometric abnormalities support the hypothesis that neuronal degeneration in the prefrontal cortex is not a prominent feature of the neuropathological changes in schizophrenia, although an ongoing process in Huntington disease. Rather, schizophrenia appears to involve more subtle abnormalities, with the largest corticocortical projection neurons of layer IIIc expressing the greatest somal reduction.

Arch Gen Psychiatry. 1998;55:215-224

ONSIDERABLE evidence indicates that the prefrontal cortex of schizophrenic patients is subject to a pathological process, but the nature of this process is far from clear. Morphometric studies of prefrontal cortex in schizophrenic brains undertaken to date have generally focused on estimates of neuronal density and number.[1-3] Although evaluation of neuronal cell size provides a measure of the structural integrity and viability of neuronal populations, only 1 study of the prefrontal cortex (Brodmann area 10) has been undertaken previously, and no size differences were observed between schizophrenic and control brains.[3] In regions of the schizophrenic brain outside the prefrontal cortex, decreased neuronal size has been reported for pyramidal neurons in the hippocampus,[4,5] substantia nigra,[6] and locus ceruleus.[7]

Quantitative analysis of glial size is also an unexplored issue in schizophrenia; although clearly relevant to theories of pathogenesis, morphometric analyses have thus far focused on glial number or density.[6,8-12]

Whether there is active gliosis in the schizophrenic brain (ie, an increase in the number of glial cells) has become a focal point of research into causal mechanisms for the disease. Although not without exception,[8] most reports indicate that glial cell number is unchanged in the schizophrenic cortex and limbic nuclei.[6,9-12] The absence of gliotic processes has been interpreted as support for a developmental cause for the disease.[13-15] We have previously observed a trend increase in glial density in Brodmann area 9 of schizophrenic cortex in conjunction with increased neuronal density and slight cortical thinning.[2] The parallel increases in neuronal and glial density were interpreted as due to tighter cell packing as a consequence of reduced interneuronal neuropil, rather than as an indication of increased glial cell number. Despite the fact that glial enlargement is an obligatory component of

From the Departments of Psychiatry and Human Behavior (Dr Rajkowska) and Anatomy (Drs Selemon and Goldman-Rakic), University of Mississippi Medical Center, Jackson; and the Section of Neurobiology (Drs Selemon and Goldman-Rakic), Yale University School of Medicine, New Haven, Conn.

This article is also available on our Web site: www.ama-assn.org/psych.

249

MATERIALS AND METHODS

HISTOLOGICAL PREPARATION AND SAMPLING PROCEDURE

Neuronal and glial cell bodies were measured in the same 40-μm Nissl-stained sections used for our previous study of cell density in the schizophrenic and HD cortex.[2,22] From the 51 cases examined previously, 26 brains with the shortest storage time in formalin were selected. Cell sizes were analyzed in prefrontal area 9 of the left hemisphere in 9 schizophrenic, 10 neurologically normal controls, and 7 (grade 3 or 4) HD cases (**Figure 1**; **Figure 2**, A; and **Table 1**). Additionally, 7 schizophrenic and 7 control brains in which the occipital pole was available (Table 1) were selected from the original sample for analysis of cell soma size in area 17 of the left hemisphere. Prefrontal area 9 was defined according to cytoarchitectonic criteria described previously,[22,23] and area 17 was delineated according to Brodmann[24] (Figure 1). The software for the 3-dimensional image analyzer used for measuring neuronal and glial cell bodies was developed at Yale University, New Haven, Conn.[25]

In each area, cell sizes were analyzed in 3 cortical probes consisting of an uninterrupted series of 3-dimensional counting boxes (70×50×25 μm) that spanned the entire depth of the cortex from the pial surface to the white matter (Figure 1, C). Probes were analyzed in 3 coronal sections representing different rostrocaudal levels of area 9 and area 17, respectively. In each counting box, neuronal and glial cell bodies were traced manually at a magnification of ×2000, using a digitizing pad and a computer mouse. The tracings were made at the focal plane in which cell soma were maximal in size and cell nuclei were clearly visible. Distinctions between neuronal and glial somata were based on morphological criteria described in our previous article.[2] Soma sizes were estimated by calculating the diameter of every traced cell profile as an equivalent circle (D-circle) with the area measured for that individual neuron or glial cell in its equatorial plane (Figure 1, D). The measured soma size of glial cell was equal to the D-circle of the cell nucleus. In this manner, 300 to 500 neuronal and 400 to 1000 glial cell profiles were measured per brain for a total of 10 722 neurons and 19 913 glial cells overall.

STATISTICAL ANALYSIS

Four statistical analyses were performed. (1) Multiple regression analysis using cell size as the dependent variable was performed with age, postmortem interval, and time in formalin as independent variables for neuronal and glial sizes in areas 9 and 17. Correlation between cell size and neuronal density, glial density, and cortical thickness also were examined. The correlation between neuronal size and duration of illness was examined for schizophrenic brains. A Bonferroni correction was used for these analyses; the effective α=.006. (2) The mean soma size for neurons and glia measured across all cortical layers represented an average of values from 3 probes. Group means (schizophrenic vs control brains; HD vs control brains) were compared using analysis of variance (ANOVA), followed by the Dunnett test, with α=.05. (3) Mean soma size in individual layers was compared between groups by using single-factor (disease), repeated-measures (cortical layers) ANOVA. Following a significant ANOVA, individual ANOVAs were used for cortical layers to determine differences between the groups by using the Dunnett test. (4) The density (number of cells divided by 0.001 mm³) of different cell size classes was obtained by using the mean (M) and standard deviation (δ) of the control cases to segment cases into small (smaller than M−1δ), medium (M−1δ to M), large (M to M+1δ), and extra large (larger than M+1δ) classes. Differences between groups were analyzed with a repeated-measures (cell-size classes) ANOVA followed by selected contrast analyses with α=.02.

gliosis, to our knowledge there are no studies to date that have examined glial cell size in schizophrenia.

Comparison of the morphometric abnormalities observed in the schizophrenic cortex with those found in Huntington disease (HD) could provide insight into whether cellular changes in schizophrenia are the result of neuronal loss, because neurodegeneration of large pyramidal cells is a well-established feature of the cortical abnormalities in late-stage HD.[16-18] Previous analysis of cell density in HD brains revealed a pattern of cytoarchitectonic abnormality distinct from that found in the schizophrenic prefrontal cortex with markedly (50%) increased glial density accompanied by pronounced (28%) cortical thinning.[2] The morphometric pattern observed in HD brains is consistent with ongoing neurodegenerative processes and reactive gliosis. Indeed, gliosis has been described previously in both the neostriatum and the prefrontal cortex in HD brains.[18-21] However, it remains to be determined whether changes in cell size occur in association with the neuronal loss and glial proliferation described in the HD prefrontal cortex.

To further explore the cellular abnormalities underlying schizophrenia and to compare the observed abnormalities with those of an established neurodegenerative disorder, neuronal and glial cell bodies were measured in a subset of the same population of schizophrenic, HD, and control brains analyzed in Selemon et al.[2] Our results indicate a differential vulnerability of neuronal and glial cell types and involvement of different cortical layers or sublayers in the 2 diseases. Further, they provide evidence for a cellular deficiency short of degeneration in neuronal populations in schizophrenia.

RESULTS

CELL SIZES IN PREFRONTAL AREA 9 OF NORMAL HUMAN BRAIN

The cytoarchitectonic features of area 9 in normal human brain are described in detail in our previous article.[22] Briefly, the presence of large pyramidal neurons in sublayers IIIc and Va and layer VI intermixed with medium and small pyramids is the most prominent feature of prefrontal area 9 (Figure 2, B). Glial architecture is more homogeneous than neuronal architecture. Mean glial size in area 9 was very similar in all cortical layers.

250

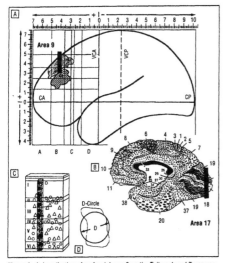

Figure 1. A, Localization of prefrontal area 9 on the Taliarach and Tournoux stereotaxic atlas of the human brain according to Rajkowska and Goldman-Rakic[23] (with modifications). B, The position of area 17 plotted according to the Brodmann map.[24] Dark bars indicate loci in areas 9 and 17 where measurements were taken. C, Schematic drawing of a cortical probe consisting of an uninterrupted series of 3-dimensional counting boxes. Cell sizes were measured in counting boxes and then divided into individual cortical layers according to cytoarchitectonic criteria established previously.[22] D, Schematic drawing of diameter circle (D-circle), the parameter used to estimate soma size.

NEURONAL SIZES IN AREA 9 OF SCHIZOPHRENIC AND HD CORTEX

Mean Values

Analysis of variance revealed a significant effect of disease ($F[2,127]=4.532$, $P=.01$) on neuronal size. Overall mean neuronal soma size and neuronal sizes in layers III through VI were 4% to 9% smaller in area 9 of schizophrenic brains, reaching significant levels ($P=.05$) only in layer III (**Table 2** and **Figure 3**). Although mean neuronal size was smaller for the schizophrenic group compared with the control group, individual variability in soma sizes was evident. Six of 9 schizophrenic brains used for our study had smaller-than-normal neuronal sizes, while 3 schizophrenic brains fell within the normal range in at least some prefrontal layers (Figure 3, A).

In HD prefrontal cortex, overall mean neuronal size was significantly smaller compared with normal control brains (9%; $P=.004$). However, significant 10% reductions in soma size were not confined to layer III but also extended to layers V (Vb) and marginally to layer VI of the HD cortex (Table 2; Figure 2, B; and Figure 3, A). No significant differences in mean soma size were found in granular layers II and IV of HD prefrontal cortex. Individual variability was high in HD brains in layers III and V while neurons of layer VI exhibited more consistent decreases in neuronal sizes (Figure 3, A).

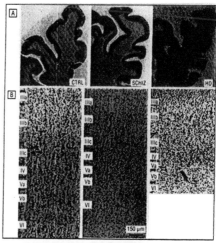

Figure 2. A, Photographs of coronal sections taken at the same magnification from the dorsolateral prefrontal cortex of control (CTRL) (N729), schizophrenic (SCHIZ) (B1702), and Huntington disease (HD) (B194) brains. The positions of cortical probes on the superior frontal gyrus (area 9) are marked by dark bars. B, Photomicrographs of Nissl-stained coronal sections of area 9 from the same 3 brains revealing their cytoarchitectonic features. Note that large pyramidal cells in sublayers IIIc and Va of control area 9 are not present in corresponding layers of the 2 diseased groups.

Multiple regression analyses of relationships between neuronal somal size and age, postmortem interval, time in formalin, and duration of illness were not significant in any layer or sublayer of area 9 in the 26 brains examined in this study (**Figure 4**). However, there was a significant correlation between neuronal size and cortical thickness in sublayers IIIb ($r^2=0.288$, $P=.003$) and IIIc ($r^2=0.378$, $P<.001$); sublayer Vb ($r^2=0.328$, $P=.001$); and layer VI ($r^2=0.345$, $P=.001$). Significant inverse correlations were found between neuronal size and neuronal density in sublayers IIIb and IIIc ($r^2=0.290$, $P=.003$ and $r^2=0.538$, $P<.001$, respectively); sublayer Vb ($r^2=0.287$, $P=.003$); and layer VI ($r^2=0.320$, $P=.002$); as well as between neuronal size and glial density in layer II ($r^2=0.254$, $P=.005$); sublayer IIIc ($r^2=0.278$, $P=.003$); and sublayer Vb ($r^2=0.308$, $P=.002$). Thus, smaller neuronal size was associated with higher neuronal and glial density and with reduced cortical thickness.

Neuronal Size Distribution

Comparison of histograms of somal size distribution for individual cortical layers revealed departures from the normal distribution of different cell size classes in both schizophrenic and HD brains (**Figure 5**). The curve of the normal distribution was shifted toward smaller sizes in cortical layers III and V of both the schizophrenic and HD brains compared with that of the controls. A marked shift of the normal distribution for layer VI was observed only in HD brains.

To determine more precisely which population of neurons was most susceptible to changes in soma size, the whole

251

Table 1. Description of Subjects Studied*

Brain	Age, y/Sex/Race	PMI, h	TF, mo	Cause of Death	Diagnosis	Symptoms
			Controls†			
B1638‡	34/F/W	7.5	...	Heart failure/burns	...	...
B1823‡	40/F/W	24	26.0	Pulmonary embolism	...	...
B1824‡	29/M/W	24.0	7.5	Cardiac arrhythmia	...	...
C0133	47/M/W	12.0	7.5	Myocardial infarction	...	...
C0176	33/M/W	16	13.5	Duodenal rupture	...	...
C0188	71/F/W	24	5.5	Myocardial infarction	...	...
MU169‡	58/M/W	6.0	...	Myocardial infarction	...	...
N113‡	19/M/B	13.5	81.0	Homicide	...	...
N129‡	50/F/B	20.0	80.5	Cardiovascular disease	...	...
N729‡	59/M/W	20.5	31.7	Cardiovascular disease	...	...
		Subjects With Schizophrenia (SCHIZ)§				
B840‡	22/M/HS	...	45.5	Suicide by jumping	Probable	a-d‖
B1138‡	27/M/W	8.0	26.0	Suicide, asphyxiation	Paranoid	a, c, d‖
B1702‡	62/M/W	21.0	2.3	Adenocarcinoma	SCHIZ	a-d‖
B1932‡	33/M/W	9.7	4.5	Suicide, asphyxiation	Paranoid	a, b‖
C0237	48/F/W	27.0	2.0	Suicide, drinking hydrochloride	SCHIZ	a, c‖
N29	55/F/B	27.5	70.3	Cardiovascular disease	Undifferentiated	a-d‖
N164‡	54/M/B	10.0	86.6	Tuberculosis	SCHIZ	a-d‖
C0234	23/M/W	19.5	10.0	Suicide	SCHIZ	a‖
N72	46/M/B	16.2	76.0	Cardiovascular disease	Undifferentiated	a-d‖
		Subjects With Huntington Disease (HD)¶				
B194	40/M/W	21.25	106.3	Pneumonia	Grade 4	...
B1135	41/F/W	...	21.3	Respiratory arrest	Grade 3	...
B1593	63/M/W	2.5	8.9	Complications of HD	Grade 4	...
B1641	55/M/W	1.9	16.5	Colitis sepsis	Grade 4	...
B1701	32/M/W	4.5	3.0	Respiratory arrest	Grade 3	...
B1940	75/F/W	15.0	1.0	Complications of HD	Grade 4	...
B1947	35/M/W	18.5	0.6	Pneumonia	Grade 4	...

*PMI indicates postmortem interval; TF, time in formalin solution; ellipses, data not available; and HS, Hispanic.
†The mean age of the controls was 44 years; PMI was 17 hours; and TF was 32 months.
‡Cases for which area 17 was analyzed. In addition to the 5 schizophrenic brains in which area 17 was analyzed, area 17 of 2 other schizophrenic brains—N207 (age,y/sex/race, 60/F/W; PMI, 13.5 hours; and TF, 164.3 months) and N371 (age, y/sex/race, 48/F/B; PMI, 26 hours; and TF, 136.3 months)—from our previous study were analyzed.
§The mean age of the subjects with schizophrenia was 41 years; PMI was 17 hours; and TF was 36 months.
‖a indicates hallucinations and/or delusions; b, flat affect; c, thought disorder; and d, depression, ie, sleep or appetite loss, hopelessness, social withdrawal, or multiple suicide attempts.
¶The mean age of subjects with HD was 49 years; PMI was 11 hours; and TF was 23 months.

Table 2. Mean Neuronal Soma Sizes in Prefrontal Area 9*

Layers	Control (n=10)	SCHIZ (n=9)	P	HD (n=7)	P
II	11.8±0.4	11.7±0.4	...	10.8±0.5	...
III	15.5±0.4	14.4±0.4	↓.047	13.9±0.4	↓.008
IIIa	13.7±0.3	13.6±0.4	...	12.8±0.4	...
IIIb	15.0±0.3	14.4±0.4	...	13.9±0.4	↓.04
IIIc	16.1±0.5	15.0±0.5	...	14.5±0.5	↓.04
IV	12.4±0.4	11.9±0.4	...	11.5±0.4	...
V	15.7±0.4	14.6±0.6	...	14.2±0.5	↓.04
Va	16.0±0.6	14.5±0.6	↓.07	14.5±0.7	...
Vb	15.6±0.5	14.7±0.5	...	13.5±0.5	↓.009
VI	15.7±0.5	14.9±0.5	...	14.3±0.6	↓.05
All cortical layers	14.2±0.3	13.5±0.3	↓.07	12.9±0.3	↓.004

*Values represent the mean±SE of 10 brains from control subjects, 9 brains from patients with schizophrenia (SCHIZ), or 7 brains from patients with Huntington disease (HD), expressed in micrometers. P<.05 is boldfaced, whereas values close to significant (.05<P<.07) are in regular typeface. Arrows next to P values indicate decreases in neuronal soma sizes in both diseased groups compared with control subjects. Ellipses indicate not applicable.

population of measured neurons was divided into 4 cell-size classes (small, medium, large, and extra large; see "Materials and Methods" section). In the schizophrenic cortex, the density of small and/or medium neurons was significantly increased by 70% to 140% in cortical layers II, Va, and Vb, and marginally in layers IV and VI (**Table 3**). In contrast, the population of large and extra large neurons in the schizophrenic cortex did not exhibit significant changes in packing density in any of the cortical layers except sublayer IIIc. In this sublayer, containing the largest pyramidal neurons, the density of extra large neurons was decreased by 40% (P=.02) compared with control brains. Further sublaminar analyses revealed an increase in the density of large neurons in sublayer IIIa, where the size of large neurons was more like that of medium neurons in other sublayers of layer III and V. We interpret this finding to be consistent with the increases in the density of medium neurons in sublayers Va and Vb.

Statistical analysis of the same prefrontal layers of HD cortex revealed a different pattern of change in the density of the 4 cell-size classes. In all cortical layers of the HD cortex except layers II and IV, the density of ex

252

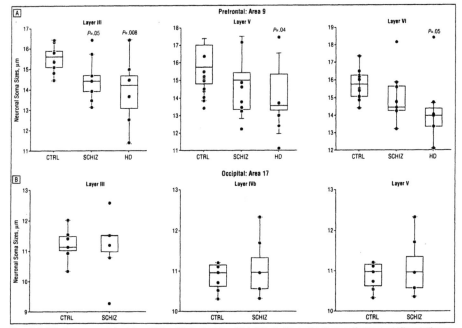

Figure 3. A, Plots of mean neuronal sizes in layers III, V, and VI of prefrontal area 9 in individual brains revealing the range of individual variability and differences between the groups in soma size. Note that significantly smaller neurons are found in pyramidal layer III of schizophrenic (SCHIZ) brains and in layers III and V and marginally in layer VI of Huntington disease (HD) brains. B, Plots of mean neuronal sizes in layers III, IVb, and V in occipital area 17 in individual brains of the control (CTRL) and the schizophrenic group. Sublayer IVb was chosen to be presented because neurons in this sublayer are among the largest cells in area 17. Note that mean soma size does not differ between schizophrenic and control brains (t = -.062, df = 82, P = .95). Note the similarity in soma sizes in layers III and V of area 17 and the reduction in soma size in corresponding cortical layers of prefrontal area 9 (A) in schizophrenic brains.

tra large or large neurons was dramatically (50%-80%) decreased in comparison with control brains (Table 3). In addition, in layer VI, the 23% decrease in the density of large neurons was accompanied by a significant 150% increase in the density of small neurons. The above statistical descriptions are consistent with our microscopic observations that pyramidal neurons are smaller in the prefrontal cortex in both schizophrenic and HD brains (Figure 2, B).

GLIAL SIZES IN AREA 9 OF SCHIZOPHRENIC AND HD CORTEX

Mean Values

Analysis of variance revealed a significant effect of disease on glial size (F[2,153]=3.879, P=.02). Post hoc contrast analyses revealed that mean glial sizes were not statistically different between schizophrenic and control prefrontal cortexes (**Table 4**). In contrast, glial cell bodies were significantly larger (P=.006) in the same cortical area of HD brains as compared with control brains.

Multiple regression analysis revealed no significant interactions between glial size and age, postmortem interval, time in formalin, neuronal density, glial den-

sity, or cortical thickness in area 9 in the 26 brains examined in this study.

Glial Size Distribution

Analysis of histograms of glial size distribution followed the paradigm used for analysis of neuronal size distribution. The analysis did not reveal significant differences in glial size in any of the 4 size classes between normal and schizophrenic prefrontal cortexes (Table 4). In contrast, in all cortical layers (I-VI) of the HD brains there was a marked and significant 100% to 150% increase in the density of large and/or extra large glial cells compared with control brains. These statistical findings confirmed our microscopic observations of the presence of enlarged, chromatin-light glial cell nuclei in all cortical layers of the HD brains and only in these cases.

SOMA SIZES IN OCCIPITAL AREA 17 OF SCHIZOPHRENIC AND CONTROL BRAINS

In contrast to the prefrontal cortex, no significant differences in mean neuronal size or size-dependent density were found between schizophrenic and control brains in any cortical layers in area 17 (Figure 3, B). In addition to the 6 main

ARCH GEN PSYCHIATRY/VOL 55, MAR 1998
219

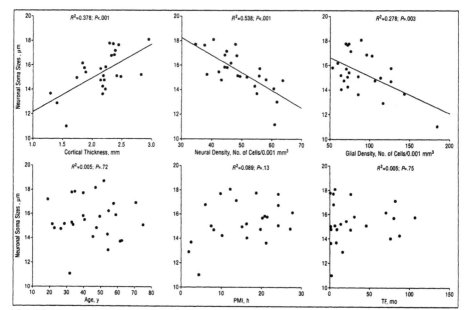

Figure 4. *Plots summarizing results of regression analyses in prefrontal area 9. Correlation between neuronal soma size in sublayer IIIc and cortical thickness, neuronal density, glial density, age, postmortem interval (PMI), and time in formalin (TF) is shown on individual plots. Note that in layer IIIc there were significant positive correlations between soma size and cortical thickness and negative correlations between mean soma size and neuronal and glial density. No significant interactions between age, PMI, or TF and neuronal sizes was found in this sublayer.*

cortical layers, neuronal sizes were compared in the 3 sublayers of layer IV (IVa, IVb, and IVc) in area 17; again, no significant differences in neuronal sizes were found. Glial sizes also did not differ between the 2 groups.

In area 17, there were no significant correlations between neuronal or glial size and age, postmortem interval, or time in formalin. Neuronal size was, however, related to neuronal density in layers III ($P=.005$) and sublayers IVa ($P=.003$) and IVb ($P=.001$; $r^2=0.854$, n=13). Glial size was not correlated with neuronal density, and neither neuronal nor glial size correlated with glial density or cortical thickness in area 17.

COMMENT

REDUCED NEURONAL SIZE IN SCHIZOPHRENIA: IMPLICATIONS FOR CYTOPLASMIC ATROPHY

To our knowledge, this is the first report of a significant reduction in neuronal size in the schizophrenic prefrontal cortex, size-dependent changes in neuronal density, and quantitative analysis of glial size. In the schizophrenic prefrontal cortex, a downward shift in neuronal size was observed in all layers with a significant reduction in layer III. Despite an overall 17% elevation in neuronal density in area 9,[2] only the density of small and medium neurons was increased by 70% to 140%; neuron density was not increased for large neurons in schizophrenic brains. If large cells had degenerated, the 70% to 140% increases in lami-

nar density of smaller size classes would have been comparable to those observed for the entire neuronal population (11%-24%)[2]; instead they were orders of magnitude larger. Therefore, the reduction in neuronal size can be attributed to a downward shift, specifically in the size of large and extra large neurons, such that they inflated the smaller size classes. The observed reduction in mean neuronal size in the context of dramatic increases in the density of smaller neurons suggests that subtle cellular changes, rather than neuronal loss, may be present in the schizophrenic prefrontal cortex. In the present study, the reduction in neuronal sizes averaged across all layers was not significant in the schizophrenic prefrontal cortex, replicating previous negative findings with respect to mean neuronal size.[3,26]

Our findings of smaller neurons, revealed only by layer-by-layer analysis, are concordant with earlier qualitative ultrastructural observations on prefrontal cortical neurons in schizophrenic brain biopsy specimens and are indicative of previously unsuspected size-dependent vulnerabilities with respect to cortical architecture and circuitry. In a unique study,[27] abnormalities were limited to intracellular alterations in organelle structure, eg, prominent and irregular Golgi apparatus, the presence of small dense granules in the cytoplasm, and synapses without synaptic vesicles. We interpret the smaller neurons observed in our study as consistent with our previous evidence of diminution of neuropil in schizophrenic cortex, as cells with reduced dendritic arbors may have reduced metabolic needs and therefore require less somal cytoplasmic volume.

254

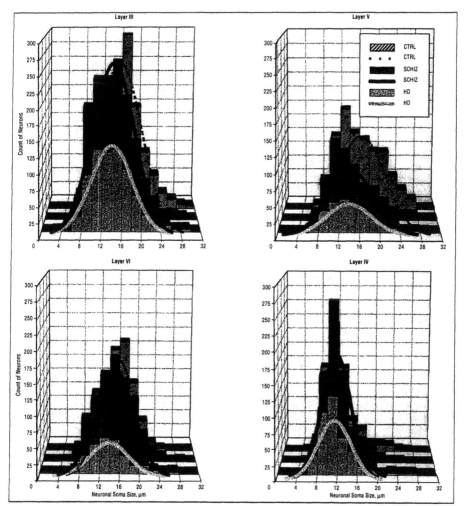

Figure 5. *Histogram comparison of the neuronal soma size distribution between control (CTRL), schizophrenic (SCHIZ), and Huntington diseased (HD) brains in layers III, IV, V, and VI of prefrontal area 9. Solid lines represent curves of normal distribution in diseased brains whereas dotted lines depict control brains. Solid bars represent the number of soma in specific size ranges in diseased brains. Hatched bars represent soma size in control brains. Notice that in cortical layers III and V of both schizophrenic and HD brains, the curves of normal distribution are shifted toward smaller sizes when compared with controls. In layer VI, a pronounced shifting of the normal distribution curve is observed only in HD but not schizophrenic brains. In contrast, no departures from the control group's normal distribution were observed in either schizophrenic or HD brains in layer IV.*

PRONOUNCED ATROPHY OF LARGE PYRAMIDAL CELLS IN LAYER III IN SCHIZOPHRENIA

Differences in mean neuronal size between schizophrenic and control brains, though present in other layers, were significant only for layer III. Furthermore, layer III was the only compartment in the schizophrenic brains in which the increase in density of smaller neurons was accompanied by a significant decrease in the density of extra large cells. These observations suggest that the large pyramidal neurons of layer III (IIIc) may undergo more severe pathological changes in the schizophrenic cortex than large neurons in other layers. It is unclear, however, whether the prominent pathological characteristics of pyramidal cells in layer III of area 9, which are among the largest neurons in the prefrontal cortex,[22]

ARCH GEN PSYCHIATRY/VOL 55, MAR 1998
221

Table 3. Neuronal Density of Different Size Classes in Area 9 in the 3 Groups*

Cell Classes	Neuronal Size, µm	Control ND	SCHIZ ND	P	HD ND	P
Layer II						
Small	4.7-9.1	19±5	18±5	...	26±6	...
Medium	9.2-12.1	32±4	49±4	↑.007	38±5	...
Large	12.2-15.2	29±3	28±3	...	20±3	...
Extra large	15.3-22.4	13±3	11±3	...	5±3	...
Layer III						
Small	5.0-10.5	9±2	11±2	...	12±2	...
Medium	10.6-15.0	16±2	21±2	...	22±2	...
Large	15.1-19.5	16±2	17±1	...	15±1	↓.01
Extra large	19.6-35.4	7±1	6±1	...	3±1	↓.004
IIIa						
Small	5.3-9.8	12±3	11±3	...	14±4	...
Medium	9.9-13.6	19±4	24±4	...	27±4	...
Large	13.7-17.3	18±3	28±3	↑.01	19±3	...
Extra large	17.4-23.4	12±2	9±2	...	4±2	...
IIIb						
Small	6.1-10.8	11±2	12±2	...	11±2	...
Medium	10.9-14.9	18±3	18±3	...	20±4	...
Large	15.0-19.1	19±2	16±2	...	15±3	...
Extra large	19.2-28.7	8±1	6±1	...	3±2	↓.02
IIIc						
Small	5.0-10.9	7±2	11±2	...	12±3	...
Medium	11.0-16.0	18±3	22±3	...	22±4	...
Large	16.1-21.1	14±2	14±2	...	10±2	...
Extra large	21.2-35.5	8±1	5±1	↓.02	3±1	↓.002
Layer IV						
Small	5.5-8.9	6±4	9±4	...	17±5	...
Medium	9.0-12.1	38±5	56±6	↑.03	51±6	...
Large	12.2-15.3	22±3	27±3	...	19±4	...
Extra large	15.4-27.7	11±2	11±2	...	10±2	...
Layer V						
Small	6.5-11.5	9±3	18±3	↑.04	14±3	...
Medium	11.6-16.2	22±2	25±3	...	19±3	...
Large	16.2-20.8	14±2	12±2	...	8±3	...
Extra large	20.9-36.7	9±2	5±2	...	3±2	...
Va						
Small	7.5-11.1	9±3	18±3	↑.05	16±4	...
Medium	11.2-16.0	22±2	30±3	↑.02	24±3	...
Large	16.0-20.9	17±2	15±2	...	13±3	...
Extra large	21.0-36.7	10±2	5±2	...	3±2	↓.02
Vb						
Small	6.9-11.6	9±3	13±3	...	12±3	...
Medium	11.7-15.7	22±2	30±3	↑.02	22±3	...
Large	15.8-19.9	17±2	15±2	...	13±3	...
Extra large	20.0-27.4	10±2	5±2	...	4±2	↓.04
Layer VI						
Small	7.5-12.2	6±2	12±2	↑.05	14±2	↑.01
Medium	12.3-15.6	11±2	15±2	...	16±2	...
Large	15.7-19.0	13±1	12±1	...	8±1	↓.002
Extra large	19.1-34.8	5±1	7±1	...	3±2	...

*Values represent mean±SE neuronal densities (ND) (calculated as the number of cells/0.001 mm³). Significant P values (P<.03) are boldfaced, whereas values close to significant (.03<P<.05) are in regular typeface. Arrows next to P values indicate increases or decreases in ND of specific cell size classes in both diseased groups compared with controls. Analysis of variance showed significant differences between schizophrenic (SCHIZ) brains vs control brains and Huntington diseased (HD) brains vs controls in the ND in different size classes. These differences were dependent on the cortical layer (F[3,381]=94.936, P<.001) and size class (F[6,381]=5.316, P<.001) in which neuronal size was analyzed. Ellipses indicate not applicable.

represent a selective vulnerability of these cells alone or a vulnerability of large neurons in general. The finding that reductions in the largest prefrontal neurons of layer Va were nearly significant (P=.07) would be compatible with a size-dependent process. However, whether general or selective, the large cell vulnerability observed in the present study was not observed in the visual cortex, and thus appears specific to prefrontal cortex.

In patients with Alzheimer disease, large pyramidal neurons have been found to be susceptible to degenerative changes as decreases in the number of large SMI32-immunoreactive neurons have been found in layers III and V of prefrontal area 9.[28] As layer III pyramidal cells are one of the major sources of corticocortical connections,[29-32] our results and evidence for reduction of spine density on layer III pyramidal neurons[33,34] suggest a prominent role of corticocortical circuitry in schizophrenia.

256

ARCH GEN PSYCHIATRY/VOL 55, MAR 1998
223

Table 4. Glial Cell Density of Different Size Classes in Area 9 in the 3 Groups*

Cell Classes	Size, μm	Control GCD	SCHIZ GCD	HD GCD	P
Layer I					
Small	2.6-4.2	9±2	8±3	6±3	...
Medium	4.3-5.2	23±5	29±5	22±6	...
Large	5.3-6.1	18±4	23±4	33±5	↑.03
Extra large	6.2-8.7	8±4	18±4	23±5	↑.04
Layer II					
Small	3.0-4.4	9±4	10±4	8±4	...
Medium	4.5-5.4	19±5	25±5	25±6	...
Large	5.5-6.3	17±4	17±5	34±5	↑.02
Extra large	6.4-8.4	8±2	9±2	18±3	↑.004
Layer III					
Small	1.3-4.3	12±4	11±5	10±5	...
Medium	4.4-5.2	35±7	33±8	39±9	...
Large	5.3-6.1	24±4	21±4	48±5	↑.001
Extra large	6.2-9.9	12±3	13±3	24±4	↑.01
Layer IV					
Small	2.9-4.2	11±4	14±5	12±5	...
Medium	4.3-5.1	37±11	45±12	55±13	...
Large	5.2-6.0	27±6	31±6	57±7	↑.003
Extra large	6.1-9.6	13±4	13±4	27±4	↑.03
Layer V					
Small	2.3-4.3	11±4	15±5	6±5	...
Medium	4.4-5.2	39±12	45±13	63±14	...
Large	5.3-6.1	28±7	29±7	64±8	↑.002
Extra large	6.2-9.9	13±3	14±3	21±4	...
Layer VI					
Small	1.1-4.4	14±5	15±5	14±6	...
Medium	4.5-5.3	41±9	41±9	65±11	...
Large	5.4-6.1	28±7	32±7	74±8	↑<.001
Extra large	6.2-10.9	15±4	14±4	25±5	...
Mean sizes for all layers		5.26±.07	5.38±.07	5.55±.08	↑.006

*Values represent mean±SE. Significant P values (P<.03) are boldfaced, whereas values close to significant (.02<P<.05) are in regular typeface. Arrows next to P values indicate increase in the large and/or very large glial cell density (GCD) in Huntington diseased (HD) brains compared with controls. Glial cell density was calculated as the number of cells/0.001 mm³. SCHIZ indicates schizophrenia.

In contrast to findings in the anterior cingulate cortex and prefrontal area 10, where a reduction in the density of small neurons has been reported in layers II through VI,[35] evidence for loss of small neurons was not observed in any cortical layer in our study. Indeed, the absence of significant decreases in neuronal size in layers II and IV suggests that small nonpyramidal cells are less impaired than large pyramidal cells. Whether the apparent discrepancies in findings represent regional variation or reflect differences in methodological approaches is unclear.

REGIONAL SPECIFICITY OF NEURONAL SIZE CHANGES IN SCHIZOPHRENIA: AREA 17 VS AREA 9

Significant abnormalities in neuronal size were not found in any cortical layers in area 17 in the schizophrenic brains despite the 10% increase in neuronal density observed previously.[2] These findings suggest that the morphologic changes in the primary visual area are less marked that those in the prefrontal region. Differences in the cytoarchitectonic composition of these 2 areas may account for the lack of change in somal sizes in area 17. Primary sensory cortical areas, including area 17, have a much less prominent layer III and smaller pyramidal cells than associational cortical regions like area 9. Although it could be argued that size changes in somal diameter may be most easily detected in layer III of area 9 because the pyramids are very large, similar decreases in somal size were not detected in the very large nonpyramidal cells in layer IV of area 17, lending further weight to the hypothesis that pyramidal cells, perhaps prefrontal pyramidal cells, are selectively impaired in the disease. Corticocortical synapses, particularly afferent input from other cortical areas, also may not be as numerous in area 17 as in the associational cortical regions.

NEURONAL DEGENERATION IN HD

In the HD prefrontal cortex, mean neuronal size was decreased relative to normal controls in layers III (IIIb, IIIc), Vb, and VI, and in addition, the density of extra large or large neurons was decreased by 50% to 80% in all cortical layers except layers II and IV. Because these decreases were not accompanied by comparable increases in the density of smaller neurons, the reductions cannot be easily attributed to a mere shift in cell size like that observed in the schizophrenic cortex. It is likely that large cells degenerate in HD. Even in layer VI, which exhibited a 150% increase in the density of small neurons, greater cell packing of the small neuron population can be mostly explained by the dramatic thinning of infragranular layers[2] rather than by the addition of "new" small neurons that have shrunk from the large neuron population. These findings of reduced density of large neurons are in accord with previous observations of loss of large pyramidal neurons in layers III, V, and VI of area 10[18] and in layers V and VI of areas 8 and 9[17] in HD brains. Reductions in somal size and density of large neurons in layers III, V, and VI of the HD prefrontal cortex suggests that corticocortical, corticostriatal, and corticothalamic projection neurons all are compromised in the advanced stages of HD.

GLIAL ENLARGEMENT IN HD BUT NOT SCHIZOPHRENIA

In our study, mean glial size and the density of large and extra large glial cells was greatly increased in HD brains relative to normal brains. In addition, increased glial density was found in the same HD brains in our previous study.[2] These findings concur with reports of increased numbers of oligodendrocytes and density of astrocytes in the prefrontal cortex for all HD grades.[18] Enlarged glial size and increased glial density strongly indicate that neurodegenerative processes and gliotic reactions are present in the HD prefrontal cortex. Whereas glial proliferation in the cortex and reactive gliosis in the striatum have been reported before,[19-21] glial enlargement has not been well-documented in prior studies of HD.

In contrast to HD brains, in schizophrenic brains only a trend increase in mean glial size was observed in area 9 and in occipital area 17; mean glial size was virtually identical in schizophrenic and control brains. Prior to this study, glial cell size has not been examined despite the fact that glial enlargement is an obligatory component of gliosis. Glial density was estimated previously in the schizophrenic prefrontal cortex and was found to be indistinguishable from normal control brains,[2,3] although in the latter study there was a trend elevation in the schizophrenic brains with storage time less than 5 years. Thus, the observation of normal glial somal sizes in conjunction with modest and variable increases in glial density suggest that glial cell reactions are not a cardinal feature of the cortical pathophysiology of schizophrenia. The lack of reactive gliosis also provides further evidence that cell loss does not occur in prefrontal and occipital cortexes of the schizophrenic brain.

Although the absence of gliotic reactions in the schizophrenic cortex has been interpreted as evidence for neuronal loss during early development,[13-15] our findings suggest that degenerative changes in all layers of cortex, with the possible exception of sublayer IIIc, stop short of neuronal loss and therefore would probably not trigger gliosis even in an adult brain. It is unclear whether the smaller neuronal volumes are due to a developmental failure or to cytoplasmic atrophy occurring early in the course of the disease. While it is not entirely possible to rule out cell loss for the select population of very large cells in layer IIIc as cell size changes in this sublayer are similar in schizophrenic and HD brains, absence of gliosis in the schizophrenic brain indicates that if neuronal loss occurred, it was very limited in scope and occurred either developmentally or at the onset of illness, because there is no evidence of ongoing neurodegeneration in the schizophrenic cortex.

Accepted for publication September 22, 1997.

This work was supported by grant 44866 from the National Institute of Mental Health (Center for the Neuroscience of Mental Disorders), Rockville, Md.

Presented at the International Congress on Schizophrenia Research, Hot Springs, Va, April 10, 1995.

The authors thank F. M. Benes, MD; J. E. Kleinman, MD, PhD; M. M. Herman, MD; and I. Delalle, MD, for the donation of postmortem brain tissue. We also acknowledge F. M. Benes, MD; J. E. Kleinman, MD, PhD; I. Delalle, MD; and E. Radonic, MD, for psychiatric diagnoses of these cases. We thank J. Coburn, J. Enwright, J. Paquette, and J. Musco for excellent technical assistance, and M. Richmond and S. Pittman for help in analyzing data. Finally, we are grateful to I. Paul, PhD, and Michael Andrew, PhD, for valuable comments on statistical analyses.

Reprints: Grazyna Rajkowska, PhD, Department of Psychiatry and Human Behavior, University of Mississippi Medical Center, 2500 N State St, Jackson, MS 39216 (e-mail: grazyna@fiona.umsmed.edu).

REFERENCES
---

1. Colon EJ. Quantitative cytoarchitectonics of the human cerebral cortex in schizophrenic dementia. *Acta Neuropathol.* 1972;20:1-10.
2. Selemon LD, Rajkowska G, Goldman-Rakic PS. Abnormally high neuronal density in the schizophrenic cortex: a morphometric analysis of prefrontal area 9 and occipital area 17. *Arch Gen Psychiatry.* 1995;52:805-818.
3. Benes FM, Davidson J, Bird ED. Quantitative cytoarchitectural studies of the cerebral cortex of schizophrenics. *Arch Gen Psychiatry.* 1986;43:31-35.
4. Benes FM, Sorensen I, Bird ED. Reduced neuronal size in posterior hippocampus of schizophrenic patients. *Schizophr Bull.* 1991;17:597-608.
5. Arnold SE, Franz BR, Trojanowski JQ. Decreased neuronal size in hippocampal subfields that mediate cortical-hippocampal interactions in schizophrenia. *Soc Neurosci Abstr.* 1994;20:621.
6. Bogerts B, Hantsch J, Herzer M. A morphometric study of the dopamine-containing cell groups in the mesencephalon of normals, parkinson patients, and schizophrenics. *Biol Psychiatry.* 1983;18:951-969.
7. Karson CN, Garcia-Rill E, Biedermann J, Mrak RE, Husain MM, Skinner RD. The brainstem reticular formation in schizophrenia. *Psychiatry Res.* 1991;40:31-48.
8. Stevens JR. Neuropathology of schizophrenia. *Arch Gen Psychiatry.* 1982;39:1131-1139.
9. Casanova MF, Stevens JR, Kleinman JE. Astrocytosis in the molecular layer of the dentate gyrus: a study in Alzheimer's disease and schizophrenia. *Psychiatry Res.* 1990;35:149-166.
10. Falkai P, Bogerts B, Rozumek M. Limbic pathology in schizophrenia, the entorhinal region: a morphometric study. *Biol Psychiatry.* 1988;24:515-521.
11. Roberts GW, Colter N, Lofthouse R, Johnstone EC, Crow TJ. Is there gliosis in schizophrenia? investigation of the temporal lobe. *Biol Psychiatry.* 1987;22:1459-1468.
12. Stevens CD, Altshuler LL, Bogerts B, Falkai P. Quantitative study of gliosis in schizophrenia and Huntington's chorea. *Biol Psychiatry.* 1988;24:697-700.
13. Weinberger DR. Implications of normal brain development for the pathogenesis of schizophrenia. *Arch Gen Psychiatry.* 1987;44:660-669.
14. Benes FM. Evidence for neurodevelopment disturbances in anterior cingulate cortex of post-mortem schizophrenic brain. *Schizophr Res.* 1987;5:187-188.
15. Benes FM. Neurobiological investigations in cingulate cortex of schizophrenic brain. *Schizophr Bull.* 1993;19:537-549.
16. Cudkowicz M, Kowall NW. Degeneration of pyramidal projection neurons in Huntington's disease cortex. *Ann Neurol.* 1990;27:200-204.
17. Hedreen JC, Peyser CE, Folstein SE, Ross CA. Neuronal loss in layers V and VI of cerebral cortex in Huntington's disease. *Neurosci Lett.* 1991;133:257-261.
18. Sotrel A, Paskevich PA, Kiely DK, Bird ED, Williams RS, Myers RH. Morphometric analysis of the prefrontal cortex in Huntington's disease. *Neurology.* 1991;41:1117-1123.
19. Bruyn GW, von Wolferen WJ. Pathogenesis of Huntington's chorea. *Lancet.* 1973;1:1382.
20. Myers RH, Vonsattel JP, Paskevich PA, Kiely DK, Stevens TJ, Cupples LA, Richardson EPJ, Bird ED. Decreased neuronal and increased oligodendroglial densities in Huntington's disease caudate nucleus. *J Neuropathol Exp Neurol.* 1991; 50:729-742.
21. Vonsattel JP, Myers RH, Stevens TJ, Ferrante RJ, Bird ED, Richardson EJ. Neuropathological classification of Huntington's disease. *J Neuropathol Exp Neurol.* 1985;44:559-577.
22. Rajkowska G, Goldman-Rakic PS. Cytoarchitectonic definition of prefrontal areas in the normal human cortex, I: quantitative criteria for distinguishing areas 9 and 46. *Cereb Cortex.* 1995;4:307-322.
23. Rajkowska G, Goldman-Rakic PS. Cytoarchitectonic definition of prefrontal areas in the normal human cortex, II: variability in locations of areas 9 and 46. *Cereb Cortex.* 1995;4:323-337.
24. Brodmann K. *Vergleichende localisationslehre Der Grosshirnrinde in ihren prinzipien dargestellt auf grund des Zellenbaues.* Leipzig, Germany: Barth; 1909.
25. Williams RW, Rakic P. Three-dimensional counting: an accurate and direct method to estimate numbers of cells in sectioned material. *J Comp Neurol.* 1988;278:344-352.
26. Lewis DA, Woo T-U, Miller JL, Soloway A. Schizophrenia and subclasses of local circuit neurons in the prefrontal cortex. *Schizophr Res.* 1997;24:38-39.
27. Miyakawa T, Sumiyoshi S, Deshimaru M, Suzuki T, Tomonari H, Yasuoka F, Tatetsu S. Electron microscopic study on schizophrenia. *Acta Neuropathol.* 1972;20:67-77.
28. Hof PR, Cox K, Morrison JH. Quantitative analysis of a vulnerable subset of pyramidal neurons in Alzheimer's disease, I: superior frontal and inferior temporal cortex. *J Comp Neurol.* 1990;301:44-54.
29. Schwartz ML, Goldman-Rakic PS. Callosal and intrahemispheric connectivity of the prefrontal association cortex in rhesus monkeys: relation between intraparietal and principal sulcal cortex. *J Comp Neurol.* 1984;226:403-420.
30. Selemon LD, Goldman-Rakic PS. Common cortical and subcortical target areas of the dorsolateral prefrontal and posterior parietal cortices in the rhesus monkey: evidence for a distributed neural network subserving spatially guided behavior. *J Neurosci.* 1988;8:4049-4068.
31. Rajkowska G, Kosmal A. Organization of cortical afferents to the frontal association cortex in the dog. *Acta Neurobiol (Warsz).* 1987;47:137-162.
32. Rajkowska G, Kosmal A. Intrinsic connections and cytoarchitectonic data of the frontal association cortex in the dog. *Acta Neurobiol (Warsz).* 1988;48:169-192.
33. Garey LJ, Ong WY, Kanani TSPM, Davis A, Hornstein C, Bauer M. Reduction in dendritic spine number in cortical pyramidal neurons in schizophrenia. *Soc Neurosci Abstr.* 1995;21:237.
34. Glantz LA, Lewis DA. Assessment of spine density on layer III pyramidal cells in the prefrontal cortex of schizophrenic subjects. *Soc Neurosci Abstr.* 1995;21:239.
35. Benes FM, McSparren J, Bird ED, SanGiovanni JP, Vincent SL. Deficits in small interneurons in prefrontal and cingulate cortices of schizophrenic and schizoaffective patients. *Arch Gen Psychiatry.* 1991;48:996-1001.

258

The Reduced Neuropil Hypothesis: A Circuit Based Model of Schizophrenia

Lynn D. Selemon and Patricia S. Goldman-Rakic

In recent years, quantitative studies of the neuropathology of schizophrenia have reignited interest in the cerebral cortex and focused attention on the cellular and subcellular constituents that may be altered in this disease. Findings have ranged from compromised circuitry in prefrontal areas to outright neuronal loss in temporal and cingulate cortices. Herein, we propose that a reduction in interneuronal neuropil in the prefrontal cortex is a prominent feature of cortical pathology in schizophrenia and review the growing evidence for this view from reports of altered neuronal density and immunohistochemical markers in various cortical regions. The emerging picture of neuropathology in schizophrenia is one of subtle changes in cellular architecture and brain circuitry that nonetheless have a devastating impact on cortical function. Biol Psychiatry 1999;45:17–25 © 1999 Society of Biological Psychiatry

Key Words: Human, postmortem, frontal, cerebral cortex, neuropathology, morphometry

Introduction

Schizophrenia is a disease in which morphologic abnormalities have proven to be both subtle and elusive. Indeed, the most notable observation is the normal appearance of the schizophrenic brain, accounting in large part for the skepticism that reigned throughout most of this century concerning a structural basis for the disorder (Plum 1972). Over the past 2 decades, quantitative approaches in neuroanatomy have opened a new era in the study of neuropathology in schizophrenia (Weinberger and Wyatt 1982; Roberts and Crow 1987; Andreasen 1988; Benes 1988). Volumetric measurements on computerized tomography (CT) and magnetic resonance imaging (MRI) scans have provided convincing evidence that the ventricular spaces are enlarged and the cerebral cortex is

smaller than normal in brains from schizophrenic patients (Weinberger et al 1983; Cannon and Marco 1994). Cell counting and planimetric analysis on postmortem specimens have revealed regions of cell loss and volumetric decrease in the cortex, findings which are not at all obvious from visual inspection in the light microscope (Benes 1993; Bogerts 1993; Shapiro 1993; Heckers 1997; Dwork 1997). In the past few years, morphometric findings in the dorsolateral prefrontal cortex have uncovered a form of cortical pathology in schizophrenia in which impoverished neuronal connectivity appears to be a sufficient substrate for cognitive dysfunction (Selemon et al 1995, 1998; Rajkowska et al 1998). In this article, we review the evidence for the reduced neuropil hypothesis (Selemon et al 1995) and speculate on how this hypothesis may be integrated with reports of cell loss in the temporal and cingulate cortices and with newer findings of subcellular pathology in the prefrontal cortex. This article focuses mainly on studies that have used quantitative measures of anatomic parameters and therefore does not review reports of altered cortical cytoarchitecture or other qualitative observations. Consideration of etiologic mechanisms, i.e., whether the pathology arises from degenerative processes or developmental perturbations, is also beyond the scope of this discussion (for reviews of this subject, see Weinberger 1987; Benes 1993; Chua and Murray 1996; Harrison 1997).

The Reduced Neuropil Hypothesis: Compromised Circuitry with Preservation of Cell Number

Recent morphometric analyses of the dorsolateral prefrontal cortex in brains from schizophrenic patients have revealed a profile of increased neuronal density in the prefrontal and occipital cortices in schizophrenic brains relative to normal control brains (Selemon et al 1995; 1998). With a direct, 3-dimensional counting method (Williams and Rakic 1988), studies in our laboratory revealed that neuronal density in prefrontal area 9 is 17% higher than normal in brains from schizophrenic patients and 10% higher in primary visual cortical area 17 (Selemon et al 1995). More recently, we extended this

From the Section of Neurobiology, Yale University School of Medicine, New Haven, CT.

Address requests for reprints to Lynn D. Selemon, PhD, Section of Neurobiology, Yale University School of Medicine, 333 Cedar Street, Rm. C-303 SHM, New Haven, CT 06510.

Received May 12, 1998; revised August 24, 1998; accepted August 26, 1998.

0006-3223/99/$19.00
PII S0006-3223(98)00281-9

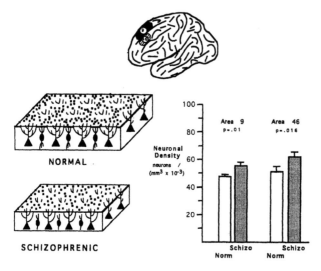

Figure 1. *Top center*: The approximate locations of prefrontal areas 9 (magnocellular) and 46 are shown on a lateral view of the human brain. *Lower right*: Neuronal density is elevated in areas 9 and 46 by 17% and 21%, respectively (Selemon et al 1995; 1998). *Lower left*: This schematic diagram illustrates the "reduced neuropil hypothesis," i.e., the schizophrenic cortex contains the same number of neurons as the normal cortex; reduced cortical volume is due to a decrease in interneuronal neuropil, dendritic trees, and cortical afferents (stippling on top of boxes). Some sizes are smaller as well (Rajkowska et al 1998).

observation to prefrontal area 46 where a 21% elevation in neuronal density was found in a new cohort of schizophrenic brains (Selemon et al 1998). At first glance, these findings seem paradoxical in light of the fact that most neurologic diseases, e.g., Alzheimer's and Huntington's, are associated with cell loss. However, measurement of neuronal density is not in itself informative regarding cell number. While increased neuronal density could be a reflection of an actual increase in the number of neurons, elevation in neuronal density could also be consistent with unaltered cell number if cortical volume were reduced, or with cell loss if the reduction in cortical volume were greatly in excess of the reduction in cell number. In light of the evidence for volumetric reduction of the schizophrenic cortex in the range of 3 to 13% (Brown et al 1986; Pakkenberg 1987, 1993; Zipursky et al 1992; Andreasen et al 1994b; Ward et al 1996; Sullivan et al 1996; Lim et al 1996), increased neuronal density in the cortex seems most consistent with a model in which the distance between neurons is diminished while the number of neurons is not changed (Figure 1). Given that the interneuronal space contains the neuronal processes and synaptic contacts between neurons, we hypothesized that the disturbances in prefrontal cognitive functioning in schizophrenia may be mediated by a process which involves atrophy of neuronal processes but stops short of actual neuronal loss, i.e., the reduced neuropil hypothesis (Selemon et al 1995).

The reduced neuropil hypothesis is supported by other quantitative studies of neuronal density in Nissl-stained sections of brains from schizophrenic patients. For exam-

ple, Benes et al (1991) reported an increase in pyramidal cell density in layer V in area 10. In a major study of Danish brains, Pakkenberg (1993) found increased neuronal density in conjunction with volumetric decreases throughout the cortex in brains from schizophrenic patients. This study is also notable for generating the only estimate of total cell number in schizophrenic cortex based on data from serial sections of the entire cortical mantle. The study revealed that the schizophrenic brain has the same number of cortical neurons as a normal brain. These and other findings to be discussed in this article lend support to the premise that neuronal loss is not an obligatory finding in the pathology of the schizophrenic cortex. To date, increased neuronal density coupled with decreased volume has been found in two regions of the dorsolateral prefrontal cortex (Selemon et al 1995; 1998) that have been widely implicated in the cognitive dysfunction in schizophrenia (Goldman-Rakic 1991; Goldman-Rakic and Selemon 1997). However, similar findings in the visual cortex (Selemon et al 1995), and in the cortical mantle as a whole (Pakkenberg 1993), suggest that the reduced neuropil form of pathology (i.e., without concomitant cell loss) may be characteristic of widespread regions of the schizophrenic cortex.

A deficit in neuronal connections as the structural correlate of schizophrenia is not a new concept. Feinberg (1982), for one, has speculated that an abnormality in synaptic pruning during adolescence might be causally related to the pathophysiology of schizophrenia. Others have postulated that the connections linking the frontal

BIOL PSYCHIATRY   19
1999;45:17-25

and temporal lobes might be disrupted or dysfunctional in schizophrenia (Weinberger et al 1992; Friston and Frith 1995; Andreasen et al 1997). A slightly different model of alteration in circuitry, one that involves rearrangement of connections, has been proposed based on findings which suggest that dopaminergic contacts have shifted from pyramidal to nonpyramidal neurons perhaps to compensate the loss of nonpyramidal targets (Benes 1997; Benes et al 1995). Although the concept of altered circuitry in schizophrenia is not new, direct evidence has been lacking. The morphometric findings described above have now provided the empirical evidence for a reduction of neuronal connections and reignited interest in circuitry-based models of neuropathology in the disease.

Further Evidence for Increased Neuronal Density: Analysis of Immunocytochemically Defined Populations of Neurons

The reduced neuropil hypothesis leads to the expectation that the density of immunocytochemically identified subsets of neurons in any given area would parallel the increases in density of the pooled population as a whole. In accord with this expectation, the calretinin-binding neurons in schizophrenic prefrontal cortex show a 9 to 19% increase in density while calbindin-reactive neurons increase by 50 to 70% (Daviss and Lewis 1995). The elevation in density of calretinin-positive cells is remarkably similar in magnitude to the increase in neuronal density measured in Nissl-stained sections (Selemon et al 1995; 1998); the increase in density of calbindin-reactive neurons, which greatly exceeds the overall increase in cell packing density, may in part be due to upregulation of expression of the protein in these cells. Increased density of nicotinamide-adenine dinucleotide phosphate-diaphorase (NADPH-d) containing (Akbarian et al 1993) and microtubule associated protein-2 (MAP-2) immunoreactive neurons (Anderson et al 1996) has been described in the white matter underlying area 9 in schizophrenic subjects as well. Akbarian et al (1995) found *diminished* density of glutamic acid decarboxylase (GAD)-positive neurons in area 9, but analysis of adjacent Nissl-stained sections failed to reveal any alteration in overall cell number. Therefore, consistent with the reduced neuropil hypothesis, the authors interpreted their findings as evidence of a downregulation of GAD expression without any change in overall neuronal number. Woo et al (1997) reported that densities of parvalbumin-reactive neurons in the dorsolateral prefrontal cortex in schizophrenic and control brains are not significantly different whereas an independent study of a more anterior region, the frontopolar cortex, indicated that parvalbumin-positive neurons are decreased in density in schizophrenic patients (Beasley

and Reynolds 1997). However, neither study provided measures of neuronal density of the unlabeled cell populations so these findings are difficult to interpret with respect to the reduced neuropil hypothesis. Overall, studies of chemically defined neurons in dorsolateral prefrontal areas are consistent with previous findings of increased neuronal density in the general population of cortical neurons as defined by Nissl staining. Reports of unaltered or decreased density of immunoreactive neurons either have been attributed to decreased expression of antigen or are indeterminate with respect to this issue.

Further Evidence for Neuronal Preservation in Schizophrenic Cortex: Comparison with a Neurodegenerative Disorder

It is instructive to compare the neuropathologic findings in schizophrenia with Huntington's disease (HD), a classic example of a neurodegenerative disorder. As mentioned, gross pathologic lesions like those present in brains from HD patients are not apparent in the schizophrenic brain as a whole, and the schizophrenic cortex is indistinguishable from that of a normal brain as well. Cortical thickness is severely reduced in HD, particularly in the infragranular layers, but only slight thinning of the cortical mantle is observed in schizophrenia (Selemon and Rajkowska 1997; Selemon et al 1995; 1998). The HD brain also exhibits pronounced reactive gliosis, a hallmark of neuronal degeneration, throughout the cortical mantle (Selemon and Rajkowska 1997). In schizophrenic cortex, on the other hand, increases in glial density are roughly commensurate with the increase in neuronal cell packing and therefore not suggestive of cell loss (Selemon et al 1995; 1998). In comparison to HD, the cytologic abnormalities observed in schizophrenia are much less pronounced and provide no overt signal that cell loss has occurred. Finally, there is a reduction in mean neuronal somal size in both diseases; however, the decrease observed in the schizophrenic cortex appears to represent a selective reduction in cell size for large neurons whereas in HD, the decrease in somal size directly reflects the loss of a population of large neurons in the HD cortex resulting in a greater proportion of small neurons contributing to the mean (Rajkowska et al 1998).

Further Evidence for Reduced Neuropil: Studies of Cellular Integrity and Synaptic Markers

A large component of the neuropil is comprised of the dendritic processes of cortical neurons and/or presynaptic terminal input onto cortical neurons. One expectation from the reduced neuropil hypothesis is that these processes would be reduced. A recent study of cell size in prefrontal area 9 provides indirect support for this hypothesis as neurons, particularly large pyramidal neurons, were found to have reduced somal sizes in the schizophrenic cortex (Rajkowska et al 1998). Since somal size generally correlates with the extent and complexity of dendritic arborization, this reduction suggests that pyramidal cells undergo atrophic changes in the schizophrenic cortex that may impair intercellular communication. Analyses of cell size in the prefrontal and cingulate cortices in previous studies failed to observe a reduction in somal size in the schizophrenic cohort. However, these studies were based on much smaller samples and were performed in thin sections where measurement of the soma at maximal diameter cannot be assured (Benes et al 1992; 1996). Pettegrew et al (1991) reported a shift in phospholipid metabolism in the dorsolateral prefrontal cortex of schizophrenic patients that is consistent with membrane degradation and a decrease in neuropil. Recent magnetic resonance spectroscopy of N-acetyl aspartate (NAA) in the frontal and temporal lobes indicates that this marker of neuronal viability is reduced in both cortices in schizophrenic patients (Bertolino et al 1996; 1998). However, the finding of decreased NAA levels does not distinguish between neuronal loss and reduction of neuropil since the metabolite is concentrated throughout all portions of the neuron, processes as well as cell bodies. The reported reduction in spine density on pyramidal cells in layer III in prefrontal cortex and widespread areas of the cerebral mantle adds further weight to the hypothesis that synaptic contacts, particularly onto pyramidal cells, are relatively impoverished in the cortex (Glantz and Lewis 1995; Garey et al 1995). Indeed, immunocytochemical staining with GAT-1, a gamma-aminobutyric acid (GABA) membrane transporter, revealed a 40% decrease in the specialized "cartridge" terminals of chandelier interneurons onto pyramidal cells in the prefrontal cortex (Woo et al 1998). In addition, a reduction in synaptophysin staining, a more general marker for synaptic terminals, has been reported in prefrontal cortex (Glantz and Lewis 1997). Decreases in synaptophysin mRNA but not immunoreactivity has also been found in medial temporal cortices (Eastwood et al 1995). These studies support the concept that presynaptic elements, i.e., cortical terminal fields, are smaller than normal in the schizophrenic brain. One explanation for the dissociation between mRNA and protein concentrations in the temporal lobe is that the reduction in synaptophysin mRNA is indicative of a decrease in distant terminals of neurons located within the temporal cortex (Eastwood et al 1995). Thus, the evidence for depletion of presynaptic terminal fields in the cortex, as well as atrophic changes in cell soma, dendritic membranes, and synaptic spines, are all consistent with the reduced neuropil hypothesis. It

should be kept in mind, however, that immunocytochem ical evidence for alterations in synaptic markers, as fo changes in cell number, could represent altered expression of the antigen.

There is still much work to be done in determining th precise nature of the alteration in neuropil. For example ultrastructural analysis would provide more direct evi dence for loss of synaptic contacts and would be highl informative in terms of laminar and cellular localization o the anatomic deficit in schizophrenia. However, becaus EM studies in human postmortem tissue are at the limit o technical feasibility due to the short postmortem interval necessary for adequate tissue preservation, only one EM study of the synaptic contacts in the schizophrenic brai has been reported. This analysis, which was confined t the neostriatum, determined that dendritic spines wer smaller in the schizophrenic sample (Roberts et al 1996) Alternatively, other anatomic approaches including stan dard Golgi impregnation and Golgi-like staining of iden tified neurons would be useful in determining whic morphologic cell types undergo dendritic changes i schizophrenia. In addition, molecular and biochemica analysis of pre- and postsynaptic markers in cortex coul distinguish which cellular components in these compart ments contribute to the reduction in cortical neuropil.

Consideration of the Cortical Connections a Risk in Schizophrenia

The proposed deficiency in prefrontal cortical circuitr could involve local, modulatory, or long tract connections At least one source of prefrontal afferent input, that from the thalamus, may be reduced in the schizophrenic brain a reductions in number of medial dorsal thalamic neurons volume and metabolic activity of the thalamus, and vol ume of thalamocortical afferent fiber bundles have bee reported in schizophrenic brains (Pakkenberg 1990; An dreasen et al 1994a; Buchsbaum et al 1996). Moreover thalamic volume has been correlated with enlargement o the lateral ventricles and expression of positive symptom in schizophrenic patients (Portas et al 1998). However, i seems unlikely that a deficit in the thalamocortical inpu alone can account for the reduction in neuropil, which i not restricted to the laminae (IIIc and IV) which receiv thalamic input, but spans many layers of cortex. Prelimi nary data from immunocytochemical studies suggest tha there may be a diminished complement of dopaminergi or GABAergic terminal fields in the prefrontal corte (Akil and Lewis 1996; Lewis et al 1997; Woo et al 1998) however, further studies are needed to verify whethe these findings represent actual terminal loss or, instead downregulation of neurotransmitters or enzymes. Th largest compliment of cortical synapses belong to the clas of local connections between glutaminergic pyramidal cells. While these connections are less easily studied with the methodologies presently available, experimental production of hypoglutaminergic states by administration of glutamate receptor antagonists has been shown to replicate psychotic features of schizophrenia (Krystal et al 1994) and to reproduce some of the anatomic deficits as well (Farber et al 1995) leading to a glutamate hypothesis for the disease (Javitt and Zukin 1991; Olney and Farber 1995). Indeed, given the associative nature of the cognitive deficit, it seems highly likely that cortico-cortical connections are compromised in schizophrenia.

Over the past decade, Crow et al (1989; 1990; 1997a,b) hypothesized that schizophrenia is a manifestation of disturbance in the processes that lead to normal brain asymmetry and lateralization of language capacity in the human. It is certainly possible that reduction of neuropil reflects a loss of interhemispheric cortico-cortical connections. In this manner, selective loss of neuropil in the normally larger left temporal lobe might account for an absence of the normal volumetric asymmetry. However, presently there are no studies which have addressed the question of selective reduction of neuropil in one hemisphere. Indeed, most studies including our own have purposely been confined to one hemisphere, usually the left, to avoid the confounding effects of hemispheric specialization and asymmetry in the human brain.

Is Cell Loss Present in the Schizophrenic Cortex? A Critical Examination of the Evidence for Reduction in Neuronal Number

The reduced neuropil hypothesis represents a departure from the currently dominant view of the schizophrenic cortex in which the major neuropathologic disturbance is depletion of cell populations whether due to degenerative processes or to developmental failure to generate them (e.g., Weinberger 1987; Benes et al 1991; Benes 1993; Chua and Murray 1996). This model of cortical pathology in schizophrenia is based on seminal quantitative studies showing reductions in density or in cell number of neuronal populations in the schizophrenic cortex (Falkai and Bogerts 1986; Jeste and Lohr 1989; Benes et al 1986; 1991). The most extensive evidence for cell loss comes from studies of the anterior cingulate cortex and, to a lesser degree, of the frontopolar cortex (area 10). These studies have shown a reduction in the density of small interneurons, particularly those of layer II, suggesting that schizophrenia is associated with a loss of GABA containing neurons (Benes et al 1986; 1991; Benes 1993). Evidence of increased GABA$_A$ receptor binding in the cingulate (Benes et al 1992) and frontopolar cortices in

schizophrenic brains supports this hypothesis (Benes et al 1996). A decrease in density of parvalbumin-containing neurons in area 10 is also supportive (Beasley and Reynolds 1997). However, comparable decreases in this neuronal population have not been uncovered in dorsolateral prefrontal cortex (Woo et al 1997). Additionally, Rajkowska et al (1998), in an analysis of neurons classified by size, actually found increases in the density of smaller sized neurons, which undoubtedly include the majority of interneurons.

In the temporal lobe, results have been inconsistent as well. Some studies reported reductions in neuronal density in the entorhinal cortex, hippocampus, and superior temporal cortex (Falkai and Bogerts 1986; Jeste and Lohr 1989; Hollinger et al 1995; 1997; Benes et al 1998) but as many studies failed to detect differences in cell density (Kovelman and Scheibel 1984; Heckers et al 1991; Arnold et al 1995; Krimer et al 1997) and a recent study of hippocampus reported an increase in neuronal density in this medial temporal lobe structure (Zaidel et al 1997).

Definitive evidence for cell loss in a given structure can only be provided by measurement of total cell number, as this parameter is not affected by tissue shrinkage (Braendgaard and Gundersen 1986; Williams and Rakic 1988; West 1993). Only a few studies examined total cell number in cerebral cortical areas, as this requires that the area under examination have clearly defined boundaries. Falkai and Bogerts (1986) examined total cell number in the entorhinal cortex, where the borders with surrounding cytoarchitectonic areas are clear-cut. The number of neurons in the entorhinal cortex was found to be diminished in the schizophrenic group relative to the control groups. A more recent analysis found only a trend decrease in total cell number in two subareas of the entorhinal cortex (Krimer et al 1997) and Heckers et al (1991) found no difference in total cell number in the hippocampus of schizophrenic and control subjects. Likewise, Pakkenberg's (1993) analysis of total cell number in the temporal lobe, as well as the cortex as a whole, revealed comparable numbers of neurons in brains from schizophrenic patients and control subjects. Analogous studies of total cell number are not available for the cingulate and dorsolateral cortices. Thus, cell loss is not present or detectable in many areas of the cortex and may be regionally specific. If present at all in prefrontal areas, for example, it is minimal.

Regional heterogeneity in the pathology of schizophrenia could possibly explain evidence from neuroimaging studies of a dissociation of prefrontal, cingulate, and temporal cortical activation that is related both to cognitive performance and various symptom clusters in schizophrenia (Friston and Frith 1995; Fletcher et al 1996; Liddle et al 1992; Weinberger et al 1992). Weinberger et al

(1992) has shown that failure to activate prefrontal cortex during the Wisconsin Card Sort Task (WCST) is associated with greater hippocampal pathology. Fletcher et al (1996) have shown that schizophrenic patients do not show the normal pattern of cingulate activation and temporal deactivation on a verbal fluency task, suggesting a disturbance of the normal frontal-temporal balance in the task. More recently, Andreasen et al (1997) found reduced blood flow in a cortical circuit including the prefrontal, inferior temporal, and parietal cortices in a group of neuroleptic-naive schizophrenic patients at rest, while other cortical and subcortical areas, such as the retrosplenial cingulate cortex, thalamus, and cerebellum, exhibited enhanced blood flow. The association between deficits in prefrontal white matter and reductions in hippocampal-amygdala volumes also supports the concept that limbic-frontal connections may be altered in schizophrenia (Breier et al 1994). Despite the growing evidence for disruption of widespread cortical networks as a principal component of pathology in schizophrenia, the concept has yet to be explained on a neurobiologic basis. Dissociation of cortical activity could arise from structural pathology in the output neurons of the prefrontal cortex or in the dendritic arbors of their limbic targets, or the converse, or both. For any of a number of possible neuropathologic scenarios, the end result would be an impairment in transmission within long-tract cortico-cortical circuits. Deficient circuitry could also lie in the local intrinsic connections within these areas, compatible with both the reduced neuropil hypothesis as well as the hypothesis of interneuron loss in limbic regions. Further studies in which frontal, temporal, and cingulate cortices are examined in the same cohort of brains with the same methods are needed to determine whether cell loss and neuropil reduction coexist in the schizophrenic cortex and represent regional heterogeneity of the pathology, or if instead, there is a unitary pathologic process in the schizophrenic brain. The reduced neuropil hypothesis does not exclude cell loss in the cortex; it emphasizes only that neuron loss is not a prominent feature of the neuropathology of schizophrenia.

Functional Implications of the Reduced Neuropil Hypothesis

One question that arises is whether the debilitating symptoms of schizophrenia can result from subtle changes in neuropil without cell degeneration. In this regard, recent anatomic and physiologic findings from nonhuman primates indicate that even small changes in neural circuitry have serious functional consequences. The cerebral cortex is comprised of neurons in local circuits that are essential for, among other functions, sensory gating (Braff 1993), ideation or working memory (Goldman-Rakic 1995), and

willed action (Frith et al, 1991), all functions which are highly relevant to the cognitive deficits associated with schizophrenia. In the prefrontal cortex, neurons are engaged in "on-line" processing of information critical to spatial mnemonic functioning: each prefrontal neuron is tuned for a particular spatial location, and its activation in response to a stimulus in its receptive field is modulated by dopamine through action at dopamine receptors (Williams and Goldman-Rakic 1995). Indeed, it has been shown that small changes in the level of dopamine D1 receptor stimulation in the dorsolateral prefrontal cortex can alter a neuron's spatial tuning and responsivity to its extrinsic input (Williams and Goldman-Rakic 1995) as well as an animal's ability to perform accurately on working memory tasks (Arnsten et al 1994). Anatomic evidence suggests that the spines and distal dendrites of pyramidal neurons are a key locus for dopamine modulation (Smiley et al 1994). Dysregulation of dopamine receptors has been observed in the prefrontal cortex in schizophrenia (Sedvall and Farde 1996; Okubo et al 1997; Joyce and Meador-Woodruff 1997). Thus, even a small alteration in the dendritic arbor, particularly at its vulnerable distal portions, would be detrimental to a prefrontal neuron's encoding of a sensory event, maintenance of sustained discharges in the absence of the stimulus, or return of activity to baseline when an action is initiated. Any or all of these component processes are presumably critical for the continuity of the thought process and each could be detuned by slight neural compromise. Similar deficits in other neurotransmitter receptors in this and other cortical areas and other deficits in neurotransmission and signaling can also be imagined. Thus, subtle changes in morphology could have profound functional consequences, particularly for those psychological functions which are impaired in schizophrenia.

Summary

Taken together, recent findings indicate that cell loss is not an obligatory feature of the pathologic process in the schizophrenic cortex. Although neuronal loss may be present in circumscribed regions of the cortex, it need not be the pathologic substrate for dysfunction in dorsolateral prefrontal areas that have been implicated in memory and cognitive dysfunction in schizophrenia or in the cortex as a whole. In these regions, the schizophrenic cortex may be characterized as essentially normal, i.e., having normal numbers of neurons and normal patterns of connectivity, except lacking the exuberance and redundancy of connections that enable the normal brain to function at full capacity.

The pathologic process in schizophrenia is not that of a classical neurodegenerative disease. Even those studies

BIOL PSYCHIATRY 23
1999;45:17-25

which report cell loss, do not find evidence of overwhelming degenerative changes in cortex. Thus, there is a growing consensus in the literature that a subtle pathology characterizes the cortex in schizophrenia. In the dorsolateral prefrontal cortex, and perhaps in more widespread areas, this pathology involves compromised cell structure, impoverishment of neuronal connectivity, and presumed loss of functional communication between neurons. Sparing of the vast majority of neurons offers a ray of hope for revival of normal cell function in the psychoses. If cortical neurons are preserved in schizophrenia, then there is a possibility, however remote, that treatments can be developed for remodeling neuronal processes given the growing evidence for plasticity of neurons in the adult mammalian brain. While this prospect is currently out of reach, detailed knowledge of cortical pathology in cells and circuits, however subtle these changes may be, is a critical step on the path to understanding the causes and course of schizophrenia.

This work was supported by grant 44866 from the Center for Neuroscience of Mental Disorders, National Institute of Mental Health, Rockville, MD.

References

Akbarian S, Bunney, WE Jr, Potkin SG, et al (1993): Altered distribution of nicotinamide-adenine dinucleotide phosphate-diaphorase cells in frontal lobe of schizophrenic implies disturbances of cortical development. *Arch Gen Psychiatry* 50:169–177.

Akbarian S, Kim JJ, Potkin SG, et al (1995): Gene expression for glutamic acid decarboxylase is reduced without loss of neurons in the prefrontal cortex of schizophrenics. *Arch Gen Psychiatry* 52:258–266.

Akil M, Lewis DA (1996): Reduced dopaminergic innervation of the prefrontal cortex in schizophrenia. *Soc Neurosci Abst* 22:1679.

Anderson SA, Volk DA, Lewis DA (1996): Increased density of microtubule associated protein 2-immunoreactive neurons in the prefrontal white matter of schizophrenic subjects. *Schizophr Res* 19:111–119.

Andreasen NC (1988): Brain imaging: Applications in psychiatry. *Science* 239:1381–1388.

Andreasen NC, Arndt S, Swayze V II, et al (1994a): Thalamic abnormalities in schizophrenia visualized through magnetic resonance imaging. *Science* 266:294–298.

Andreasen NC, Flashman L, Flaum M, et al (1994b): Regional brain abnormalities in schizophrenia measure with magnetic resonance imaging. *JAMA* 272:1763–1769.

Andreasen NC, O'Leary DS, Flaum M, et al (1997): Hypofrontality in schizophrenia: Distributed dysfunctional circuits in neuroleptic naive patients. *Lancet* 349:1730–1734.

Arnold SE, Franz BR, Gur RC, et al (1995): Smaller neuron size in schizophrenia in hippocampal subfields that mediate cortical-hippocampal interactions. *Am J Psychiatry* 152:738–748.

Arnsten AFT, Cai JX, Murphy BL, Goldman-Rakic, PS (1994): Dopamine D1 receptor mechanisms in the cognitive performance of young adult and aged monkeys. *Psychopharmacology* 116:143–151.

Beasley CL, Reynolds GP (1997): Parvalbumin-immunoreactive neurons are reduced in the prefrontal cortex of schizophrenics. *Schizophr Res* 24:349–355.

Benes FM (1997): The role of stress and dopamine-GABA interactions in the vulnerability for schizophrenia. *J Psychiat Res* 31:257–275.

Benes FM (1993): Neurobiological investigations in cingulate cortex of schizophrenic brain. *Schizophr Res.* 19:537–549.

Benes FM, Davison J, Bird ED (1986): Quantitative cytoarchitectural studies of the cerebral cortex of schizophrenics. *Arch Gen Psychiatry* 43:31–35.

Benes FM, Kwok EW, Vincent SL, Todtenkopf MS (1998): A reduction of nonpyramidal cells in schizophrenics and manic depressives. *Biol Psychiatry* 44:88–97

Benes FM, McSparren J, Bird ED, SanGiovanni JP, Vincent SL (1991): Deficits in small interneurons in prefrontal and cingulate cortices of schizophrenic and schizoaffective patients. *Arch Gen Psychiatry* 48:996–1001.

Benes FM (1998) Post-mortem structural analyses of schizophrenic brain. Study designs and the interpretation of data. *Psychiatric Developments* 6:213–226.

Benes FM, Todtenkopf MS, Taylor JB (1995): A shift in tyrosine hydroxlase-immunoreactive varicosities (TH-IRv) from pyramidal (PN) to nonpyramidal (NP) neurons occurs in layer II of the anterior cingulate cortex of schizophrenics. *Soc Neurosci Abst* 21:259.

Benes FM, Vincent SL, Marie A, Khan Y (1996): Up-regulation of $GABA_A$ receptor binding on neurons of the prefrontal cortex in schizophrenic subjects. *Neuroscience* 75:1021–1031.

Benes FM, Vincent SL, Alsterberg G, Bird ED, SanGiovanni JP (1992): Increased $GABA_A$ receptor binding in superficial layers of cingulate cortex in schizophrenics. *J Neurosci* 12:924–929.

Bertolino A, Callicott JH, Elman I, et al (1997): Regionally specific neuronal pathology in untreated patients with schizophrenia: A proton magnetic resonance spectroscopic study. *Biol Psychiatry* 43:641–648.

Bertolino A, Nawroz S, Mattay VS, et al (1996): Regionally specific pattern of neurochemical pathology in schizophrenia as assessed by multislice proton magnetic resonance spectroscopic imaging. *Am J Psychiatry* 153:1554–1563.

Bogerts B (1993): Recent advances in the neuropathology of schizophrenia. *Schizophr Bull* 19:431–445.

Braendgaard H, Gundersen HJG (1986): The impact of recent stereological advances on quantitative studies of the nervous system. *J Neurosci Meth* 18:39–78.

Braff DL (1993): Information processing and attention dysfunctions in schizophrenia. *Schizophr Bull* 19:233–259.

Breier A, Buchanan W, Elkashef A, Munson RC, Kirkpatrick B, Gellard F (1994): Brain morphology and schizophrenia. A magnetic resonance imaging study of limbic, prefrontal cortex, and caudate structures. *Arch Gen Psychiatry* 49:921–926.

Brown R, Colter N, Corsellis JAN, et al (1986): Postmortem evidence of structural brain changes in schizophrenia: Differences in brain weight, temporal horn area, and parahippocampal gyrus compared with affective disorder. *Arch Gen Psychiatry* 43:36–42.

Buchsbaum MS, Someya T, Teng CY, et al (1996): PET and MRI of thalamus in never-medicated patients with schizophrenia. *Am J Psychiatry* 153:191–199.

Cannon TD, Marco E (1994): Structural brain abnormalities as indicators of vulnerability to schizophrenia. *Schizophr Bull* 20:89–101.

Chua SE, Murray RM (1996): The neurodevelopmental theory of schizophrenia: Evidence concerning structure and neurophysiology. *Ann Med* 28:547–555.

Crow TJ (1997a): Is schizophrenia the price that homo sapiens pays for language? *Schizophr Res* 28:127–141.

Crow TJ (1997B): Schizophrenia as a failure of hemispheric dominance for language. *Trend Neurosci* 20:339–343.

Crow TJ (1990): Temporal lobe asymmetries as the key to the etiology of schizophrenia. *Schizophr Bull* 16:433–443.

Crow TJ, Ball J, Bloom SR, et al (1989): Schizophrenia as an anomaly of development of cerebral asymmetry. A postmortem study and a proposal concerning the genetic basis of the disease. *Arch Gen Psychiatry.* 46:1145–1150.

Daviss SR, Lewis DA (1995): Local circuit neurons of the prefrontal cortex in schizophrenia: Selective increase in the density of calbindin-immunoreactive neurons. *Psychiatry Res* 59:81–96.

Dwork AJ (1997): Postmortem studies of the hippocampal formation in schizophrenia. *Schizophr Bull* 23:385–402.

Eastwood SL, Burnet PWJ, Harrison PJ (1995): Altered synaptophysin expression as a marker of synaptic pathology in schizophrenia. *Neuroscience* 66:309–319.

Falkai P, Bogerts B (1986): Cell loss in the hippocampus of schizophrenics. *Eur Arch Psychiatry Neurol Sci* 236:154–161.

Farber NB, Wozniak DF, Price MT, et al (1995): Age-specific neurotoxicity in the rat associated with NMDA receptor blockade: Potential relevance to schizophrenia? *Soc Biol Psychiatry* 38:788–796.

Feinberg I (1982): Schizophrenia: Caused by a fault in programmed synaptic elimination during adolescence? *J Psychiat Res* 17:319–330.

Fletcher PC, Frith CD, Grasby PM, Friston KJ, Dolan RJ (1996): Local and distributed effects of apomorphine on frontotemporal function in acute unmedicated schizophrenia. *J Neurosci* 16:7055–7062.

Friston KJ, Frith CD (1995): Schizophrenia: A disconnection syndrome? *Clin Neurosci* 3:89–97.

Frith CD, Friston KJ, Liddle PF, Frackowiak RS (1991) Willed action and the prefrontal cortex in man. Proc R Sec Lend (B) 244:241–246.

Garey LJ, Ong WY, Patel TS, et al (1995): Reduction in dendritic spine number on cortical pyramidal neurons in schizophrenia. *Soc Neurosci Abst* 21:237.

Glantz LA, Lewis DA (1997): Reduction of synaptophysin immunoreactivity in the prefrontal cortex of subjects with schizophrenia. *Arch Gen Psychiatry* 54:943–952.

Glantz LA, Lewis DA (1995): Assessment of spine density on layer III pyramidal cells in the prefrontal cortex of schizophrenic subjects. *Soc Neurosci Abst* 21:239.

Goldman-Rakic PS (1995): Cellular basis of working memory. *Neuron* 14:477–485.

Goldman-Rakic PS (1991): Prefrontal cortical dysfunction in schizophrenia: The relevance of working memory. In: Carroll BJ, Barrett JE, editors. *Psychopathology and the Brain.* New York: Raven Press, pp 1–23.

Goldman-Rakic PS, Selemon LD (1997): Functional and anatomical aspects of prefrontal pathology in schizophrenia. *Schizophr Bull.* 23:437–458.

Harrison PJ (1997): Schizophrenia: A disorder of neurodevelopment? *Current Opin Neurobiol* 7:285–289.

Heckers S (1997): Neuropathology of schizophrenia. *Schizophr Bull* 23:403–422.

Heckers S, Heinsen H, Geiger B, Beckmann H (1991): Hippocampal neuron number in schizophrenia. A stereological study. *Arch Gen Psychiatry* 48:1002–1008.

Hollinger DP, Mori C, Galaburda AM (1997): Schizophrenia: Neuronal measures in left and right language and visual cortices. *Soc Neurosci Abst* 23:2198.

Hollinger DP, Rosen GD, Galaburda AM (1995): Decreased neuronal density in supragranular layers of area TPT of the superior temporal gyrus of schizophrenics. *Soc Neurosci Abst.* 21:238.

Javitt DC, Zukin SR (1991): Recent advances in the phencyclidine model of schizophrenia. *Am J Psychiatry* 148:1301–1308.

Jeste DV, Lohr JB (1989): Hippocampal pathologic findings in schizophrenia: A morphometric study. *Arch Gen Psychiatry* 46:1019–1024.

Joyce JN, Meador-Woodruff JH (1997): Linking the family of D2 receptors to neuronal circuits in human brain: Insight into schizophrenia. *Neuropsychopharmacol.* 16:375–384.

Kovelman JA, Scheibel AB (1984): A neurohistological correlate of schizophrenia. *Biol Psychiatry* 19:1601–1621.

Krimer L, Herman MM, Saunders RC, et al (1997): A qualitative and quantitative analysis of the entorhinal cortex in schizophrenia. *Cereb Cortex* 7:732–739.

Krystal JH, Karper LP, Seibyl JP, et al (1994): Subanesthetic effects of the noncompetitive NMDA antagonist, ketamine, in humans: Psychotomimetic, perceptual, cognitive and neuroendocrine responses. *Arch Gen Psychiatry* 51:199–214.

Lewis DA, Woo T-U, Miller JL, Soloway AS (1997): Schizophrenia and subclasses of local circuit neurons in the prefrontal cortex. *Schizophr Res.* 24:38–39.

Liddle PF, Friston KJ, Frith CD, Hirsch SR, Jones T, Frackowiak RS (1992): Patterns of cerebral blood flow in schizophrenia. *Br J Psychiatry* 160:179–186.

Lim KO, Tew W, Kushner M, Chow K, Matsumoto B, DeLisi LE (1996): Cortical gray matter volume deficit in patients with first episode schizophrenia. *Am J Psychiatry* 153:1548–1553.

Okubo Y, Suhara T, Suzuki K, et al (1997): Decreased prefrontal D1 receptors in schizophrenia revealed by PET. *Nature* 385:634–635.

Olney JW, Farber NB (1995): Glutamate receptor dysfunction and schizophrenia. *Arch Gen Psychiatry* 52:998–1007.

Pakkenberg B (1993): Total nerve cell number in neocortex in chronic schizophrenic and controls estimated using optical disectors. *Biol Psychiatry* 34:768–772.

Pakkenberg P (1990): Pronounced reduction of total neuron number in mediodorsal thalamic nucleus and nucleus accumbens in schizophrenics. *Arch Gen Psychiatry* 47:1023–1028.

Pakkenberg B (1987): Post-mortem study of chronic schizophrenic brains. *Brit J Psychiatry* 151:744–752.

Pettegrew JW, Keshavan MS, Panchalingam K, et al (1991): Alterations in brain high-energy phosphate and membrane phospholipid metabolism in first-episode, drug-naive schizophrenics: A pilot study of the dorsal prefrontal cortex by in vivo phosphorus 31 nuclear magnetic resonance spectroscopy. *Arch Gen Psychiatry* 48:563–568.

Plum F (1972): Neuropathological findings. *Neurosci Res Prog Bull* 10:384–388.

Portas CM, Goldstein JM, Shenton ME, et al (1998): Volumetric evaluation of the thalamus in schizophrenic male patients using magnetic resonance imaging. *Biol Psychiatry* 43:649–659.

Rajkowska G, Selemon LD, Goldman-Rakic PS (1998): Neuronal and glial somal size in the prefrontal cortex: A postmortem study of schizophrenia and Huntington's disease. *Arch Gen Psychiatry* 55:215–224.

Roberts GW, Crow TJ (1987): The neuropathology of schizophrenia—A progress report. *Brit Med Bull* 43:599–615.

Roberts RC, Conley R, Kung L, Peretti FJ, Chute DJ (1996): Reduced striatal spine size in schizophrenia: A postmortem ultrastructural study. *Neuroreport* 7:1214–1218.

Sedvall G, Farde L (1996): Dopamine receptors in schizophrenia. *Lancet* 347:264.

Selemon LD, Rajkowska G (1997): Deep layer degeneration in prefrontal cortical area 46 in advanced-stage Huntington's diseased brains. *Soc Neurosci Abst* 23:1912.

Selemon LD, Rajkowska G, Goldman-Rakic PS (1998): Elevated neuronal density in prefrontal area 46 in brains from schizophrenic patients: Application of a 3-dimensional, stereologic counting method. *J Comp Neurol* 392:402–412.

Selemon LD, Rajkowska G, Goldman-Rakic PS (1995): Abnormally high neuronal density in the schizophrenic cortex: A morphometric analysis of prefrontal area 9 and occipital area 17. *Arch Gen Psychiatry* 52:805–818.

Shapiro RM (1993): Regional neuropathology in schizophrenia: Where are we? Where are we going? *Schizophr Res* 10:187–239.

Smiley JF, Levey AI, Ciliax BJ, Goldman-Rakic PS (1994): D1 dopamine receptor immunoreactivity in human and monkey cerebral cortex: Predominant and extrasynaptic localization in dendritic spines. *Proc Natl Acad Sci USA* 91:5720–5724.

Sullivan EV, Shear PK, Lim KO, Zipursky RB, Pfefferbaum A (1996): Cognitive and motor impairments are related to gray matter volume deficits in schizophrenia. *Biol Psychiatry* 39:234–240.

Ward KE, Friedman L, Wise A, Schulz SC (1996): Meta-analysis of brain and cranial size in schizophrenia. *Schizophr Res* 22:197–213.

Weinberger DR (1987): Implications for normal brain development for the pathogenesis of schizophrenia. *Arch Gen Psychiat* 44:660–669.

Weinberger DR, Berman KF, Suddath R, Torrey EF (1992): Evidence of dysfunction of a prefrontal-limbic network in schizophrenia: A magnetic resonance imaging and regional blood flow study of discordant monozygotic twins. *Am J Psychiatry* 149:890–897.

Weinberger DR, Wyatt RJ (1982): Brain morphology in schizophrenia: In vivo studies. In: Henn F, Nasrallah H, editors. *Schizophrenia as a Brain Disease.* Oxford: Oxford Univ Press, pp 148–175.

Weinberger DR, Wyatt RL, Wyatt RJ (1983): Neuropathological studies of schizophrenia: A selective review. *Schizophr Bull* 9:193–212.

West MJ (1993): New stereological methods for counting neurons. *Neurobiol Aging* 14:275–285.

Williams GV, Goldman-Rakic PS (1995): Modulation of memory fields by dopamine D1 receptors in prefrontal cortex. *Nature* 376:572–575.

Williams RW, Rakic P (1988): Three-dimensional counting: An accurate and direct method to estimate numbers of cells in sectioned material. *J Comp Neurol* 278:344–352.

Woo T-U, Miller JL, Lewis DA (1997): Schizophrenia and the parvalbumin-containing class of cortical local circuit neurons. *Am J Psychiatry* 154:1013–1015.

Woo T-U, Whitehead RE, Melchitzky DS, Lewis DA (1998): A subclass of prefrontal gamma-aminobutyric acid axon terminals are selectively altered in schizophrenia. *Proc Natl Acad Sci USA* 95:5341–5346.

Zaidel DW, Esiri MM, Harrison PJ (1997): The hippocampus in schizophrenia: Lateralized increase in neuronal density and altered cytoarchitectural asymmetry. *Psychol Med* 27:703–713.

Zipursky RB, Lim KO, Sullivan EV, Brown BW, Pfefferbaum A (1992): Widespread cerebral gray matter volume deficits in schizophrenia. *Arch Gen Psychiatry* 42:195–205.

The New England
Journal of Medicine

| Volume 322 | MARCH 22, 1990 | Number 12 |

ANATOMICAL ABNORMALITIES IN THE BRAINS OF MONOZYGOTIC TWINS DISCORDANT FOR SCHIZOPHRENIA

Richard L. Suddath, M.D., George W. Christison, M.D., E. Fuller Torrey, M.D.,
Manuel F. Casanova, M.D., and Daniel R. Weinberger, M.D.

Abstract Recent neuroradiologic and neuropathological studies indicate that at least some patients with schizophrenia have slightly enlarged cerebral ventricles and subtle anatomical abnormalities in the region of the anterior hippocampus. Using magnetic resonance imaging (MRI), we studied 15 sets of monozygotic twins who were discordant for schizophrenia (age range, 25 to 44 years; 8 male and 7 female pairs). For each pair of twins, T_1-weighted contiguous coronal sections (5 mm thick) were compared blindly, and quantitative measurements of brain structures were made with a computerized image-analysis system.

In 12 of the 15 discordant pairs, the twin with schizophrenia was identified by visual inspection of cerebrospinal fluid spaces. In two pairs no difference could be discerned visually, and in one the twin with schizophrenia was misidentified. Quantitative analysis of sections through the level of the pes hippocampi showed the

hippocampus to be smaller on the left in 14 of the 15 affected twins, as compared with their normal twins, and smaller on the right in 13 affected twins (both P<0.001). In the twins with schizophrenia, as compared with their normal twins, the lateral ventricles were larger on the left in 14 (P<0.003) and on the right in 13 (P<0.001). The third ventricle also was larger in 13 of the twins with schizophrenia (P<0.001). None of these differences were found in seven sets of monozygotic twins without schizophrenia who were studied similarly as controls.

We conclude that subtle abnormalities of cerebral anatomy (namely, small anterior hippocampi and enlarged lateral and third ventricles) are consistent neuropathologic features of schizophrenia and that their cause is at least in part not genetic. Further study is required to determine whether these changes are primary or secondary to the disease. (N Engl J Med 1990; 322: 789-94.)

D URING the first half of this century, numerous claims of pathologic findings in the brains of patients with schizophrenia were reported, but most of these findings turned out to be artifacts, the results of poorly controlled studies, or impossible to replicate.[1] During the past decade, studies using new imaging techniques, such as computerized tomography (CT) and magnetic resonance imaging (MRI), have repeatedly demonstrated that many patients with schizophrenia have slightly enlarged cerebral ventricles.[2-6] This finding, as well as slight reductions in size and subtle dysmorphic changes of medial temporal-lobe structures, has also been reported in recent controlled postmortem studies.[7-12]

Although these results implicate a neuropathologic process in at least some cases of schizophrenia, little is

known about the relation of this process to the pathogenesis of the illness. Data from both the in vivo and the postmortem studies are primarily quantitative (e.g., the area of the ventricles,[2,3,5-8] the volume of the hippocampus,[10] and the width of the parahippocampal gyrus[7,11] were measured) and describe overall comparisons between groups. Since the differences between patients and control subjects in any of these measurements are slight and there is considerable normal variation, the groups overlap to a large degree. As a result, it has been argued that the putative neuropathologic process affects only a small subgroup and is not characteristic of most patients with schizophrenia.

One way to reduce variation between patients and controls and to enhance the power of morphologic measurements to discriminate subtle neuropathologic deviations is to compare monozygotic twins discordant for schizophrenia. Since monozygotic twins share a common genome and similar socioeconomic, developmental, and psychological backgrounds, the degree to which these factors contribute to morphometric variance is greatly reduced. We report here the results of a study of the anatomy of the brain in schizophre-

From the Clinical Brain Disorders Branch (G.W.C., E.F.T., M.F.C., D.R.W.) and the Neuropsychiatry Branch (R.L.S.), Intramural Research Program, National Institute of Mental Health, Neuroscience Center at Saint Elizabeths, 2700 Martin Luther King, Jr., Ave., SE, Washington, DC 20032, where reprint requests should be addressed to Dr. Weinberger.

Supported in part by a grant (MH 41176) from the National Institute of Mental Health to the Friends Medical Science Research Center and by funds from the Theodore and Vada Stanley Foundation.

nia based on analysis of MRI scans of sets of monozygotic twins who were discordant for schizophrenia.

METHODS

Subjects

Sets of monozygotic twins from the United States and Canada were recruited as part of a multidimensional study of monozygotic twins discordant and concordant for schizophrenia. Zygosity was determined by physical similarity and by a likeness questionnaire[13] and confirmed by analysis of 19 red-cell antigens and, when necessary, by fingerprinting and HLA typing. We chose four years as the minimal length of discordance on the basis of low reported rates of conversion beyond four years.[14] The diagnosis in both the discordant and normal sets of twins was established according to criteria of the *Diagnostic and Statistical Manual*, third edition, revised, as assessed by Parts 1 and II of the structured clinical interview described by Spitzer et al.[15]

The study groups consisted of 15 sets of monozygotic twins discordant for schizophrenia (8 male and 7 female pairs) whose mean age (±SD) was 32.4±5.3 years (range, 25 to 44). The mean age at the onset of schizophrenia was 22.1±4.9 years (range, 14 to 31), and the mean duration of illness was 10.5±5.5 years (range, 4 to 24). In all cases the affected twin met the diagnostic criteria for schizophrenia, whereas the unaffected twin did not meet the criteria for schizophrenia or the schizophrenia spectrum disorder. We also studied seven normal sets of monozygotic twins (three male and four female pairs) whose mean age was 30.6±7.7 years (range, 19 to 44); none of these subjects fulfilled the criteria for a schizophrenia spectrum disorder. Among the affected index twins, 11 were given a diagnosis of chronic undifferentiated schizophrenia; 3, of chronic paranoid schizophrenia; and 1, of schizoaffective disorder (schizophrenia type). One member each of two control pairs had had a single self-limited episode of depression as a young adult. None of the study participants met criteria for substance abuse either at the time of testing or in recent years. All were in excellent general health without evidence of dehydration or malnutrition.

In the families of two of the discordant twins, there was a history of definite schizophrenia in a first- or second-degree relative. Ten of the affected twins had been born first, and 5 had been born second (P>0.35, by Fisher's exact test for deviation from chance order). The affected twins had been hospitalized an average of 8.7 times (range, 3 to 28). At the time of testing, only two of the twins with schizophrenia were inpatients, another had been recently discharged, and two others were living in group homes. None of the patients with schizophrenia were self-supporting or living completely on their own. All unaffected twins were functioning independently and were employed, except for one who was attending graduate school. All but two of the patients were being treated with neuroleptic medications at the time of the study (mean dose, 20.3±22.6 mg of fluphenazine equivalents; range, 2.5±80).[16] A review of the medical records indicated that the mean lifetime exposure to neuroleptic agents was 39,164±32,440 mg of fluphenazine equivalents (range, 10,000 to 103,000). Only two patients had ever received a course of electroconvulsive therapy.

Magnetic Resonance Imaging

We used the same 1.5-T (tesla) General Electric scanner and the same scanning sequence for MRI of all subjects. T_1-weighted coronal and sagittal slices and T_2-weighted transverse slices were obtained with spin echo-pulse sequences. The coronal slices were contiguous and 5 mm thick, with a repetition time of 800 msec and an echo time of 20 msec. The coronal slices were oriented so that they were parallel to the floor of the fourth ventricle, as determined on a midsagittal image. The slices began at the frontal pole and extended rostrally 15 cm (30 slices); this approach generally resulted in the inclusion of most of the occipital lobe.

Anatomical Measurements

All MRI scans were reviewed in pairs by an investigator who did not know which of the twins in each pair had schizophrenia. The

investigator knew that at least one member of the pair was affecte or that the pair was unaffected. The entire MRI study of each tw was compared visually with that of his or her sibling in an effort identify the affected twin according to the presence of larger cer brospinal fluid spaces, including cerebral ventricles and major fi sures.

Quantitative measurements of regions of interest were made wi an off-line computerized image-analysis system. The system and th method used have been described in detail elsewhere.[6] Area mea urements of gray and white matter and of the cerebral ventricle were made in each coronal section after fourfold magnification. Th values were then summed and multiplied by the thickness of th slice (0.5 cm) to produce estimates of the volume. The measure ments were made by other investigators who did not know th identity of the subjects of the scans. Measurements of both mem bers of a pair were made by the same person.

The volumes of the following structures were determined in th discordant sets of twins: total prefrontal region, prefrontal whi matter, prefrontal gray matter, total temporal lobe, temporal-lob white matter, and temporal-lobe gray matter (including cortic and subcortical gray matter). Neuroanatomical structures wer identified with the assistance of brain and MRI atlases.[17,18] Th prefrontal region was defined as all sections (range, 7 to 8 slices anterior to the genu of the corpus callosum. The temporal-lob sections (range, 10 to 14 slices) were considered to begin at th anterior pole and to extend posteriorly to the last section in whic the sylvian fissure was visualized, usually two slices posterior to th pulvinar nuclei. Our manner of defining the temporal lobe in cor onal sections has been described elsewhere.[6] Each structure wa measured bilaterally.

A more focal examination was then performed on six contiguou slices through the temporal lobe (Fig. 1). Bilateral area measure ments were made on these slices after an eightfold magnification A cursor was used to outline the amygdala, anterior hippocampu third ventricle, and temporal horns on the following slices: the thir ventricle, slices 1 through 4; temporal horns, slices 1 and 2; amyg dala, slice 1; and hippocampus, slices 2 through 4. When the margi of a structure was indistinct (e.g., the border of the hippocampu and subiculum), we estimated the boundary on the basis of ana tomical atlases.[17,18] The volumes of these structures and of th lateral ventricles in slices 1 through 6 were then determined by summing the areas and multiplying by the thickness of the slice. Anatomical differences between normal twins were examined for all structures measured on slice 2, corresponding to the level of the pes hippocampi, where maximal differences between the discordant twins were found (see below). To establish the reliability of these measurements, both raters made bilateral measurements of the area of the prefrontal lobe, temporal lobe, and white matter (a total of 48 measurements). The intraclass correlation coefficient was 0.99 (P<0.0001).

RESULTS

Visual Inspection

In 12 of the 15 discordant sets of twins, the affected twin was identified by visual inspection of the MRI scan alone, even when the ventricles of the affected twin were small (P = 0.06 by Fisher's exact test) (Fig. 2). Among these 12 pairs were the 2 with a family history of schizophrenia. In 3 of the 15 sets of twins, the affected twin could not be determined. In two pairs the scans were similar and could not be readily distinguished. The third set was the only instance in which the affected twin was incorrectly identified because the lateral ventricles of the unaffected twin were clearly larger than those of the twin with schizophrenia. Two anatomical levels were found to be consistently useful in visually differentiating the affected from the unaffected twin: the level of the anterior hippocampus immediately posterior to the amygdala

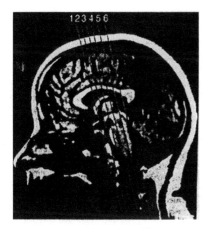

Figure 1. MRI Midsagittal View Showing the Location of the Coronal Slices Used in Area and Focal-Volume Measurements of Temporal-Lobe Structures.

and the level of the posterior thalamus. Inspection of T_2-weighted scans revealed only one or two punctate, high-intensity "lesions" in subcortical white matter in both members of two sets of discordant twins. In five of the normal sets of twins, ventricles were considered to be visually indistinguishable. Slight differences were noted in one pair. In another pair, the right lateral ventricle of one twin was grossly enlarged, and the septum was deviated. This finding could not be explained by the available clinical history.

Global Volume Measurements

Among the discordant sets of twins, affected and unaffected twins were compared by matched-pair t-tests (two-tailed). The total volume of the gray matter in the left temporal lobe was smaller in 13 of the patients with schizophrenia than in their twins (26.77±5.37 vs. 28.43±5.99 cm³; P<0.002). There were no significant differences between the affected and unaffected twins in the total volume of the right prefrontal gray matter (27.63±5.86 vs. 27.72±7.40 cm³), left prefrontal gray matter (25.13±6.22 vs. 25.29±7.46 cm³), right prefrontal white matter (24.00±4.95 vs. 25.07±5.60 cm³), left prefrontal white matter (22.08±5.32 vs. 22.89±5.80 cm³), right-temporal-lobe white matter (20.80±2.76 vs. 20.39±3.45 cm³),

left-temporal-lobe white matter (18.57±1.73 vs. 18.62±3.24 cm³), or right-temporal-lobe gray matter (30.21±4.97 vs. 30.53±6.24 cm³) (P>0.38 for all comparisons).

Area Measurements

As shown in Table 1, there were significant differences between the patients with schizophrenia and their unaffected twins in the areas of most of the structures measured in slices 1 through 3 (Fig. 1) and in the ventricles in slice 4. In slice 2, the area of the left hippocampus was smaller in 14 of the affected twins than in their unaffected siblings; in slice 3, the right hippocampus was smaller in 13 of the affected twins. In slices 1 through 4, no differences could be distinguished in the measurements of the entire cerebral area, or of the right and left temporal horns of the lateral ventricles. No significant differences were found in the measurements of the amygdala in slice 1 or in any measure in slices 5 and 6.

Each member of the normal sets of twins was randomly assigned to one of two groups, and matched-pair t-tests were performed on each of the structures examined. No significant differences were found between these two groups (right hippocampus, P>0.53; left hippocampus, P>0.65; right lateral ventricle, P>0.52; left lateral ventricle, P>0.23; and third ventricle, P>0.89). Because the low level of probability

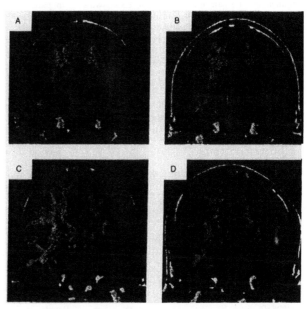

Figure 2. MRI Coronal Views from Two Sets of Monozygotic Twins Discordant for Schizophrenia Showing Subtle Enlargement of the Lateral Ventricles in the Affected Twins (Panels B and D) as Compared with the Unaffected Twins (Panels A and C), Even When the Affected Twin Had Small Ventricles.

Table 1. Area Measurements in MRI Slices through the Temporal Lobe in Monozygotic Twins Discordant for Schizophrenia.*

STRUCTURE	UNAFFECTED TWIN	AFFECTED TWIN	PERCENT DIFFERENCE	P VALUE	PREDICTIVE ACCURACY
	cubic centimeters				
Right lateral ventricle					
Slice 1	1.09±0.60	1.33±0.55	21	0.005	13
Slice 2	0.96±0.63	1.20±0.59	25	0.001	13
Slice 3	0.85±0.67	1.00±0.53	16	0.09	12
Slice 4	0.78±0.61	0.95±0.61	22	0.03	13
Left lateral ventricle					
Slice 1	1.10±0.61	1.27±0.64	16	0.005	14
Slice 2	1.01±0.65	1.19±0.65	18	0.003	14
Slice 3	0.92±0.73	1.05±0.59	14	0.08	12
Slice 4	0.85±0.72	0.97±0.68	14	0.03	12
Third ventricle					
Slice 1	0.33±0.12	0.37±0.10	12	0.04	11
Slice 2	0.34±0.12	0.42±0.13	23	0.001	13
Slice 3	0.36±0.21	0.39±0.23	8	0.33	8
Slice 4	0.38±0.21	0.43±0.19	13	0.02	11
Right hippocampus					
Slice 2	1.50±0.26	1.35±0.25	10	0.02	12
Slice 3	1.21±0.28	1.09±0.20	10	0.001	13
Slice 4	0.76±0.27	0.72±0.19	5	0.49	7
Left hippocampus					
Slice 2	1.51±0.19	1.23±0.25	19	0.001	14
Slice 3	1.18±0.25	1.07±0.26	9	0.06	13
Slice 4	0.83±0.20	0.75±0.20	10	0.13	8

*Slices refer to those illustrated in Figure 1. Predictive accuracy indicates the number of pairs out of 15 in which the measurement predicted which twin had schizophrenia. Plus–minus values are means ±SD.

might reflect the sample size, we also used the Mann–Whitney U test to compare the differences between each member of a pair in the discordant sets of twins and the normal sets of twins. This analysis revealed significantly greater differences between twins in the discordant sets in the measurements of the right hippocampus (P<0.003) and left hippocampus (P<0.02); the difference approached significance in the measurement of the left lateral ventricle (P<0.07).

Focal Volume Measurements

As shown in Table 2, affected and unaffected twins differed in the volumes of most of the structures contained in slices 1 through 6 (Fig. 1). The volume of the left hippocampus was smaller in 14 of the affected

Table 2. Volume Measurements in the Brains of Monozygotic Twins Discordant for Schizophrenia.*

STRUCTURE	UNAFFECTED TWIN	AFFECTED TWIN	PERCENT DIFFERENCE	P VALUE	PREDICTIVE ACCURACY
	cubic centimeters				
Right lateral ventricle	2.78±1.84	3.33±1.62	20	0.02	11
Left lateral ventricle	2.88±1.98	3.30±1.98	15	0.03	13
Third ventricle	0.81±0.31	0.71±0.28	12	0.001	13
Right hippocampus	1.73±0.36	1.58±0.26	9	0.01	13
Left hippocampus	1.76±0.24	1.56±0.30	11	0.006	14
Gray matter					
Right anterior temporal lobe	8.47±1.27	8.57±1.33	2	0.37	7
Left anterior temporal lobe	7.86±1.20	7.61±1.36	3	0.11	10

*Volumes were determined from the slices shown in Figure 1. Predictive accuracy indicates the number of pairs out of 15 in which the measurement predicted which twin had schizophrenia. Plus–minus values are means ±SD.

twins than in their unaffected siblings, and in 13 affected twins the volume of the right hippocampus was smaller.

Correlations

None of the anatomical measurements that distinguished affected from unaffected twins correlated significantly with the age at the onset of schizophrenia (maximal r<−0.28, P>0.30 for the left hippocampus, slice 2), duration of illness (maximal r<0.28, P>0.30 for the focal volume of the left hippocampus), or the extent of exposure to neuroleptic agents (maximal r<−0.50, P>0.06 for the right hippocampus, slice 5).

DISCUSSION

The chief finding of this study was that evidence of anatomical changes in the brain was present in almost every twin with schizophrenia. Although the differences were subtle, relatively enlarged cerebral ventricles were visually apparent in most cases, even if the ventricles were small. Significant quantitative differences between affected and unaffected twins were found in the lateral ventricles, third ventricle, and temporal lobe, including both sides of the anterior hippocampus, and in the total volume of the gray matter in the left temporal lobe. None of these differences were found in normal pairs of twins. These findings are consistent with previous reports of enlarged lateral and third ventricles[2,3,5-7] and smaller hippocampi in patients with schizophrenia.[10] Comparing schizophrenic twins with their unaffected twins controls for variation in cerebral anatomy due to genetic causes and, to a great degree, for variation due to nonspecific environmental causes.

The use of pairs of discordant monozygotic twins makes it possible to address the question of whether subtle neuroanatomical findings are an occasional or a consistent pathologic correlate of schizophrenia. In the current study, 14 of the 15 affected twins had a smaller left anterior hippocampus, and 13 had a smaller right hippocampus and enlargement of the third and lateral ventricles. These results suggest that the observed abnormalities are not confined to a minority of patients. In fact, the data suggest that when appropriate controls are available, subtle anatomical changes can be detected in most patients with schizophrenia and are probably characteristic of the disease. Similar results have been described in other studies that have used sibling controls. Weinberger et al.[19] used CT to examine 11 sibling groups and found that the affected family member had larger cerebral ventricles in each case, even if the size of the ventricles appeared to be normal. DeLisi et al.[20] also observed larger ventricles in patients with schizophrenia than in their unaffected siblings. In a CT study of 12 sets of monozygotic twins discordant for schizophrenia, Reveley et al.[21] found that in all but 1 pair the affected twin had larger lateral cerebral ventricles than the unaffected twin.

The fact that an affected monozygotic twin can be differentiated from an unaffected twin on the basis of tructural differences in the central nervous system probably means that the cause of the underlying neuropathologic process is at least partly not genetic. This may seem at odds with a number of studies showing that the risk of schizophrenia involves genetic factors. Our study does not directly address the question of whether there is a genetic factor associated with schizophrenia. We cannot rule out, for example, a genetic predisposition to the changes we observed. Clearly, however, something extragenetic must occur as well.

We also cannot rule out the possibility that our findings may be due primarily not to the illness itself but to nonspecific aspects of schizophrenia or its treatment. For instance, affected twins differ from unaffected twins in their exposure to neuroleptic medications, history of hospitalization, and possibly, nutritional status and level of stress. We doubt, however, that these secondary factors have a primary role in our findings for the following reasons: the absence of correlations with the extent of exposure to neuroleptic agents or with the duration of illness in our patients — findings that are consistent with those of numerous other studies[3-5,23-27] — and the reports of identical findings of large lateral and third ventricles[28-31] and small hippocampi[32] at the time of patients' initial hospitalizations for schizophrenia.

Our quantitative in vivo findings in anteromedial limbic structures are consistent with the results of several controlled postmortem studies[7,10-12] that implicate subtle pathologic changes in the anatomy of the limbic system in schizophrenia. Despite interest in the role of the limbic system in this illness and evidence of somewhat localized pathologic changes of the temporal lobe, findings involving other areas of the brain have also been reported. Decreased volume of the cerebral hemispheres, including cortex and central gray matter, has been described by Pakkenberg.[8] Benes et al[33] have reported reduced numbers of neurons in prefrontal, cingulate, and motor cortices. Other studies have observed smaller vermis cerebelli.[34,35] The findings in the present study and in previous ones that cerebral ventricular enlargement is often observed at some distance from limbic structures and that the third ventricle is also enlarged suggest that the underlying changes are not limited to a single site. Further work is needed to characterize the extent and localization of the pathologic anatomy in schizophrenia.

Several studies have suggested that morphologic abnormalities of the brain in schizophrenia occur more commonly in the left hemisphere. When unilateral changes are observed, including structural,[36,37] chemical,[38,39] and electrophysiologic differences,[40] left-sided changes predominate. Although most anatomical studies using CT, MRI, or postmortem techniques have found bilateral changes in schizophrenia, morphologic changes of the left hemisphere, and particularly of the left temporal lobe, appear to be slightly more obvious. In the current study, we noted bilateral increases in the size of the lateral ventricles and decreases in the size of the anterior hippocampus. However, the reduction in the total volume of the gray matter in the temporal lobe was significant only on the left side. At present, it seems reasonable to conclude that although changes in the left temporal lobe may be slightly more obvious in schizophrenia, the pathologic process is not confined to the left hemisphere.

The abnormal MRI findings we identified are not specific histopathological observations, and their implications for the pathogenesis of schizophrenia are unclear. Reduced parenchymal volume usually suggests degeneration of brain tissue. In the case of schizophrenia, however, the research data do not support the existence of a progressive degenerative condition. For instance, most studies have failed to show the expected correlation between ventricular size and the duration of schizophrenia.[3-6,25-29,31] Moreover, several studies suggest that pathologic structural changes, as demonstrated by increased ventricular size, predate the onset of psychotic symptoms[27,28,31,41,42] and remain static during the course of the illness.[43-45] Some subtle failure of development, such as abnormal neuronal migration,[12] may better explain the changes. The conspicuous absence of gliosis in most of the postmortem studies reporting decreased tissue volume[46] and abnormal cytoarchitecture[12] is also consistent with an early developmental neuropathologic process. The mechanism by which this process may result in an illness of adult onset is the subject of considerable speculation and ongoing research.[47]

We are indebted to Dr. Irving I. Gottesman, Dr. Stanley Perl, Mr. Alex Terrazas, who assisted with the project, and Ms. Gail A. Miller, who assisted in the preparation of the manuscript.

REFERENCES

1. Kirch DG, Weinberger DR. Anatomical neuropathology in schizophrenia: post-mortem findings. In: Nasrallah HA, Weinberger DR, eds. The neurology of schizophrenia. Vol. 1 of Handbook of schizophrenia. Amsterdam: Elsevier, 1986:325-48.
2. Johnstone EC, Crow TJ, Frith CD, Husband J, Kreel L. Cerebral ventricular size and cognitive impairment in chronic schizophrenia. Lancet 1976; 2:924-6.
3. Weinberger DR, Torrey EF, Neophytides AN, Wyatt RJ. Lateral cerebral ventricular enlargement in chronic schizophrenia. Arch Gen Psychiatry 1979; 36:735-9.
4. Shelton RC, Weinberger DR. X-ray computerized tomography studies in schizophrenia: a review and synthesis. In: Nasrallah HA, Weinberger DR, eds. The neurology of schizophrenia. Vol. 1 of Handbook of schizophrenia. Amsterdam: Elsevier, 1986:207-50.
5. Kelsoe JR Jr, Cadet JL, Pickar D, Weinberger DR. Quantitative neuroanatomy in schizophrenia: a controlled magnetic resonance imaging study. Arch Gen Psychiatry 1988; 45:533-41.
6. Suddath RL, Casanova MF, Goldberg TE, Daniel DG, Kelsoe JR Jr, Weinberger DR. Temporal lobe pathology in schizophrenia: a quantitative magnetic resonance imaging study. Am J Psychiatry 1989; 146:464-72.
7. Brown R, Colter N, Corsellis JA, et al. Postmortem evidence of structural brain changes in schizophrenia: differences in brain weight, temporal horn area, and parahippocampal gyrus compared with affective disorder. Arch Gen Psychiatry 1986; 43:36-42.
8. Pakkenberg B. Post-mortem study of chronic schizophrenic brains. Br J Psychiatry 1987; 151:744-52.
9. Scheibel AB, Kovelman JA. Disorientation of the hippocampal pyramidal cell and its processes in the schizophrenic patient. Biol Psychiatry 1981; 16:101-2.
10. Bogerts B, Meertz E, Schonfeldt-Bausch R. Basal ganglia and limbic system pathology in schizophrenia: a morphometric study of brain volume and shrinkage. Arch Gen Psychiatry 1985; 42:784-91.
11. Falkai P, Bogerts B, Rozumek M. Limbic pathology in schizophrenia: the entorhinal region — a morphometric study. Biol Psychiatry 1988; 24:515-21.
12. Jakob H, Beckmann H. Prenatal developmental disturbances in the limbic allocortex in schizophrenics. J Neural Transm 1986; 65:303-26.

13. Cederlöf R, Friberg L, Jonsson E, Kaij L. Studies on similarity diagnosis in twins with the aid of mailed questionnaires. Acta Genet Stat Med 1961; 11:338-62.
14. Belmaker R, Pollin W, Wyatt RJ, Cohen S. A follow-up of monozygotic twins discordant for schizophrenia. Arch Gen Psychiatry 1974; 30:219-22.
15. Spitzer RL, Williams JBW, Gibbon M. Structured clinical interview for DSM-III-R-non-patient version (SCID NP 4/1/87). New York: Biometrics Research Department, New York State Psychiatric Institute, 1987.
16. Torrey EF. Surviving schizophrenia: a family manual. New York: Harper & Row, 1988:188.
17. DeArmond SJ, Fusco MM, Dewey MM. Structure of the human brain: a photographic atlas. 2nd ed. New York: Oxford University Press, 1976.
18. Schnitzlein HN, Murtagh FR. Imaging anatomy of the head and spine: a photographic color atlas of MRI, CT, gross, and microscopic anatomy in axial, coronal, and sagittal planes. Baltimore: Urban & Schwarzenberg, 1985.
19. Weinberger DR, DeLisi LE, Neophytides AN, Wyatt RJ. Familial aspects of CT scan abnormalities in chronic schizophrenia patients. Psychiatry Res 1981; 4:65-71.
20. DeLisi LE, Goldin LR, Hamovit JR, Maxwell ME, Kurtz D, Gershon ES. A family study of the association of increased ventricular size with schizophrenia. Arch Gen Psychiatry 1986; 43:148-53.
21. Reveley AM, Reveley MA, Clifford CA, Murray RM. Cerebral ventricular size in twins discordant for schizophrenia. Lancet 1982; 1:540-1.
22. Kendler KS. Overview: a current perspective on twin studies of schizophrenia. Am J Psychiatry 1983; 140:1413-25.
23. Golden CJ, Graber B, Coffman J, Berg RA, Newlin DB, Bloch S. Structural brain deficits in schizophrenia: identification by computed tomographic scan density measurements. Arch Gen Psychiatry 1981; 38:1014-7.
24. Frangos E, Athanassenas G. Differences in lateral brain ventricular size among various types of chronic schizophrenics: evidence based on a CT scan. Acta Psychiatr Scand 1982; 66:459-63.
25. Nasrallah HA, Jacoby CG, McCalley-Whitters M, Kuperman S. Cerebral ventricular enlargement in subtypes of chronic schizophrenia. Arch Gen Psychiatry 1982; 39:774-7.
26. Schulsinger F, Parnas J, Petersen ET, et al. Cerebral ventricular size in the offspring of schizophrenic mothers: a preliminary study. Arch Gen Psychiatry 1984; 41:602-6.
27. Williams AO, Reveley MA, Kolakowska T, Ardern M, Madelbrote BM. Schizophrenia with good and poor outcome. II. Cerebral ventricular size and its clinical significance. Br J Psychiatry 1985; 146:239-46.
28. Weinberger DR, DeLisi LE, Perman GP, Targum S, Wyatt RJ. Computed tomography in schizophreniform disorder and other acute psychiatric disorders. Arch Gen Psychiatry 1982; 39:778-83.
29. Nyback H, Wiesel F-A, Berggren B-M, Hindmarsh T. Computed tomography of the brain in patients with acute psychosis and in healthy volunteers. Acta Psychiatr Scand 1982; 65:403-14.

30. Schulz SC, Koller MM, Kishore PR, Hamer RM, Gehl JJ, Friedel M. Ventricular enlargement in teenage patients with schizophrenia spectra disorder. Am J Psychiatry 1983; 140:1592-5.
31. Iacono WG, Smith GN, Moreau M, et al. Ventricular and sulcal size at onset of psychosis. Am J Psychiatry 1988; 145:820-4.
32. Bogerts B, Ashtari M, Degreet G, Alvir JM, Bilder RM, Lieberman. Reduced temporal limbic structure volumes on magnetic resonance ima in first episode schizophrenia. Psychiatry Res (in press).
33. Benes FM, Davidson J, Bird ED. Quantitative cytoarchitectural studies the cerebral cortex of schizophrenics. Arch Gen Psychiatry 1986; 43:31
34. Weinberger DR, Torrey EF, Wyatt RJ. Cerebellar atrophy in chro schizophrenia. Lancet 1979; 1:718-9.
35. Weinberger DR, Kleinman JE, Luchins DJ, Bigelow LB, Wyatt RJ. Ce bellar pathology in schizophrenia: a controlled postmortem study. Am Psychiatry 1980; 137:359-61.
36. Largen JW Jr, Calderon M, Smith RC. Asymmetries in the densities white and gray matter in the brains of schizophrenic patients. Am J Psych try 1983; 140:1060-2.
37. Reveley MA, Reveley AM, Baldy R. Left cerebral hemisphere hypodens in discordant schizophrenic twins: a controlled study. Arch Gen Psychia 1987; 44:625-32.
38. Losonczy MF, Song IS, Mohs RC, et al. Correlates of lateral ventricu size in chronic schizophrenia. 1. Behavioral and treatment response mea ures. Am J Psychiatry 1986; 143:976-81.
39. Reynolds GP. Increased concentrations and lateral asymmetry of amygda dopamine in schizophrenia. Nature 1983; 305:527-9.
40. Reite M, Teale P, Zimmerman J, Davis K, Whalen J, Edrich J. Sour origin of a 50-msec latency auditory evoked field component in you schizophrenic men. Biol Psychiatry 1988; 24:495-506.
41. Weinberger DR, Cannon-Spoor E, Potkin SG, Wyatt RJ. Poor premorb adjustment and CT scan abnormalities in chronic schizophrenia. Am J Ps chiatry 1980; 137:1410-3.
42. DeLisi EI, Schwartz CC, Targum SD, et al. Ventricular brain enlargeme and outcome of acute schizophreniform disorder. Psychiatry Res 198 9:169-71.
43. Nasrallah HA, Olson SC, McCalley-Whitters M, Chapman S, Jacoby CC Cerebral ventricular size in schizophrenia: a preliminary follow-up stud Arch Gen Psychiatry 1986; 43:157-9.
44. Illowsky BP, Juliano DM, Bigelow LB, Weinberger DR. Stability of CT scan findings in schizophrenia: results of an eight year follow-up stud J Neurol Neurosurg Psychiatry 1988; 51:209-13.
45. Vita A, Sacchetti E, Valvassori G, Cazzullo CL. Brain morphology i schizophrenia: a 2- to 5-year CT scan follow-up study. Acta Psychiatr Scan 1988; 78:618-21.
46. Roberts GW, Colter N, Lofthouse R, Bogerts B, Zech M, Crow TJ. Glios in schizophrenia: a survey. Biol Psychiatry 1986; 21:1043-50.
47. Weinberger DR. Implications of normal brain development for the patho genesis of schizophrenia. Arch Gen Psychiatry 1987; 44:660-9.

The Psychosocial Treatment of Schizophrenia: An Update

Juan R. Bustillo, M.D.

John Lauriello, M.D.

William P. Horan, M.S.

Samuel J. Keith, M.D.

Objective: The authors sought to update the randomized controlled trial literature of psychosocial treatments for schizophrenia.

Method: Computerized literature searches were conducted to identify randomized controlled trials of various psychosocial interventions, with emphasis on studies published since a previous review of psychosocial treatments for schizophrenia in 1996.

Results: Family therapy and assertive community treatment have clear effects on the prevention of psychotic relapse and rehospitalization. However, these treatments have no consistent effects on other outcome measures (e.g., pervasive positive and negative symptoms, overall social functioning, and ability to obtain competitive employment). Social skills training improves social skills but has no clear effects on relapse prevention, psychopathology, or employment status. Supportive employment programs that use the place-and-train vocational model have important effects on obtaining competitive employment. Some studies have shown improvements in delusions and hallucinations following cognitive behavior therapy. Preliminary research indicates that personal therapy may improve social functioning.

Conclusions: Relatively simple, long-term psychoeducational family therapy should be available to the majority of persons suffering from schizophrenia. Assertive community training programs ought to be offered to patients with frequent relapses and hospitalizations, especially if they have limited family support. Patients with schizophrenia can clearly improve their social competence with social skills training, which may translate into a more adaptive functioning in the community. For patients interested in working, rapid placement with ongoing support offers the best opportunity for maintaining a regular job in the community. Cognitive behavior therapy may benefit the large number of patients who continue to experience disabling psychotic symptoms despite optimal pharmacological treatment.

(Am J Psychiatry 2001; 158:163–175)

Antipsychotic medications have been repeatedly shown to be effective for the treatment of acute psychosis and the prevention of relapse for persons suffering from schizophrenia. Novel antipsychotics with fewer neuromotoric side effects are a clear therapeutic advancement. However, with the exception of clozapine for treatment-resistant psychosis, the newer agents have not been clearly shown to have clinical advantages in other domains of outcome, such as social adjustment and obtaining competitive employment (1). Thus, the majority of persons with schizophrenia, even those who benefit from medication, continue to have disabling residual symptoms and impaired social functioning and will most likely experience a relapse despite medication adherence. Hence, it is necessary to integrate empirically validated psychosocial treatments into the standard of care for this population.

In this article, we present an updated review of the various forms of psychosocial interventions that have been studied in methodologically sound clinical trials, with a special emphasis on studies published since the 1996 review by Penn and Mueser (2). Randomized controlled trials currently assess relevant outcomes in patients with schizo-

phrenia beyond the traditional measures of psychopathology and rates of rehospitalization. Other domains of outcomes include cognitive performance, social skills and adjustment, overall quality of life, competitive employment, and comorbid substance abuse as well as less usual clinical measures such as negative, depressive, and deficit symptoms. As we describe different psychosocial interventions, we will define the primary targeted outcome measure addressed in each study. We will not address the important area of treatment research concerning schizophrenia and comorbid substance abuse (the reader is referred to the paper by Drake and colleagues [3]).

Research into psychosocial treatment strategies exists at varying stages of development, some modalities having been studied more often and with better-designed randomized controlled trials. The majority of the randomized controlled trials reviewed assumed that optimal antipsychotic medication management was provided. From the available literature, whenever possible, we will address the following questions. What is the efficacy of the specific intervention for the primary outcome measure? For secondary outcomes? Is a particular kind of psychosocial intervention more efficacious for certain outcomes? (If so, what is the evidence for an "active ingredient"?). What evidence exists for effectiveness and transferability, i.e., effectiveness in more usual clinical settings? What data exist regarding cost-effectiveness?

Because family therapy is the most extensively studied psychosocial intervention, a reasonable attempt can be made to address most of these questions for this modality. For other forms of treatment, some of the questions may not be addressed because of limited data.

Method

We selected articles for review by conducting MEDLINE and PsychInfo computerized searches of the English language literature for the period 1966 to March 2000. For the MEDLINE searches, the following key words were used in conjunction with the terms "schizophrenia," "randomized control trial," and "human": "psychotherapy," "psychosocial rehabilitation," "social adjustment," "social support," "cognitive therapy," "family therapy," and "social skills training." From these searches, 155 separate references were found. For the PsychInfo searches, the following key words were used in conjunction with the terms "schizophrenia," "empirical study," "human," and "journal articles": "group psychotherapy," "psychotherapy," "family therapy," "social adjustment," "social skills," and "cognitive therapy." From these searches, 12 additional references not included in the initial MEDLINE search were identified. We primarily selected randomized controlled trials that used standardized rating instruments, but some pertinent less rigorously conducted studies were also included. We also checked the references in the articles obtained to ensure that other relevant articles that had not been identified with the initial searches were included, and we consulted some experts in the field in order to identify other recent studies.

Results

In total we identified 18 new studies since the review by Penn and Mueser (2): two for family therapy, two for case management, five for social skills training, three for supported employment programs, five for cognitive behavior therapy, and one for individual therapy (which also had a family therapy arm).

Family Therapy

Brown and Rutter (4) demonstrated, and Butzlaff and Hooley (5) have recently supported the concept, that schizophrenia patients who returned to families that were originally rated as being high in expressed emotion (an empirically derived index of criticism, overinvolvement, and hostility) were more likely to experience a relapse during the following year despite adequate pharmacotherapy. Although high expressed emotion environments are not specific to families of patients with schizophrenia (5), the expressed emotion literature provided the background for most of the initial randomized controlled trials of family therapy that attempted to reduce psychotic relapse.

Efficacy with regard to primary outcome. A large body of evidence has demonstrated the superiority of a variety of family therapy interventions that employ behavioral

and psychoeducational techniques over customary outpatient care or individual therapy in terms of the primary outcome measures of psychotic relapse and rehospitalization (2). On average, relapse rates among schizophrenic patients whose treatment involves family therapy are approximately 24% as compared to about 64% among those who receive routine treatment (6). Additionally, the beneficial effects of long-term family interventions (i.e., greater than 9 months) appear to be quite durable and may be maintained for up to 2 years (6) or longer (7).

However, the few studies published since the 1996 review by Penn and Mueser (2) are remarkable for their lack of relapse prevention findings (Table 1). Linszen and colleagues (8, 9) studied adolescent patients early in their illness and found a very low (16%–20%) overall relapse rate at 1 year, with no advantage for the patients whose treatment included family therapy. It is worth noting that the comparison intervention involved a fairly intensive individual treatment approach rather than "standard" services. The personal therapy trial of Hogarty et al. (10) included a family therapy arm for patients residing with their families. Unlike the subjects in the previous study, these subjects were mostly chronic patients. Family therapy offered no advantage over supportive therapy in preventing relapse (the overall relapse rate was only 29% at 3 years). The supportive therapy group received biweekly sessions, minimum effective medication dosage, and case management—an enriched package of care compared to most community standards. These studies illustrate that if the base relapse rate is low (either because of the population selected or the use of a comprehensive control care program), the potential advantages of family therapy may not be realized.

Are some interventions more efficacious? Considerable attention has focused on the reduction of expressed emotion levels as an active mediator for the efficacy of family therapy interventions. In studies that selected families with high levels of expressed emotion, patients who did not experience a relapse were more likely to reside in a family household in which the expressed emotion environment had changed from high to low during the treatment (13–16). However, the number of subjects/families reassessed was very small, and there were no reports of a clear correlation between relapse and reductions in expressed emotion levels. Because it is possible that a high level of expressed emotion may be a consequence of the relapse itself (or of patients being more severely ill), proving a causal role of expressed emotion for psychotic relapse requires a controlled study that includes interim expressed emotion assessments. Only Tarrier et al. (16) assessed expressed emotion levels at baseline, 4.5 months, and 9 months. Although they found that the level of expressed emotion changed from high to low in the relatives in the experimental treatment, similar changes occurred for the control condition. They concluded that "...this latter result would not be expected if expressed emotion is a

276

TABLE 1. Studies on Treatment of Schizophrenia With Family Therapy[a]

Study	Subjects	Length of Follow-Up	Treatment Group		Relapse Rates	Secondary Outcomes
			Experimental Condition	Control Condition		
Linszen et al. (8) and Nugter et al. (9)	Patients with recent-onset schizophrenic disorders (N=76)	12 months	Individual treatment plus 18 sessions of family therapy over 12 months that focused on education, communication, and problem-solving skills	Individual treatment alone	Equivalent	
Hogarty et al. (10, 11)	Patients with schizophrenia or schizoaffective disorder (N=48)	36 months	Biweekly family therapy for first year; biweekly to monthly family therapy for years 2 and 3	Biweekly supportive therapy	Equivalent	There was tentative evidence for greater improvement in social functioning for patients in the experimental group
McFarlane et al. (12)	Patients with schizophrenia (N=68) at high risk for relapse[b]	24 months	Biweekly multifamily psycho-educational group therapy plus assertive community treatment	Family intervention in times of crisis only plus assertive community treatment	Equivalent	Patients in both groups reported equivalent reductions in symptom severity; family members in both conditions reported reduced burden; higher overall (but not competitive) employment was achieved by patients in the experimental group

[a] Reports of randomized controlled trials published since the 1996 review by Penn and Mueser (2).
[b] History of poor compliance, violence, or homelessness.

stable dimension with a simple causal role in relapse" (16, p. 540).

Direct comparisons of two forms of family treatment (with one usually more intensive than the other) have failed to demonstrate differential efficacy for the experimental intervention (16–20). Because these studies did not include a no-treatment group, interpretations regarding the efficacy of the different forms of family therapy are problematic. However, the reported relapse rates at 2 years for these studies were low (under 36%) and comparable to the rates reported in previous comparison studies of active family intervention versus standard treatment (between 14% and 33% versus 40%–83%, respectively) (6). This suggests that in studies comparing two forms of family treatment, both interventions were efficacious.

McFarlane et al. (12) studied schizophrenia patients at high risk for relapse (Table 1). Half received biweekly multifamily group treatment, and half received family therapy only during times of crisis. There were no differences in relapse for the two treatment groups (27% at 2 years). Thus, research has failed to identify the relative superiority of any particular form of family therapy and suggests that treatment intensity (i.e., beyond moderate intensity with sustained availability) or format does not differentially effect outcome.

Efficacy with regard to secondary outcomes. Some studies have reported improvement in such factors as family burden, coping, and knowledge of schizophrenia (12, 21–23). However, these studies do not separate the effect that reduced relapse rates due to the family therapy intervention might have on these other outcome measures. The effect on social functioning independent of the effect on relapse has been assessed in two studies (11, 20) in which relapsed subjects reentered their original treat-

ment group once stabilized. Social functioning was assessed between relapse episodes. Neither study found an advantage in social functioning for the experimental family treatment group (11 and Mueser, personal communication, 1999).

Effectiveness and transferability. Many randomized controlled trials have employed treatment manuals to guide the family therapy, which would facilitate implementation in alternate settings. The model of Falloon et al. (13) (behaviorally oriented problem-solving in the home) has been repeatedly transferred to other research settings (8, 9, 20, 24). Unfortunately, the evidence for effectiveness in a more typical nonresearch setting is very limited, primarily because family therapy has not become the standard of care in the community (25). Some studies from China show that a relatively simple psychoeducational approach can be implemented in the community with large numbers of patients and have an important effect on relapse (23, 26, 27). However, the control condition in these studies (usual care) failed to include scheduled medication management follow-up (clearly suboptimal care by Western standards). Therefore, it is not surprising that the family management groups (which encouraged family members to actively pursue medication follow-up) had substantially better outcomes (relapse rates of 15%–44% versus 31%–64%, respectively). These Chinese studies also suggest that cultural differences are not necessarily an impediment to successfully applying existing family therapy interventions to diverse cultural groups. However, Telles et al. (28) applied the model of Falloon et al. (13) to a group of Hispanic families and found no differences between behavioral family therapy and standard treatment. Thus, the impact of more complex models of family treatments to non-Caucasian cultures is unclear.

Cost-effectiveness. Although a large effect of family therapy on prevention of relapse and rehospitalizations could potentially result in important cost savings, only a few studies report cost-benefit analyses. In an analysis that compared home-based family treatment versus individual management over a 12-month period, Cardin et al. (29) reported that the total costs of family management were 19% less than those of individual treatment, with overall benefits favoring the family therapy intervention. Tarrier et al. (30) documented a favorable cost-benefit ratio for patients from high expressed emotion environments who received a 9-month family therapy intervention as compared to a control group from high expressed emotion environments who received routine treatment. Despite the extra costs associated with therapist time, the family therapy intervention resulted in a mean cost savings of 27% per patient. The study by Xiong et al. (26) reported significant cost savings associated with family therapy ($170 per patient per year, a large savings by contemporary Chinese standards). However, as stated before, a replication study that applies Western standards of community care is required.

Case Management

Patients with schizophrenia are often ill-prepared to find and maintain the multiple services they need in order to function in the community. Traditionally, case managers have functioned as brokers of services, being contacted by other professionals who have identified a new need for the patient and then referring the patient to the provider able to deliver these services. Unfortunately, many patients with schizophrenia lack the level of cognitive and social competence to consistently follow-through and get their needs met, which further increases their risk of relapsing.

A different approach to case management and service delivery is exemplified by the assertive community treatment program (31). Patients are assigned to one multidisciplinary team (case manager, nurse, etc.). The team has a fixed caseload and a high staff/patient ratio and delivers all services when and where needed by the patient, 24 hours a day, 7 days a week. Mueser et al. (32) reviewed the literature on assertive community treatment programs for patients with chronic mental illness, and two more randomized controlled trials have since been published (33, 34). There are now 32 studies of assertive community treatment programs with a true experimental design.

Efficacy with regard to primary outcome. The main goal of assertive community treatment programs is to prevent rehospitalization in patients at risk for relapse through provision of comprehensive integrated community services. The most consistent effects have been a reduction of time spent in the hospital (demonstrated in 14 of 24 studies; nine reported no differences) and an improvement in housing stability (demonstrated in nine of 13 studies; four reported no differences) (32–34). These ef-

fects are clinically meaningful and more robust among patients with high service utilization rates. It is of interest that the two most recent studies (33, 34) did not find an effect on rehospitalizations. Both studies included an intensive clinical case management approach as a control treatment and did not provide 24-hour coverage as a component of assertive community treatment. Also, Issakidis et al. (34) did not restrict subject inclusion to those who were high service utilizers (only one-third of their study group were high service utilizers). These characteristics may explain the negative findings.

Efficacy with regard to secondary outcomes. Only a minority of studies have found advantages in social adjustment (four of 16) or employment (three of nine, and these jobs represented mostly sheltered rather than competitive employment) (32–34). The disappointing effects on functioning are perhaps accounted for by the emphasis of assertive community treatment in directly assisting patients with their immediate needs, without a formal component of rehabilitation directed toward either social or vocational skills. If a reasonable goal for some patients is self-sufficiency, more systematic efforts aimed at rehabilitation may need to be incorporated into assertive community treatment.

Are some interventions more efficacious? In general, programs that more closely resemble the original assertive community treatment model tend to have a more reliable effect on rehospitalization (35). However, because assertive community treatment is so complex and there have been no studies that systematically assess the impact of each component, it is not known which components are essential. Hence, the effect on hospitalization could be due to improved medication compliance, continuity of caregivers, 24-hour coverage, site of service, intensity of services, or a combination of some of these elements.

Effectiveness and transferability. The original assertive community treatment program has been successfully transferred to many communities by other teams of clinical researchers. Also, assertive community treatment programs have been successfully implemented as part of routine clinical care and have been shown to be effective at reducing rehospitalizations (36).

Cost-effectiveness. In patients with high service utilization rates, assertive community treatment may result in some net savings, since expensive inpatient treatments are reduced by employing less costly community services (31, 37). Rosenheck and Neale (36) documented the cost savings associated with assertive community treatment compared to the cost of standard care at a Veterans Administration (VA) facility, but only for the sickest of the high inpatient service users who were treated at neuropsychiatric hospitals. However, a recently published analysis (38) of a previous study (33) that compared assertive community treatment with another high-quality case management system that did not use multidisciplinary teams with constant availability did not support the cost savings advantages of assertive community treatment.

Social Skills Training

Social skills are those "...specific response capabilities necessary for effective social performance" (39). Social skills training uses learning theory principles to improve social functioning by working with patients to remediate problems in activities of daily living, employment, leisure, and relationships. It is hoped that the improved skills (primary outcome) will generalize to better community functioning and have a downstream effect on relapse and psychopathology. Following the framework described by Bellack and Mueser (39), there are three forms of social skills training: the basic model, the social problem-solving model, and the cognitive remediation model.

In the basic model, complex social repertoires are broken down into simpler steps, subjected to corrective learning, practiced through role playing, and applied in natural settings. The social problem-solving model focuses on improving impairments in information processing that are assumed to be the cause of social skills deficits. The model targets domains needing changes including medication and symptom management, recreation, basic conversation, and self-care. Each domain is taught as part of a module, with the purpose of correcting deficits in receptive, processing, and sending skills. In the cognitive remediation model, the corrective learning process begins by targeting more fundamental cognitive impairments, like attention or planning. The assumption is that if the underlying cognitive impairment can be improved, this learning will be transferred to support more complex cognitive processes, and the traditional social skills models can be better learned and generalized in the community.

Efficacy with regard to the primary outcome. The basic model has been repeatedly demonstrated to have an effect on improving specific social skills, and this learning is maintained for up to 12 months (2). However, the outcomes measured in most of these studies closely resembled those assessed in the skills training setting, and there is little evidence that this learning translates into improved social competence in the community (40). In the most extensive study of the basic social skills training model, Hogarty et al. (41) failed to demonstrate a significant impact on social adjustment after 2 years of treatment, despite a very intensive intervention (1 hour weekly for 21 months plus medication compared to medication only). The lack of generalization in this study and others that used the basic model has been a significant limitation.

The social problem-solving model has also been demonstrated an effect on skill enhancement (42–44). Two studies have examined the long-term impact of this model. Marder et al. (45) assigned schizophrenic outpatients to problem-solving group therapy or supportive group therapy for 2 years. Both groups received the same intensity, frequency, and overall length of intervention (90 minutes

twice weekly for the first 6 months, then weekly). There was a small but statistically significant advantage for the problem-solving intervention in two out of six measures of social adjustment after 2 years. Thus, the experimental treatment had modest benefits.

Liberman et al. (46) compared the problem-solving group model to equally intensive occupational therapy. Subjects received the psychosocial interventions for 6 months (3 hours a day, four times a week) and were followed for 2 years. The experimental condition had a significant effect in three out of 10 independent living skills (more personal possessions, more skilled food preparation, and improved money management) that were maintained up to 18 months after completing the intervention. The authors posited that the effect on independent living skills generalization of skills learned and attributed this effect to the fact that all subjects were assigned a case manager who actively encouraged them to apply the skills learned in the community.

Although initial studies of the cognitive remediation model demonstrated some improvement of elementary cognitive processes (47), studies that have evaluated more complex cognitive and social skills have provided mixed results. Hodel and Brenner (48) failed to find in a program that started with cognitive remediation before skills training (N=10) the predicted advantage on social adjustment over a program that followed the opposite order (N=11). Wykes et al. (49) found that 17 patients treated with an intensive cognitive remediation approach (1-hour daily sessions for up to 3 months) that targeted executive functioning deficits showed improvement on three of 12 cognitive measures as compared to 16 patients who received a comparison intervention (occupational therapy) matched for therapist contact and treatment duration. The cognitive remediation intervention did not result in any direct improvements in social functioning or symptoms.

A recent report by Spaulding et al. (50) from their large study (total N=90) comparing cognitive remediation plus the social problem-solving modules with equally intensive supportive therapy plus the modules presents a more hopeful outlook. Subjects were very ill, mostly with schizophrenia, and were referred for long-term hospital treatment because of inability to sustain community living. The experimental and control interventions were matched for intensity (3 hours per week for 6 months). The cognitive remediation group did better in two out of four measures of social competence and demonstrated better acquisition of skills for two out of four of the social problem-solving modules. This study suggests that the cognitive remediation approach can enhance response to more standard skills training in very ill, institutionalized patients.

Efficacy with regard to secondary outcomes. The study by Hogarty et al. (15, 41) is the only large social skills training study to find an effect on relapse prevention (46% for social skills training versus 30% for the control condition

TABLE 2. Studies on Treatment of Schizophrenia With Supported Employment Intervention Programs[a]

Study	Subjects	Length of Follow-Up	Treatment Group		Rate of Competitive Employment[b]	Secondary Outcomes
			Experimental Condition	Control Condition		
Bond et al. (54)	Patients with severe psychiatric disabilities (N=74)	12 months	Accelerated supported employment (no screening for job readiness, no prevocational training)	Gradual supported employment that followed job coach model; at least 4 months of prevocational work readiness training	Greater for the experimental group	Rates of rehospitalization were equivalent
Drake et al. (55)	Patients with severe mental illness (N=143)	18 months	Interpersonal placement and support: clinical and vocational services integrated within the mental health center	Group skills training: pre-employment skills training and support in obtaining and maintaining jobs provided by a professional rehabilitation agency outside of the mental health center	Greater for the experimental group despite approximately equivalent personnel and direct contact hours	Rates of rehospitalization were equivalent; the two groups had similar improvements in global functioning, self-esteem, quality of life, and symptoms
Drake et al. (56)	Patients with severe mental illness (N=152)	18 months	Individual placement and support: help obtaining competitive jobs provided by employment specialists within the mental health center	Enhanced vocational rehabilitation: stepwise vocational services delivered by rehabilitation agency	Greater for the experimental group despite same amount of job support	Rates of rehospitalization were equivalent; the two groups had similar improvements in symptoms, global adjustment, self-esteem, quality of life, and satisfaction

[a] Reports of randomized controlled trials published since the 1996 review by Penn and Mueser (2).
[b] Regular community jobs as opposed to those owned by a rehabilitation agency.

after 1 year), but there is an important caveat to this finding: the relapse prevention effect was lost in the second year, 3 months after the social skills training was reduced from weekly to biweekly. Thus, it is not clear whether the effect on relapse was due to the higher patient contact rather than a specific advantage of social skills training. Two studies that used the social problem-solving model (45, 46) and controlled for the nonspecific effects of patient contact failed to find an effect on relapse prevention, which suggests that some nonspecific aspects of social skills training (e.g., improved symptom monitoring) may reduce relapse rates. For other outcomes such as psychopathology and employment there have been no consistent effects reported for any of the social skills training modalities.

Effectiveness and transferability. The problem-solving model has been standardized into well-defined modules with printed manuals, making it easy to transfer to other settings. In a pre-post design, Wallace et al. (51) documented learning of skills in seven nonresearch settings as implemented by regular staff trained through a 2-day workshop. The study by Liberman (46) also documented the effectiveness of intervention implemented by paraprofessionals in a typical VA clinical setting.

Vocational Rehabilitation

Competitive employment (holding a regular community job as opposed to being employed in a program overseen by a rehabilitation agency) has been estimated at less than 20% for severely mentally ill persons and is probably lower for patients with schizophrenia (52). In an effort to keep patients as functional and autonomous as possible in the community, various programs have been implemented to help patients find jobs and maintain them. Supported employment programs, the most recent approach to enhancing outcomes beyond those associated with traditional vocational rehabilitation (like transitional or sheltered employment), aims to improve opportunities for competitive employment.

The implementation of supported employment programs differs along a number of dimensions. However, several common components across models may be identified, including a goal of permanent competitive employment, minimal screening for employability, avoidance of preoccupational training, individualized placement (i.e., not enclaves or mobile work crews), time-unlimited support, and consideration of client preferences (53).

Efficacy with regard to the primary outcome. We identified three randomized controlled trials for supported employment programs (54–56) that had competitive employment as the primary targeted outcome (Table 2). The results were consistent in demonstrating significant advantages for supported employment programs over control interventions. The unweighted mean among patients in supported employment programs for obtaining competitive employment was 65% (range=56%–78%), whereas the corresponding rate for patients in the control conditions was 26% (range=9%–40%). Thus, in contrast to traditional vocational-rehabilitation approaches, these results provide encouraging evidence for the efficacy of supported employment programs in terms of increasing rates of competitive employment.

These positive results must be interpreted in light of the small number of trials that have been conducted and a number of methodological limitations (described in detail

168

280

by Bond et al. [53]). Retention is a particularly important issue to consider, since dropout rates over 40% are not uncommon (53). Although supported employment programs appear to be efficacious in helping patients attain entry-level positions, there are no data to evaluate whether supported employment programs confer longer-term benefits for patients who may be capable of progressing beyond these positions. For patients who have poor work histories and limited premorbid skills (perhaps the majority of persons with schizophrenia), attainment of entry-level positions may be a reasonable outcome.

Efficacy with regard to secondary outcomes. Supportive employment programs do not appear to result in benefits for nonvocational outcomes (Table 2). For example, despite the belief that employment may produce such secondary benefits as improved self-esteem, improved quality of life, and reductions of symptoms and relapses, the studies reviewed provide little to no evidence to support these assumptions. However, it is possible that employment per se, apart from the vocational rehabilitation strategy implemented, could lead to improvement in other outcomes (57).

Are some interventions more efficacious? Drake et al. (56) compared two types of supported employment interventions, one with early placement plus integration of vocational and mental health services (interpersonal placement and support) and the other with initial training and later placement (and no integration of services). The interpersonal placement and support group achieved higher rates of competitive employment, but it is not clear whether the effect was due to early placement or integration of services.

Effectiveness and transferability. The efficacy of interpersonal placement and support, which was originally demonstrated in two small cities in New Hampshire (55), was subsequently replicated in a Washington, D.C., patient group with a very different ethnic composition (83% African American) (56). These results provide some evidence that supported employment programs are transferable to urban settings and to diverse ethnic and socioeconomic populations. Additionally, Drake et al. (56) documented the effectiveness of supported employment programs compared to standard vocational services available in the Washington, D.C., area. The availability of a treatment manual for interpersonal placement and support (58) should facilitate research into the transferability of this treatment modality.

Cognitive Behavior Therapy

Over the past decade, there has been a growing interest in applying cognitive behavior therapy techniques to persons with schizophrenia, particularly those who continue to experience psychotic symptoms despite optimal pharmacological treatment. The principal aims of cognitive behavior therapy for medication-resistant psychosis are to reduce the intensity of delusions and hallucinations (and the related distress) and promote active participation of the individual in reducing the risk of relapse and levels of social disability. Interventions focus on rationally exploring the subjective nature of the psychotic symptoms, challenging the evidence for these, and subjecting such beliefs and experiences to reality testing.

Efficacy with regard to the primary outcome. We identified five randomized controlled trials of cognitive behavior therapy for the treatment of psychotic symptoms as compared to standard or control treatment in patients with chronic psychoses (Table 3). For four of these studies, a reduction in delusions and hallucinations was the primary targeted outcome; one trial targeted reduced rehospitalization rates.

Three studies examined the effects of cognitive behavior therapy on medication-resistant psychotic symptoms in schizophrenic outpatients and included follow-ups of up to 1 year posttreatment. Kuipers et al. (59) found that patients receiving cognitive behavior therapy demonstrated a significant reduction in overall symptoms as compared to standard treatment alone but did not find a specific reduction in psychotic symptoms.

Tarrier et al. (60) found a reduction of delusions and hallucinations with cognitive behavior therapy compared to supportive counseling (of equal intensity) and routine care alone. The effects were clinically meaningful: 11 out of 33 of the patients treated with cognitive behavior therapy had reductions in delusions and hallucinations of at least 50% (compared to four out of 26 subjects who received supportive counseling). A particular effort was made in this study to ensure that symptoms were rated blindly. The advantage for cognitive behavior therapy was maintained at 12-month follow-up (61). A methodologically rigorous study by Sensky et al. (62) found that patients treated with cognitive behavior therapy or a befriending intervention (of equal intensity) plus routine care both experienced a reduction of psychotic symptoms following 9 months of treatment. At the end of treatment, there were no advantages for cognitive behavior therapy. However, at 9-month follow-up the treatment gains were sustained in the cognitive behavior therapy group but were not in the comparison condition. These studies suggest that the therapeutic benefit of cognitive behavior therapy is not simply attributable to nonspecific benefits of a psychological intervention.

In acutely psychotic inpatients, Drury et al. (63) found that cognitive behavior therapy adjunctive to antipsychotic medication resulted in a significantly faster and more complete recovery from the psychotic episode. At 9-month follow-up, 95% of the patients in the cognitive behavior therapy group reported no or only minor hallucinations or delusions as compared to 44% of patients in the control condition. A limitation of this study was that the raters of psychopathology also provided the experimental treatment.

TABLE 3. Psychosocial Treatment of Schizophrenia With Cognitive Behavior Therapy[a]

Study	Subjects	Length of Follow-Up	Treatment Group		Change in Positive Symptoms[b] or Rehospitalization Rate	Secondary Outcomes
			Experimental Condition	Control Condition		
Kuipers et al. (59, 65)	Psychiatric outpatients with psychosis (N=60)	18 months	Weekly cognitive behavior therapy for up to 9 months plus standard care	Standard care	Only the experimental group exhibited significant improvement in BPRS total scores	Both groups had similar improvements in psychotic symptoms and social functioning; the experimental group had greater reductions in delusional distress and the frequency of delusions
Tarrier et al. (60, 61)	Outpatients with schizophrenia (N=87)	12 months	Two sessions of cognitive behavior therapy a week for 10 weeks plus routine care	1) Two supportive counseling sessions a week for 10 weeks or 2) routine care	The experimental group reported psychotic symptom improvements that were greater than those for both control conditions at 3 months and the routine care condition at 12 months	All groups had similar improvements in negative symptoms; the experimental group experienced fewer exacerbations and days in the hospital than patients in the routine care condition
Sensky et al. (62)	Outpatients with schizophrenia (N=90)	9 months	Approximately one 45-minute cognitive behavior therapy session a week for 2 months, reduced session frequency for remaining 7 months plus routine care	Befriending intervention plus routine care	Both groups exhibited significant reductions in positive symptoms after 9 months of treatment; continued improvement at 9-month follow-up was reported for the experimental group only	The experimental group exhibited greater reductions in negative symptoms and depression
Drury et al. (63)	Patients with acute nonaffective psychosis (N=40)	9 months	Eight hours a week of cognitive behavior therapy administered in individual, group, and family formats	Matched hours of informal therapist support and structured activities	Patients in the experimental group exhibited greater reductions in positive symptoms by the 7th week, maintained at the 9-month follow-up	The two groups had similar reductions in disorganization and negative symptoms
Buchkremer et al. (64)	Outpatients with schizophrenia (N=124)	24 months	1) Fifteen sessions of cognitive psycho-therapy (7 weekly, 8 biweekly); 10 sessions of psychoeducational medication management (5 weekly, 5 biweekly); and 20 sessions of key-person counseling, or 2) cognitive psychotherapy and psychoeducational medication management only	Routine care	Rates of rehospitalization were equivalent for all three groups; post hoc analyses suggested reduced rehospitalization rates for the first experimental condition	Evidence suggested greater improvements in social functioning for patients in the first experimental group

[a] Reports of randomized controlled trials published since the 1996 review by Penn and Mueser (2).
[b] Delusions, hallucinations.

Buchkremer et al. (64) compared four programs of care (two that included cognitive behavior therapy) to routine care. The interventions were delivered over 8 months and were assessed after 1 and 2 years of follow-up. The predicted reduction in rehospitalizations with cognitive behavior therapy was not found, but the group that received the most intensive intervention (cognitive behavior therapy plus individual and family psychoeducational psychotherapy) showed a trend toward fewer hospitalizations. In addition, cognitive behavior therapy failed to demonstrate an effect on psychotic symptoms.

Overall, the few available randomized controlled trials provide some preliminary evidence for the efficacy of cognitive behavior therapy in reducing delusions and hallucinations in medication-resistant patients and for its use as a complement to pharmacotherapy in acute psychosis.

Efficacy with regard to secondary outcomes. Cognitive behavior therapy failed to improve social functioning (59, 65) or relapse rates (60), both of which have been targeted outcomes in medication-resistant patients. Studies that have reported negative symptom effects have generally not found significant improvements associated with

170

cognitive behavior therapy (60, 63, 64). However, the recent study by Sensky et al. (62) reported improvements in negative and depressive symptoms that were sustained up to 9 months following completion of treatment. A brief cognitive behavior therapy intervention based on motivational interviewing techniques that targeted compliance with antipsychotic medication showed significant improvements in compliance and patient attitudes toward drug treatment and insight into their illness as compared to standard treatment (66). However, the effects of this intervention were not translated into improvements in social functioning or symptoms.

Are some interventions more efficacious? Only one study has compared two forms of cognitive behavior therapy for medication-resistant psychotic symptoms. Tarrier et al. (67) found that coping strategy enhancement or problem-solving interventions both led to targeted reductions in psychotic symptoms, with no between-group differences. The lack of a no-treatment group limits conclusions that may be drawn regarding "active ingredients."

Cost-effectiveness. Kuipers et al. (65) reported some evidence that the monthly cost per patient was not higher for the cognitive behavior therapy group (£ 958) than for the standard treatment (£ 1,139) during an 18-month follow-up period. Because of the small study group size, this difference did not reach statistical significance.

Individual Therapy

Before the 1960s, individual psychoanalytically oriented therapy was considered by many the optimal treatment for schizophrenia. Following the negative findings in the landmark studies of May et al. (68) and Gunderson et al. (69), psychoanalytically oriented individual psychotherapy for most patients with schizophrenia has been practically eliminated in the United States. Only recently has a different form of intensive individual treatment been examined.

Hogarty et al. (10, 11) compared individual personal therapy for schizophrenia to family therapy, combined treatment, and supportive therapy in a 3-year trial. Personal therapy was conducted weekly (for 30 to 45 minutes) following an incremental approach individualized for the patients' stage of recovery: the initial phase focused on the relationship between stress and symptoms; the intermediate phase emphasized learning to use relaxation and cognitive reframing techniques when stressed; the advanced phase (which generally started 18 months into treatment) focused on seeking social and vocational initiatives in the community and applying what was learned in personal therapy.

For the primary outcome measure of relapse prevention, personal therapy was no different than the other conditions. However, the personal therapy group was clearly favored in a composite measure of social adjustment (with an effect size that was over twice as large as that seen with non-personal-therapy), with the greatest differential im-

provement occurring in the last 2 years. Adjustment data were derived from various sources: patient interview, therapist assessments, and relatives' perception, which argues for its validity. Limitations were that 40% of the patients assigned to personal therapy did not move on to the advanced phase of the treatment, and adjustment ratings were not blind to treatment conditions.

Conclusions

Summary of Findings

Over the last 4 years, research on psychosocial treatments for schizophrenia has continued to develop. We reviewed randomized controlled trials with a special emphasis on those published since the last update by Penn and Mueser (2). For the more extensively studied interventions (family therapy and assertive community treatment), the recent studies have had largely negative findings (8–10, 12, 33, 34). In our view, this does not so much put in doubt the large body of research supporting the efficacy of these treatments but rather is consistent with the level of evolution of research into these modalities. These findings reflect more sophisticated studies of either special populations (e.g., patients very early in their illness [8, 9]) or inclusion of enriched packages of care as control conditions (10, 12, 33, 34). In contrast, studies of two relatively new modalities, supported employment programs (54, 56) and cognitive behavior therapy (59–64), have shown mostly positive findings. Also, the few social skills training studies of interventions designed to increase generalization of skills (the social problem-solving [45, 46] and cognitive remediation models [50]) have reported promising results.

On the whole, the literature is consistent in that the various interventions have been largely successful for the primary outcome measures they were designed to target (i.e., family therapy and assertive community treatment for prevention of psychotic relapse and rehospitalization, social skills training for learning specific social behaviors, supported employment programs for obtaining competitive employment, and cognitive behavior therapy for reducing delusions and hallucinations). However, these effects tend to be domain specific and do not result in improvements in other clinically important secondary outcomes. For some interventions, this lack of an effect on other measures is not a serious limitation. With supported employment programs, attainment of competitive employment is clearly worthwhile, regardless of a limited effect on social adjustment or psychopathology. Likewise, with cognitive behavior therapy, reduction in the distress associated with psychotic symptoms is a highly desirable outcome, especially when other available treatments have failed. However, for the social skills training modalities, even if learning of skills is robust in most patients and can be maintained over time with relatively few resources, demonstrating some degree of generalizability and improved community functioning is crucial. Direct demonstration of use of learned skills in the community is a daunting methodological challenge yet to be accomplished.

The identification of "active ingredients" for different interventions has had very limited success. Beyond the general advantage of sustained over brief interventions in terms of primary outcomes, little is known regarding the specificity of the various treatments. Even for family interventions, the construct of "expressed emotion" has not been clearly shown to underlie the efficacy for relapse prevention. Also, when two forms of family interventions are compared, the literature is consistent that no advantages are evident. Similarly, recent studies of assertive community treatment suggest that "more is not necessarily better" and that for many patients, even those with high relapse rates, high-quality clinical case management with adequate service availability is equally effective. Because the effects of these interventions are mainly on relapse prevention, in populations of patients in which the base rate of relapse is already low (such as medication compliant persons early in their illness), there may be no advantage of adding family therapy, as the most recent studies suggest. With novel antipsychotic medications becoming the standard of care, compliance will hopefully improve, and relapse rates may be lowered; this could result in the amelioration of the effects of family treatment and assertive community treatment programs on relapse.

Transferability of efficacious treatments to more usual clinical settings has been documented for only a minority of interventions (like assertive community treatment and perhaps the social skills training problem-solving model). Cost-effectiveness has been documented for assertive community treatment when compared to usual community care but not when compared to another high-resource model of clinical case management.

Future Research

For the newer interventions such as supported employment programs, cognitive behavior therapy, cognitive remediation, and personal therapy, replication of the initial positive findings is necessary in large samples, in different settings, and by investigators not directly involved in the development of these treatment modalities. For family interventions and assertive community treatment, future research should concentrate on 1) identifying the minimal intensity of services that will maintain the relapse-preventing effects and 2) examining whether some subgroups of patients may benefit in particular. In the services research arena, it is necessary to demonstrate whether assertive community treatment programs effective in the community result in cost savings. Likewise, studies are needed of the cost-effectiveness of sustained psychoeducational family interventions added to adequate standard care.

Since effective interventions tend to be domain specific, it is important to investigate when to apply particular

treatments. Because the majority of patients will relapse, sustain deficits in social competence, and fail to attain competitive employment (and many will experience persistent psychosis), research is needed to guide the optimum sequencing and combination of specific services to be delivered. For example, should social skills training precede, follow, or be implemented concurrently with cognitive behavior therapy in patients with persistent psychosis and limited social skills? And for what subgroups of patients and at what stage of the illness should a particular intervention be implemented?

For the supported employment approach, future studies should address the issue of the extent of ongoing support required to maintain efficacy and changes in the social security disability system such as retention of benefits despite competitive employment that might foster these vocational gains.

Finally, because of the continued development of newer and hopefully better antipsychotic agents, the interactions between different psychosocial and pharmacological modalities should be investigated. We are aware of only two (20, 45) randomized trials that controlled the psychosocial as well as the pharmacological intervention (neither involved novel antipsychotic agents). One study (45) found an interaction between psychosocial and pharmacological treatments, which suggested that the problem-solving social skills training approach may provide protection against relapse among patients suboptimally medicated. The other study (20) found no interaction between two forms of family treatment and three antipsychotic medication dose regimens.

Clinical Recommendations

What implications can be drawn for the use of the psychosocial interventions described in this review, for the standard of care for persons suffering from schizophrenia? For frequent relapsers who reside with family, a relatively simple but sustained psychoeducational family approach should be offered (for example, monthly visits in a single or multifamily group setting). Additionally, for the majority of patients, the family should be viewed as a natural ally that can provide crucial early information regarding relapse, substance abuse, community functioning, and compliance. For patients with high service utilization rates, assertive community treatment programs should be considered, especially if family involvement is not available. With the large majority of schizophrenia patients living in the community and hospital stays becoming progressively shorter as a result of managed care, a comprehensive system of delivery of services based on assertive community treatment principles will continue to be necessary for a large proportion of patients.

Once stable community living is achieved, a systematic rehabilitation effort for the majority of persons with schizophrenia is necessary. Beyond allowing patients to make use of previously learned social skills once the psychotic process is sufficiently controlled, there is no compelling evidence that medications (even the novel drugs) offer additional benefits in terms of social competence (1). Specific strategies to teach social skills are available. Of these, the social problem-solving model not only has resulted in the acquisition of skills but also is the approach with some evidence that suggests generalization of skills to community functioning and of effectiveness in more routine clinical settings. The requirement of social skills training for clinicians specifically trained in these techniques presently limits their use, but the availability of printed manuals with well-defined modules targeting different areas of social functioning is a fundamental step towards disseminating these interventions.

Patients who wish to work should be referred to a vocational rehabilitation agency with resources for supported employment. No other psychosocial or pharmacological treatment has been shown to promote competitive employment. However, for many patients a traditional sheltered form of employment or no employment will remain the best option. Because presently there is no evidence to identify these patients in advance, the majority of persons suffering from schizophrenia should be offered the supported employment approach when available.

A large number of patients will continue to experience disturbing delusions and hallucinations despite the best available medications. Persistent symptoms after an adequate trial with one antipsychotic agent generally predict little response to other medications. Superiority for previously resistant psychotic symptoms has been demonstrated only for clozapine (1), but a recent meta-analysis of efficacy for this agent suggests that the effects, although important, are smaller than originally found (70). Therefore, the results from cognitive behavior therapy interventions are particularly encouraging. Currently, these strategies are in their infancy, there are few clinicians with the expertise to implement them, and it is not clear that even in the best hands these strategies will result in clinically meaningful sustained effects. Nevertheless, cognitive behavior therapy has become established for the treatment of depressive and anxiety disorders and may prove to be a valuable resource for clinicians helping persons with chronic psychotic disorders as well.

Received Feb. 1, 2000; revision received May 26, 2000; accepted June 5, 2000. From the Departments of Psychiatry and Psychology, University of New Mexico School of Medicine. Address reprint requests to Dr. Bustillo, Department of Psychiatry, University of New Mexico School of Medicine, 2400 Tucker NE, Albuquerque, NM 87131; jbustillo@salud.unm.edu (e-mail).

References

1. Bustillo JR, Lauriello J, Keith SJ: Schizophrenia: improving outcome. Harv Rev Psychiatry 1999; 6:229–240
2. Penn DL, Mueser KT: Research update on the psychosocial treatment of schizophrenia. Am J Psychiatry 1996; 153:607–617
3. Drake RE, Mercer-McFadden C, Mueser KT, McHugo GJ, Bond GR, Kosten TR, Ziedonis DM: A review of integrated mental health and substance abuse treatment for patients with dual disorders. Schizophr Bull 1998; 24:589–608
4. Brown GW, Rutter M: The measurement of family activities and relationships: a methodological study. Human Relations Suppl 1966; 2:10–15
5. Butzlaff RL, Hooley JM: Expressed emotion and psychiatric relapse: a meta-analysis. Arch Gen Psychiatry 1998; 55:547–552
6. Mueser KT, Glynn SM: Family intervention for schizophrenia, in Best Practice: Developing and Promoting Empirically Supported Interventions. Edited by Dobson KS, Craig KD. Newbury Park, Calif, Sage Publications, 1998, pp 157–186
7. Tarrier N, Barrowclough C, Fitzpatrick E: The Salford Family Intervention Project: relapse rates of schizophrenia at five and eight years. Br J Psychiatry 1994; 165:829–832
8. Linszen D, Dingemans P, Van Der Does JW, Nugter A, Scholte P, Lenior R, Goldstein MJ: Treatment, expressed emotion and relapse in recent onset schizophrenic disorders. Psychol Med 1996; 26:333–342
9. Nugter A, Dingemans P, Van der Does JW, Linszen D, Gersons B: Family treatment, expressed emotion and relapse in recent onset schizophrenia. Psychiatry Res 1997; 72:23–31
10. Hogarty GE, Kornblith SJ, Greenwald D, DiBarry AL, Cooley S, Ulrich RF, Carter M, Flesher S: Three-year trials of personal therapy among patients living with or independent of family, I: description of study and effects on relapse rates. Am J Psychiatry 1997; 154:1504–1513
11. Hogarty GE, Greenwald D, Ulrich RF, Kornblith SJ, DiBarry AL, Cooley S, Carter M, Flesher S: Three-year trials of personal therapy among schizophrenic patients living with or independent of family, II: effects on adjustment of patients. Am J Psychiatry 1997; 154:1514–1524
12. McFarlane WR, Dushay RA, Stastny P, Deakins SM, Link B: A comparison of two levels of family-aided assertive community treatment. Psychiatr Serv 1996; 47:744–750
13. Falloon IR, Boyd JL, McGill CW, Razani J, Moss HB, Gilderman AN: Family management in the prevention of exacerbations of schizophrenia: a controlled study. N Engl J Med 1982; 306:437–440
14. Leff J, Kuipers L, Berkowitz R, Berlein-Vries R, Sturgeon D: A controlled trial of social intervention in the families of schizophrenic patients. Br J Psychiatry 1982; 141:121–134
15. Hogarty GE, Anderson CM, Reiss DJ, Kornblith SJ, Greenwald DP, Javna CD, Madonia MJ: Family psychoeducation, social skills training, and maintenance chemotherapy in the aftercare treatment of schizophrenia, I: one-year effects of a controlled study on relapse and expressed emotion. Arch Gen Psychiatry 1986; 43:633–642
16. Tarrier N, Barrowclough C, Vaughn C, Bamrah JS, Porceddu K, Watts S, Freeman H: The community management of schizophrenia: a controlled trial of a behavioural intervention with families to reduce relapse. Br J Psychiatry 1988; 153:532–542
17. Zastowny TR, Lehman AF, Cole RE, Kane C: Family management of schizophrenia: a comparison of behavioral and supportive family treatment. Psychiatr Q 1992; 63:159–186
18. Leff J, Berkowitz R, Shavit N, Strachan A, Glass I, Vaughn C: A trial of family therapy versus a relatives group for schizophrenia. Br J Psychiatry 1989; 154:58–66
19. McFarlane WR, Lukens E, Link B, Dushay R, Deakins SA, Newmark M, Dunne EJ, Horen B, Toran J: Multiple-family groups and psychoeducation in the treatment of schizophrenia. Arch Gen Psychiatry 1995; 52:679–687
20. Schooler NR, Keith SJ, Severe JB, Matthews SM, Bellack AS, Glick ID, Hargreaves WA, Kane JM, Ninan PT, Frances A, Jacobs M, Lieberman JA, Mance R, Simpson GM, Woerner MG: Relapse and rehospitalization during maintenance treatment of schizo-

phrenia: the effects of dose reduction and family treatment. Arch Gen Psychiatry 1997; 54:453–463

21. Falloon IRH, McGill CW, Boyd JL, Pederson J: Family management in the prevention of morbidity of schizophrenia: social outcome of a two-year longitudinal study. Psychol Med 1987; 17:59–66

22. Barrowclough C, Tarrier N: Social functioning in schizophrenic patients, I: the effects of expressed emotion and family intervention. Soc Psychiatry Psychiatr Epidemiol 1990; 25:125–129

23. Zhang M, Yan H: Effectiveness of psychoeducation of relatives of schizophrenic patients: a prospective cohort study in five cities of China. Int J Ment Health 1993; 22:47–59

24. Randolf ET, Eth S, Glynn SM, Paz GG, Leong GB, Shaner AL, Strachan A, Van Vort W, Escobar JI, Liberman RP: Behavioural family management in schizophrenia: outcome of a clinic-based intervention. Br J Psychiatry 1994; 164:501–506

25. Lehman AF, Steinwachs DM (Survey Coinvestigators of the PORT Project): Patterns of usual care for schizophrenia: initial results from the Schizophrenia Patient Outcomes Research Team (PORT) client survey. Schizophr Bull 1998; 27:11–19

26. Xiong W, Phillips MR, Xiong H, Wang R, Dai Q, Kleinman J, Kleinman A: Family-based intervention for schizophrenic patients in China: a randomised controlled trial. Br J Psychiatry 1994; 165: 239–247

27. Zhang M, Wang M, Li J, Phillips MR: Randomised-control trial of family intervention for 78 first-episode male schizophrenic patients: an 18-month study in Suzhou, Jiangsu. Br J Psychiatry Suppl 1994; 165:96–102

28. Telles C, Karno M, Mintz J, Paz G, Arias M, Tucker D, Lopez S: Immigrant families coping with schizophrenia: behavioral family intervention v case management with a low-income Spanish-speaking population. Br J Psychiatry 1995; 167:473–479

29. Cardin VA, McGill CW, Falloon IRH: An economic analysis: costs, benefits, and effectiveness, in Family Management of Schizophrenia. Edited by IRH Falloon. Baltimore, Johns Hopkins University Press, 1986, pp 115–123

30. Tarrier N, Lowson K, Barrowclough C: Some aspects of family interventions in schizophrenia, II: financial considerations. Br J Psychiatry 1991; 159:481–484

31. Stein LI, Test MA: Alternative to mental hospital treatment, I: conceptual model, treatment program and clinical evaluation. Arch Gen Psychiatry 1980; 37:392–397

32. Mueser KT, Bond GR, Drake RE, Resnick SG: Models of community care for severe mental illness: a review of research on case management. Schizophr Bull 1998; 24:37–74

33. Holloway F, Carson J: Intensive case management for the severely mentally ill: controlled trial. Br J Psychiatry 1998; 172: 19–22

34. Issakidis C, Sanderson K, Teesson M, Johnston S, Buhrich N: Intensive case management in Australia: a randomized controlled trial. Acta Psychiatr Scand 1999; 99:360–367

35. Teague GB, Bond GR, Drake RE: Program fidelity in assertive community treatment: development and use of a measure. Am J Orthopsychiatry 1998; 68:216–232

36. Rosenheck RA, Neale MS: Cost-effectiveness of intensive psychiatric community care for high users of inpatient services. Arch Gen Psychiatry 1998; 55:459–466

37. Latimer E: Economic impacts of assertive community treatment: a review of the literature. Can J Psychiatry 1999; 44:443–454

38. Johnston S, Salkeld G, Sanderson K, Issakidis C, Teesson M, Buhrich N: Intensive case management: a cost-effectiveness analysis. Aust NZ J Psychiatry 1998; 32:551–559

39. Bellack A, Mueser K: Psychosocial treatment of schizophrenia. Schizophr Bull 1993; 19:317–336

40. Dilk MN, Bond GR: Meta-analytic evaluation of skills training research for individuals with severe mental illness. J Consult Clin Psychol 1996; 6:1337–1346

41. Hogarty G, Anderson C, Reiss D, Kornblith S, Greenwald D, Ulrich R, Carter M: Family psychoeducation, social skills training and maintenance chemotherapy in the aftercare treatment of schizophrenia, II: two-year effects of a controlled study on relapse and adjustment. Arch Gen Psychiatry 1991; 48:340–347

42. Wallace CJ, Liberman RP: Social skills training for patients with schizophrenia: a controlled clinical trial. Psychiatry Res 1985; 15:239–247

43. Brown MA, Munford AM: Life skills training for chronic schizophrenics. J Nerv Ment Dis 1983; 171:466–470

44. Eckman TA, Wirshing WC, Marder SR, Liberman RP, Johnston-Cronk K, Zimmerman K, Mintz J: Technique for training schizophrenic patients in illness self-management: a controlled trial. Am J Psychiatry 1992; 149:1549–1555

45. Marder SR, Wirshing WC, Mintz J, McKenzie J, Johnston K, Eckman TA, Lebell M, Zimmerman K, Liberman R: Two-year outcome of social skills training and group psychotherapy for outpatients with schizophrenia. Am J Psychiatry 1996; 153:1585–1592

46. Liberman RP, Wallace CJ, Blackwell G, Kopelowicz A, Vaccaro JV, Mintz J: Skills training versus psychosocial occupational therapy for persons with persistent schizophrenia. Am J Psychiatry 1998; 155:1087–1091

47. Brenner H, Hodel B, Roder V, Corrigan P: Treatment of cognitive dysfunctions and behavioral deficits in schizophrenia. Schizophr Bull 1992; 18:21–26

48. Hodel B, Brenner HD: Cognitive therapy with schizophrenic patients: conceptual basis, present state, future directions. Acta Psychiatr Scand Suppl 1994; 90:108–115

49. Wykes T, Reeder C, Corner J, Williams C, Everitt B: The effects of neurocognitive remediation on executive processing in patients with schizophrenia. Schizophr Bull 1999; 25:291–307

50. Spaulding WD, Reed D, Sullivan M, Richardson C, Weiler M: The effects of cognitive treatment in psychiatric rehabilitation. Schizophr Bull 1999; 25:291–307

51. Wallace CJ, Liberman RP, MacKain SJ, Blackwell, G, Eckman TA: Effectiveness and replicability of modules for teaching social and instrumental skills to the severely mentally ill. Am J Psychiatry 1992; 149:654–658

52. Lehman A: Vocational rehabilitation in schizophrenia. Schizophr Bull 1995; 21:645–656

53. Bond GR, Drake RE, Mueser KT, Becker DR: An update on supported employment for people with severe mental illness. Psychiatr Serv 1997; 48:335–346

54. Bond GR, Dietzen LL, McGrew JH, Miller LD: Accelerating entry into supported employment for persons with severe psychiatric disabilities. Rehab Psychol 1995; 40:91–111

55. Drake RE, McHugo GJ, Becker DR, Anthony WA, Clark RE: The New Hampshire study of supported employment for people with severe mental illness. J Consult Clin Psychol 1996; 64:391–399

56. Drake RE, McHugo GJ, Bebout RR, Becker DR, Harris M, Bond GR, Quimby E: A randomized clinical trial of supported employment for inner-city patients with severe mental disorders. Arch Gen Psychiatry 1999; 56:627–633

57. Bell MD, Lysaker PH, Milstein RM: Clinical benefits of paid work activity in schizophrenia. Schizophr Bull 1996; 22:51–67

58. Becker DR, Drake RE: A Working Life: The Individual Placement and Support (IPS) Program. Concord, New Hampshire-Dartmouth Psychiatric Research Center, 1993

59. Kuipers E, Garety P, Fowler D, Dunn G, Bebbington P, Freeman D, Hadley C: London-East Anglia randomised controlled trial of cognitive-behavioural therapy for psychosis, I: effects of treatment phase. Br J Psychiatry 1997; 171:319–327

286

60. Tarrier N, Yusupoff L, Kinney C, McCarthy E, Gledhill A, Haddock G, Morris J: Randomised controlled trial of intensive cognitive behaviour therapy for patients with chronic schizophrenia. Br Med J 1998; 317:303–307

61. Tarrier N, Wittkowski A, Kinney C, McCarthy E, Morris J, Humphreys L: Durability of the effects of cognitive-behavioural therapy in the treatment of schizophrenia: 12-month followup. Br J Psychiatry 1999; 174:500–504

62. Sensky T, Turkington D, Kingdon D, Scott JL, Scot J, Siddle R, O'Carroll M, Barnes TRE: A randomized controlled trial of cognitive-behavioral therapy for persistent symptoms in schizophrenia resistant to medication. Arch Gen Psychiatry 2000; 57: 165–172

63. Drury V, Birchwood M, Cochrana R, MacMillan F: Cognitive therapy and recovery from acute psychosis: a controlled trial, I: impact on psychotic symptoms. Br J Psychiatry 1996; 169: 593–601

64. Buchkremer G, Klingberg S, Holle R, Schulze Monking H, Hornung WP: Psychoeducational psychotherapy for schizophrenic patients and their key relatives or care-givers: results of a 2-year follow-up. Acta Psychiatr Scand 1997; 96:483–491

65. Kuipers E, Fowler D, Garety P, Chisholm D, Freeman D, Dunn G, Bebbington P, Hadley C: London-East Anglia randomised controlled trial of cognitive-behavioural therapy for psychosis, III: follow-up and economic evaluation at 18 months. Br J Psychiatry 1998; 173:61–68

66. Kemp R, Hayward P, Applewhaite G, Everitt B, David A: Compliance therapy in psychotic patients: randomised controlled trial. Br Med J 1996; 312:345–349

67. Tarrier N, Beckett R, Harwood S, Baker A, Yusupoff L, Ugarteburu I: A trial of two cognitive-behavioural methods of treating drug-resistant psychotic symptoms in schizophrenic patients, I: outcome. Br J Psychiatry 1993; 162:524–532

68. May PRA, Tuma AH, Dixon WJ, Yale C, Thiele DA, Kraude WH: Schizophrenia: a follow-up study of the results of five forms of treatment. Arch Gen Psychiatry 1981; 38:776–784

69. Gunderson JG, Frank AF, Katz HM, Vannicelli ML, Frosch JP, Knapp PH: Effects of psychotherapy in schizophrenia, II: comparative outcome of two forms of treatment. Schizophr Bull 1984; 10:564–598

70. Wahlbeck K, Cheine M, Essali A, Adams C: Evidence of clozapine's effectiveness in schizophrenia: a systematic review and meta-analysis of randomized trials. Am J Psychiatry 1999; 156: 990–999

Reversal of Antipsychotic-Induced Working Memory Deficits by Short-Term Dopamine D1 Receptor Stimulation

Stacy A. Castner, Graham V. Williams, Patricia S. Goldman-Rakic*

Chronic blockade of dopamine D2 receptors, a common mechanism of action for antipsychotic drugs, down-regulates D1 receptors in the prefrontal cortex and, as shown here, produces severe impairments in working memory. These deficits were reversed in monkeys by short-term coadministration of a D1 agonist, ABT 431, and this improvement was sustained for more than a year after cessation of D1 treatment. These findings indicate that pharmacological modulation of the D1 signaling pathway can produce long-lasting changes in functional circuits underlying working memory. Resetting this pathway by brief exposure to the agonist may provide a valuable strategy for therapeutic intervention in schizophrenia and other dopamine dysfunctional states.

The efficacy with which typical neuroleptics block D2 receptors is positively correlated with their ability to alleviate positive symptoms in schizophrenia (1). Chronic D2 antagonism, which is characteristic of neuroleptic therapy, up-regulates these receptors in both the striatum and prefrontal cortex (2). However, long-term D2 receptor blockade also induces a coincident down-regulation of D1-type receptors in the prefrontal cortex in non-human primates (3). D1 receptors are present in high concentrations in this region (4), and optimal stimulation at these sites potentiates signaling in neurons that are essential to the working memory process (5). Thus, we hypothesized that chronic haloperidol treatment in monkeys should induce working memory impairments due to insufficient stimulation at D1 receptors in the prefrontal cortex and, if so, that these deficits might be reversed by a D1 receptor agonist.

Six young adult female monkeys (6) were trained on delayed response (7) and delayed nonmatch-to-sample (DNMS) (8) tasks in order to assess spatial and object working memory, respectively. After establishing a consistent baseline performance, haloperidol, a typical neuroleptic commonly used in the treatment of schizophrenia, was administered twice daily [0.07 to 0.20 mg per kilogram body weight (mg/kg) per day] throughout all phases of the experiment (9). These doses approximate clinically effective doses (~5 to 15 mg/day) used in patients and compensate for the more rapid metabolism of the drug in monkeys. Performance on the tasks was assessed in alternate test sessions 3 to 5 days per week.

Section of Neurobiology, Yale University School of Medicine, 333 Cedar Street, New Haven, CT 06510, USA.

*To whom correspondence should be addressed. E-mail: Patricia.Goldman-Rakic@yale.edu

By the end of the pre-drug baseline testing period of 6 to 12 or more months, all six monkeys reached a consistent (~75%) level of performance on each task (Table 1 and Fig. 1, A and E; delayed response: $R = 0.01$, $F[1,159] = 0.03$, $P = 0.86$; two-object DNMS: $R = 0.19$, $F[1,97] = 3.47$, $P = 0.07$). After 1 to 4 months of chronic haloperidol administration, performance decrements emerged in five monkeys. A sixth monkey refused to leave the home cage at the lowest dose of haloperidol and had to be dropped from the group analysis. Regression analysis on data obtained from the five other monkeys revealed a highly significant impairment in performance on both working memory tasks (Fig. 1, B and F; delayed response: $R = -0.2$; $F[1,195] = 8.73$; $P = 0.003$; DNMS: $R = -0.48$; $F[1,103] = 29.82$; $P = 0.0000004$) (also see Table 1, Fig. 2, A and B, and Fig. 3A). In the spatial task, there was a significant effect of delay across all conditions; that is, monkeys made more errors at longer delays, independent of drug treatment (delay: $F[4,80] = 13.369$, $P = 0.0001$; treatment: $F[3,80] = 0.088$, $P = 0.9664$).

To determine the cognitive specificity of the haloperidol-induced deficits, we also tested the monkeys on two control tasks—object retrieval and fine motor performance—which required sensorimotor integrative skills but lacked a working memory requirement (10). Neither chronic haloperidol nor D1 agonist treatment affected the monkeys' performance on these tasks (fine motor: $F[3,19] = 0.35$, $P = 0.7906$, Fig. 3B; object retrieval: $F[3,15] = 1.36$, $P = 0.3302$ (11)), which indicates that the working memory deficits were not due to the sensory and motor components required to perform these tasks. With the exception of the monkey that refused to test, the monkeys showed no change in appetite, motivation, or sedation, nor did they display any extrapyramidal symptoms during haloperidol treatment.

Because the emergence of cognitive deficits falls within the time frame in which the D1 receptor in the prefrontal cortex has been shown to be down-regulated in previous studies (3), it seemed highly probable that the monkeys in the present study also experienced similar down-regulation of D1 receptors, and that their working memory impairments could be due to suboptimal stimulation at these prefrontal receptors.

To examine this possibility, the selective full D1 agonist ABT 431 [0.00001 to 0.0001mg/kg, intramuscular (i.m.)] was co-administered for five to six blocks of five consecutive days per week with a minimum washout period of 2 weeks between blocks (9). Across 3 to 7 months of this intermittent coadministration of D1 agonist, all monkeys displayed a significant improvement in their performance on the spatial working memory task (Fig. 1C; $R = 0.27$, $F[1,241] = 18.50$, $P =$

Table 1. Spatial and object working memory performance across all test conditions. Shown are the mean ± SEM for all five monkeys across baseline, the "impaired" haloperidol dose, the last two rounds of D1 agonist coadministration, and the post-D1 testing periods. Symbols indicate that performance under a particular condition differs significantly from that under another condition at an alpha level of 0.05, as indicated by factorial analysis of variance with Scheffe post-hoc comparisons.

Monkey	Baseline	Haloperidol	Haloperidol +D1 agonist	Haloperidol post-D1
		Delayed response		
ROS	66.00 ± 3.23	48.86 ± 2.30*	61.82 ± 2.70†	67.77 ± 1.14†
NOE	74.29 ± 2.24	56.47 ± 2.45*	65.46 ± 1.86	72.82 ± 1.26†
AUD	88.75 ± 1.58	74.35 ± 1.87*	80.00 ± 1.68*	83.81 ± 1.10†
DOR	76.94 ± 2.29	64.80 ± 2.13*	72.33 ± 2.43	78.00 ± 1.38†
RUP	81.55 ± 1.89	68.42 ± 2.42*	71.17 ± 1.45*	73.48 ± 1.11*
		Two-object DNMS		
ROS	78.00 ± 3.00	66.50 ± 3.58	78.75 ± 2.80	75.63 ± 1.97
NOE	66.88 ± 3.27	58.33 ± 2.36	61.88 ± 3.27	65.16 ± 2.08
AUD	76.25 ± 2.02	73.09 ± 2.99	74.17 ± 4.56	82.80 ± 2.14
DOR	74.09 ± 2.32	63.07 ± 2.16	69.00 ± 2.08	63.28 ± 3.25
RUP	72.86 ± 2.30	58.85 ± 2.54*	68.33 ± 1.74†	73.33 ± 1.55†

*Significant versus baseline.   †Significant versus haloperidol.

288

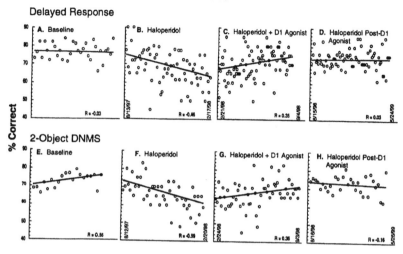

Delayed Response

A. Baseline   B. Haloperidol   C. Haloperidol + D1 Agonist   D. Haloperidol Post-D1 Agonist

2-Object DNMS

E. Baseline   F. Haloperidol   G. Haloperidol + D1 Agonist   H. Haloperidol Post-D1 Agonist

Test Sessions

Fig. 1. Circles represent the average performance of five monkeys on the spatial (top) and object working memory (bottom) tasks for individual test sessions across baseline, haloperidol, D1 agonist, and post-D1 testing periods. Baseline performance was stable before haloperidol treatment (A and E). Performance declined on haloperidol for both tasks (B and F). D1 agonist coadministration produced a significant (C) or near-significant (G) reversal of deficits. After D1 coadministration, the monkeys' performance on both tasks has remained stable for periods of up to 1 year (D and H). R values in the graphs reflect the mean performance of all five monkeys on given test sessions.

0.000025) and a nonsignificant but strong trend for improvement on the object working memory task (Fig. 1G; $R = 0.15$, $F[1,139] = 3.22$, $P = 0.075$) (see Table 1 for individual means). Upon repeated exposure to the agonist, the monkeys showed increasingly extended periods of sustained improvement on the working memory tasks, which carried over into the washout periods between coadministrations (Fig. 1, C and G, and Fig. 2, C and D), despite continued haloperidol treatment. Indeed, after the final treatment with D1 agonist, performance did not differ significantly from pre-haloperidol baseline for all monkeys on the object working memory task and for four monkeys on the spatial task (Table 1). This reversal has persisted, in some cases, for more than 1 year (Fig. 1, D and H; delayed response: $R = 0.03$, $F[1,293] = 0.32$, $P = 0.57$; DNMS: $R = -0.07$, $F[1,134] = 0.57$, $P = 0.45$). Further, the sixth monkey that stopped testing when given chronic haloperidol treatment began to test again on the first day of D1 agonist coadministration and has continued to test for more than a year since.

The present findings provide evidence that chronic haloperidol treatment can induce cognitive impairment and that these impair-

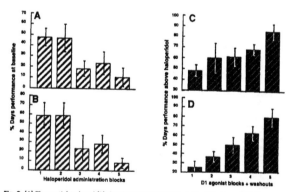

Fig. 2. (A) The spatial task and (B) the object task show the gradual emergence of haloperidol-induced cognitive deficits in five monkeys across 6 months. The period has been divided into five blocks of approximately equivalent numbers of test sessions per block. Data are expressed as the percent of test days on which cognitive performance did not differ significantly from baseline. (C) The spatial task and (D) the object task reveal that D1 coadministration progressively reverses the cognitive deficits. Each D1 agonist block includes test performance under D1 coadministration and during the subsequent washout. Data are expressed as the percentage of days on which cognitive performance was significantly above that shown under haloperidol treatment alone.

289

ments can be reversed by short-term D1 stimulation. This result is consistent with previous evidence about the behavioral effects of D1 agonists, both in monkeys and in patients with schizophrenia (12). However, because D2 up-regulation is also produced by chronic haloperidol treatment (3), the possibility exists that this change alone or in combination with D1 could also contribute to the cognitive deficits observed.

The developing pattern of cognitive enhancement evoked by intermittent D1 agonist administration is reminiscent of the phenomenon of behavioral sensitization to drugs that elevate dopamine release, such as amphetamine and cocaine (13). However, the present findings suggest a potentially beneficial role for selective stimulation of this receptor in altered dopaminergic states, such as we produced by blocking the D2 receptor (14). It remains to be determined whether a similar state exists in patients with schizophrenia

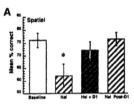

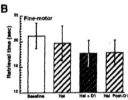

Fig. 3. Average performance of five monkeys on the spatial working memory (A) and fine motor (B) tasks for baseline (open bars), haloperidol (Hal) alone (white cross-hatched bars), D1 agonist coadministration (black cross-hatched bars), and up to 1 year of continued haloperidol after the final D1 washout period (white cross-hatched bars at right). Chronic haloperidol produced a significant impairment in delayed response performance [(A); $F[3, 20] = 4.36$, $P = 0.0189$; asterisk indicates $P < 0.05$ by Scheffe post-hoc comparison]. This deficit was improved during the 3 to 6 months of D1 agonist coadministration. In the 8- to 12-month period after D1, the monkeys exhibited sustained enhancement of cognitive performance as compared to the 6-month period of haloperidol alone ($P < 0.05$ by Scheffe post-hoc comparison). Conversely, all monkeys displayed only continued improvement, as indicated by decreased retrieval times, on the fine motor task (B) across treatment conditions (see text for statistics).

treated with a variety of neuroleptic drugs.

The enduring improvement in performance suggests that the agonist treatment induced a fundamental change in the circuits involved in working memory. These long-lasting changes may involve alterations in the D1 signal transduction pathway. Cyclic adenosine monophosphate (cAMP) production is stimulated by D1 agonists but inhibited by D2 agonists, particularly from the down-regulated state (15). It could be the case that cognitive improvement requires synergistic interactions between D1 stimulation and D2 blockade to achieve a high degree of activation of the cAMP cascade. An additional pathway may involve the novel protein calcyon, which has recently been shown to enable D1 potentiation of intracellular calcium release (16). Morphological changes could also be involved. Chronic haloperidol treatment in rodents decreases the density of dendritic spines in prefrontal neurons (17), whereas indirect dopamine agonists have been shown to increase the density of dendritic spines (18). Another strong possibility is that D1 agonist treatment may normalize D2 receptor sensitivity, and this may be the mechanism that reinstates and maintains normal cognitive performance.

The present findings have potential relevance for the treatment of cognitive deficits and/or negative symptoms in a variety of conditions, including schizophrenia, Parkinson's disease, and age-related memory decline. D1 down-regulation in the prefrontal cortex has recently been reported in both drug-naïve and medicated schizophrenic patients (19). Thus, the persistent recovery produced by brief periods of coadministration of D1 agonist revealed here suggests that schizophrenic patients now treated with D2 antagonist drugs may show substantial improvements in their cognitive abilities from a limited adjuvant exposure to a D1 agonist.

References and Notes
1. P. Seeman, *Synapse* 1, 133 (1987).
2. W. J. Florijn, F. I. Tarazi, I. Creese, *J. Pharmacol. Exp. Ther.* 280, 561 (1997); J. R. Goss, A. B. Kelly, D. G. Morgan, *Life Sci.* 48, 1015 (1991); P. R. Buckland, M. C. O'Donovan, P. McGuffin, *Neurosci Lett.* 150, 25 (1993).
3. M. S. Lidow and P. S. Goldman-Rakic, *Proc. Natl. Acad. Sci. U.S.A.* 91, 4353 (1994); M. S. Lidow, J. D. Elsworth, P. S. Goldman-Rakic, *J. Pharmacol. Exp. Ther.* 281, 597 (1997); M. S. Lidow, G. V. Williams, P. S. Goldman-Rakic, *Trends Pharmacol. Sci.* 19, 136 (1998).
4. M. S. Lidow et al., *Neuroscience* 40, 657 (1991); P. S. Goldman-Rakic et al., *J. Neural Transm. Suppl.* 36, 163 (1992).
5. T. Sawaguchi and P. S. Goldman-Rakic, *Science* 251, 947 (1991); A. F. T. Arnsten and P. S. Goldman-Rakic, *Arch. Gen. Psychiatry* 55, 362 (1998); J. X. Cai and A. F. T. Arnsten, *J. Pharmacol. Exp. Ther.* 282, 1 (1997); G. V. Williams and P. S. Goldman-Rakic, *Nature* 376, 572 (1995).
6. Monkeys received a maintenance number of biscuits, fruit, and peanuts each day. They were housed individually and maintained in accordance with Yale Animal Use and Care Committee guidelines for nonhuman primates.
7. Delayed response was measured as follows: A well was
baited in the monkey's view, then all the wells (two to four) were covered with identical plaques and an opaque screen was lowered for a randomized delay. After the delay, the animal had to move the correct plaque to obtain the reward. Performance was maintained at 75% by increasing the delays or the number of wells. The maximal delay set for a given number of wells included 0-, 10-, 20-, 30-, and 40-s delays. Monkeys were required to perform 20 trials.
8. Monkeys were trained on a traditional DNMS task (20). Next, they were trained to 75% performance on two-object DNMS, where only two objects were randomly selected as the "original" and "novel" stimuli for 20 trials during a given test session.
9. Haloperidol (in powder form) was obtained from RBI (Natick, MA). Daily doses were weighed out from a haloperidol:sucrose (1:99) mixture. Haloperidol was always administered (twice daily, 8 to 12 hours apart) after testing and disguised in fruit. The selective D1 agonist ABT 431 (provided by Hoechst Marion Roussel) was dissolved in nitrogen-percolated double-distilled water under dark conditions with 0.2% ascorbic acid. Individual aliquots were stored in light-protected containers at −70°C. This drug was always administered (i.m.) 30 min before testing.
10. For the object retrieval task, a three-dimensional clear Plexiglas box (4 inches by 4 inches) with an opening on one side was used. Animals performed nine trials per session, with the location of the opening (left, right, or front) randomized across trials. All trials were baited in the view of the monkey. The retrieval time and the number of barrier reaches were recorded. The fine motor task required the monkeys to use only the thumb and index finger to retrieve 20 treats from recessed wells on a clear Plexiglas board. The retrieval time and the number of drops were recorded.
11. S. A. Castner, G. V. Williams, P. S. Goldman-Rakic, unpublished observations.
12. J. X. Cai and A. F. T. Arnsten, *J. Pharmacol. Exp. Ther.* 282, 1 (1997); A. F. T. Arnsten et al., *Psychopharmacology* 116, 143 (1994); G. L. Wenk et al., *Neurobiol. Aging* 10, 11 (1989); J. de Keyser et al., *Brain Res.* 528, 308 (1990); T. Suhara et al., *Psychopharmacology* 103, 41 (1991); J. O. Rinne, P. Lonneberg, P. Marjamaki, *Brain Res.* 508, 349 (1990); C. Marin and T. N. Chase, *Eur. J. Pharmacol.* 231, 191 (1993); M. Davidson et al., *Arch. Gen. Psychiatry* 47, 190 (1990); J. S. Schneider, Z.-Q. Sun, D. P. Roeltgen, *Brain Res.* 663, 140 (1994).
13. T. E. Robinson and J. B. Becker, *Brain Res.* 396, 157 (1986); P. W. Kalivas and J. Stewart, *Brain Res. Rev.* 16, 223 (1991); J. Stewart and P. Vezina, *Brain Res.* 495, 401 (1989); P. Vezina, *J. Neurosci.* 16, 2411 (1996); Y. Bijjou et al., *J. Pharmacol. Exp. Ther.* 277, 1177 (1996); C. A. Crawford et al., *Neuroreport* 8, 2523 (1997).
14. H. Criswell, R. A. Mueller, G. R. Breese, *J. Neurosci.* 9, 125 (1989); *Brain Res.* 512, 282 (1990).
15. O. Civelli, J. R. Bunzow, D. K. Grandy, *Annu. Rev. Pharmacol. Toxicol.* 32, 281 (1993).
16. Lezcano et al., *Science* 287, 1660 (2000).
17. J. J. Kelley et al., *Exp. Neurol.* 146, 471 (1997); S. L. Vincent et al., *Neuropsychopharmacology* 5, 147 (1991).
18. T. E. Robinson and B. Kolb, *Eur. J. Neurosci.* 11, 1598 (1999); *J. Neurosci.* 17, 8491 (1997).
19. G. Sedvall and L. Farde, *Lancet* 346, 743 (1995); Y. Okubo, T. Suhara, Y. Sudo, M. Toru, *Molec. Psychiatry* 2, 291 (1997); T. Suhara et al., *Psychopharmacology* (Berlin) 106, 14 (1992); Y. Okubo et al., *Nature* 385, 634 (1997); H. Y. Meltzer and S. R. McGurk, *Schizophr. Bull.* 25, 233 (1999).
20. J. Bachevalier and M. Mishkin, *Behav. Neurosci.* 98, 770 (1984).
21. We thank T. A. Trakht and H. A. Findlay for their expert technical assistance and Hoechst Marion Roussell for funding this work and for their kind gift of ABT-431. Additional funding was provided by grants from the National Institutes of Mental Health (P50MH44866) and the National Institute of Drug Abuse (P01DA10160).

8 November 1999; accepted 25 January 2000

Clozapine for the Treatment-Resistant Schizophrenic

A Double-blind Comparison With Chlorpromazine

John Kane, MD; Gilbert Honigfeld, PhD; Jack Singer, MD; Herbert Meltzer, MD; and the Clozaril Collaborative Study Group

• The treatment of schizophrenic patients who fail to respond to adequate trials of neuroleptics is a major challenge. Clozapine, an atypical antipsychotic drug, has long been of scientific interest, but its clinical development has been delayed because of an associated risk of agranulocytosis. This report describes a multicenter clinical trial to assess clozapine's efficacy in the treatment of patients who are refractory to neuroleptics. DSM-III schizophrenics who had failed to respond to at least three different neuroleptics underwent a prospective, single-blind trial of haloperidol (mean dosage, 61 ± 14 mg/d) for six weeks. Patients whose condition remained unimproved were then randomly assigned, in a double-blind manner, to clozapine (up to 900 mg/d) or chlorpromazine (up to 1800 mg/d) for six weeks. Two hundred sixty-eight patients were entered in the double-blind comparison. When a priori criteria were used, 30% of the clozapine-treated patients were categorized as responders compared with 4% of chlorpromazine-treated patients. Clozapine produced significantly greater improvement on the Brief Psychiatric Rating Scale, Clinical Global Impression Scale, and Nurses' Observation Scale for Inpatient Evaluation; this improvement included "negative" as well as positive symptom areas. Although no cases of agranulocytosis occurred during this relatively brief study, in our view, the apparently increased comparative risk requires that the use of clozapine be limited to selected treatment-resistant patients.

(Arch Gen Psychiatry 1988;45:789-796)

The efficacy of antipsychotic drugs in short-term and maintenance treatment of schizophrenia has been well established in numerous double-blind placebo controlled trials over the past 30 years.[1,2] However, despite the considerable magnitude of the medication effect in this condition, most controlled trials continue to find a subgroup of 10% to 20% of patients who derive little benefit from typical neuroleptic drug therapy.[1] The treatment of this

refractory subgroup remains a major public health problem—these individuals require more intensive care and are subject to the persistent disabilities associated with chronic schizophrenia. In addition, the continued presence of psychotic signs and symptoms makes these patients less available to psychosocial and vocational rehabilitation.

It is estimated that about 1 million Americans suffer from schizophrenia. While there are no definitive data available on how many do not respond to neuroleptics, extrapolations from clinical trial data suggest that there may be 100 000 to 200 000 such patients.

Data from maintenance medication trials indicate that even among patients initially responsive to antipsychotic drugs, 20% to 30% may relapse during the first year or two of maintenance drug treatment.[3] A proportion of these patients contributes to the number in the subgroup of patients refractory to treatment. Since many of these patients remain ill, there is a cumulative increase in the number of people in the treatment-refractory category.

See also p 865.

The recognition that some patients do not benefit from typical neuroleptics has resulted in research along two fronts: (1) to identify phenomenologic, demographic, and/ or biologic factors that may be associated with poor treatment response and (2) to explore alternative treatment strategies that might be beneficial to this subgroup. With regard to the former, there are no consistently replicated findings providing clues about why patients are refractory to treatment. There are countless reports of anecdotal or pilot study experiences with a variety of alternative treatments for poor responders. However, no particular strategy has been found to be more than occasionally useful; with controlled studies, the usual result is that the experimental treatment proves to be no more effective than conventional treatments.

Since the introduction of chlorpromazine, numerous other chemical classes and compounds with antipsychotic activity have been used. Despite considerable differences in chemical structures, these agents seem to share an ability to bind to dopamine receptors. When in vitro binding assays are used, antidopaminergic (specifically, dopamine D_2 receptor antagonism) and therapeutic potency are highly correlated.[4] To a greater or lesser degree these are all "neuroleptics," ie, associated with short-term extrapyramidal side effects (including dystonias) and share the longer-term liability of inducing tardive dyskinesia. Despite numerous comparative trials, there are no consistent data suggesting that any specific antipsychotic drug or drug class is superior to any other in treating schizophrenia.[1,2]

Over the past decade, considerable effort has gone into the development and testing of potential antipsychotic compounds designated *atypical*. The concept of atypicality, however, is a working concept rather than a well-delineated

Accepted for publication March 9, 1988.

From the Department of Psychiatry, Hillside Hospital–Long Island Jewish Medical Center, Glen Oaks, NY (Dr Kane); the Department of Psychiatry, State University of New York at Stony Brook (Dr Kane); the Department of Medical Research, the Sandoz Research Institute, East Hanover, NJ (Drs Honigfeld and Singer); the Department of Psychiatry, University of Medicine and Dentistry of New Jersey–Robert Wood Johnson Medical School, Piscataway (Dr Singer); and the Department of Psychiatry, Case Western Reserve School of Medicine, Cleveland (Dr Meltzer). The members of the Clozaril Collaborative Study Group are as follows: Joyce Small, MD, Indianapolis; Richard Borison, MD, Augusta, Ga; Rob Conley, MD, Pittsburgh; Richard Wagner, MD, Providence, RI; Jan Volavka, MD, New York; John Rotrosen, MD, New York; Donald Seidel, MD, San Antonio, Tex; Larry Ereshefsky, PharmD, San Antonio, Tex; Jerome Costa, MD, Norwalk, Calif; John Herrera, PhD, Norwalk, Calif; Samuel Gershon, MD, Detroit; Neil Hartman, MD, Los Angeles; George Simpson, MD, Philadelphia; Richard Abrams, MD, Chicago; Benjamin Graber, MD, Omaha; and Martha Martin, MD, Washington, DC.

Read in part before the 140th Annual Meeting of the American Psychiatric Association, Chicago, May 14, 1987.

Reprint requests to Department of Psychiatry, Hillside Hospital, Long Island Jewish Medical Center, PO Box 38, Glen Oaks, NY 11004 (Dr Kane).

291

and validated classification. In general, this term has been used to describe drugs that appear to have limited short-term extrapyramidal effects in animals or human subjects. Most are more selective in their dopamine D_2 antagonist properties (eg, sulpiride or raclopride) and/or more broadly active, with marked antiserotonergic, antinoradrenergic, or other effects as well (eg, clozapine).

Clozapine (8-chloro-11-(4-methyl-1-piperazinyl)-5H-dibenzo[b,e][1,4]diazepine) belongs to the chemical class of dibenzodiazepines, related chemically to the antipsychotic dibenzoxazepine drug loxapine. However, its pharmacologic characteristics are different from those of loxapine. Clozapine has serotonin (S_2), adrenergic (α_1), and histaminergic (H_1) blocking activity. It is also a potent muscarinic acetylcholine receptor antagonist.[4-7] Its binding to D_1 and D_2 receptors is relatively weak and more equivalent than that of most typical neuroleptics.[8] The relationship between these characteristics and clozapine's clinical effects remains highly speculative, and a full review of this topic is beyond the scope of this report.[9]

Unlike "typical" neuroleptics, clozapine produces only slight, transient elevations in serum prolactin levels in patients, even when moderate to high doses are given.[10,11] Its profile of extrapyramidal side effects appears to be very different from those of typical neuroleptics. In both US and foreign studies, it has been reported that clozapine does not induce dystonia when administered on a short-term basis, and although akinesia or akathisia develops in some patients, the incidence appears to be low.[12]

Thirteen cases of "dyskinesia" were reported from a sample of 12 000 patients in Europe, but the nature of these cases is not clear (unpublished results, P. Krupp, MD, and C. Monka, Sandoz Ltd, Basel, Switzerland, 1987). There has been one report of clozapine apparently exacerbating preexisting tardive dyskinesia.[13] One case of apparent neuroleptic malignant syndrome has been reported in a patient receiving clozapine and lithium.[14]

Previous controlled clinical trials have been conducted with clozapine. Claghorn et al[15] reported a six-center double-blind comparison of clozapine and chlorpromazine in 151 hospitalized schizophrenic patients who had experienced either extrapyramidal side effects or tardive dyskinesia with at least two different neuroleptics. Clozapine was significantly superior to chlorpromazine according to the major efficacy measures, and it produced fewer side effects. The dosage ratio of chlorpromazine to clozapine in this study was approximately 2:1. Fischer-Cornelssen and Ferner[16] conducted a five-center double-blind comparison of clozapine and chlorpromazine in 223 hospitalized schizophrenic patients; they found clozapine to be superior in efficacy, particularly among the more severely ill patients. In this study, however, the mean chlorpromazine dose at six weeks was only 360 mg compared with 310 mg of clozapine. In a similar two-center European study,[16] clozapine was compared with haloperidol in a sample of 79 schizophrenic inpatients. The average dosage of clozapine was 397 mg/d at day 40 compared with a dosage of 7.6 mg/d of haloperidol. Though clozapine was found to be more efficacious, the latter two comparisons could be criticized on the basis of inadequate dosing of the reference drug. The results of these clinical trials suggested that clozapine is an effective antipsychotic drug and also provided some suggestions of potential benefit in patients who are more severely ill or refractory to treatment.

However, in 1975, granulocytopenia developed in 16 patients in Finland, and agranulocytosis developed in 13 of these patients (eight fatalities resulted from secondary infection).[17,18] Worldwide experience now reveals over 100 cases of agranulocytosis in patients receiving clozapine. Because of this, the use of clozapine was curtailed in many countries, and the drug was withdrawn for a time from clinical research by its US sponsor. For humanitarian reasons, some countries (including the United States) allowed continued use of the drug for carefully selected patients who were resistant to treatment, sensitive extrapyramidal side effects, or dyskinetic; these patients underwent intensive precautionary monitoring of white blood cell and differential counts. Since the introduction of restrictions in use and intensive hematologic monitoring, the overall incidence of agranulocytosis has declined, and has the lethal risk for patients in whom this reaction develops. Overall estimates continue to indicate that the risk of agranulocytosis with clozapine exceeds that associated with other antipsychotic drugs. In the United States, this problem developed in ten patients of 894 treated, and all of these patients recovered without any apparent long-term effect. Using the life-table method of calculating risk, data from the US experience indicate a 2% cumulative incidence after 52 weeks of clozapine treatment (95% confidence limits, 0.2% and 4%).[19] Based on US and worldwide experience, the risk of this adverse effect does not appear to be related to age, sex, or dose. The risk of "benign" neutropenia, however, does not appear to be any higher than with marketed neuroleptics.

Given clozapine's apparently greater risk and its promise of benefit for patients unresponsive to neuroleptics, the decision was made to initiate a controlled trial in carefully selected treatment-resistant patients. In considering the benefit-to-risk ratio of a therapeutic trial of clozapine, the time course of the development of agranulocytosis was also considered. The majority of agranulocytosis cases worldwide have occurred between the sixth and 18th weeks of clozapine treatment. Previous data also suggest that six weeks would provide a reasonably accurate test of the drug's therapeutic potential in individual patients. Exposure beyond that time was therefore limited in the present study to only those patients who had already shown significant therapeutic benefit from clozapine.

METHODS
Study Design

This study was designed to test the comparative efficacy of clozapine in schizophrenic inpatients who by history and prospective study would be considered to be resistant to treatment. Sixteen participating centers contributed data on a total of 319 patients. Patients had to meet DSM-III[20] criteria for schizophrenia. The criteria for being classified as refractory to treatment included the following: (1) at least three periods of treatment in the preceding five years with neuroleptic agents (from at least two different chemical classes) at dosages equivalent to or greater than 1000 mg/d of chlorpromazine for a period of six weeks, each without significant symptomatic relief, and (2) no period of good functioning within the preceding five years.

Subjects had to meet the following psychopathologic severity criteria: total Brief Psychiatric Rating Scale (BPRS) score of at least 45 (18-item version, in which 1 indicates absent and 7 indicates severe) plus a minimum Clinical Global Impressions (CGI) Scale rating of 4 (moderately ill). In addition, item scores of at least 4 (moderate) were required on two of the following four BPRS items: conceptual disorganization, suspiciousness, hallucinatory behavior, and unusual thought content.

All patients who met both the historical criteria for treatment resistance and the initial severity criteria and gave their informed consent entered a prospective period of treatment with haloperidol (up to 60 mg/d or higher) and benztropine mesylate (6 mg/d) for a period of six weeks to confirm the lack of drug responsiveness. Improvement in this context was defined a priori as a 20% decrease in the BPRS total score plus either a post-treatment CGI Scale

292

rating of mildly ill (≤3) or a post-treatment BPRS score of 35 or less. Any haloperidol responders (ie, those who met the improvement criteria) were dropped from further study.

Patients who met the multiple psychiatric symptom criteria were then randomly assigned to a six-week double-blind treatment trial with either clozapine (up to 900 mg/d) or chlorpromazine and benztropine mesylate (up to 1800 mg/d of chlorpromazine hydrochloride and up to 6 mg/d of benztropine mesylate). All medications were coded and administered under double-blind conditions; in addition to coded active antipsychotic medication in blue capsules, patients received either white benztropine tablets (chlorpromazine group) or identical white placebo tablets (clozapine group). The use of prophylactic benztropine mesylate (up to 6 mg/d) for all patients receiving chlorpromazine was designed to enhance the double-blind condition, in light of clozapine's previously established profile of reduced extrapyramidal side effects. In addition, this strategy was thought to minimize the potential for behaviorally manifest adverse effects to confound assessment of the relative clinical efficacy of the two drugs.

Before the start of the study, a priori criteria for supporting the superiority of clozapine in this patient population were determined. These criteria required proof of statistical superiority in all of three predetermined areas: the CGI Scale, changes in BPRS total score, and improvement in at least two of the following four BPRS items (or the cluster score derived from summing these four items): conceptual disorganization, hallucinatory behavior, suspiciousness, and unusual thought content.

Treatment

Patients entering the double-blind phase of the study were treated for six weeks. During the first two weeks, the dosage was titrated upward, if well tolerated, to dosage levels of either 500 mg/d of clozapine or 1000 mg/d of chlorpromazine (plus 6 mg/d of benztropine mesylate for chlorpromazine patients only). Dosing during the final four weeks was flexible, to maximum allowable dosages of 900 mg/d of clozapine and 1800 mg/d of chlorpromazine (plus up to 6 mg/d of benztropine mesylate). The number of patients entering each study period was as follows:

Period No.	Description	Duration, d	No. of Patients
1	Baseline placebo	≤14	319
2	Haloperidol	≤42	305
3	Placebo washout	≤7	272
4	Double-blind	≤42	268

Of the patients who entered period 4, 126 were randomized to clozapine, and 142 were randomized to chlorpromazine and benztropine mesylate.

Evaluation of Efficacy

Patients were interviewed by physicians or psychologists weekly during the course of double-blind treatment, and their assessments were recorded on the BPRS and on a seven-point CGI Scale (in which 1 indicates no mental illness and 7 indicates severe mental illness). In addition, patients were regularly evaluated in terms of ward behavior by the nursing staff, using the 30-item Nurses' Observation Scale for Inpatient Evaluation (NOSIE-30).[21]

Evaluation of Safety

Adverse reactions were evaluated by systematic patient query and observation by both medical and nursing personnel. Reactions were graded for severity and evaluated as to attribution to study drug, and the course of the reaction was documented. Regular clinical laboratory tests were performed, as were physical examinations, an electrocardiogram, and vital sign determinations. Systematic assessments of extrapyramidal symptoms and abnormal involuntary movements were made weekly using the Simpson-Angus Scale for Extrapyramidal Side Effects[22] and the Abnormal Involuntary Movements Scale (AIMS).[23]

SUBJECTS

Three hundred nineteen inpatients entered this study; their demographic and treatment history characteristics are summarized in Tables 1 and 2. Only 20% of the patients were female, largely due to the high proportion of Veterans Administration

Table 1. — Sex, Race, and Diagnosis of Patients Entering the Study (N = 319)

Characteristic	No. (%) of Patients
Sex	
M	256 (80)
F	63 (20)
Race	
White	208 (65)
Black	74 (23)
Hispanic	31 (10)
Oriental	2 (1)
Other	4 (1)
Diagnosis (DSM-III schizophrenic subtypes)	
Undifferentiated	160 (50)
Paranoid	107 (34)
Disorganized	25 (8)
Residual	11 (3)
Unspecified	10 (3)
Catatonic	6 (2)

medical centers among the participating institutions and possibly also because women were less likely to have received 1000-mg chlorpromazine equivalents of three different neuroleptics.

The typical patient was a 35-year-old male chronic undifferentiated schizophrenic first hospitalized for psychosis at age 20 years, after which seven or eight additional periods of hospitalization ensued. The median duration of the current hospitalization was about two years.

RESULTS

Over 80% of the patients completed the six-week prospective haloperidol phase of the study. A complete tabulation of patient outcomes after haloperidol treatment is provided in Table 3. Of those patients who completed the full six weeks of haloperidol treatment (dosages up to 60 mg/d and greater; mean [SD], 61 [14] mg/d), 80% were nonresponders. Fewer than 2% were classified as haloperidol responders. In the balance of the patients, haloperidol was terminated early for a variety of reasons, the most prominent of which was intolerance to haloperidol. On average, haloperidol-treated patients showed no change during the course of six weeks of treatment in any areas of the BPRS or NOSIE-30. Twenty-two patients were unable to tolerate the complete haloperidol phase due to adverse effects, but since they met all retrospective criteria for treatment resistance, they were allowed to continue into the double-blind comparison. (Thirteen of these patients received chlorpromazine, and nine received clozapine. Efficacy analyses excluding these patients were also carried out and did not alter the results.)

Two hundred sixty-eight patients entered the critical clozapine vs chlorpromazine and benztropine double-blind phase. The diagnostic composition of each treatment subgroup in the double-blind phase was similar to that seen initially: approximately half of the patients in each treatment group were in the "undifferentiated" category and about one third were in the "paranoid" category. From the point of view of psychiatric history, the subgroups did not differ in any significant way in major characteristics of patient history and treatment, including age at first hospitalization for psychosis, number of hospitalizations, duration of illness, duration of current episode, and duration of present hospitalization.

Average daily doses of active antipsychotic medication received during double-blind treatment are shown by treatment week in Fig 1. Adequate dose levels of each drug were attained with mean peak dosages exceeding 1200 mg/d of chlorpromazine and 600 mg/d of clozapine. The decrease in average dosage for both treatment groups at week 6 reflects the mandated taper-down at the end of the treatment period for all patients, designed to avoid abrupt discontinuation.

Review of dispositions at the end of each patient's double-blind participation indicated high overall completion rates for both clozapine- and chlorpromazine-treated patients (88% and 87%, respectively). Early terminations occurred for the following reasons: adverse reactions (6%), illness not related to drugs (1%),

293

Table 2.—General Characteristics of Patients Entering the Study (N = 319)

Characteristic	No. of Patients*	Median	Mean (SD)	Range
Age, y	318	35.0	35.7 (8.87)	20-59
Duration of current symptoms, wk	307	212.0	314.7 (316.76)	5-1976
Age at first hospitalization, y	294	20	20.4 (4.61)	8-40
No. of hospitalizations	245	7.0	9.2 (7.26)	1-50
Duration of current hospitalization, wk	304	104.0	215.9 (321.41)	0-1976

*The number of patients varies because of "missing" or "unknown" data elements.

Table 3.—Patient Classification After Treatment With Haloperidol and Benztropine

Patient Classification	No. (%) of Patients (n = 305)
Haloperidol responder	5 (1.6)
Haloperidol nonresponder	248 (81.3)
Terminated early	52 (17.0)
Intolerant of haloperidol	22 (7.2)
Uncooperative	15 (4.9)
Protocol violated	4 (1.3)
Physical conditions not related to drug	5 (1.6)
Other (eg, seizure, electrocardiographic changes, withdrew consent)	6 (2.0)

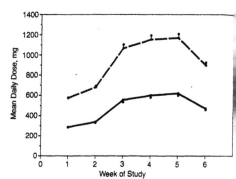

Fig 1.—Mean daily doses of clozapine (solid line) and chlorpromazine (broken line) during double-blind phase of study (period 4). For clozapine, at week 1, n = 126; week 2, n = 126; week 3, n = 122; week 4, n = 120; week 5, n = 119; and week 6, n = 116. For chlorpromazine, at week 1, n = 141; week 2, n = 140; week 3, n = 137; week 4, n = 133; week 5, n = 128; and week 6, n = 125.

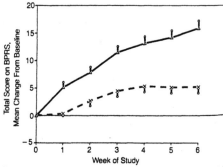

Fig 2.—Mean change from baseline in total score on Brief Psychiatric Rating Scale (BPRS) for patients treated with clozapine (solid line, n = 126) or chlorpromazine and benztropine mesylate (broken line, n = 139). $P<.001$ during each week of study.

uncooperativeness (2.9%), protocol violations (1%), symptom exacerbation (1%), and other causes (1%). Rates of early termination for all reasons were comparable for patients in both treatment groups.

Clinical Efficacy

Analyses of covariance of posttreatment change scores conducted for week 6 vs baseline (using pretreatment scores as covariates) were performed for all efficacy variables. An "intent to treat" analysis[34] was carried out for all patients who had a baseline assessment and at least one assessment following randomization, with the last observation carried forward, yielding essentially equal numbers of patients in each cell.

Figures 2 and 3 display findings for two of the predetermined critical variables, the two overall indexes of improvement: BPRS total score and the CGI Scale. The improvement in both the BPRS total score and the CGI Scale was approximately three times greater in the clozapine-treated patients. Differences favoring clozapine were statistically significant by the first week of treatment and continued to be present each week over the entire course of study. Similarly, four "positive" BPRS items determined a priori to be central to the assessment of therapeutic response (conceptual disorganization, hallucinatory behavior, suspiciousness, and unusual thought content) all demonstrated significant differences favoring clozapine over chlorpromazine and benztropine. These items were combined into a cluster score, which also yielded significant differences favoring clozapine. The mean scores at baseline and end point are presented in Table 4. Clozapine was superior to chlorpromazine in the treatment of negative signs and symptoms as well, as evidenced by statistically significant differences on the BPRS items of emotional withdrawal, blunted affect, psychomotor retardation, and disorientation. These items in combination form the BPRS "anergia" factor, displayed in Fig 5.

Analysis of variance and analysis of covariance results for all BPRS variables, including the a priori criteria, are shown in Table 5. Therapeutic response was assessed by the nursing staff as well, who rated patients' ward behavior on the NOSIE-30 (Table 5). For all six factors (social competence, social interest, personal neatness, irritability, manifest psychosis, and retardation), the nursing staff, blind to treatment assignment, judged clozapine effects superior to those of chlorpromazine and benztropine. Weekly

changes on the composite score, "total patient assets," are presented in Fig 6.

Concerning the onset of therapeutic effects, Figs 2 to 6 indicated significant differences favoring clozapine over chlorpromazine as early as the first week. Analysis of variance of the comparative rates of improvement for these treatment groups (analysis of slopes) found that clozapine produced more rapid onset of activity.

Clozapine—Kane et al

294

Table 4.—Comparative Drug Efficacy and Neurologic Ratings

Scale*	Drug	No. of Patients†	Score (Mean ± SD) Baseline	Score (Mean ± SD) End Point	Two-Tailed Analysis of Covariance, P
BPRS total score	Clozapine	126	61 ± 12	45 ± 13	<.001
	Chlorpromazine	139	61 ± 11	56 ± 12	
BPRS cluster of four key items	Clozapine	126	19 ± 4	14 ± 5	<.001
	Chlorpromazine	139	19 ± 4	17 ± 4	
CGI Scale	Clozapine	126	5.6 ± 0.7	4.4 ± 1.1	<.001
	Chlorpromazine	139	5.7 ± 0.7	5.3 ± 0.8	
AIMS total score	Clozapine	126	8.8 ± 6.8	5.1 ± 5.4	.09
	Chlorpromazine	139	6.5 ± 5.4	5.8 ± 5.5	
Simpson-Angus Scale for Extrapyramidal Side Effects	Clozapine	126	3.2 ± 3.6	1.8 ± 2.1	.03
	Chlorpromazine	139	3.3 ± 3.5	2.9 ± 3.2	

*BPRS indicates Brief Psychiatric Rating Scale; CGI, Clinical Global Impressions; and AIMS, Abnormal Involuntary Movements Scale.
†Three patients were excluded from these analyses. One patient did not undergo rating after randomization, and one study site had only two patients, both of whom received chlorpromazine.

Table 5.—Comparative Efficacy of Clozapine vs Chlorpromazine and Benztropine

Criterion Variable*	Drug(s) Proved Effective†	Drug Proved Superior/P‡	Week of Onset of Superior Drug Activity‡	Drug Proved Faster§
BPRS positive symptoms Conceptual disorganization	Clozapine and chlorpromazine	Clozapine/<.001	1	Clozapine
Mannerisms/posturing	Clozapine	Clozapine/<.001	1	Clozapine
Hostility	Clozapine and chlorpromazine	Clozapine/<.001	1	Clozapine
Suspiciousness	Clozapine and chlorpromazine	Clozapine/<.001	2	...
Hallucinatory behavior	Clozapine and chlorpromazine	Clozapine/<.001	2	...
Excitement	Clozapine and chlorpromazine	Clozapine/<.001	3	...
Unusual thought	Clozapine and chlorpromazine	Clozapine/<.001	1	Clozapine
Grandiosity	Clozapine	...	...	...
BPRS negative symptoms Emotional withdrawal	Clozapine	Clozapine/<.001	2	Clozapine
Uncooperativeness	Clozapine	Clozapine/<.001	1	Clozapine
Blunted affect	Clozapine	Clozapine/<.001	3	Clozapine
Disorientation	Clozapine	Clozapine/<.001	2	Clozapine
Motor retardation	...	Clozapine/<.05	6	...
BPRS general symptoms Somatic concern	Clozapine	Clozapine/<.01	6	Clozapine
Anxiety	Clozapine and chlorpromazine	...	...	...
Guilt	Clozapine and chlorpromazine	...	...	...
Tension	Clozapine and chlorpromazine	Clozapine/<.001	1	...
Depressed mood	Clozapine and chlorpromazine	...	...	...
BPRS total score	Clozapine and chlorpromazine	Clozapine/<.001	1	Clozapine
CGI Scale	Clozapine and chlorpromazine	Clozapine/<.001	1	Clozapine
NOSIE-30 factors Social competence	Clozapine and chlorpromazine	Clozapine/<.001	2	Clozapine
Social interest	Clozapine	Clozapine/<.001	1	Clozapine
Personal neatness	Clozapine	Clozapine/<.001	2	Clozapine
Irritability	Clozapine and chlorpromazine	Clozapine/<.01	2	...
Manifest psychosis	Clozapine and chlorpromazine	Clozapine/<.001	2	...
Motor retardation	...	Clozapine/<.05	2	Clozapine
NOSIE total assets	Clozapine and chlorpromazine	Clozapine/<.001	2	Clozapine

*BPRS indicates Brief Psychiatric Rating Scale; CGI, Clinical Global Impression; and NOSIE-30; 30-item Nurses' Observation Scale for Inpatient Evaluation.
†Significant pre-post change by within-group t tests.
‡Significant pre-post change by between-group analysis of covariance.
§Analysis of variance of rates of improvement.

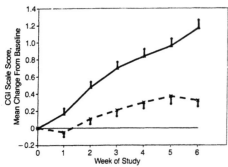

Fig 3.—Mean change from baseline in score on Clinical Global Impressions (CGI) Scale for patients treated with clozapine (solid line, n = 126) or chlorpromazine and benztropine mesylate (broken line, n = 139). For week 1, $P = .003$; weeks 2 through 6, $P < .001$.

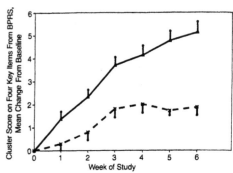

Fig 4.—Mean change from baseline in cluster score on four key items from Brief Psychiatric Rating Scale (BPRS) for patients treated with clozapine (solid line, n = 126) or chlorpromazine and benztropine mesylate (broken line, n = 139). For week 1, $P = .011$; week 2, $P = .001$; weeks 3 through 6, $P < .001$.

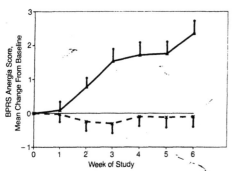

Fig 5.—Mean change from baseline in score on anergia item from Brief Psychiatric Rating Scale (BPRS) for patients treated with clozapine (solid line, n = 125) or chlorpromazine and benztropine mesylate (broken line, n = 139). For week 1, $P < .544$; week 2, $P = .002$; weeks 3 through 6, $P < .001$.

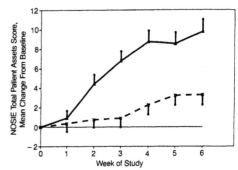

Fig 6.—Mean change from baseline in score on total patient assets item from Nurses' Observation Scale for Inpatient Evaluation (NOSIE) for patients treated with clozapine (solid line, n = 126) or chlorpromazine and benztropine mesylate (broken line, n = 139). For week 1, $P = .356$, weeks 2 through 6, $P < .001$.

in 16 of 27 tests performed; this was never true for chlorpromazine (Table 5).

To test for differential effects among centers, mean improvement scores (total BPRS) by treatment group were individually arrayed for each of the 16 centers. The data were homogeneous: in 14 of 16 centers, greater improvement was found for clozapine-treated patients.

The interpretations allowed by the parametric data are limited by the fact that clinically unimportant changes in rating-scale scores can be statistically significant if a large enough sample of patients is studied. The critical test from a clinical perspective is the extent to which a treatment produces a clinically meaningful response; ie, is the patient believed to have truly benefited from the medication? This issue underscores the importance of the a priori criteria for clinical improvement that provide the critical outcome measures in this investigation.

Patients were classified as having "improved" to a clinically significant extent or not over the course of double-blind treatment. The a priori criteria for defining a patient as improved included a reduction greater than 20% from baseline in the BPRS total score plus either a posttreatment CGI Scale score of 3 (mild) or less or a posttreatment BPRS total score of 35. or lower. When these criteria were applied to all patients who completed at least one

week of the double-blind phase of treatment, it was found that only 4% of patients treated with chlorpromazine and benztropine had improved, while 30% of clozapine-treated patients had improved ($P < .001$) (Table 6). These results provide the most cogent evidence of clozapine's superiority.

Evaluation of Safety

Comparative incidences of adverse reactions (the number of patients reporting a new or worsened effect one or more times during double-blind treatment) are presented in Table 7 for the more frequent adverse reactions. This table is ordered by descending frequency of occurrence for patients receiving clozapine compared with chlorpromazine and benztropine.

Extrapyramidal side effects during the chlorpromazine and haloperidol treatment periods were largely masked by the prophylactic administration of benztropine. Rating-scale evidence of relative extrapyramidal side effects of the three active drug conditions (clozapine, chlorpromazine and benztropine, and haloperidol and benztropine) was provided by weekly assessments using the Simpson-Angus Scale for Extrapyramidal Side Effects. Figure 7 provides mean ratings for these patients throughout the entire course of study, showing a rise in such symptoms (excluding

Table 6.—No. of Patients Whose Condition Improved*			
Drug	No. (%) of Patients Whose Condition Improved	All Others, No. (%)	Total, No. (%)
Ciozapine	38 (30)	88 (70)	126 (100)
Chlorpromazine	5 (4)	136 (96)	141 (100)
Total	43 (16)	224 (84)	267 (100)

*The categorization is based on the last evaluation completed for each patient. P<.001 by two-tailed Fisher's exact test.

Table 7.—Most Frequent Adverse Reactions			
Adverse Reaction	Clozapine (n = 126), No. (%) of Patients	Chlorpromazine (n = 142), No. (%) of Patients	P*
Drowsiness	26 (21)	18 (13)	.098
Tachycardia	21 (17)	16 (11)	.218
Constipation	20 (16)	17 (12)	.380
Dizziness	18 (14)	23 (16)	.735
Hypotension	16 (13)	54 (38)	<.001
Fever (hyperthermia)	16 (13)	6 (4)	.014
Salivation	17 (13)	2 (1)	<.001
Hypertension	15 (12)	7 (5)	.045
Headache	13 (10)	14 (10)	.999
Nausea/vomiting	12 (10)	17 (12)	.560
Dry mouth	6 (5)	28 (20)	<.001

*Based on two-tailed Fisher's exact test.

salivation) during the haloperidol and benztropine phase followed by a decrease during washout, with little subsequent benefit for patients treated with chlorpromazine and benztropine. However, clozapine-treated patients continued to improve further until the end of the six-week study period. This improvement was statistically significant at weeks 4, 5, and 6.

Although the impact of these treatments on tardive dyskinesia was not a focus of this study, changes in scores on the AIMS were also examined. The clozapine-treated patients had a significantly higher mean baseline score on the AIMS (8.8 vs 6.5). Analyses of covariance showed a trend for clozapine-treated patients to improve more on this measure ($P = .09$ by total test).

Dry mouth was more prominent in patients receiving chlorpromazine and benztropine (20%), while salivation was more characteristic of patients receiving clozapine (13%). In the cardiovascular area, hypotensive reactions occurred in 38% of patients treated with chlorpromazine and benztropine compared with 13% of clozapine-treated patients. However, tachycardia was more prevalent in clozapine-treated patients (17%).

In terms of miscellaneous adverse effects, benign temperature elevations not associated with laboratory test abnormalities were more frequent in clozapine-treated patients (13%). Three cases of hepatic enzyme elevations were judged to be clinically significant in the clozapine group compared with one in the chlorpromazine group. There were no reports of agranulocytosis in this cohort. (The cases that occurred in the United States were among individuals being treated according to an open-label "humanitarian" protocol.)

The two treatments did not differ in the proportion of patients who experienced a drop in total white blood cell count below 3.9×10^9/L (4.9% for clozapine and 3.3% for chlorpromazine). Thirteen percent of the clozapine-treated patients experienced a drop in neutrophils to below 0.50 of the total white blood cells compared with 20% of the patients receiving chlorpromazine.

COMMENT

The results of this 16-center investigation of 319 patients have implications for the understanding of chronic schizophrenia both methodologically and clinically. From the viewpoint of methodology, this study suggests some validity for a set of historical and prospective criteria defining refractoriness to treatment in schizophrenia—the conditions of fewer than 2% of patients selected improved after six weeks of treatment with haloperidol at daily dosages averaging over 60 mg/d at peak, and the conditions of fewer than 5% of patients treated with chlorpromazine improved with a peak dosage averaging 1200 mg/d. At several of the 16 collaborating sites, many patients who were initially judged to be refractory to treatment had not in fact received adequate trials of three different neuroleptic drugs in recent years, and some patients did respond to a change in pharmacologic treatment; those patients became ineligible for the trial. Obviously, the clinician treating the nonresponsive patient must strive for a balanced approach, avoiding both therapeutic nihilism and overzealous utilization of every imaginable pharmacologic or somatic treatment. Even patients who are apparently hopelessly ill deserve periodic reevaluation of ongoing pharmacotherapy and consideration of shifts to alternative treatments.

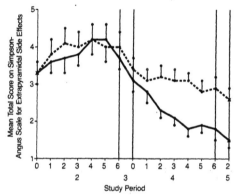

Fig 7.—Mean total scores (lower scores are better) on Simpson-Angus Scale for Extrapyramidal Side Effects, excluding salivation, for patients treated with clozapine (solid line, n = 116) or chlorpromazine and benztropine mesylate (broken line, n = 125) during period 2 (haloperidol and benztropine mesylate), period 3 (placebo washout phase), period 4 (double-blind phase), and period 5 (placebo washout phase).

The response to clozapine demonstrates that this subgroup of severely ill schizophrenic patients, previously considered by many to be beyond the reach of conventional therapy, does remain capable of experiencing substantial medication response. This further argues for the importance and feasibility of conducting carefully controlled, large-scale treatment trials in this patient population.

We believe that this is the first time any specific antipsychotic drug has been shown to be superior to another in a well-defined group of treatment-resistant patients who are unresponsive to haloperidol and other traditional neuroleptics. In addition, given the use of prophylactic benztropine in the chlorpromazine group, the evident superiority of clozapine cannot be attributed simply to a reduction in or lack of extrapyramidal side effects.

Much consideration went into the choice of haloperidol and chlorpromazine in this study design. Both drugs are among the most widely used antipsychotic agents, and they represent the high- and low-potency ends of the spectrum. Chlorpromazine was believed to be the best comparison drug for the double-blind phase, because, in combination with prophylactic antiparkinsonian medication, its adverse-effect profile would be more similar to that of clozapine than the adverse-effect profile of haloperidol. Undoubtedly, one or both of these medications might have failed in the past in some patients included in this study, but this in no way diminishes the importance of clozapine's superiority in this design, since the intent was to identify patients who were unresponsive to available compounds.

Much deliberation also went into the decision to include prophylactic benztropine along with chlorpromazine and haloperidol. We believed that the potential advantages in enhancing the double-blind character of the study (by reducing the possibility of extrapyramidal side effects) argued for the use of benztropine, given that clozapine is relatively free from extrapyramidal side effects.

The superiority of clozapine in this clinical trial is impressive both because of the rigorous manner in which patients were defined and selected and because the superiority was consistent across such a full range of items and factors on the BPRS as well as the CGI Scale. These findings were confirmed and extended by the nurses' ratings. This superiority was not confined to a particular aspect or dimension of psychopathologic characteristics (eg, hallucinations, delusions, or suspiciousness) but involved all the major psychotic signs and symptoms associated with this patient group, including such negative items as blunted affect, emotional withdrawal, apathy, and disorientation. It might be suggested that the antimuscarinic potency of combined chlorpromazine and benztropine produced a cognitive dysfunction leading to disorientation or a worsening of some psychotic signs; however, the superiority of clozapine on the disorientation item resulted from improvement among patients receiving clozapine, not from a worsening among patients treated with chlorpromazine and benztropine.

Given these findings, there is an obvious need for further research to explore the mechanisms by which clozapine accomplishes its clinical effects and to identify possible predictors that might help to select, if possible, the subgroup of patients most likely to benefit. Since drug refractoriness probably occurs for various reasons, however, even this carefully chosen sample of schizophrenic patients remains heterogeneous.

There were no reports of agranulocytosis during this relatively brief study. At present, however, we believe that the apparently increased comparative risk of agranulocytosis requires that the use of clozapine be limited to selected treatment-resistant patients for whom the potential benefits are judged to outweigh the risks.

At the same time, research is under way that attempts to identify risk factors that might predispose certain individuals to the development of hematopoeitic suppression. Careful, regular monitoring of blood cell counts is necessary in patients receiving clozapine, and only those individuals who demonstrate significant benefits within the first four to six weeks should enter the period during which there is increased risk for the development of agranulocytosis (between the sixth and 18th weeks of treatment). With prompt drug discontinuation and proper medical treatment, this problem appears to be reversible within about two weeks, with no physical sequelae. For individuals suffering from treatment-resistant schizophrenia, the availability of clozapine, a potentially helpful

treatment, is, in our view, a useful therapeutic advance. even a small proportion of these patients can go on adjust to life in the community, with the associated reduc need for long-term hospitalization, this has signi cance for public health and health financing.

This study was supported by grants from the Sandoz Research Institu East Hanover, NJ. Dr Kane is also supported by grant MH41960 from Public Health Service, and Dr Meltzer is also supported by grants MH41 and MH 47808 from the Public Health Service.
Statistical analyses were performed by John Patin, MS.

References

1. Davis JM, Schaffer CB, Killian GA, Kinard C, Chan C: Import issues in the drug treatment of schizophrenia. Schizophr Bull 1980;6:70-
2. Klein DF, Davis JM: Diagnosis and Drug Treatment of Psychia Disorders. Baltimore, Williams & Wilkins, 1969.
3. Kane JM, Lieberman J: Maintenance pharmacotherapy in schizoph nia, in Meltzer HY (ed): Psychopharmacology, the Third Generation Progress: The Emergence of Molecular Biology and Biological Psychiat New York, Raven Press, 1987, pp 1103-1109.
4. Creese I, Burt DR, Snyder SH: Dopamine receptor binding predi clinical and pharmacological potencies of antischizophrenic drugs. Scien 1976;192:481-483.
5. Peroutka SJ, Snyder SH: Relationship of neuroleptic drug effects brain dopamine, serotonin, adrenergic, and histamine receptors to clini potency. Am J Psychiatry 1980;137:1518-1522.
6. Richelson E: Neuroleptics and neurotransmitter receptors. Psychic Ann 1980;10:21-26.
7. Richelson E: Neuroleptic affinities for human brain receptors a their use in predicting adverse effects. J Clin Psychiatry 1984;45:331-3
8. Hyttel J, Larsen JJ, Christensen AV, Arnt J: Receptor-binding profi of neuroleptics, in Casey DE (ed): Dyskinesia: Research and Treatme New York, Springer-Verlag NY Inc, 1985, pp 9-18.
9. Meltzer HY: Clozapine: Clinical advantages and biological mech nisms, in Schulz C, Tamminga C, Chase TN, Christensen AV, Gerlach (eds): Schizophrenia: A Scientific Focus. New York, Oxford Universi Press Inc, in press.
10. Meltzer HY, Goode DJ, Schyve PM, Young M, Fang VS: Effect clozapine on human serum prolactin levels. Am J Psychiatry 1979;136:155 1555.
11. Kane JM, Cooper TB, Sachar EJ, Halpern FS, Bailine S: Clozapir Plasma levels and prolactin response. Psychopharmacology 1981;73:18 187.
12. Juul Povlsen U, Noring U, Fog R, Gerlach J: Tolerability a therapeutic effect of clozapine: A retrospective investigation of 216 patien treated with clozapine for up to 12 years. Acta Psychiatr Scand 1985;71:17 185.
13. Doepp S, Muddeberg C: Extrapyramidale Symptome unter Clozapi Nervenarzt 1975;46:589-590.
14. Pope HG, Cole JO, Choras PT, Fulwiler CE: Apparent neurolept malignant syndrome with clozapine and lithium. J Nerv Ment Dis 198 174:493-495.
15. Claghorn J, Honigfeld G, Abuzzahab FS, Wans R, Steinbook Tuason V, Klerman G: The risks and benefits of clozapine versus chlorpror azine. J Clin Psychopharmacol 1987;7:377-384.
16. Fischer-Cornelssen KA, Ferner UJ: An example of European mult center trials: Multispectral analysis of clozapine. Psychopharmacol B 1976;12:34-39.
17. Griffith RW, Saameli K: Clozapine and agranulocytosis. Lanc 1975;2:657.
18. De la Chapelle A, Kari C, Nurminen M, Hernberg S: Clozapin induced agranulocytosis. Hum Genet 1977;37:183-194.
19. Lieberman JA, Johns CA, Kane JM, Rai K, Pisciotta AV, Saltz DI Howard A: Clozapine induced agranulocytosis: Non-cross reactivity wit other psychotropic drugs. J Clin Psychiatry 1988;49:271-277.
20. American Psychiatric Association, Committee on Nomenclature a Statistics: Diagnostic and Statistical Manual of Mental Disorders, ed Washington, DC, American Psychiatric Association, 1980.
21. Honigfeld G, Klett G: The nurses' observation scale for inpatie evaluation (NOSIE): A new scale for measuring improvement in chron schizophrenia. J Clin Psychol 1965;21:65-71.
22. Simpson G, Angus JSW: A rating scale for extrapyramidal sid effects. Acta Psychiatr Scand 1970;212(suppl):9-11.
23. Guy W: ECDEU Assessment Manual for Psychopharmacology. U Dept of Health and Human Services publication (ADM) 76-338. Rockvill Md, 1976, pp 534-535.
24. Sackett DL, Gent M: Controversy in counting and attributing event in clinical trials. N Engl J Med 1979;301:1410-1412.

298

Clinical and Theoretical Implications of 5-HT$_2$ and D$_2$ Receptor Occupancy of Clozapine, Risperidone, and Olanzapine in Schizophrenia

Shitij Kapur, M.D., Ph.D., F.R.C.P.C.,
Robert B. Zipursky, M.D., F.R.C.P.C., and Gary Remington, M.D., Ph.D., F.R.C.P.C.

Objective: Dopamine D$_2$ receptor occupancy measurements provide a valid predictor of antipsychotic response, extrapyramidal side effects, and elevation of prolactin levels. The new antipsychotics clozapine, risperidone, and olanzapine obtain antipsychotic response with few extrapyramidal side effects and little prolactin elevation. The purpose of this study was to compare the D$_2$ and serotonin 5-HT$_2$ receptor occupancies of these drugs in patients receiving multiple-dose, steady-state regimens. **Method:** Forty-four patients with schizophrenia (16 taking risperidone, 2–12 mg/day; 17 taking olanzapine, 5–60 mg/day; and 11 taking clozapine, 75–900 mg/day) had their D$_2$ and 5-HT$_2$ occupancies determined with the use of [^{11}C]raclopride and [^{18}F]setoperone, respectively, and positron emission tomography imaging. **Results:** Clozapine showed a much lower D$_2$ occupancy (16%–68%) than risperidone (63%–89%) and olanzapine (43%–89%). Risperidone and olanzapine gave equal D$_2$ occupancies at doses of 5 and 20 mg/day, respectively. All three drugs showed greater 5-HT$_2$ than D$_2$ occupancy at all doses, although the difference was greatest for clozapine. **Conclusions:** Clozapine, at doses known to be effective in routine clinical settings, showed a D$_2$ occupancy clearly lower than that of typical antipsychotics, while risperidone and olanzapine at their usual clinical doses gave the same level of D$_2$ occupancy as low-dose typical antipsychotics. The results also suggest that some previous clinical comparisons of antipsychotics may have been confounded by different levels of D$_2$ occupancy. Clinical comparisons of these drugs, matching for D$_2$ occupancy, may provide a better measure of their true "atypicality" and will help in understanding the contribution of non-D$_2$ receptors to antipsychotic effects.

(Am J Psychiatry 1999; 156:286–293)

Every known antipsychotic blocks dopamine D$_2$ receptors. While this does not prove a causal relationship between D$_2$ blockade and antipsychotic response, the association between the two is undeniable. Thus, it is

Received April 6, 1998; revision received July 29, 1998; accepted Aug. 10, 1998. From the Schizophrenia Division and PET Centre, The Clarke Institute of Psychiatry, Department of Psychiatry, University of Toronto; and the Rotman Research Institute, Baycrest Centre, University of Toronto. Address reprint requests to Dr. Kapur, PET Centre, The Clarke Institute of Psychiatry, 250 College St., Toronto, ON, Canada M5T 1R8; kapur@clarke-inst.on.ca (e-mail).
Supported by an award from the Medical Research Council of Canada to Dr. Kapur. Astra Arcus, A.B., provided the precursor used in the synthesis of [^{11}C]raclopride, and Janssen-Cilag (France) provided the precursor for the radiochemical synthesis of [^{18}F]setoperone. Some of the data in this report were collected with the support of Janssen Pharmaceutica, Inc. (makers of risperidone) and Eli Lilly & Co. (makers of olanzapine).
The authors thank Erin Toole, Doug Hussey, Kevin Cheung, and Terry Bell for technical assistance; Dr. Alan Wilson, Dr. Jean DaSilva, Armando Garcia, and Li Jin for radiochemical synthesis; and Dr. Sylvain Houle for interpretation of PET data.

of obvious interest to compare the relative D$_2$ receptor occupancies of the available antipsychotics. Farde and colleagues (1) proposed that one needs a "threshold" of D$_2$ occupancy to induce antipsychotic response. Prospective studies have largely confirmed this notion, although it is unclear whether this threshold is 60% or 70% and whether the threshold for inducing response is the same as the one for maintaining it (2, 3). Nonetheless, there is a mechanism of antipsychotic response that relies on D$_2$ occupancy alone (4). Furthermore, it has been noted that as D$_2$ occupancy increases, especially as it rises above 80%, the incidence of extrapyramidal side effects increases (1). Elevation of prolactin levels may also show a threshold relationship with respect to D$_2$ occupancy (5, 6, and unpublished data from our laboratory). While D$_2$ occupancy may be necessary for response, it is not always sufficient, as there are patients who do not respond despite adequate D$_2$ occupancy (7). However, it would be fair to claim that D$_2$ occupancy provides a reliable (and perhaps the best) pharmacological predictor of response to antipsychotic medication, extrapyramidal side effects, and elevation of prolactin levels.

There are now several antipsychotics that have a lower propensity than typical antipsychotics to cause extrapyramidal side effects and prolactin elevation: clozapine, risperidone, olanzapine, sertindole, and quetiapine (8–12). The first three have been used most extensively in patients and are the focus of this study. Given the relevance of D_2 occupancy for response to antipsychotics, extrapyramidal side effects, and prolactin elevation, it is of obvious interest how these antipsychotics compare on this index. The main purpose of this study was to compare the D_2 occupancy of these three drugs in patients receiving multiple-dose, steady-state regimens of the drugs across their usual range of clinical use.

It has been suggested that drugs may demonstrate atypical clinical features (i.e., low extrapyramidal side effects and prolactin elevation) if they have at least a 10 times higher affinity for serotonin $5\text{-}HT_2$ receptors than D_2 receptors in vitro (13, 14). In patients this translates into a preferential occupancy of $5\text{-}HT_2$ receptors as opposed to D_2 receptors (15). Clozapine, risperidone, and olanzapine all show a higher affinity for $5\text{-}HT_2$ receptors than D_2 receptors but the amount by which $5\text{-}HT_2$ exceeds D_2 is unclear. In animal tissue or cloned human receptors, clozapine shows a much higher $5\text{-}HT_2/D_2$ ratio (20 times higher affinity for $5\text{-}HT_2$ than for D_2) than either risperidone (11 times) or olanzapine (12 times) (16). On the other hand, occupancy measurements in rats following subcutaneous injection showed that risperidone had the highest $5\text{-}HT_2/D_2$ affinity ratio (19 times) as compared with clozapine (5.1 times) and olanzapine (7.5 times) (16). Therefore, a second purpose of this study was to systematically compare the $5\text{-}HT_2$ occupancies and the $5\text{-}HT_2/D_2$ occupancy ratios in patients.

Several previous reports have presented data on one or two of these antipsychotics separately. However, these studies used different imaging modalities (positron emission tomography [PET; 17–21] or single photon emission computed tomography [SPECT; 22, 23]); different radioligands ([^{11}C]raclopride [17–20], [^{11}C]-NMSP [21], or [^{123}I][IBZM [22, 23]); and different imaging analysis models (cerebellum as reference [17–21] or frontal cortex as reference [22, 23]). As a result, it is not valid to compare the occupancy of, say, risperidone obtained with [^{123}I]IBZM SPECT to that of clozapine derived by using [^{11}C]NMSP PET. It is essential, when comparing drugs, that the data be obtained on all of the drugs in the same fashion. Furthermore, dose of a drug is a central determinant of its receptor occupancy, and some previous studies have compared occupancies without adequately controlling for dose (23). Any systematic comparison across drugs must compare not just the occupancy but also the dose-occupancy relationships over the clinically relevant dose range. To provide the first such comparison, we present data on the relation between dose, plasma level, and $5\text{-}HT_2$ and D_2 oc-

cupancies in 44 patients with schizophrenia who were receiving a wide range of steady-state doses of clozapine, risperidone, and olanzapine.

METHOD

The procedures for this study were approved by the Human Subjects Review Committee of the University of Toronto. Patients participated after receiving detailed written information about the study and signing a consent document. Patients receiving ongoing treatment in our inpatient and outpatient clinic were recruited over a period of 4 years. We studied 44 patients (36 male and eight female) aged 19–54 years; 43 had a DSM-IV diagnosis of schizophrenia, and one had a diagnosis of atypical psychosis. Sixteen patients were receiving risperidone (2–12 mg/day), 17 were receiving olanzapine (5–60 mg/day), and 11 were receiving clozapine (75–900 mg/day). The patients were not randomly assigned to the three drugs, and the limitations of this are discussed later. Most of the patients were chosen from a clinic population so as to provide a representative range of doses for each drug, which is a sufficient study design for obtaining the in vivo $5\text{-}HT_2/D_2$ profile of the three drugs in patients. However, because of inadequate prospective control over drug and dose assignment and the fact that patients were in various degrees of remission at the time of scanning, the design was limited in its ability to obtain reliable associations between receptor occupancy and clinical outcome. Nonetheless, to ensure a valid comparison of the action of the three drugs on the receptors, the patients in this report conformed to the following criteria.

1. All patients were on multiple-dose, steady-state levels (at least 5 days on the particular dose) of the medication for which they were assessed.

2. All patients were free of any confounding major medical or neurological illness. None of the patients had received any depot antipsychotics in the year before this PET examination, and none had received any other antipsychotics for a minimum of 14 days before the PET examination. None of the patients had concurrent substance abuse or substance dependence (nicotine excepted).

3. Patients were not receiving any other psychotropic medication that might confound the findings for D_2 occupancy, with the exception of benzodiazepines and/or an antiparkinsonian agent, as indicated in table 1. It has been shown that the addition of lorazepam does not alter the measurement of D_2 occupancy with [^{11}C]raclopride (24).

4. All patients had a scan for dopamine D_2 receptors, and most received a scan for serotonin $5\text{-}HT_2$ receptors. All patients had their [^{11}C]raclopride examinations done 12–13 hours after their last nightly drug dose (the usual scan start was at 9:00 a.m.). The [^{18}F]setoperone PET examination for $5\text{-}HT_2$ receptors, if done, followed the [^{11}C]raclopride examination on the same day and started 14–15 hours after the last nightly drug dose.

PET data on some of the patients have appeared in previous reports (19, 20); these patients are identified in table 1. To carry out a systematic comparison, data on all of the subjects in the study were analyzed (those reported before were reanalyzed) with the methods described below, and all patient data were compared with the same baseline data to eliminate any across-drug bias. As a result, there may be a slight variation in the occupancy reported here and that reported before.

The PET scans to estimate D_2 occupancy were obtained after the injection of 10 mCi of high specific activity [^{11}C]raclopride (300–1600 Ci/mmol) according to a bolus-plus-infusion protocol. The scanning methods used have been described in a previous report in this journal (2). The pertinent aspects are the following. Striatal and cerebellar regions of interest were drawn on two contiguous PET slices on a composite PET image with reference to a coregistered magnetic resonance imaging (MRI) scan (GE Signa 1.5-T scanner; T_2-weighted spin-echo sequence coregistered to the PET scan with a surface-matching algorithm). An estimate of the D_2 binding potential (D_2 BP) of raclopride (which represents the B_{max}/K_d of [^{11}C]-raclopride for D_2 receptors, where B_{max} is the total number of receptors available to a ligand, and K_d is the affinity of the ligand for the

301

TABLE 1. Relationship Between Drug Dose, Plasma Level, and D_2 and 5-HT$_2$ Receptor Occupancies in Subjects Taking Risperidone, Olanzapine, and Clozapine

Subject	Age (years)	Sex	Dose (mg/day)	Plasma Level (ng/ml)	Other Medications	D_2 Occupancy (%)	5-HT$_2$ Occupancy (%)
Risperidone group							
1[a]	36	M	2	17.4	Benzodiazepine	64	—[b]
2[a]	19	M	2	8.3	None	67	—[b]
3[a]	28	M	2	11.6	None	71	—[b]
4	24	M	2	21.5	None	63	72
5[a]	19	M	4	11.9	None	70	—[b]
6[a]	33	M	4	20.5	Benzodiazepine	79	—[b]
7[a]	24	M	4	15.7	None	74	—[b]
8[a]	20	M	4	19.8	Benzodiazepine	81	—[b]
9	45	F	4	21.5	None	76	~100
10	33	M	5	32.0	Benzodiazepine	79	96
11[a]	28	M	6	84.4	Benzodiazepine	85	—[b]
12[a]	20	M	6	17.1	None	73	—[b]
13	31	M	6	39.5	Benzodiazepine	81	~100
14	37	M	8	50.2	Benzodiazepine	82	~100
15	26	F	10	72.2	Thyroxine, benzodiazepine	89	95
16	20	M	12	71.0	Antiparkinsonian agent	87	97
Olanzapine group							
1[a]	25	M	5	8.9	Benzodiazepine	43	93
2[a]	24	M	5	15.8	Benzodiazepine	64	~100
3[a]	25	F	5	8.5	Benzodiazepine	59	91
4[a]	20	M	10	38.1	None	75	93
5[a]	38	F	10	19.7	Benzodiazepine	71	~100
6[a]	24	M	10	36.4	None	74	99
7	28	M	10	22.1	None	66	—[b]
8[a]	29	M	15	20.9	None	75	~100
9[a]	23	F	15	62.2	None	76	~100
10[a]	36	M	15	32.4	None	73	~100
11[a]	44	M	20	38.4	Benzodiazepine	74	~100
12[a]	30	F	20	29.6	None	76	~100
13[a]	19	M	20	37.5	None	80	~100
14[a]	21	M	30	78.4	Benzodiazepine and antiparkinsonian agent	84	—[b]
15[a]	25	M	30	61.0	None	82	—[b]
16[a]	24	M	40	181.5	Antiparkinsonian agent	88	—[b]
17	20	M	60	—[b]	None	89	—[b]
Clozapine group							
1	54	F	75	255	None	16	~100
2	25	M	150	107	None	28	97
3	37	M	200	191	Benzodiazepine	64	~100
4	20	M	250	427	None	53	—[b]
5	31	M	300	859	Benzodiazepine	60	90
6	24	M	350	394	None	64	~100
7	25	M	500	442	None	56	93
8	20	M	500	285	None	52	—[b]
9	36	F	600	430	None	65	~100
10	41	M	850	362	Benzodiazepine	47	~100
11	43	M	900	205	Benzodiazepine	68	~100

[a] Subject was reported on in previous articles (19, 20).
[b] Data not available.

receptors) was obtained from the ratio of the striatum to the cerebellum during the 30- to 75- minute interval, a period of prolonged pseudo equilibrium afforded by the bolus-plus-infusion protocol. As used in our laboratory, this method yields a test-retest standard deviation of 6% and has been standardized to have an interrater and intrarater reliability, as measured by the intraclass correlation coefficient (ICC-III), of >0.95.

To estimate receptor occupancy, we used an age-corrected baseline value derived from a pool of 16 normal subjects and 12 antipsychotic-naive patients with schizophrenia. Since the illness had no statistically discernible effect on D_2 receptors as measured with [^{11}C]raclopride in this sample (F=0.66, df=1, 25, p=0.42) and in a previous report by others (25), data from the antipsychotic-naive patients and normal subjects were pooled to provide a more robust effect of age on D_2 binding potential. Drug-induced D_2 receptor occupancy was determined as $(D_2 \; BP_{Base}–D_2 \; BP_{Drug})/(D_2 \; BP_{Base})$, where

$D_2 \; BP_{Base}$ is the age-corrected D_2 baseline binding potential, and D_2 BP_{Drug} is the D_2 binding potential for patients taking the antipsychotic drug. The absence of the patient's own baseline values introduces a potential error; the error as calculated on the basis of variance in the data from antipsychotic-naive persons is expected to vary from 0% to 9% for patients with 50% occupancy and from 0% to 4% for patients with 80% occupancy (26).

The 5-HT$_2$ scans were obtained with the use of a bolus injection of 5 mCi of high specific activity [^{18}F]setoperone (360–6210 Ci/mmol), according to the method developed and standardized by Blin et al. (27, 28). The 5-HT$_2$ occupancy was determined in the prefrontal cortex regions of interest drawn on the [^{18}F]setoperone scan with reference to a coregistered MRI (as described above). An index of the 5-HT$_2$ receptors was obtained from the prefrontal cortex/cerebellar ratio over the 65- to 90-minute time period. The cerebellum is practically devoid of 5-HT$_2$ receptors (29), and studies in baboons as

302

well as humans report no displaceable [^{18}F]setoperone binding in this region (27, 28, 30). It can be shown that at a time when the binding of the radioligand is at pseudo equilibrium, the prefrontal/cerebellum ratio represents 5-HT$_2$ BP + 1 (31). The details of this method as applied here have been described elsewhere (32). We have shown that this method yields an average test-retest deviation of 6%–7% and an acceptably high interrater reliability (ICC-III >0.95) (32).

Since these patients were already receiving treatment, it was not possible to measure their baseline 5-HT$_2$ binding potential. In the absence of this baseline, we used the age-corrected 5-HT$_2$ binding potential obtained from 11 antipsychotic-free patients with schizophrenia and 26 age-matched normal subjects. The pooling of normal subjects and patients results in a more robust age-corrected regression and is justified because there was neither a main effect of diagnosis (F=1.20, df=1, 33, p=0.28) nor a significant effect of diagnosis on the age regression (F=0.59, df=1, 33, p=0.45) (33). Occupancy was calculated in the same way as for dopamine D$_2$ occupancy.

The patients had blood drawn at the time of the D$_2$ PET scan; the samples were analyzed in batches by drug. Clozapine plasma levels were measured by means of high-performance liquid chromatography with electrochemical detection by a method based on previously published techniques (34). Risperidone plasma levels were measured by means of a radioimmunoassay for the active moiety, which reflects both risperidone and 9-OH risperidone, by the Janssen Research Foundation, Beerse, Belgium (35). Olanzapine plasma levels were measured by means of high-performance liquid chromatography with electrochemical detection by BAS Analytics (West Lafayette, Ind.).

Since the patients were, by design, taking the drugs at different dose and plasma levels, a direct comparison of the occupancies without reference to dose is not very informative. To provide a valid comparison, we characterized the dose-occupancy relationship for each drug and compared these profiles across the three drugs. The expected relationship between a drug level and occupancy of the receptors should conform to a rectangular hyperbola, assuming bimolecular (drug-receptor) interactions and negligible occupancy by the endogenous ligand. A rectangular hyperbola, in this context, is defined by equation 1:

$$\%Occ = Occ_{max} \times \frac{D_{Conc}}{ED_{50} + D_{Conc}} ,$$

where %Occ is the observed occupancy, Occ$_{max}$ is the theoretically maximum occupancy for that particular drug, D$_{Conc}$ is the amount of the drug (expressed either as dose or plasma level), and ED$_{50}$ is a constant equivalent to the amount of the drug required to occupy 50% of Occ$_{max}$. If there is reason to believe that all of the [^{11}C]raclopride can be displaced by the drug in question, Occ$_{max}$ can be replaced by 100 in equation 1. In its truest form, D$_{Conc}$ should represent the concentration of the drug in the synapse. Since there is no easy way to measure the synaptic concentration of the drug in patients, one can use dose and plasma level as functional surrogates. However, it should be kept in mind that dose and plasma level only indirectly reflect synaptic concentrations. Noncompliance with the medication regimen or changes in metabolism may lead to different plasma levels for a given dose, and there may be significant differences in the levels of the freely available drug in the synapse if there is a change in protein binding. The observed receptor occupancy was related to the administered dose and measured plasma level with the use of equation 1 implemented in SPSS for Windows (SPSS Inc., Chicago).

RESULTS

For all three drugs, increasing doses led to increasing plasma levels, consistent with expectations and affirming reasonable compliance (table 1). A simple comparison of the occupancies shows that clozapine had a significantly lower D$_2$ occupancy than risperidone and olanzapine (main analysis of variance, F=13.05, df=2, 39, p<0.001; post hoc comparison with risperidone: p<0.001; with

olanzapine: p<0.001), which were themselves indistinguishable (Tukey's honestly significant difference post hoc test, risperidone versus olanzapine: p=0.80).

The D$_2$ occupancies in response to increasing doses and plasma levels are presented in figure 1 and figure 2. In each case, a rectangular hyperbola provided a better fit (i.e., explained a greater degree of variance) than a simple linear fit. The parameters for the curves relating occupancy to dose were as follows: for risperidone, Occ$_{max}$=91%, ED$_{50}$=0.8 mg/day, with 77% variance explained; for olanzapine, Occ$_{max}$=92%, ED$_{50}$=3.2 mg/day, with 81% variance explained; for clozapine, Occ$_{max}$=71%, ED$_{50}$=112 mg/day, with 55% variance explained. The parameters for the curves relating occupancy to plasma level were as follows: for risperidone, Occ$_{max}$=88%, ED$_{50}$=3.2 ng/ml, with 59% variance explained; for olanzapine, Occ$_{max}$=90%, ED$_{50}$=6.4 ng/ml, with 84% variance explained; for clozapine, Occ$_{max}$=68%, ED$_{50}$=88 mg/day, with 18% variance explained. It is important to note that clozapine does not saturate the D$_2$ receptors, and the theoretical maximum occupancy (Occ$_{max}$) is 68%–71%. This is in contrast to risperidone and olanzapine, where we observed occupancies of up to 83% and where Occ$_{max}$ was 91% and 92%, respectively.

Curves relating dose and occupancy for risperidone and olanzapine had the same shape (a near-saturating rectangular hyperbola) and differed only in the dose axis. The amount of drug required to occupy 50% of the available D$_2$ receptors is 3.2 mg/day for olanzapine and 0.8 mg/day for risperidone if the equation is fitted with two parameters (and 4.5 versus 1.2 mg/day if Occ$_{max}$ is assumed to be 100%). This suggests that D$_2$-occupancy-equipotent doses of risperidone and olanzapine are in the ratio of 5:20 mg/day.

All three drugs showed a preferential occupancy of 5-HT$_2$ receptors versus D$_2$ receptors and the ability to completely occupy 5-HT$_2$ receptors, as measured by [^{18}F]setoperone (figures 1 and 2). The lowest doses tested—75 mg/day of clozapine, 2–4 mg/day of risperidone, and 5–10 mg/day of olanzapine—all led to more than 95% occupancy of frontal 5-HT$_2$ receptors in most patients. It should be noted that once occupancy goes beyond 90%, the signal available for analysis is less than 10%, and the precision of data beyond this point is limited. Since there were few patients who had midrange 5-HT$_2$ occupancies, it was not valid to try to fit the data to rectangular-hyperbola relationships. Nonetheless, clozapine possesses a greater degree of separation between its 5-HT$_2$ and D$_2$ occupancies than either risperidone or olanzapine (F=12.67, df=2, 25, p< 0.0002; clozapine was different at p<0.05, according to Tukey's post hoc unequal-N test, while risperidone and olanzapine were not different, p>0.10).

DISCUSSION

The data show that clozapine differs from risperidone and olanzapine in its D$_2$ occupancy profile. Ris-

FIGURE 1. Relationships Between Drug Dose and 5-HT₂ and D₂ Receptor Occupancies for Risperidone, Olanzapine, and Clozapine[a]

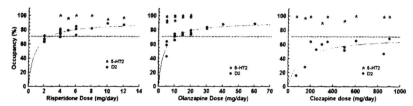

[a] The curves conform to equation 1 in the text. The horizontal line across the three graphs shows the theoretically maximum occupancy expected with the highest dose of clozapine. Even doses of 2 mg/day of risperidone and 10 mg/day of olanzapine gave higher occupancies than those expected with the highest dose of clozapine.

FIGURE 2. Relationships Between Plasma Drug Level and 5-HT₂ and D₂ Receptor Occupancies for Risperidone, Olanzapine, and Clozapine[a]

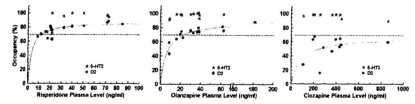

[a] The curves conform to equation 1 in the text. The horizontal line across the three graphs displays the theoretically maximum occupancy expected with the highest dose of clozapine. Levels of 10 ng/ml of risperidone and 20 ng/ml of olanzapine gave higher occupancies than those expected with the highest dose of clozapine.

peridone and olanzapine have similar profiles but differ in potency. All three of the antipsychotics are complete blockers of 5-HT₂ receptors, although clozapine shows the greatest difference between its 5-HT₂ and D₂ occupancies. We discuss how these findings relate to previous published work, discuss the limitations of our results, and then present the implications of these findings for comparisons between antipsychotics.

Differences in ligand selection, imaging modality, and analysis procedures make comparisons of numbers obtained by different centers difficult. Therefore, our results are best compared with those reported by groups that have data, at least on one of the two receptors, on all three drugs. Pilowsky et al. (23) compared the D₂ occupancies of clozapine, risperidone, and olanzapine using IBZM SPECT imaging. They concluded that the D₂ occupancy of olanzapine is statistically indistinguishable from that of clozapine and that the D₂ occupancy of risperidone is higher than that of both clozapine and olanzapine. Our data disagree with regard to olanzapine. The Pilowsky et al. study had several limitations. First, the spatial resolution, quantification, and signal/noise characteristics of IBZM SPECT imaging are inferior to those of [¹¹C]raclopride PET. Second, their study had a smaller total number of

subjects (N=22, versus N=44 in this study), a restricted dose range (10–20 mg/day for olanzapine, while we report on 5–60 mg/day), and fewer subjects taking olanzapine (six, while we report on 17). Third, Pilowsky et al. compared the occupancies without reference to the dose of the drug—the average dose for olanzapine patients was 12.5 mg/day, while that for risperidone patients was 8.7 mg/day, a confounding factor that might explain their finding of a lower occupancy for olanzapine and a higher one for risperidone (see below). Finally, they found no relation between dose and occupancy, questioning the internal consistency of the data. The present study overcomes these limitations.

The Karolinska PET group has provided data on a series of patients taking 125–600 mg/day of clozapine (18), four patients taking 6 mg/day of risperidone (17), and three normal control subjects taking a single dose of 10 mg/day of olanzapine (36). Our data on clozapine confirm theirs. We observed a maximal D₂ occupancy of 68%, and Nordström et al. (18) reported 67%; the theoretical maximum occupancy when plasma levels were related to D₂ occupancy was 68% in our study and 61% in theirs. Farde et al. (17) reported that 6 mg/day of risperidone led to 75%–80% D₂ occupancy; our data show an average of 79%

290

(range=73%–85%). Finally, on the basis of their study of single-dose olanzapine in normal volunteers, these investigators predicted that 10 mg/day of olanzapine should lead to 70% D_2 occupancy (36), which is consistent with our observed average of 72% (range= 66%–75%). Thus, our results are consistent with previous PET data and provide a more valid basis for comparison of the D_2 occupancies of the three drugs.

In addition, we made a comparison of the 5-HT_2 and D_2 occupancies of these drugs, which has never been reported before. It has been reported previously that low doses of clozapine lead to complete saturation of the 5-HT_2 receptors (18). The new finding here is that risperidone and olanzapine also completely block 5-HT_2 receptors. The results refute the findings of the occupancy studies in rats done by Schotte et al. (16) in which risperidone showed a greater separation of 5-HT_2 and D_2 occupancies. In our data, clozapine showed the greatest separation, with risperidone and olanzapine being similar.

Our study is not without its limitations. An important one is that the subjects were not randomly assigned to the drugs and to different doses of each drug. Since clozapine is used in patients who do not respond satisfactorily to other typical and atypical antipsychotics, there is a systematic selection bias here. While, clearly, a prospective randomized assignment to the three drugs would have been preferable, no study has yet been able to achieve this. Furthermore, while the clozapine patients do represent a more treatment-refractory group, there are no data to suggest that D_2 occupancy varies systematically as a function of lack of response; in fact, a previous study suggested that responders and nonresponders do not differ in D_2 occupancy (7). [^{11}C]raclopride provides only striatal D_2 occupancy. The exact site of antipsychotic response is not known, but it is speculated that the mesolimbic D_2 receptors may be crucial. However, it is worth noting that a recent study comparing striatal to mesolimbic D_2 occupancy, using [^{11}C]raclopride and [^{11}C]FLB (37), found no significant regional differences in D_2 occupancy between the striatum and the temporal cortex. It should be pointed out that preferential mesolimbic D_2 blockade is not a necessary precondition for mesolimbic selectivity. While there was no evidence for limbic selectivity of receptor blockade for any typical or atypical antipsychotics in ex vivo animal receptor occupancy studies (16), there is clear evidence for preferential functional antagonism of the limbic as opposed to the striatal dopamine system with several of the atypical antipsychotics (38).

Another limitation of our work, as of all the previous studies, is that the individual's own pretreatment binding potential was not available; therefore, the estimate of occupancy carries an inherent error. However, this error is likely to be small and randomly distributed (39). Furthermore, since the main focus of this study was the difference between the three drugs, all compared with the same baseline values, any such error is unlikely to account for the observed pattern of differ-

ences. Finally, it has been demonstrated in animals (40) and suggested in humans (5) that antipsychotics lead to an up-regulation of dopamine D_2 receptors. If so, a pretreatment baseline D_2 value may result in a lower estimate of D_2 occupancy. However, most animal data show that clozapine does not result in receptor up-regulation (40, 41), while the situation with respect to olanzapine and risperidone is not clear. Even if up-regulation occurs, it is more likely with risperidone and olanzapine than with clozapine, and this would have decreased, rather than increased, our chances of finding the difference we report.

What do these results tell us about the pharmacological mechanisms of antipsychotic action? Farde and colleagues (1) have suggested that one needs a threshold of D_2 receptor occupancy to obtain a satisfactory antipsychotic response. This threshold lies in the range of 65%–70% (2, 4). It is interesting, then, that both risperidone and olanzapine become effective antipsychotics only at doses which cross these levels of D_2 occupancy. Doses of risperidone and olanzapine that do not reach these levels (i.e., <2 mg/day of risperidone and <10 mg/day of olanzapine) are not reliably antipsychotic in most clinical situations. Clozapine, on the other hand, is able to obtain an antipsychotic response with levels of D_2 occupancy (usually 30%–60%) that would be insufficient to cause antipsychotic response by themselves (4). Thus, clozapine does not call on the typical D_2 occupancy mechanism for inducing antipsychotic response; risperidone and olanzapine do. This raises the possibility that despite some similarities in their receptor profile in vitro, the fundamental mechanism of response of clozapine may be different from that of olanzapine and risperidone in patients. While this question can ultimately be resolved only in a clinical arena in crossover studies, the data on D_2 occupancy provide a rationale for why patients who do not respond to risperidone/olanzapine may respond to clozapine and the other way around.

The 5-HT_2 receptor data show that all of these drugs are potent antagonists at that receptor. The fact that clozapine saturates 5-HT_2 receptors at such a low dose and that one continues to see an increasing response to clozapine in doses up to 350–400 mg/day (42) makes it unlikely that 5-HT_2 is the primary source of the antipsychotic effect of clozapine. A similar conclusion was reached by Trichard et al. (43) in their study of chlorpromazine and clozapine. It does not rule out the possibility that high levels of 5-HT_2 blockade may modulate or enhance the ability of D_2 blockade to induce response or to delay the onset of D_2-related side effects (14, 15). However, any benefit provided by a mixed 5-HT_2/D_2 model must express itself in a narrow range. Patients taking risperidone and olanzapine who have high D_2 occupancies experience extrapyramidal side effects and prolactin elevation despite a concomitantly high 5-HT_2 occupancy (19, 20).

These findings also raise interesting questions regarding the comparison of risperidone and olanzapine with each other and with typical antipsychotics. All of

305

the currently published "pivotal" studies that have compared olanzapine and risperidone with the reference drug haloperidol have used 10–20 mg/day of haloperidol (9, 10, 44). Thus, doses of olanzapine and risperidone that lead to 70%–80% D_2 occupancy have been compared with doses of haloperidol that result in more than 90% D_2 occupancy (3, 19). It is increasingly being realized that the optimal dose of haloperidol for treatment of most patients may be less than 6 mg/day, while higher doses may result in greater extrapyramidal side effects without extra efficacy (45). Since extrapyramidal side effects can also influence measurement of negative symptoms (46), this raises an interesting question: would risperidone/olanzapine demonstrate superior benefits for extrapyramidal side effects, prolactin levels, and negative symptoms if they were compared with a typical antipsychotic that has the same D_2 occupancy? Such D_2-occupancy-matched studies will be very valuable for discerning the true components of atypicality.

These data are also of interest in interpreting the comparison between risperidone and olanzapine. In a recently published trial (47), olanzapine, 17.2 mg/day, was compared with risperidone, 7.2 mg/day, and risperidone showed a higher propensity for extrapyramidal side effects and prolactin elevation. According to the equations derived from our data, the study compared an average of 77%–79% D_2 occupancy induced by olanzapine with an average of 82%–86% D_2 occupancy induced by risperidone. Because both extrapyramidal side effects and prolactin elevation are related to the amount of D_2 occupancy, and because as occupancy rises beyond 80%, extrapyramidal side effects become more prominent (1), this raises the question of whether the higher incidence of extrapyramidal side effects/prolactin elevation with risperidone is a function of the choice of dose (and resulting D_2 occupancy) rather than a qualitative difference between the two drugs. On the other hand, since the design of the Tran et al. study (47) permitted a clinical titration of the dose, it could also be true that olanzapine is able to muster a greater clinical response with a slightly lower level of D_2 occupancy (possibly because of the synergism of its multiple-receptor-blocking profile), and that if D_2-equipotent doses of risperidone and olanzapine were compared (e.g., 4–5 mg of risperidone versus 17.2 mg of olanzapine), risperidone might have lower extrapyramidal side effects/prolactin elevation, but olanzapine might then show superior efficacy.

In conclusion, this study provides the first systematic comparison of the D_2 and 5-HT$_2$ receptor occupancies of the three most commonly used atypical antipsychotics. Clozapine is able to induce an antipsychotic response with a D_2 occupancy lower than that of typical antipsychotics, and this may explain its freedom from extrapyramidal side effects and prolactin elevation. Risperidone and olanzapine become effective antipsychotics only when their D_2 occupancy is in the range obtained by low-dose typical antipsychotics (2, 3). They occupy equal numbers of D_2 receptors when used in the

dose ratio of 1:4 mg/day, respectively. All three drugs saturate the 5-HT$_2$ receptors at subtherapeutic doses, suggesting that 5-HT$_2$ occupancy alone is an unlikely explanation for their antipsychotic effects. The data also have implications for clinical comparison studies. Most studies comparing atypical antipsychotics with haloperidol have compared doses of risperidone/olanzapine that give 65%–80% D_2 occupancy with doses of haloperidol that give more than 90% D_2 occupancy. This may have biased these comparisons to produce higher extrapyramidal side effects and prolactin elevation with haloperidol. D_2-occupancy-matched trials of atypical antipsychotics versus haloperidol and atypical versus atypical antipsychotics would be more informative with regard to the true superiority of one drug over another and would also help in distinguishing the clinical role of receptors other than D_2.

REFERENCES

1. Farde L, Nordstrom AL, Wiesel FA, Pauli S, Halldin C, Sedvall G: Positron emission tomographic analysis of central D1 and D2 dopamine receptor occupancy in patients treated with classical neuroleptics and clozapine: relation to extrapyramidal side effects. Arch Gen Psychiatry 1992; 49:538–544
2. Kapur S, Remington G, Jones C, Wilson A, DaSilva J, Houle S, Zipursky R: High levels of dopamine D2 receptor occupancy with low-dose haloperidol treatment: a PET study. Am J Psychiatry 1996; 153:948–950
3. Nyberg S, Farde L, Halldin C, Dahl M-L, Bertilsson L: D2 dopamine receptor occupancy during low-dose treatment with haloperidol decanoate. Am J Psychiatry 1995; 152:173–178
4. Nordstrom AL, Farde L, Wiesel FA, Forslund K, Pauli S, Halldin C, Uppfeldt G: Central D2-dopamine receptor occupancy in relation to antipsychotic drug effects—a double-blind PET study of schizophrenic patients. Biol Psychiatry 1993; 33: 227–235
5. Baron JC, Martinot JL, Cambon H, Boulenger JP, Poirier MF, Caillard V, Blin J, Huret JD, Loc'h C, Maziere B: Striatal dopamine receptor occupancy during and following withdrawal from neuroleptic treatment: correlative evaluation by positron emission tomography and plasma prolactin levels. Psychopharmacology (Berl) 1989; 99:463–472
6. Schlegel S, Schlosser R, Hiemke C, Nickel O, Bockisch A, Hahn K: Prolactin plasma levels and D2-dopamine receptor occupancy measured with IBZM-SPECT. Psychopharmacology (Berl) 1996; 124:285–287
7. Wolkin A, Barouche F, Wolf AP, Rotrosen J, Fowler JS, Shiue C-Y, Cooper TB, Brodie JD: Dopamine blockade and clinical response: evidence for two biological subgroups of schizophrenia. Am J Psychiatry 1989; 146:905–908
8. Kane JM, Freeman HL: Towards more effective antipsychotic treatment. Br J Psychiatry 1994; 165:22–31
9. Marder SR, Meibach RC: Risperidone in the treatment of schizophrenia. Am J Psychiatry 1994; 151:825–835
10. Tollefson GD, Beasley CM Jr, Tran PV, Street JS, Krueger JA, Tamura RN, Graffeo KA, Thieme ME: Olanzapine versus haloperidol in the treatment of schizophrenia and schizoaffective and schizophreniform disorders: results of an international collaborative trial. Am J Psychiatry 1997; 154:457–465
11. Zimbroff DL, Kane JM, Tamminga CA, Daniel DG, Mack RJ, Wozniak PJ, Sebree TB, Wallin BA, Kashkin KB, Sertindole Study Group: Controlled, dose-response study of sertindole and haloperidol in the treatment of schizophrenia. Am J Psychiatry 1997; 154:782–791
12. Arvanitis LA, Miller BG, Seroquel Trial 13 Study Group: Multiple fixed doses of "Seroquel" (quetiapine) in patients with acute exacerbation of schizophrenia: a comparison with haloperidol and placebo. Biol Psychiatry 1997; 42:233–246

13. Meltzer HY, Matsubara S, Lee JC: The ratios of serotonin-2 and dopamine-2 affinities differentiate atypical and typical antipsychotic drugs. Psychopharmacol Bull 1989; 25:390–392

14. Meltzer HY, Matsubara S, Lee JC: Classification of typical and atypical antipsychotic drugs on the basis of dopamine D-1, D-2 and serotonin-2 pKi values. J Pharmacol Exp Ther 1989; 251:238–246

15. Kapur S: A new framework for investigating antipsychotic action in humans: lessons from PET imaging. Mol Psychiatry 1998; 3:135–140

16. Schotte A, Janssen PFM, Gommeren W, Luyten WHML, VanGompel P, Lesage AS, DeLoore K, Leysen JE: Risperidone compared with new and reference antipsychotic drugs: in vitro and in vivo receptor binding. Psychopharmacology (Berl) 1996; 124:57–73

17. Farde L, Nyberg S, Oxenstierna G, Nakashima Y, Halldin C, Ericsson B: Positron emission tomography studies on D-2 and 5-HT2 receptor binding in risperidone-treated schizophrenic patients. J Clin Psychopharmacol 1995; 15:S19–S23

18. Nordström A-L, Farde L, Nyberg S, Karlsson P, Halldin C, Sedvall G: D$_1$, D$_2$, and 5-HT$_2$ receptor occupancy in relation to clozapine serum concentration: a PET study of schizophrenic patients. Am J Psychiatry 1995; 152:1444–1449

19. Kapur S, Remington G, Zipursky RB, Wilson AA, Houle S: The D2 dopamine receptor occupancy of risperidone and its relationship to extrapyramidal symptoms: a PET study. Life Sci 1995; 57:PL103–PL107

20. Kapur S, Zipursky RB, Remington G, Jones C, DaSilva J, Wilson AA, Houle S: 5-HT$_2$ and D$_2$ receptor occupancy of olanzapine in schizophrenia: a PET investigation. Am J Psychiatry 1998; 155:921–928

21. Goyer PF, Berridge MS, Morris ED, Semple WE, Compton-Toth BA, Schulz SC, Wong DF, Miraldi F, Meltzer HY: PET measurement of neuroreceptor occupancy by typical and atypical neuroleptics. J Nucl Med 1996; 37:1122–1127

22. Kufferle B, Brucke T, Topitz-Schratzberger A, Tauscher J, Gossler R, Vesely C, Asenbaum S, Podreka I, Kasper S: Striatal dopamine-2 receptor occupancy in psychotic patients treated with risperidone. Psychiatry Res Neuroimaging 1996; 68:23–30

23. Pilowsky LS, Busatto GF, Taylor M, Costa DC, Sharma T, Sigmundsson T, Ell PJ, Nohria V, Kerwin RW: Dopamine D-2 receptor occupancy in vivo by the novel atypical antipsychotic olanzapine—a I-123 IBZM single photon emission tomography (SPET) study. Psychopharmacology (Berl) 1996; 124: 148–153

24. Hietala J, Kuoppamaki M, Nagren K, Lehikoinen P, Syvalahti E: Effects of lorazepam administration on striatal dopamine D-2 receptor binding characteristics in man—a positron emission tomography study. Psychopharmacology (Berl) 1997; 132:361–365

25. Farde L, Wiesel FA, Stone-Elander S, Halldin C, Nordstrom AL, Hall H, Sedvall G: D2 dopamine receptors in neuroleptic-naive schizophrenic patients. Arch Gen Psychiatry 1990; 47: 213–219

26. Kapur S, Zipursky R, Jones C, Remington G, Wilson A, DaSilva J, Houle S: The D2 receptor occupancy profile of loxapine determined using PET. Neuropsychopharmacology 1996; 15:562–566

27. Blin J, Pappata S, Kiyosawa M, Crouzel C, Baron JC: [18F]Setoperone: a new high-affinity ligand for positron emission tomography study of the serotonin-2 receptors in baboon brain in vivo. Eur J Pharmacol 1988; 147:73–82

28. Blin J, Sette G, Fiorelli M, Bletry O, Elghozi JL, Crouzel C, Baron JC: A method for the in vivo investigation of the serotonergic 5-HT2 receptors in the human cerebral cortex using positron emission tomography and 18F-labeled setoperone. J Neurochem 1990; 54:1744–1754

29. Pazos A, Probst A, Palacios JM: Serotonin receptors in the human brain, IV: autoradiographic mapping of serotonin-2 receptors. Neuroscience 1987; 21:123–139

30. Petit-Taboue MC, Landeau B, Osmont A, Tillet I, Barre L, Baron JC: Estimation of neocortical serotonin-2 receptor binding potential by single-dose fluorine-18-setoperone kinetic PET data analysis. J Nucl Med 1996; 37:95–104

31. Mazoyer B: Investigation of the dopamine system with positron emission tomography: general issues in modelling, in Brain Dopaminergic Imaging With Positron Emission Tomography. Edited by Baron JC. Dordrecht, The Netherlands. Kluwer Academic, 1991, pp 65–83

32. Kapur S, Jones C, DaSilva J, Wilson A, Houle S: Reliability of a simple non-invasive method for the evaluation of 5-HT2 receptors using [18F]-setcperone PET imaging. Nucl Med Commun 1997; 18:395–399

33. Kapur S, Kapur S, Jones C, DaSilva J, Brown GM, Wilson AA, Houle S, Zipursky RB: Serotonin 5-HT$_2$ receptors in schizophrenia: a PET study using [^{18}F]setoperone in neuroleptic-naive patients and normal subjects. Am J Psychiatry 1999; 156: 72–78

34. Lovdahl MJ, Perry PJ, Miller DD: The assay of clozapine and N-desmethylclozapine in human plasma by high-performance liquid chromatography. Ther Drug Monit 1991; 13:69–72

35. Huang ML, Van Peer A, Woestenborghs R, De Coster R, Heykants J, Jansen AA, Zylicz Z, Visscher HW, Jonkman JH: Pharmacokinetics of the novel antipsychotic agent risperidone and the prolactin response in healthy subjects. Clin Pharmacol Ther 1993; 54:257–268

36. Nyberg S, Farde L, Halldin C: A PET study of 5-HT2 and D-2 dopamine receptor occupancy induced by olanzapine in healthy subjects. Neuropsychopharmacology 1997; 16:1–7

37. Farde L, Suhara T, Nyberg S, Karlsson P, Nakashima Y, Hietala J, Halldin C: A PET study of [C-11]FLB 457 binding to extrastriatal D-2-dopamine receptors in healthy subjects and antipsychotic drug-treated patients. Psychopharmacology (Berl) 1997; 133:396–404

38. Arnt J, Skarsfeldt T: Do novel antipsychotics have similar pharmacological characteristics? a review of the evidence. Neuropsychopharmacology 1998; 18:63–101

39. Kapur S, Zipursky R, Remington G, Jones C, McKay G, Houle S: PET evidence that loxapine is an equipotent blocker of 5-HT2 and D2 receptors: implications for the treatment of schizophrenia. Am J Psychiatry 1997; 154:1525–1529

40. Burt DR, Creese I, Snyder SH: Antischizophrenic drugs: chronic treatment elevates dopamine receptor binding in brain. Science 1977; 196:326–328

41. Lidow MS, Goldman-Rakic PS: Differential regulation of D2 and D4 dopamine receptor mRNAs in the primate cerebral cortex vs neostriatum: effects of chronic treatment with typical and atypical antipsychotic drugs. J Pharmacol Exp Ther 1997; 283:939–946

42. VanderZwaag C, McGee M, McEvoy JP, Freudenreich O, Wilson WH, Cooper TB: Response of patients with treatment-refractory schizophrenia to clozapine within three serum level ranges. Am J Psychiatry 1996; 153:1579–1584

43. Trichard C, Paillère-Martinot M-L, Attar-Levy D, Recassens C, Monnet F, Martinot J-L: Binding of antipsychotic drugs to cortical 5-HT$_{2A}$ receptors: a PET study of chlorpromazine, clozapine, and amisulpride in schizophrenic patients. Am J Psychiatry 1998; 155:505–508

44. Chouinard G, Jones B, Remington G, Bloom D, Addington D, MacEwan GW, Labelle A, Beauclair L, Arnott W: A Canadian multicenter placebo-controlled study of fixed doses of risperidone and haloperidol in the treatment of chronic schizophrenic patients. J Clin Psychopharmacol 1993; 13:25–40

45. Bollini P, Pampallona S, Orza MJ, Adams ME, Chalmers TC: Antipsychotic drugs: is more worse? a meta-analysis of the published randomized control trials. Psychol Med 1994; 24: 307–316

46. Carpenter WT Jr, Heinrichs DW, Wagman AMI: Deficit and nondeficit forms of schizophrenia: the concept. Am J Psychiatry 1988; 145:578–583

47. Tran PV, Hamilton SH, Kuntz AJ, Potvin JH, Andersen SW, Beasley C, Tollefson GD: Double-blind comparison of olanzapine versus risperidone in the treatment of schizophrenia and other psychotic disorders. J Clin Psychopharmacol 1997; 17: 407–418

ORIGINAL ARTICLES

Antipsychotic Treatment Induces Alterations in Dendrite- and Spine-Associated Proteins in Dopamine-Rich Areas of the Primate Cerebral Cortex

Michael S. Lidow, Zan-Min Song, Stacy A. Castner, Patrick B. Allen, Paul Greengard, and Patricia S. Goldman-Rakic

Background: *Mounting evidence indicates that long-term treatment with antipsychotic medications can alter the morphology and connectivity of cellular processes in the cerebral cortex. The cytoskeleton plays an essential role in the maintenance of cellular morphology and is subject to regulation by intracellular pathways associated with neurotransmitter receptors targeted by antipsychotic drugs.*

Methods: *We have examined whether chronic treatment with the antipsychotic drug haloperidol interferes with phosphorylation state and tissue levels of a major dendritic cytoskeleton–stabilizing agent, microtubule-associated protein 2 (MAP2), as well as levels of the dendritic spine–associated protein spinophilin and the synaptic vesicle–associated protein synaptophysin in various regions of the cerebral cortex of rhesus monkeys.*

Results: *Among the cortical areas examined, the prefrontal, orbital, cingulate, motor, and entorhinal cortices displayed significant decreases in levels of spinophilin, and with the exception of the motor cortex, these regions also exhibited increases in the phosphorylation of MAP2. No changes were observed in either spinophilin levels or MAP2 phosphorylation in the primary visual cortex. Also, no statistically significant changes were found in tissue levels of MAP2 or synaptophysin in any of the cortical regions examined.*

Conclusions: *Our findings demonstrate that long-term haloperidol exposure alters neuronal cytoskeleton– and spine–associated proteins, particularly in dopamine-rich regions of the primate cerebral cortex, many of which have been implicated in the psychopathology of schizophrenia. The ability of haloperidol to regulate cytoskeletal proteins should be considered in evaluating the mechanisms of both its palliative actions and its side effects. Biol Psychiatry 2001;49:1–12 © 2001 Society of Biological Psychiatry*

Key Words: Antipsychotic drugs, dendrite, spine, synapse, microtubule-associated protein 2, spinophilin, synaptophysin

Introduction

Since the introduction of antipsychotic medications nearly 40 years ago, the main emphasis of studies on the effects of these drugs in brain tissue has been on alterations in neurotransmitters and their receptors (for a review, see Csernansky 1996). There is, however, mounting evidence that antipsychotics may produce morphological changes in cellular elements in several regions of the brain, particularly in the association areas of the cerebral cortex (Benes et al 1985; Klinzova et al 1989, 1990; Meshul et al 1992; Uranova et al 1991; Vincent et al 1991, 1994). It has even been suggested that these slow-developing morphological changes might explain why the pharmacologic treatment of psychosis typically requires several weeks to attain its full effect and why it may take months to reverse this effect after cessation of treatment (Benes et al 1985). It has also been proposed that antipsychotic-induced morphological alterations may underlie the side effects produced by these drugs (Kelley et al 1997; Seeman 1988). Interest in the effects of antipsychotic medications on the morphology of cortical cells is further reinforced by the discovery of alterations in the volume and organization of the neuropil in postmortem cortical tissue from schizophrenic patients (Anders 1978; Garey et al 1998; Glantz and Lewis 1997; Selemon et al 1996; Uranova et al 1996), raising the question as to whether these changes are associated with the disease itself or its treatment.

The ability of antipsychotic drugs to affect cell morphology can be predicted from their binding to dopaminergic and other neurotransmitter receptors (Seeman 1990), which are coupled to second messengers that regulate the activity of kinases and phosphatases (Kebabian and Greengard 1971; Roth et al 1998; Walsh et al 1972; Yurko-Mauro and Friedman 1995). These enzymes control the phosphorylation states of such proteins as

From the Department of Oral and Craniofacial Biological Sciences, University of Maryland, Baltimore (MSL, Z-MS), Section of Neurobiology, Yale University School of Medicine, New Haven, Connecticut (SAC, PSG-R), and Laboratory of Molecular and Cellular Neuroscience, The Rockefeller University, New York, New York (PBA, PG).

Address reprint requests to Michael S. Lidow, Ph.D., University of Maryland, Baltimore, OCBS Department, Room 5-A-12, HHH, 666 W. Baltimore Street, Baltimore MD 21201.

Received June 15, 2000; revised August 25, 2000; accepted August 28, 2000.

0006-3223/01/$20.00
PII S0006-3223(00)01058-1

microtubule-associated protein 2 (MAP2; Goldenring et al 1985; Sloboda et al 1975; Tsuyama et al 1986; Walaas and Nairn 1989). MAP2 contains multiple phosphorylatable residues, and the levels of phosphorylation of this protein are inversely proportional to its ability to stabilize dendritic microtubules (Cleveland and Hoffman 1991; Maccioni and Cambiazo 1995; Tsuyama et al 1986, 1987; Wiche et al 1991). As microtubules are among the major cytoskeletal constituents involved in the maintenance of dendritic processes (Cleveland and Hoffman 1991; Keith 1990; Shea and Beermann 1994; Yamada et al 1970), any changes in their stability could affect major cellular compartments of neurons—their dendrites, spines, and synapses. Despite the obvious importance of understanding the effects of antipsychotic drugs on the cytoskeleton of cortical cells, their effects on the phosphorylation of MAP2 and other cytoskeletal proteins in the cortex are not known.

During the past several years our laboratories have been involved in an analysis of the effects of chronic antipsychotic treatment on the integrity of the primate cortex. We have previously reported a significant upregulation of D_2 receptors and downregulation of D_1 receptors in the prefrontal and temporal cortical regions of the rhesus monkey brain following chronic treatment with several typical and atypical antipsychotic drugs (Lidow et al 1997; Lidow and Goldman-Rakic 1994). The cortex of these monkeys also exhibits increased glial density (Selemon et al 1999), although this increase was not induced by all of the antipsychotic drugs examined. In particular, haloperidol was not among the drugs that induced significant gliosis.

This study extends our investigations to the influence of chronic treatment with antipsychotic drugs—in this instance, haloperidol—on tissue levels and degree of phosphorylation of the dendritic cytoskeleton–stabilizing protein MAP2 in multiple regions of the monkey cerebral cortex. In addition, we examined the impact of this treatment on cortical levels of spinophilin, the dendritic spine–affiliated protein that has been implicated in linking plasma membrane–associated synaptic components, such as dopamine D_1 and D_2 receptors, to the actin cytoskeleton (Allen et al 1997; Smith et al 1999; Yan et al 1999). We also evaluated cortical levels of synaptophysin, a synaptic marker commonly associated with synaptic vesicles (Eastwood et al 1995; Masliah et al 1990) presumed to act as an exocytotic fusion pore (Bajjalieh and Scheller 1995; Edelmann et al 1995). Effects of haloperidol treatment on spinophilin and synaptophysin were examined because alterations in the density of spines and synapses containing these proteins have previously been noted in the cortex of haloperidol-exposed animals (Benes et al 1985; Klinzova et al 1989, 1990; Meshul et al 1992; Vincent et al 1991).

In this investigation we studied monkeys that were 1 years of age or older to model the effects of drug treatmen on brain cells in a population of older patients. A parall study is currently in progress on a younger cohort c monkeys. We report the findings on the older animals no because of the insight they provide for neural vulnerabi ities in aged individuals as well as for possible implica tions for chronic medication in clinical practice.

Methods and Materials

Animals

This study included four haloperidol-treated and four drug-nai control female rhesus monkeys (*Macaca mulatta*). The monke in the drug-exposed group were 15, 19, 19, and 20 years of ag whereas the animals in the control group were 15, 16, 19, and 2 years of age. The animals were kept in individual cages accordance with Yale Animal Use and Care Committee guid lines for nonhuman primates. All monkeys were fed High Prote Monkey Chow (Ralston Purina, Saint Louis), were given fru twice a day, and had fresh water available ad libitum. Th animals were also provided with standard enrichment device logs, dog toys, plastic chains, and mirrors.

Drug Treatment and Tissue Collection

Haloperidol (in powder form) was obtained from RBI (Natic MA). For administration, a stock solution of haloperidol:sucro (1:50) was prepared, from which daily doses were portioned o and given to animals within fruit treats such as pieces of banan prune, apple, or marshmallow. The animals received the dr twice a day for a period of 1 year. During the first month c treatment the daily dose was 0.07 mg/kg. During the secor month it was increased to 0.14 mg/kg. After that, the daily do was increased to 0.20 and 0.27 and finally to 0.35 mg/kg 2-week intervals. The latter dose was maintained throughout th rest of the treatment period. For one monkey, the final daily do was 0.42 mg/kg, which was dictated by requirements of testir for cognitive impairments, also conducted in these animals. Th final doses of haloperidol employed in this study fall within t therapeutic range given to psychiatric patients during maint nance treatment (Physicians' Desk Reference 1999). The contr animals received fruit treats only. During the entire period treatment the animals displayed no signs of extrapyramidal sic effects.

Between 12 and 18 hours after the last treatment, the anima were anesthetized with sodium pentobarbital. Their brains we rapidly removed, dissected, and immersed in liquid nitrogen f storage.

The female monkeys used in this study were cycling. Since w cannot exclude the possibility that the biochemical paramete examined may also fluctuate with the estrous cycle, vagin smears were taken from all the animals for several days befo the end of the treatment and the perfusions were conducted c the next day after the appearance of the menstrual bleeding. Th assured a reasonable uniformity of the hormonal state of tl animals at the time of perfusion. Also, since the estrous cycles in rhesus monkeys display seasonal variations (Hutz et al 1985; Walker et al 1983), all the animals were perfused in the period from November through February, which is within the breeding season for these species.

Samples from the following cortical areas were analyzed: frontal pole (cortical area 10; Walker 1940), dorsolateral prefrontal cortex (area 46; Walker 1940), dorsomedial prefrontal cortex (area 9; Walker 1940), anterior orbital cortex (area 11; Walker 1940), posterior orbital cortex (area 13; Walker 1940), anterior cingulate cortex (area 24; Walker 1940), prelimbic cortex (area 25; Walker 1940), premotor cortex (lateral portion of area 6; Brodmann 1994), primary motor cortex (area 4; Brodmann 1994), primary visual cortex (area 17; Brodmann 1994), and entorhinal cortex (area 28; Brodmann 1994). The cortical regions examined are shown in Figure 1. Samples of all brain regions were collected from both hemispheres, but those from each hemisphere were processed separately.

Tissue Levels of MAP2, Spinophilin, and Synaptophysin

TISSUE HOMOGENATES. Tissue samples were homogenized for 3 min on a TriR Homogenizer (Cole-Palmer, Vernon Hill, IL) in 100 volumes of ice-cold TBS buffer (0.5 mol/L Tris base [pH 8.0] containing 0.1 mol/L NaCl and 0.8 mmol/L phenymethylsulfonyl fluoride).

SLOT BLOTS FOR PROTEIN ANALYSIS. Comparative levels of specific proteins in the sample homogenates were examined using slot blots on NitroPure membranes (Osmonics, Westbrough, MA) prepared with Bio-Dot SF Microfiltration Apparatus (Bio-Rad, Hercules, CA). Before the blotting, each tissue homogenate was diluted 1:100 with the TBS buffer, and 200 µL of the resultant solution were used per blot.

For immunolabeling, membranes were preincubated for 1 hour at room temperature in blocking solution containing 5% dry milk and 0.2% Tween, in PBS buffer (137 mmol/L NaCl, 2.7 mmol/L KCl, 4.3 mmol/L Na_2HPO_4, and 1.4 mmol/L KH_2PO_4; pH 7.3). Incubation with protein-specific antibodies diluted in the same buffer was conducted overnight at 4°C. The dilution of MAP2 and spinophilin antibodies was 1:2500; for synaptophysin antibodies, the dilution was 1:1000. After incubation, the membranes were washed 2 × 5 min in PBS buffer and exposed for 1.5 hours to the secondary peroxidase-conjugated antibodies diluted 1:62500 in the blocking solution described above. Visualization of labeling was conducted with the Super Signal Chemiluminescence Substrate (Pierce, Rockford, IL). The images were produced by opposing transparent plastic-wrapped chemiluminescence-soaked membranes to an X-Omat AR Film (Kodak, Rochester, NY) for a period of 2–25 min. For analysis with Universal Software (Advanced American Biotechnology, Fullerton, CA), the film images of slot blots were digitized on a UC 1260 flat bed scanner (U-Max, Hsinchy, Taiwan). For examination of the levels of each specific protein, the tissue samples from the same brain region of the same hemisphere of all eight animals used in this study were always processed simultaneously on a single membrane and blots for every sample were done in

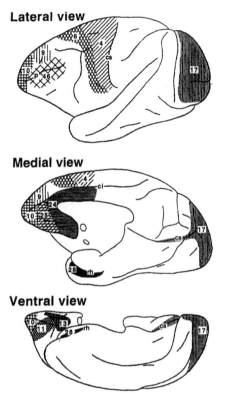

Lateral view

Medial view

Ventral view

Figure 1. Diagrams of the lateral, medial, and ventral surfaces of the rhesus monkey cerebral hemisphere on which the positions of the regions examined in this study have been indicated. These include the frontal pole (cortical area 10; Walker 1940), dorsolateral prefrontal cortex (area 46; Walker 1940), dorsomedial prefrontal cortex (area 9; Walker 1940), anterior orbital cortex (area 11; Walker 1940), posterior orbital cortex (area 13; Walker 1940), anterior cingulate cortex (area 24; Walker 1940), prelimbic cortex (area 25; Walker 1940), premotor cortex (lateral part of area 6; Brodmann 1994) primary motor area (area 4; Brodmann 1994), primary visual cortex (area 17; Brodmann 1994), and entorhinal cortex (area 28; Brodmann 1994). p, principal sulcus; cs, central sulcus; ci, cingulate sulcus; ca, calcarine sulcus; rh, rhinal sulcus.

triplicate (Figure 2B). This assured the similarity of the blot formation and immunolabeling allowing the gray values of the resultant film images to be used in the comparative analysis of the levels of specific proteins in individual blots, as long as the measured gray values had linear relationship to the amounts of the blotted antigen. To verify the linearity of the relationship between the amounts of antigen in the blots and the gray values of the resultant film images, each membrane also included

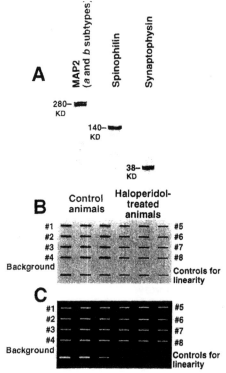

A MAP2 (a and b subtypes), Spinophilin, Synaptophysin

280– KD

140– KD

38– KD

B Control animals   Haloperidol-treated animals

#1   #5
#2   #6
#3   #7
#4   #8
Background   Controls for linearity

C
#1   #5
#2   #6
#3   #7
#4   #8
Background   Controls for linearity

Figure 2. Representative examples of the images of the Western blots and slot blots generated in this study. (A) Film images produced by the Western blots of the proteins examined in this study. These images show only bands with the molecular weight appropriate for the specific protein being visualized. (B) Film images generated by the spinophilin immunolabeling of slot blot samples from tissue homogenates of the right dorsolateral prefrontal cortex from four control and four haloperidol-treated animals. (C) Fluorescent images of DNA-specific–labeled slot blots from the same homogenates. 1–4, control animals from which the triplicate blots were made; 5–8, haloperidol-treated animals from which the triplicate blots were made. The background blots contained bovine serum albumin. The controls for linearity for spinophilin immunolabeling were six serial dilutions of the monkey brain tissue collected and stored for this purpose. The controls for linearity for DNA labeling were six serial dilutions of a herring sperm DNA.

controls for linearity, represented by six blots generated by a serial dilution of monkey brain prepared for this purpose (Figure 2B). The film images of the sample blots from a membrane were accepted for analysis only if all of them had gray value within the range of those produced by the controls for linearity and if the relationship between the gray values of the images of the

linearity control blots and the tissue dilution in these blots was in the linear range. In addition, every membrane included a line of six blots produced by bovine serum albumin (BSA), prepared as the tissue samples, to check the level of background immunolabeling. The BSA blots produced no detectable images on any of the films examined in this study (Figure 2B).

ANTIBODIES. Specific proteins were labeled with the following antibodies: monoclonal antibodies to the high–molecular weight a and b isoforms of MAP2 (Sigma, Saint Louis), the rabbit polyclonal antibodies RU 144 to spinophilin (Allen et al 1997), and the mouse monoclonal antibodies EP10 to synaptophysin (StressGen Biotechnology, Victoria, Canada). The secondary goat antimouse and goat–antirabbit peroxidase–conjugated antibodies were purchased from Jackson Immunoresearch (West Grove, PA). The specificity of the primary antibodies was tested on Western blots of monkey cortical and striatal tissues. The homogenates were mixed 5:1, with the loading buffer containing1.0 mol/L Tris-HCl (pH 6.8), 20% sodium dodecyl sulfate (SDS), 50% glycerol, 0.2% Bromophenol blue, and 4.9% DTT. Thirty microliters of this mixture were loaded per well in Ready-made 4–15% Gradient SDS Gels (Bio-Rad). The gels were run for 1.5 hours at 100 V using a Bio-Rad Ready Gel Cell with Bio-Rad Tris/Glycine/SDS Running Buffer. The transfer on a PVDF-Plus membrane (Osmonics) was performed at 100 A, overnight at 4°C also using a Bio-Rad Ready Gel Cell with Bio-Rad Tris/Glycine Buffer. Immunolabeling of the membranes was performed as described above for the slot blots. The specificity of all the antibodies used in this test was demonstrated by the observation that they produced labeling only in bands with molecular weight in the appropriate range (Figure 2A): MAP2 ~ 280 kd (two bands of close molecular weight that represented a and b isoforms of this protein were visualized; Johnson and Jope 1992), spinophilin ~ 140kD (Allen et al 1997), and synaptophysin ~ 38 kD (Honer et al 1992).

SLOT BLOTS FOR ANALYSIS OF THE DNA LEVELS. The slot blots were used for measurement of the comparative levels of DNA in the sample homogenates. Similar to the blots for the protein analysis, the blots for analysis of DNA were prepared using a Bio-Dot SF Microfiltration Apparatus (Bio-Rad, Hercules, CA). However, here it was loaded with the Hybond-N Nylon membrane (Amersham, Piscataway, NJ). Also, before blotting, the tissue homogenates were diluted 1:20 in 90 mmol/L citrate buffer (pH 7.0) containing 0.9 mol/L NaCl, 3.0 mmol/L EDTA, and 40 μg/mL RNase A. For visualization of the DNA, the dried membranes were soaked for 15 min in SYBR DX DNA-specific Blot Stain (Molecular Probe, Eugene, OR) mixed 1:1000 with 89 mmol/L Tris-H$_3$BO$_3$ buffer (pH 8.0) containing 10 mmol/L EDTA. The staining was observed with the UV Photo Viewer Illumination System (Ultra-Lum, Paramount, CA) at the wavelength of 454 nm. The system also digitized the images for densitometric analysis with Universal Software. A typical example of the digitized image of a membrane stained for DNA is presented in Figure 2C. As in the case of the blots for the protein analysis, samples from the same region of the same hemisphere were processed simultaneously for all eight animals, with blots for every sample done in triplicate. The controls for linearity consisted of slot blots of six serial dilutions of herring sperm DNA (Figure 2C). The background staining on each membrane was checked with six blots of BSA prepared in a manner identical to that of the experimental samples (Figure 2C). On all membranes used for densitometric analysis, the BSA blots generated no staining.

DETERMINATION OF PROPORTION OF NEURONS IN THE TISSUE. Since the overwhelming majority of cells in the brain are not in a process mitosis and have a single complement of identical DNA, it is reasonable to expect that the proportion of the neuronal DNA in a blot would be very close to the proportion of the neuronal cells in the tissue sample. Therefore, it was of interest to determine the proportions of the neuronal DNA in the samples collected for this study. For this purpose, three randomly cut slabs from each tissue sample were processed for direct three-dimensional counting of cell nuclei. The counting was performed as outlined in Selemon et al (1996, 1999) using a Macintosh-based computer system described in Williams and Rakic (1988b). For counting, the slabs were sliced into 80-μm sections on an HM 500 OM cryostat (Zeiss, Walldorf, Germany), and the sections were stained with cresyl violet. The counting was conducted on one section per slab. For each section, the counting was performed in two nonoverlapping randomly selected counting boxes (55 μm wide × 25 μm deep) stretching across the brain structure. Therefore, we examined six counting boxes for every tissue sample (two boxes × three separate sections). Neuronal nuclei were identified based on the criteria of Williams and Rakic (1988a). The proportions of neuronal nuclei among all the nuclei were calculated for every counting box. These data were then used for calculation of the mean proportions ± SEMs of neuronal nuclei for every brain region of each animal.

MEASUREMENT OF TOTAL PROTEIN. The measurement of total protein in the sample tissue homogenates was performed with a Modified Lowry Protein Assay Kit (Pierce) on a Hitachi U110 spectrophotometer (Hitachi USA, San Jose, CA).

EXPRESSION OF THE DATA AND STATISTICAL ANALYSIS. MAP2 and spinophilin are produced by cortical neurons, and synaptophysin, although situated presynaptically, still represents the synapses on cortical cells. Therefore, we wanted to evaluate the effects of the drug treatment on the levels of MAP2, spinophilin, and synaptophysin per neuron in every brain region examined. Since it is not possible to determine precisely the number of cells in the tissue samples used for blots, the closest representation of the quantity of a specific protein per neuron is to divide the amount of this protein by the DNA amount in the same sample and multiply by the proportion of neuronal cells in the sample tissue. In practice, the mean gray values of the images generated by the protein-specific immunostaining of the blots from each sample were divided by the mean gray value of the images generated by the DNA staining of the blots from this sample and multiplied by the mean proportion of the neurons in the counting boxes in the sections also obtained from the same sample. In addition, we expressed the levels of all specific

proteins examined (gray value of blot labeling) per unit of total protein in the sample.

While 22 cortical areas (11 areas per hemisphere) were examined in this study, the goal of the experiments did not include any comparison of protein levels between these areas. The basic analysis of the data, therefore, was a two-tailed t test comparing the levels of each protein in individual cortical area between control and treated animals. Given that four different proteins were measured in each cortical area, however, we adopted a conservative approach by applying a Bonferroni correction to the p values calculated from the t tests. Hence, the p value used in determining the statistical significance of each analysis was equal to the p value calculated from the t test divided by 4, which is the number of proteins analyzed in each cortical area.

Analysis of Phosphorylation of MAP2

PROCESSING OF THE TISSUE. The analysis of the effect of drug treatment on phosphorylation of MAP2 was conducted according to Miyamoto et al (1997) with modifications. Frozen tissue samples were homogenized for 3 min on ice (using a TriR S63C Homogenizer [Cole-Palmer, Vernon Hill, IL]) in 3 volumes of 50 mmol/L Tris-HCl buffer (pH 7.4) containing 0.8 mol/L NaCl, 5 mmol/L EDTA, 5 mmol/L EGTA, 2.5 mmol/L β-mercaptoethanol, 50 mmol/L sodium pyrophosphate, 4 mmol/L p-nitrophenyl phosphate, 1% Sigma Protease Inhibitor Cocktail for mammalian tissue, 1% Sigma Phosphatase Inhibitor Cocktail for Phosphoserine, and 1% Sigma Phosphatase Inhibitor Cocktail for Phosphothreonine and Phosphotyrosine. Immediately after homogenization, the tissue samples were centrifuged at 20000 g for 30 min at 4°C. MAP2 was precipitated from the supernatants with the IMMUNOcatcher Protein Immunoprecipitation Kit (CytoSignal, Irvine, CA). The immunoprecipitating agent (the same monoclonal antibodies that were employed in examination of the tissue levels of MAP2) was used at a concentration of 2.5 μg/100 μL of the supernatant. The resultant immunoprecipitates were mixed 1:5 with the loading buffer described above for the gels used for Western blot testing of the specificity of antibodies employed for labeling of slot blots, and boiled for 5 min. The boiled mixtures (30 μL per well) were run on a gel and blotted on a PVDF membrane as described for the Western blots used in testing of the specificity of antibodies employed for labeling of slot blots. The completeness and evenness of transfer was verified by afterstaining of gels with Comassie blue. Every run included samples of MAP2 immunoprecipitates obtained from the matching cortical regions of the same hemisphere of all eight animals used in this study. The blots were first processed for immunolabeling with antibodies for phosphoserine, phosphothreonine, or phosphotyrosine and the resultant images digitized. The membrane was then stripped of antibodies using a buffer containing 2% SDS, 100 mmol/L β-mercaptoethanol, and 62.5 mmol/L Tris (pH 6.7) at 50°C for 30 min (Wilson et al 1998) and processed for the MAP2 immunolabeling. The overall immunolabeling and signal visualization procedures were similar to those described above for the slot blots, with the exception that here we used the phosphorylated residue-free Blocking Solution from Zymed Laboratories

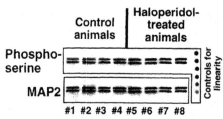

Figure 3. Film images of Western blots of a set of MAP2 immunoprecipitates from the right hemisphere dorsolateral prefrontal cortex of control animals (1–4) and haloperidol-treated (5–8) animals. The upper set is immunolabeled for phosphoserine. The lower set is the same set as above, but immunolabeled for MAP2 after the antibodies for phosphoserine had been stripped off. The controls for linearity are shown only for the phosphoserine immunolabeling. They were six serial dilutions of the monkey brain tissue collected and stored for this purpose.

(San Francisco). The antibodies for immunolabeling of MAP2 were the same as those used for immunoprecipitation (dilution 1:2500). In this case, the secondary antibodies visualized both the immunolabeling and immunoprecipitating antibodies. However, the immunolabeling of MAP2 can be easily distinguished because the molecular weights of *a* and *b* isoforms of MAP2 are in the range of 280 kd, whereas the molecular weights of the heavy and light chains of the immunoprecipitating antibodies are 50 kd and 25 kd, respectively (Alberts et al 1995). Rabbit polyclonal antibodies for phosphoserine, phosphothreonine, and phosphotyrosine were purchased from Zymed Laboratories and used at a dilution 1:500. The peroxidase-conjugated secondary antibodies were the same as those used in the immunolabeling of the slot blots. Their dilution was 1:62500. A typical example of the digitized film images of the immunoblots generated in this part of the study is presented in Figure 3. All Western blots were generated in six replicates. Also, each membrane processed for immunolabeling contained controls for linearity that, as described earlier for the slot blots, were used to ensure that the gray values obtained in the film images were in the linear range. The controls for linearity were made of six serial dilutions of the monkey brain tissue collected and stored for this purpose. The controls for linearity were placed manually, as 2-µL dot blots, on the edge of the membrane immediately upon its removal from the transfer apparatus, before the drying step (Figure 3).

EXPRESSION OF THE DATA AND STATISTICAL ANALYSIS. The residue-specific phosphorylation in every blot of a given sample was expressed as the ratio of the gray value of the film images produced by the phosphoaminoacid immunolabeling and the gray value of the images produced by the immunolabeling of the immunoprecipitated protein in this blot. For every set of blots on a single membrane, the ratios obtained were then normalized to the ratio generated by the sample from the 15-year-old control animal. Since every assay was performed in six replicates (on six separate membranes), the normalized ratios from the matching samples in all six replicates (membranes) were averaged for statistical analysis. The data obtained in this way were appropriate only for comparison of the levels of residue-specific MAP2 phosphorylation in the same region of the same hemisphere of control and experimental animals. The statistic employed for this purpose was a two-tailed *t* test. In assessing statistical significance, we used the Bonferroni correction with *p* value divided by 3, the number of specific assays performed in each brain area.

Results

Proportion of Neuronal Cells in Multiple Cortical Regions

Our calculations of the proportions of neuronal nuclei among the cell nuclei in the samples from all the cortical regions examined in this study showed that neurons constitute approximately half of the cells in these regions (Table 1). There were no statistical differences between the proportions of neuronal nuclei in the haloperidol-treated and control animals in any of the cortical regions in either hemisphere (Table 1).

Levels of Spinophilin, MAP2, and Synaptophysin

Comparative analysis of spinophilin levels in the haloperidol-treated and control animals showed that the drug induced a statistically significant downregulation of this protein in all of the frontal and temporal cortical areas examined in both hemispheres (Figure 4). These areas included the cortex of the frontal pole, dorsolateral and dorsomedial prefrontal cortices, anterior and posterior orbital cortices, anterior cingulate and prelimbic cortices, premotor and primary motor cortices, and entorhinal cortex. Among the cortical areas

Table 1. Percentages ± SEMs of Neurons in 11 Different Cortical Regions of the Right Hemisphere of the Long-Term Haloperidol-Treated and Drug-Naive Control Monkeys

	Frontal pole	Dorsolateral prefrontal	Dorsomedial prefrontal	Anterior orbital	Posterior orbital	Anterior cingulate	Prelimbic	Premotor	Primary motor	Primary visual	Entorhinal
Control animals	57.4 ± 4.2	54.8 ± 4.6	53.0 ± 2.2	57.0 ± 4.0	56.4 ± 3.0	49.9 ± 5.6	52.6 ± 2.2	49.7 ± 4.0	55.4 ± 3.8	60.9 ± 4.2	58.3 ± 4.6
Haloperidol-treated animals	55.8 ± 5.2	56.1 ± 3.2	52.3 ± 3.6	55.8 ± 3.6	55.4 ± 4.4	51.1 ± 3.6	52.6 ± 1.4	49.0 ± 3.4	54.6 ± 2.0	59.3 ± 5.0	56.9 ± 6.0
t test	*p* > .05	*p* > .05	*p* > .05	*p* > .05	*p* > .05	*p* > .05	*p* > .05	*p* > .05	*p* > .05	*p* > .05	*p* > .05

BIOL PSYCHIATRY   7
2001;49:1–12

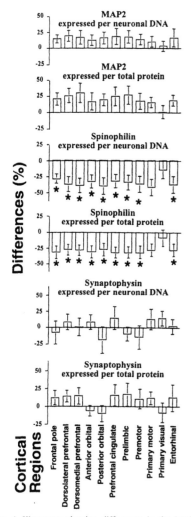

Figure 4. Histograms showing differences in the levels of MAP2, spinophilin, and synaptophysin between the control and haloperidol-treated monkeys in 11 cortical regions examined in this study. The differences are expressed as percentages ± SEMs of the mean levels of these proteins in control samples. Note that, for each protein, one set of bar graphs shows changes expressed per neuronal DNA and another set represents changes expressed per total protein. The data expressed per DNA are from the right hemisphere, whereas the data expressed per protein are from the left hemisphere. *Statistically significant change.

analyzed in this study, only the primary visual cortex did not display a statistically significant decline in this protein (Figure 4). The same results were obtained whether the levels of spinophilin were expressed per neuronal DNA or per total protein (Figure 4).

We also found that the haloperidol-treated monkeys had elevated levels of MAP2 in all cortical regions examined in both hemispheres, whether the levels of this protein were calculated per neuronal DNA or per total protein of the sample (Figure 4). However, this upregulation did not reach statistical significance in any region (Figure 4).

We detected no statistically significant differences in the levels of synaptophysin between the drug-treated and control animals in any cortical region examined (Figure 4).

Phosphorylation of MAP2

The analysis of MAP2 phosphorylation in the haloperidol-treated and control animals revealed a statistically significant drug-induced increase in the levels of phosphorylation of this protein on the serine residue in the cortex of the frontal pole, dorsolateral and dorsomedial prefrontal cortices, anterior and posterior orbital cortices, anterior cingulate and prelimbic cortices, and entorhinal cortex (Figure 5). Increases in MAP2 serine phosphorylation were also observed in the premotor, primary motor, and primary visual cortical areas, but these increases did not reach statistical significance (Figure 5). Increases in the levels of MAP2 phosphorylation were also observed on the threonine residue in all brain regions, but these increases were also not statistically significant (Figure 5). No significant effects on the tyrosine residue phosphorylation of MAP2 were found in the haloperidol-treated animals (Figure 5).

Discussion

Selective Regional Vulnerability of MAP2 and Spinophilin to Chronic Haloperidol Treatment

This study demonstrates that chronic haloperidol treatment significantly increases MAP2 phosphorylation on the serine residue and significantly downregulates spinophilin in specific regions of the primate cerebral cortex. Furthermore, the haloperidol-induced downregulation of spinophilin is detectable independent of whether the levels of this protein are expressed per neuronal DNA or per total protein in the tissue. This indicates that haloperidol treatment selectively affected spinophilin levels, without interfering with the proportion of neurons in the cortex, as demonstrated by the cell counts conducted in this study, and without altering the total protein content of the cortical cells. The protein specificity of the detected effects is also emphasized by the absence of statistically significant

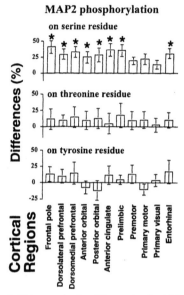

Figure 5. Histograms showing differences in microtubule-asso-ciated protein 2 (MAP2) phosphorylation on the serine, threo-nine, and tyrosine residues between control and haloperidol-treated monkeys in 11 cortical regions of the right hemisphere examined in this study. The differences are expressed as percent-ages ± SEMs of the mean levels of phosphorylation of MAP2 in the control samples. *Statistically significant change.

changes in the levels of MAP2 and synaptophysin in the haloperidol-treated animals.

A central observation of this study is that the effects of haloperidol were detectable in such cortical areas as the frontal pole; the prefrontal, anterior cingulate, prelimbic, and entorhinal regions; and the motor and premotor cortices, all of which are known to contain extensive dopaminergic innervation (Berger et al 1988; Nieuwen-huys 1985; Williams and Goldman-Rakic 1993). These areas, except the motor cortex, also contain the highest densities of D_2 receptors in the monkey cerebral cortex (Lidow et al 1998). Conversely, we detected no significant haloperidol-induced alterations in the aforementioned pro-teins in the visual cortex, which has a barely detectable dopamine innervation and is D_2 receptor poor (Berger et al 1988; Lidow et al 1989). Interestingly, in the motor cortex, which is richly innervated by dopamine fibers (Berger et al 1988; Williams and Goldman-Rakic 1993) but relatively poor in D_2 receptors (Lidow et al 1998), haloperidol interfered significantly only with spinophilin levels with-out affecting MAP2 phosphorylation. This suggests that

the cortical dopaminergic system plays an important rol in haloperidol's ability to affect both the level of spinoph lin and phosphorylation of MAP2 and that D_2 recepto may be particularly involved in regulation of the pho phorylation of the latter protein.

Also of interest is that the cortical regions in whic haloperidol treatment affected MAP2 and spinophilin hav all been implicated in the psychopathology of schizophre nia (Goldman-Rakic 1999a; Harrison 1999; Weinberger al 1994). These regions have also been suggested a possible sites for the palliative action of antipsychoti medications (Lidow and Goldman-Rakic 1997; Lidow al 1998). It is possible, therefore, that haloperidol-induce changes in MAP2 phosphorylation and spinophilin leve may underlie, at least in part, the ability of antipsychoti medications to improve the quality of life of schizophren patients. It is important to remember, however, that th results of this study pertain to older (15–25 years of ag monkeys, and that some of the drug-induced alteratior could be products of an interaction of the treatment wit an aged brain.

The Molecular Biological Findings of This Study Reflect Morphological Changes in the Cortices of the Haloperidol-Treated Animals

The molecular biological data collected in this stud correspond well with morphological findings from sever previous studies on the effects of chronic haloperid treatment. As mentioned earlier, the degree of MAP phosphorylation is inversely proportional to its ability stabilize dendritic microtubules, which are essential for th maintenance of these neuronal processes. Therefore, it reasonable to expect that increased MAP2 phosphoryla tion, which we observed in several cortical regions haloperidol-treated animals, would result in some measu of dendritic collapse in these regions. Indeed, Benes an her colleagues (Benes et al 1985; Vincent et al 199 reported a significant decrease in the number of smal caliber dendritic processes in the prefrontal cortex haloperidol-exposed rats. Furthermore, an electron micr scopic analysis (Benes et al 1985) revealed that most these processes were dendritic spines, whose necks have cytoskeletal structure identical to that of the dendritic sha proper (Bloom and Fawcett 1975). These findings are als compatible with the decrease in levels of the spin associated protein spinophilin, which we observed in th frontal lobe of the drug-treated animals. Additionally, decline in the volume of cortical neuropil (which composed largely of dendritic processes), together with reduced number of microtubules within dendritic shaf and a lower density of dendritic spines, has been found postmortem studies of the frontal cortex of schizophren patients (Garey et al 1998; Glantz and Lewis 1997; Selemon et al 1996; Uranova 1988). Our data, along with those of Benes and her colleagues (Benes et al 1985; Vincent et al 1991), indicate that antipsychotic treatments may have contributed to the generation of some of the aforementioned alterations in the schizophrenic brains.

Another observation of our study is that the levels of MAP2 in the haloperidol-treated animals, though not reaching statistical significance, were consistently elevated in the same cortical areas where increases in phosphorylation of this protein were detected. This is consistent with reports that an increase in MAP2 phosphorylation not only reduces its microtubule-stabilizing capacity but also elevates its resistance to proteolysis (Alexa et al 1996; Johnson and Foley 1993). Interestingly, studies in schizophrenic brains have suggested that this disease may be characterized by an upregulation of non-phosphorylated MAP2 and downregulation of the total MAP2 in some cortical areas (Arnold et al 1995; Cotter et al 1997; Dwork 1997). Our findings demonstrate that haloperidol can, at least partially, counteract these effects both by increasing the levels of MAP2 phosphorylation and by reducing the extent of MAP2 degradation in cortical cells. Consequently, this may be among the bases for the therapeutic benefits of antipsychotic drugs.

It has recently been demonstrated that spines are the main sites of D_1 dopamine receptors in cortical pyramidal neurons (for a review, see Goldman-Rakic 1999b). Therefore, any decrease in the number of spines in the cortex would be expected to affect the expression of D_1 receptors by these cells. This may explain a decline in the levels of D_1 receptors detected after long-term neuroleptic treatment in the primate cortex (Lidow et al 1997; Lidow and Goldman-Rakic 1994) and in the cortex of schizophrenic patients (Okubo et al 1997; Sedvall and Farde 1996).

Several studies have suggested that haloperidol treatment is accompanied by a shift in the position of synaptic contacts from dendritic spines to dendritic shafts, without significantly changing the density of synaptic contacts per se within the cortex (Benes et al 1985; Klinzova et al 1989, 1990; Meshul et al 1992). In agreement with these observations, we detected no significant changes in the levels of the synaptic marker synaptophysin in any of the cortical areas examined. Our results also support the earlier report of Nakahara et al (1998), who found no changes in the levels of synaptophysin messenger RNA in the prefrontal cortex of rats chronically treated with haloperidol. On the other hand, Eastwood et al (1997) detected an increase in the levels of this message in the frontoparietal cortex of haloperidol-treated rats. It should be noted, however, that the latter study characterized the parietal cortex, which was not analyzed by us nor by Nakahara et al (1998). Finally, the lack of haloperidol-

induced changes in synaptophysin levels observed in our study suggests that antipsychotic treatment may not be responsible for the decrease in this protein reported in the prefrontal and medial temporal cortical regions of schizophrenic patients (Eastwood and Harrison 1995; Glantz and Lewis 1997; Honer et al 1999; Karson et al 1999; Perrone-Bizzozero et al 1996).

Possible Cellular Mechanisms of Haloperidol-Induced Alterations in the Proteins Observed in This Study

One of the major pharmacologic properties of haloperidol as an antipsychotic medication is its ability to block D_2 dopaminergic receptors (for a review, see Seeman 1992). Since D_2 receptors are negatively coupled to adenylyl cyclase (Hemmings et al 1987), their blockade results in an increase in the intracellular levels of cyclic adenosine monophosphate (cAMP; Kaneko et al 1992; Nilsson and Eriksson 1993), which may persist during long-term treatments despite D_2 receptor upregulation (Lau and Gnegy 1982; Okada et al 1996). Analysis of the literature suggests that elevated intracellular cAMP levels can lead to all of the alterations detected in the haloperidol-treated animals in this study. For example, upregulation of cAMP activates protein kinase A (PKA; Walsh et al 1972), which is one of the major enzymes responsible for phosphorylation (Goldenring et al 1985; Sloboda et al 1975; Tsuyama et al 1986, 1987; Walaas and Nairn 1989). The involvement of the cAMP–PKA pathway in increasing phosphorylation of MAP2 is supported in our study by the fact that this increase reaches statistical significance only for the serine residues, the only MAP2 residues known to be susceptible to PKA-induced MAP2 phosphorylation (Goldenring et al 1985; Walaas and Nairn 1989).

Elevated levels of cAMP could also lead to a collapse of dendritic spines and, consequently, to decreases in levels of spinophilin in the affected neurons. This collapse might result from destabilization of the microtubule skeleton of spine necks due to the PKA-induced increase in MAP2 phosphorylation. Alternatively, increased intracellular levels of cAMP may affect the cAMP–PKA–CREB pathway, which has also been demonstrated to play an important role in the maintenance of dendritic spines (Martin and Kandel 1996; Murphy and Segal 1997).

Haloperidol may also generate the effects observed in this study by acting through nondopaminergic receptors because treatment with this drug affects multiple neurotransmitter systems in the brain, including noradrenergic and γ-aminobutyric acid–ergic circuitries (Borda et al 1999; Bourdelais and Deutch 1994; Nalepa 1993; Sasaki, et al 1997), which also play a role in the regulation of the neuronal cytoskeleton (Lipton and Kater 1989). In this respect, it is interesting that chronic administration of the tricyclic antidepressant desipramine, which interferes with the brain noradrenergic system, also affects phosphorylation of the cerebral cortical MAP2 on the serine residue (Miyamoto et al 1997). Of particular significance may be the ability of haloperidol to act as a noncompetitive antagonist at N-methyl-D-asparate (NMDA) receptors (Coughenour and Cordon 1997; Whittemore et al 1997). Activation of NMDA receptors has been shown to induce MAP2 dephosphorylation and increased spine formation in the cortex (Collin et al 1997; Halpain and Greengard 1990). Haloperidol-induced blockade of NMDA receptors should therefore result in increased MAP2 phosphorylation and reduced levels of spine-associated proteins, both of which were observed in our study.

This work was funded by the National Institute of Mental Health Grant No. MH44866 (PSG-R, MSL), the Hoechst Marion Roussel Co. (PSG-R), and the Essel Foundation (MSL).

The authors thank Galina Artamonova, Tatyana A. Trakht, Heather A. Findlay, and Terri A. Beattie for their excellent technical assistance; Dr. Ashiwel S. Undie for his help in designing experiments aimed at analysis of protein phosphorylation; and Dr. Lynn D. Selemon for sharing her extensive expertise in three-dimensional cell counting.

References

Alberts B, Bray D, Lewis J, Raff M, Roberts K, Watson J (1995): Molecular Biology of the Cell. New York: Garland.

Alexa A, Tompa P, Baki A, Vereb G, Friedrich P (1996): Mutual protection of microtubule-associated protein 2 (MAP2) and cyclic AMP-dependent protein kinase II against mu-calpain. J Neurosci Res 44:438–445.

Allen PB, Ouimet CC, Greengard P (1997): Spinophilin, a novel protein phosphatase 1 binding protein localized to dendritic spines. Proc Natl Acad Sci U S A 94:9956–9961.

Anders VN (1978): Ultrastructural features of cerebral synapses in schizophrenic parients. Zh Nevropatol Psikhiatr 78:1065–1070.

Arnold SE, Lee VM-F, Gur RE, Trojanowski JQ (1995): Abnormal expression of two microtubule-associated proteins (MAP2 and MAP5) in specific subfields of the hippocampal formation in schizophrenia. Proc Natl Acad Sci U S A 88:10850–10854.

Bajjalieh SM, Scheller RH (1995): The biochemistry of neurotransmitter secretion. J Biol Chem 270:1971–1974.

Benes FM, Paskevich PA, Davidson J, Domesik VB (1985): Synaptic rearrangements in medial prefrontal cortex of haloperidol-treated rats. Brain Res 348:15–20.

Berger B, Trottier C, Verney C, Gaspar P, Alvarez C (1988): Regional and laminar distribution of the in the macaque cerebral cortex: A radioautoradiographic study. J Comp Neurol 273:99–119.

Bloom W, Fawcett DW (1975): The Textbook of Histology. Philadelphia: Saunders.

Borda T, Genaro AM, Cremaschi G (1999): Haloperidol effect on

intracellular signals system coupled to alpha1-adrenergic receptor in rat cerebral frontal cortex. Cell Signal 11:293–300.

Bourdelais AJ, Deutch AY (1994): The effects of haloperidol and clozapine on extracellular GABA levels in the prefrontal cortex of the rat: An in vivo microdialysis study. Cereb Cortex 4:69–77.

Brodmann K (1994): Localization in the Cerebral Cortex [Gray LJ, translator]. London: Smith-Gordon.

Cleveland DW, Hoffman PN (1991): Neuronal and glial cytoskeleton. Curr Opin Neurobiol 1:346–353.

Collin C, Miyaguchi K, Segal M (1997): Dendritic spine density and LTP induction in cultured hippocampal slices. J Neurophysiol 77:1614–1623.

Cotter D, Kerwin R, Doshi B, Martin CS, Everall IP (1997): Alterations in hippocampal non-phosphorylated MAP2 protein expression in schizophrenia. Brain Res 765:238–246.

Coughenour LL, Cordon JJ (1997): Characterization of haloperidol and trifluperidol as subtype-selective N-methyl-D-aspartate (NMDA) receptor antagonists using [³H]TCP and [³H]ifenprodil binding in rat brain. J Pharmacol Exp Ther 280:584–592.

Csernansky JG (1996): Antipsychotics. New York: Springer Verlag.

Dwork AJ (1997): Postmortem studies of the hippocampal formation in schizophrenia. Schizophr Bull 23:385–402.

Eastwood SL, Burnet PW, Harrison PJ (1995): Altered synaptophysin expression as a marker of synaptic pathology in schizophrenia. Neuroscience 66:309–319.

Eastwood SL, Harrison PJ (1995): Decreased synaptophysin in the medial temporal lobe in schizophrenia demonstrated using immunoautoradiography. Neuroscience 69:339–343.

Eastwood SL, Heffernan J, Harrison PJ (1997): Chronic haloperidol treatment differentially affects the expression of synaptic and neuronal plasticity-associated genes. Mol Psychiatry 2:322–329.

Edelmann L, Hanson PI, Chapman ER, Jahn R (1995): Synaptobrevin binding to synaptophysin: A potential mechanism for controlling the exocytotic fusion machine. EMBO J 14:224–231.

Garey LJ, Ong WY, Patel TS, Kanani M, Davis A, Mortimer AM, et al (1998): Reduced density on cerebral cortical pyramidal neurons in schizophrenia. J Neurol Neurosurg Psychiatry 65:446–453.

Glantz LA, Lewis DA (1997): Reduction of synaptophysin immunoreactivity in the prefrontal cortex of subjects with schizophrenia. Regional and diagnostic specificity. Arch Gen Psychiatry 54:943–952.

Goldenring JR, Vallano ML, DeLorenzo RJ (1985): Phosphorylation of microtubule-associated protein 2 at distinct sites by calmodulin-dependent and cyclic-AMP-dependent kinases. J Neurochem 45:900–905.

Goldman-Rakic PS (1999a): The physiological approach: Functional architecture of working memory and disordered cognition in schizophrenia. Biol Psychiatry 26:650–661.

Goldman-Rakic PS (1999b): The "psychic" neuron of the cerebral cortex. Ann N Y Acad Sci 868:13–26.

Halpain S, Greengard P (1990): Activation of NMDA receptors induces rapid dephosphorylation of the cytoskeletal protein MAP2. Neuron 5:237–246.

Harrison PJ (1999): The neuropathology of schizophrenia. A

critical review of the data and their interpretation. *Brain* 122:593–624.

Hemmings HC, Walaas SI, Ouimet CC, Greengard P (1987): Dopamine receptors: Regulation of protein phosphorylation. In: Crees I, Fraser CM, editors. *Dopamine Receptors*. New York: Liss, 115–152.

Honer WG, Falkai P, Chen C, Arango V, Mann JJ, Dwork AJ (1999): Synaptic and plasticity-associated proteins in anterior frontal cortex in severe mental illness. *Neuroscience* 91: 1247–1255.

Honer WG, Kaufmann CA, Davies P (1992): Characterization of a synaptic antigen of interest in neuropsychiatric illness. *Biol Psychiatry* 31:147–158.

Hutz RJ, Dierschke DJ, Wolf RC (1985): Seasonal effects on ovarian folliculogenesis in rhesus monkeys. *Biol Reprod* 33:653–659.

Johnson GV, Foley VG (1993): Calpain-mediated proteolysis pf microtubule-associated protein 2 (MAP2) is inhibited by phosphorylation by cAMP-dependent protein kinase but not by CA2+/calmoduline-dependent protein kinase II. *J Neurosci Res* 34:642–647.

Johnson GVW, Jope RS (1992): The role of microtubule-associated protein 2 (MAP2) in neuronal growth, plasticity, and degeneration. *J Neurosci Res* 33:505–512.

Kaneko M, Sato K, Hirikoshi R, Yaginuma M, Yaginuma N, Shiragata M, Kumashiro H (1992): Effects of haloperidol on cyclic AMP and inositol triphosphate in rat striatum *in vivo*. *Prostaglandins Leukot Essent Fatty Acids* 46:53–57.

Karson CN, Mark RE, Schluterman KO, Sturner WQ, Sheng JG, Griffinj WS (1999): Alterations in synaptic proteins and their encoding mRNAs in prefrontal cortex in schizophrenia: A possible neurochemical basis for "hypofrontality". *Mol Psychiatry* 4:39–45.

Kebabian JW, Greengard P (1971): Dopamine-sensitive adenyl cyclase: Possible role in synaptic transmission. *Science* 174: 1346–1349.

Keith CH (1990): Neurite elongation is blocked if microtubules polymerization is inhibited in PC12 cells. *Cell Motil Cytoskeleton* 17:95–105.

Kelley JJ, Gao XM, Tamminga CA, Roberts RC (1997): The effect of chronic haloperidol treatment on dendritic spines in the rat striatum. *Exp Neurol* 146:471–478.

Klinzova AJ, Haselhorst U, Uranova NA, Schenk H, Isomin VV (1989): The effect of haloperidol on synaptic plasticity in rat medial prefrontal cortex. *J Hirnforsch* 30:51–57.

Klinzova AJ, Uranova NA, Haselhorst U, Schenk H (1990): Synaptic plasticity in rat medial prefrontal cortex under haloperidol treatment produced behavioral sensitivity. *J Hirnforsch* 2:173–179.

Lau Y-S, Gnegy ME (1982): Chronic haloperidol treatment increased calcium-dependent phosphorylation in rat striatum. *Life Sci* 30:21–28.

Lidow MS, Elthworth JD, Goldman-Rakic PS (1997): Down-regulation of the D1 and D5 dopamine receptors in the primate prefrontal cortex by chronic treatment with antipsychotic drugs. *J Pharmacol Exp Ther* 281:597–603.

Lidow MS, Goldman-Rakic PS (1994): A common action of clozapine, haloperidol and remoxipride on D1-and D2-dopamine receptors in the primate cerebral cortex. *Proc Natl Acad Sci U S A* 91:4353–4356.

Lidow MS, Goldman-Rakic PS (1997): Differential regulation of D2 and D4 dopamine receptor mRNAs in the primate cerebral cortex vs. neostriatum: Effects of chronic treatment with typical and atypical antipsychotic drugs. *J Pharmacol Exp Ther* 283:939–946.

Lidow MS, Goldman-Rakic PS, Rakic P, Innis RI (1989): Dopamine D2 receptors in the cerebral cortex: Distribution and pharmacological characterization with [³H]raclopride. *Proc Natl Acad Sci U S A* 86:6412–6416.

Lidow MS, Williams G, Goldman-Rakic PS (1998): A case for cerebral cortex as a common site of action by antipsychotic medications. *Trends Pharmacol Sci* 19:136–140.

Lipton SA, Kater SB (1989): Neurotransmitter regulation of neuronal outgrowth, plasticity and survival. *Trends Neurosci* 7:265–270.

Maccioni RB, Cambiazo V (1995): Role of microtubule-associated proteins in the control of microtubule assembly. *Physiol Rev* 75:835–864.

Martin KC, Kandel ER (1996): Cell adhesion molecules, CREB, and the formation of new synaptic connections. *Neuron* 17:567–570.

Masliah E, Terry RD, Alford M, DeTersa R (1990): Quantitative immunohistochemistry of synaptophysin in human neocortex: An alternative method to estimate density of presynaptic terminals in paraffin sections. *J Histochem Cytochem* 38:837–844.

Meshul CK, Janowsky A, Casey DE, Stallbaumer RK, Taylor B (1992): Effects of haloperidol and clozapine on the density of "perforated" synapses in caudate, nucleus accumbens, and medial prefrontal cortex. *Psychopharmacology* 106:45–52.

Miyamoto S, Asakura M, Sasuga Y, Osada K, Bodaiji N, Imafuku J, Aoba A (1997): Effects of long-term treatment with desipramine on microtubule proteins in rat cerebral cortex. *Eur J Pharmacol* 333:279–287.

Murphy DD, Segal M (1997): Morphological plasticity of dendritic spines in central neurons is mediated by activation of cAMP resdponse element binding protein. *Proc Natl Acad Sci U S A* 94:1482–1487.

Nakahara T, Nakamura K, Tsutsumi T, Hashimoto K, Hondo H, Hisatomi S, et al (1998): Effects of chronic haloperidol treatment on synaptic protein mRNAs in the rat brain. *Mol Brain Res* 61:238–242.

Nalepa I (1993): The effect of chlorpromazine and haloperidol on second messenger system related to adrenergic receptors. *Pol J Pharmacol* 45:399–412.

Nieuwenhuys R (1985): *Chemoarchitecture of the Brain*. New York: Springer Verlag.

Nilsson CL, Eriksson E (1993): Haloperidol increases prolactin release and cyclic AMP formation *in vitro*: Inverse agonism at dopamine D2 receptors? *J Neural Transm* 92:213–220.

Okada F, Ito A, Horikawa T, Tokumitsu Y, Nomura Y (1996): Long-term neuroleptic treatments counteract dopamine D2 agonist inhibition of adenylate cyclase but do not affect pertussis toxin ADP-rybosylation in the rat brain. *Neurochem Int* 28:161–168.

Okubo Y, Suhara T, Suzuki K, Kabayashi K, Inoue O, Terasaki O, et al (1997): Decreased prefrontal dopamine D1 receptors in schizophrenia revealed by PET. *Nature* 385:634–636.

Perrone-Bizzozero NI, Sower AC, Bird ED, Benowitz LI, Ivins KJ, Neve RL (1996): Levels of the growth-associated protein

GAP-43 are selectively increased in association cortices in schizophrenia. *Proc Natl Acad Sci U S A* 93:14182–14187.

Physicians' Desk Reference, 53rd ed (1999): Oradell, NJ: Medical Economics.

Roth BL, Berry SA, Kroeze WK, Willins DL, Kristiansen K (1998): Serotonin 5HT2A receptors: Molecular biology and mechanisms of regulation. *Crit Rev Neurobiol* 12:319–338.

Sasaki T, Kennedy JL, Nobrega JN (1997): Localized changes in GABA receptor-gated chloride channel in rat brain after long-term haloperidol:Relation to vacuous chewing movements. *Synapse* 25:73–79.

Sedvall G, Farde L (1996): Dopamine receptor in schizophrenia. *Lancet* 347:264.

Seeman P (1988): Tardive dyskinesia, dopamine receptors, and neuroleptic damage to cell membranes. *J Clin Psychopharmacol* 8(suppl):3S–9S.

Seeman P (1990): Atypical neuroleptics: Role of multiple receptors, endogenous dopamine, and receptor linkage. *Acta Psychiatr Scand* 358(suppl):14–20.

Seeman P (1992): Dopamine receptor sequences. Therapeutic levels of neuroleptics accupy D2 receptors, clozapine occupies D4. *Neuropsychopharmacology* 7:261–284.

Selemon LD, Lidow MS, Goldman-Rakic PS (1999): Increased volume and glial density in primate prefrontal cortex associated with chronic antipsychotic drug exposure. *Biol Psychiatry* 46:161–172.

Selemon LD, Rajkowska G, Goldman-Rakic PS (1996): Abnormally high neuronal density in the schizophrenic cortex. *Arch Gen Psychiatry* 52:805–818.

Shea TB, Beermann ML (1994): Respective roles of neurofilaments, microtubules, MAP1B and tau in neurite outgrowth and stabilization. *Mol Cell Biol* 5:863–875.

Sloboda RD, Rudolph SA, Rosenbaum JL, Greengard P (1975): Cyclic AMP-dependent endogenous phosphorylation of a microtubule-associated protein. *Proc Natl Acad Sci U S A* 72:177–181.

Smith FD, Oxford GS, Milgram SL (1999): Association of D2 dopamine receptor third cytoplasmic loop with spinophilin, a protein phosphatase-1-interacting protein. *J Biol Chem* 274: 19894–19900.

Tsuyama S, Bramblet GT, Huang KP, Flavin M (1986): Calcium/phospholipid-dependent kinase recognized sites in microtubule-associated protein 2 which are phosphorylated in living brain and are not accesible to other kinases. *J Biol Chem* 261:4110–4116.

Tsuyama S, Terayama Y, Matsuyama S (1987): Numerous phosphates of microtubule-associated protein in living rat brain. *J Biol Chem* 262:10886–10892.

Uranova NA (1988): Structural changes in the neuropil of the frontal cortex in schizophrenia. *Zh Nevropatol Psikhiatr* 88:52–58.

Uranova NA, Casanova MF, DeVaughn NM, Orlovskaya DD, Denisov DV (1996): Ultrastructural alterations of synaptic contactes and astrocytes in postmortem caudate nucleus of schizophrenic patients. *Schizophr Res* 22:81–83.

Uranova NA, Orlovskaya DD, Apel K, Klintsova AJ, Haselhorst U, Schenk H (1991): Morphometric study of synaptic patterns in the rat caudate nucleus and hippocampus under haloperidol treatment. *Synapse* 7:253–259.

Vincent SL, Adamec E, Sorensen I, Benes FM (1994): The effects of chronic haloperidol administration on GABA-immunoreactive axon terminals in rat medial prefrontal cortex. *Synapse* 17:26–35.

Vincent SL, Wang J, Wang RY, Benes FM (1991): Evidence for ultrastructural changes in cortical axodendritic synapses following long-term treatment with haloperidol or clozapine. *Neuropsychopharmacology* 5:147–155.

Walaas SI, Nairn AC (1989): Multisite phosphorylation of microtubule-associated protein 2 (MAP2) in rat brain: Peptide mapping distinguishes between cyclic AMP-, calcium/calmodulin-. and calcium/phospholipid-regulated phosphorylation mechanisms. *J Mol Neurosci* 1:117–127.

Walker E (1940): A cytoarchitectural study of the prefrontal area of the macaque monkey. *J Comp Neurol* 73:59–86.

Walker ML, Gordon TP, Wilson ME (1983): Menstrual cycle characteristics of seasonally breeding rhesus monkeys. *Biol Reprod* 29:841–848.

Walsh DA, Brostrom CO, Brostrom MA, Chen L, Corbin JD, Reimann E, et al (1972): Cyclic AMP-dependent protein kinase from skeletal muscle and liver. *Adv Cyclic Nucleotide Res* 1:33–45.

Weinberger DR, Aloia MS, Goldberg TE, Berman KF (1994): The frontal lobes and schizophrenia. *J Neuropsychiatry Clin Neurosci* 6:419–427.

Whittemore ER, Ilyin VI, Woodward RM (1997): Antagonism of N-methyl-D-aspartate receptors by σ site ligands: Potency, subtype-selectivity and mechanisms of inhibition. *J Pharmacol Exp Ther* 282:326–338.

Wiche G, Oberkanins C, Himmler A (1991): Molecular structure and function of microtubule-associated proteins. *Int Rev Cytol* 124:217–273.

Williams RW, Rakic P (1988a): Elimination of neurons from the rhesus monkey's lateral geniculate nucleus during development. *J Comp Neurol* 272:424–436.

Williams RW, Rakic P (1988b): Three-dimentional counting: An accurate and direct method to estimate numbers of cells in sectioned material. *J Comp Neurol* 278:344–352.

Williams SM, Goldman-Rakic PS (1993): Characterization of the dopaminergic innervation of the primate frontal cortex using a dopamine-specific antibody. *Cereb Cortex* 3:199–222.

Wilson JR, Ludowyke RS, Biden TJ (1998): Nutrient stimulation results in a rapid Ca^{+2}-dependent threonine phosphorylation of myosin heavy chain in rat pancreatic islets and RINm5F cells. *J Biol Chem* 273:22729–22737.

Yamada KM, Spooner BS, Wessells NK (1970): Axon growth: Role of microfilaments and microtubules. *Proc Natl Acad Sci U S A* 66:1206–1212.

Yan Z, Hsieh-Wilson L, Feng J, Komizawa K, Allen PB, Fienberg AA, et al (1999): Protein phosphatase 1 modulation of neostriatal AMPA channels: Regulation by DARPP-32 and spinophilin. *Nat Neurosci* 2:13–17.

Yurko-Mauro KA, Friedman E (1995): Dopamine receptor stimulation decreases cytosolic gamma protein kinase C immunoreactivity in rat hippocampal slices: Evidence for increased Ca(2+)-dependent proteolysis. *J Neurochem* 65:1622–1630.

Age at Onset and Gender of Schizophrenic Patients in Relation to Neuroleptic Resistance

Herbert Y. Meltzer, M.D., Jonathan Rabinowitz, D.S.W., Myung A. Lee, M.D.,
Philip A. Cola, M.A., Rakesh Ranjan, M.D.,
Robert L. Findling, M.D., and Paul A. Thompson, Ph.D.

Objective: The age at onset of schizophrenia for males has usually but not always been reported to be less than that for females. Early onset has also been associated with poor response to neuroleptic treatment and worse long-term outcome. The authors compared age at onset in neuroleptic-resistant and -responsive schizophrenic patients to determine whether the gender difference in age at onset is related to response to neuroleptic treatment. Method: The subjects were 322 patients with schizophrenia or schizoaffective disorder who were consecutively admitted to a university hospital-based research program. Results: Analysis of variance showed significant relationships between age at onset and both gender and long-term responsivity to neuroleptic drugs. The mean ages at onset in the neuroleptic-responsive men (mean=21.2 years, SD=6.1, N=75), neuroleptic-resistant men (mean=19.4 years, SD=4.7, N=119), and neuroleptic-resistant women (mean=20.1 years, SD=6.3, N=77) were fairly similar, whereas that of the neuroleptic-responsive women (mean=24.2 years, SD=8.7, N=51) was significantly greater than for all other groups. A simple effects model indicated that male and female neuroleptic-resistant patients did not differ significantly in age at onset, whereas male and female neuroleptic-responsive patients did. The effect of gender and neuroleptic responsivity on age at onset was related to schizophrenic subtype. Conclusions: These results confirm previous data indicating neuroleptic resistance is associated with early onset. The finding that the difference in age at onset between males and females is smaller in neuroleptic-resistant patients than in neuroleptic-responsive patients suggests that neuroleptic-resistant patients differ premorbidly as well as after onset of illness.

(Am J Psychiatry 1997; 154:475–482)

A ccording to the neurodevelopmental hypothesis of schizophrenia, the process(es) that lead to the development of vulnerability to schizophrenia may be initiated during the second and third trimesters of pregnancy, during the perinatal period, or during a later stage of development (1–3), including puberty (4). The symptoms of schizophrenia usually do not emerge until the second and third decades of life, but they sometimes develop earlier or even as late as the seventh decade (5), although there is some question whether the forms with late-life onset should be included within the group of schizophrenias (6). Traditionally, the age at onset has been identified as the time at which positive psychotic symptoms or disorganization first appear. This is true even though negative symptoms (7) and cognitive dysfunction (8) are now considered to be integral aspects of the illness and are likely to predate the first appearance of psychosis (9, 10).

On the basis of a review of studies of age at onset in schizophrenia, De Lisi (11) concluded that age at onset is the "single most important characteristic of schizophrenia that could yield clues to its origin." While this may be an overstatement, the striking concentration of patients' ages, between 15 and 30 years, at the initial appearance of positive psychotic symptoms or disorganization in most studies of age at onset in schizophrenia strongly suggests that pathological processes

Received Feb. 21, 1995; revisions received Oct. 6, 1995, and Jan. 3 and Oct. 11, 1996; accepted Oct. 29, 1996. From the Laboratory of Biological Psychiatry, Department of Psychiatry, Case Western Reserve University School of Medicine, Cleveland. Address reprint requests to Dr. Meltzer, Department of Psychiatry, Vanderbilt University School of Medicine, Suite 306, 1601 23rd Avenue South, Nashville, TN 37212; herbert.meltzer@mcmail.vanderbilt.edu (e-mail).

Supported in part by NIMH grant MH-41684, by grant RR-00080 from the NIH Division of Research Resources, by the National Alliance for Research on Schizophrenia and Depression, and by grants from the Sihler Foundation, the Elisabeth Severance Prentiss Foundation, and the John Pascal Sawyer Foundation. Dr. Meltzer is the recipient of Research Career Scientist Award MH-47808 from NIMH.

The authors thank Steven Schilling, Ph.D., for assistance in data analysis.

occur in the brain during that period of time. These processes, modulated by environmental and experiential factors, play the decisive role in the ultimate expression of the biological vulnerability to schizophrenia. Thus, identification of any factors that affect the age at onset of psychosis may help identify the biological basis of schizophrenia.

Relatively young age at onset, i.e., 20 years or younger, within the large group of patients with schizophrenia whose onset occurs primarily in the second to third decades of life, has been found to be related to poor outcome in schizophrenia in numerous studies. Thus, earlier onset of schizophrenia has been associated with greater impairment at follow-up (12), poorer response to treatment (13–15), and higher risk of rehospitalization, regardless of gender (16).

In an important study of predictors of poor long-term outcome in schizophrenia, defined as the presence of chronic psychiatric symptoms, social impairment, and poor response to neuroleptics in the most recent psychotic episode, Kolakowska et al. (13) found that 25 patients with good outcome (14 males, 11 females) had an average age at onset of 27.3 years (SD=6.3), which was significantly later than that of 20 patients (16 males, four females) with poor outcome (mean=22.7 years, SD=5.4) (p<0.05). These two groups did not differ significantly in age at onset from an intermediate-outcome group (N=32, 19 males, 13 females), whose mean age at onset was 24.8 years (SD=7.4). Nimgaonkar et al. (14) studied the response at 6 weeks to the equivalent of 600 mg/day of chlorpromazine in 51 schizophrenic patients (35 males, 16 females) and found that early onset was associated with unsatisfactory response. Nimgaonkar et al. suggested that early onset may herald the drug-resistant type of schizophrenia. Harvey et al. (17) reported that the onset of psychosis for 16 neuroleptic-responsive ("non-Kraepelinian") male schizophrenic patients was later by almost a year than that for eight neuroleptic-resistant ("Kraepelinian") schizophrenic patients. This difference was not statistically significant, probably because of the small group size. Loebel et al. (16) reported that early onset was inversely related to extent of improvement but not time to remission in first-episode schizophrenic patients. None of these studies addressed the issue of a gender effect on age at onset.

Response to neuroleptic treatment has become of particular interest since the development of clozapine and its designation primarily for patients with schizophrenia who have a poor response to neuroleptic drugs (18). There has been, to our knowledge, no study of age at onset in neuroleptic-resistant patients, defined as patients with persistent positive or negative symptoms despite at least three trials of typical neuroleptics of adequate dosage and duration, the criteria used in the clozapine multicenter trial (18). This group is to be distinguished from patients with "poor outcome," who may include noncompliant patients, patients with poor social function but without moderate to severe positive or negative symptoms, and patients with the deficit syndrome (19), a classification that does not depend on poor response to neuroleptic drugs (19, 20).

There is also extensive evidence that age at onset in schizophrenia is a function of gender. A review of more than 50 studies published before 1983 indicated that the onset of schizophrenia for females is later than that for males by about 3 to 5 years (21). Nine later studies (22–30) of age at onset in relation to gender that used diagnostic criteria more in keeping with current practice, i.e., DSM-III and DSM-III-R, also suggested that females have a later age at onset than males, with differences ranging from 2.9 to 5.4 years, a finding that agrees with those from earlier studies of gender and age at onset. However, another study (31) showed no gender-based difference in age at onset among 60 schizophrenic patients, of whom 35 were male and 25 were female.

There is also evidence that the effect of gender on age at onset may vary as a function of clinical subtypes of schizophrenia. In several early studies (32–35) the early onset in males was particularly evident in paranoid schizophrenia. This was confirmed in a study by Beratis et al. (24), who found a significantly earlier onset in males than females among the paranoid patients and an earlier onset in females among patients with the disorganized subtype.

The purpose of this study was to compare the ages at onset of neuroleptic-resistant and neuroleptic-responsive schizophrenic patients to test the hypothesis that there would be no difference in age at onset between male and female neuroleptic-resistant patients but that neuroleptic-responsive patients would show a significant difference. We also examined the influence of schizophrenia subtype on the relation of age at onset to neuroleptic response and gender.

METHOD

Subjects and Procedure

All 322 patients (194 men, 128 women) consecutively admitted to a university-based schizophrenia research program who gave informed consent and who had a diagnosis of schizophrenia or schizoaffective disorder by DSM-III-R criteria were included in this study. The criteria for subtyping were also those of DSM-III-R. Diagnosis was based on the results of a structured interview—the Schedule for Affective Disorders and Schizophrenia, for both lifetime and current diagnoses (36)—and all available data in medical records. A consensus conference of research psychiatrists and other clinical personnel provided the final diagnosis. Age at onset was established prospectively during the index admission by interviews of informants and patients by a social worker and research assistant and by a review of medical records. Age at onset was defined as the first report of positive psychotic symptoms.

A reliability study on the age at onset was conducted. Fifty-one patients who participated in the main study and one or both parents were interviewed an average of 4 years after the index admission by a trained research assistant who was blind to the age at onset ascertained at the limited evaluation. The age at onset was obtained independently from the proband and the family member, and each report was compared to that obtained at the index admission. Intraclass correlations were calculated to determine reliability.

In accordance with criteria developed by Kane et al. (18), patients

TABLE 1. Characteristics of Male and Female Neuroleptic-Responsive and Neuroleptic-Resistant Patients With Schizophrenia or Schizoaffective Disorder

Characteristic	Neuroleptic-Responsive				Neuroleptic-Resistant			
	Men (N=75)		Women (N=51)		Men (N=119)		Women (N=77)	
	Mean	SD	Mean	SD	Mean	SD	Mean	SD
Age (years)[a]	33.0	7.7	39.6	11.4	32.2	8.0	35.7	10.9
Duration of illness (years)[b]	11.7	6.9	15.4	9.0	12.8	6.6	15.7	8.5
Number of hospitalizations[c]	6.1	5.9	6.4	7.8	8.2	7.8	8.5	8.0
	N	%	N	%	N	%	N	%
Race[d]								
African American (N=65)	21	32.3	18	27.7	10	15.4	16	24.6
Caucasian (N=253)	52	20.6	33	13.0	107	42.3	61	24.1
Diagnostic subtype[e]								
Paranoid schizophrenia (N=120)	28	23.3	16	13.3	48	40.0	28	23.3
Schizoaffective disorder (N=46)	8	17.4	14	30.4	7	15.2	17	37.0
Undifferentiated schizophrenia (N=98)	24	24.5	12	12.2	41	41.8	21	21.4
Other types of schizophrenia (N=58)	15	25.9	9	15.5	23	39.7	11	19.0

[a]Significant difference between neuroleptic-resistant and -responsive patients (F=4.6, df=1, 318, p=0.03) and significant gender effect (F=21.5, df=1, 318, p<0.0001).
[b]Significant gender effect (F=13.7, df=1, 318, p<0.0003).
[c]Significant difference between neuroleptic-resistant and -responsive patients (F=5.4, df=1, 291, p=0.02).
[d]Significant difference between neuroleptic-resistant and -responsive patients (χ^2=114.1, df=1, p=0.0002).
[e]Significant gender effect (χ^2=15.5, df=3, p=0.001).

were considered to be neuroleptic resistant if they had either 1) persistent moderate to severe delusions, hallucinations, or thought disorder or 2) pervasive negative symptoms, such as withdrawal, anhedonia, poverty of thought content, a deficit in volition, and lack of energy, despite at least three trials of typical neuroleptic drugs for at least 6 weeks at adequate doses. Neuroleptic-responsive patients were those who had at most mild positive and negative symptoms during the most recent course of neuroleptic treatment. None of these subjects had had a trial of clozapine or risperidone before entry into the study. Many of the patients determined to be neuroleptic resistant were subsequently treated with clozapine, with an overall response rate of 60% (37). The responders to clozapine were still considered to be neuroleptic resistant.

Statistical Analysis

The main hypothesis of this study was that there would be no difference in age at onset between the male and female neuroleptic-resistant patients but that the neuroleptic-responsive patients would show a significant between-sex difference in age at onset. The effects of neuroleptic resistance and gender on age at onset were examined by using two-way analysis of variance (ANOVA) for unbalanced data (SAS GLM procedure). ANOVA typically consists of a full factorial parameterization consisting of main effects and interactions. However, in order to permit precise testing of the main hypothesis, simple effects ANOVA was also used (38). A three-way ANOVA with simple effects was also used to investigate the effect of schizophrenia subtype.

To estimate the extent to which age at onset influenced the likelihood of being treatment resistant, a Bayesian approach was used (39). The data on age at onset for the men and women who were neuroleptic resistant or responsive were divided into six age groups: ≤15, 16 to 18, 19 to 21, 22 to 24, 25 to 27, and ≥28 years old. For each age group, the conditional probability of a patient being neuroleptic resistant, given his or her age at onset, was determined by the following formula: P(TR|AG) = P(AG|TR)P(TR) / P(AG), where P(TR|AG) is the conditional probability of being treatment resistant at a given age, P(AG|TR) is the sample estimate of the proportion of ages in the treatment-resistant group (the other conditional probability), P(TR) is the overall estimate of treatment resistance, and P(AG) is the proportion of cases in each age group (estimated to be 0.30) (18, 40).

RESULTS

Table 1 presents age, duration of illness, number of hospitalizations, race, and diagnosis for the four response-by-gender groups and results of the ANOVA and log-linear models comparing these measures. The male patients were younger than the female patients at the time of index admission, and the neuroleptic-resistant patients were significantly younger than the neuroleptic responders. The women had a significantly longer duration of illness than the men. The neuroleptic-resistant patients, as would be expected, had had more hospitalizations than the neuroleptic-responsive patients, despite their much younger age. A significantly greater proportion of African Americans than Caucasians were neuroleptic responsive. There was no difference in the proportions of the neuroleptic-resistant and -responsive patients in the patients with paranoid, undifferentiated, and other types of schizophrenia. The proportions of neuroleptic-responsive and -resistant women were higher in the schizoaffective group than in any of the other three groups.

The intraclass correlation between the age at onset determined at the index admission and the independent determination based on the reinterview of the patient by a second interviewer at follow-up (for 51 patients) was significant (rho=0.72, df=44/45, p=0.02). The intraclass correlation for the age at onset reported by the informant at the follow-up was similar (rho=0.77, df=44/45, p=0.01).

Table 2 presents the means, standard deviations, and ranges of the ages at onset for the neuroleptic-responsive and neuroleptic-resistant patients by gender. The youngest ages at onset for the neuroleptic-responsive men and women were 8 and 12 years, respectively. For

TABLE 2. Age at Onset in Relation to Neuroleptic Responsivity and Gender for Patients With Schizophrenia or Schizoaffective Disorder

| | Neuroleptic-Responsive | | | | Neuroleptic-Resistant | | | | Combined | | | |
| | Age at Onset (years) | | | | Age at Onset (years) | | | | Age at Onset (years) | | | |
Gender	N	Mean	SD	Range	N	Mean	SD	Range	N	Mean	SD	Range
Total	126	22.5	7.4	8–55	196	19.7[a]	5.3	5–45	322	20.8	6.2	5–55
Men	75	21.2	6.1	8–46	119	19.4	4.7	5–45	194	20.1	5.3	5–46
Women	51	24.2[b]	8.7	12–55	77	20.1	6.3	5–39	128	21.7[c]	7.5	5–55

[a]Significant difference from neuroleptic-responsive group (F=17.1, df=1, 318, p<0.0001).
[b]Significant difference from neuroleptic-responsive men (F=6.6, df=1, 318, p<0.01), neuroleptic-resistant women (F=21.1, df=1, 318, p<0.0001), and neuroleptic-resistant men (F=21.6, df=1, 318, p=0.0001).
[c]Significant difference from men (F=6.1, df=1, 318, p<0.01).

FIGURE 1. Cumulative Age at Onset of Patients With Schizophrenia or Schizoaffective Disorder as a Function of Gender and Response to Neuroleptic Treatment

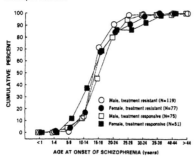

○ Male, treatment resistant (N=119)
● Female, treatment resistant (N=77)
□ Male, treatment responsive (N=75)
■ Female, treatment responsive (N=51)

AGE AT ONSET OF SCHIZOPHRENIA (years)

the neuroleptic-resistant male and female patients, the youngest age at onset was 5 years for each group. The age at onset was greater than 25 years for 10%–35% of the study group, depending on sex and neuroleptic response. Only two patients had onsets after age 45 years.

A two-way ANOVA factorial model was fit to the data in table 2. The gender-by-response interaction was not statistically significant (F=2.3, df=1, 318, p=0.13). However, age at onset was significantly lower in the neuroleptic-resistant than in the neuroleptic-responsive patients, and the women had a significantly later onset than the men.

The lack of statistically significant interaction, while appearing to indicate a lack of support for the study's main hypothesis, actually results from the lack of specificity of the full factorial ANOVA parameterization for the hypothesis of interest. The difficulty is that the large difference between the male and female neuroleptic responders and the lack of a difference between the male and female neuroleptic nonresponders in age at onset is reflected in both the overall gender effect and the gender-by-response interaction. For this hypothesis, a simple effects model (38) is more appropriate. The simple effects model decomposes the main gender effect and the gender-by-response interaction into two orthogonal

contrasts: the difference between male and female neuroleptic responders and the difference between male and female neuroleptic nonresponders. Neuroleptic response remains as a main effect. This analysis reveals a significant effect of neuroleptic response (F=17.1, df=1, 318, p<0.0001), a significant difference between the male and female responders (F=6.6, df=1, 318, p< 0.01), but no difference between the male and female neuroleptic nonresponders (F=0.6, df=1, 318, p=0.46).

A cumulative distribution of the patients' ages at onset for the four groups is presented in figure 1. As can be seen, the largest and most consistent difference was between the female neuroleptic-resistant and neuroleptic-responsive patients. The curves are virtually identical for the male and female neuroleptic-resistant patients until age 20, when the rate increases slightly for the males. The age at onset of psychosis for the neuroleptic-responsive women was nearly always higher than that for the neuroleptic-responsive men. Both of these groups had slower rates of onset of psychosis than their neuroleptic-resistant counterparts after age 15.

We examined race as a factor in age at onset, controlling for gender and neuroleptic response. There was a significant race effect (F=5.0, df=1, 310, p=0.03) but no significant two-way interactions involving race. There were gender and neuroleptic response effects, but no response-by-race-by-gender interactions. The mean age at onset for the African Americans (N=65) was 23.1 years (SD=8.2), and for the Caucasians (N=253) it was 20.2 years (SD=5.7). African Americans had a later age at onset in each of the four gender-by-response groups.

We next examined the effect of neuroleptic response, gender, and subtype of schizophrenia on age at onset (table 3). The two catatonic patients were omitted because of the small number of subjects. Furthermore, because of the small numbers of subjects in some other groups, the patients with the paranoid, residual, and schizoaffective subtypes were combined into one group (group A) and the patients with the undifferentiated and disorganized subtypes were combined into another (group B). The ANOVA revealed a significant response-by-gender-by-subtype interaction, making all other lower-order main effects and interactions uninterpretable. Significant results of a simple effects model testing male-female differences in each of the response-

478

TABLE 3. Age at Onset in Relation to Neuroleptic Responsivity, Gender, and Diagnostic Subtype for Patients With Schizophrenia or Schizoaffective Disorder

	Neuroleptic-Responsive				Neuroleptic-Resistant					
	Men		Women		Men		Women		Combined	
	Age at Onset (years)		Age at Onset (years)		Age at Onset (years)		Age at Onset (years)		Age at Onset (years)	
Diagnostic Subtype	N	Mean SD	N	Mean SD	N	Mean SD	N	Mean SD	N	Mean SD
Group A										
Paranoid schizophrenia	28	19.5 4.3	16	24.8[a] 8.0	48	20.0 4.5	28	21.6 7.5	120	— —
Residual schizophrenia	11	22.1 8.1	4	29.3 18.6	12	18.2 2.3	2	22.0 2.8	29	— —
Schizoaffective disorder	8	21.1 1.9	14	24.4 6.4	7	21.4 11.7	17	17.5 5.1	46	— —
Total	47	20.4 5.2	34	25.2[b] 8.9	67	19.9 5.3	47	20.1 6.8	195	20.9 6.6
Group B										
Disorganized schizophrenia	4	26.3 13.6	2	19.0 7.1	10	17.9 3.2	7	18.1 5.1	23	— —
Undifferentiated schizophrenia	24	22.2 5.9	12	21.3 8.6	41	19.2 3.8	21	21.1 5.2	98	— —
Total	28	22.8 7.2	14	21.0 8.2	51	18.9 3.7	28	20.4 5.2	121	20.4 5.8

[a]Significant difference from neuroleptic-responsive men with paranoid subtype (F=8.4, df=1, 116, p<0.01).
[b]Significant difference from neuroleptic-responsive men in group A (F=12.0, df=1, 308, p<0.01) and neuroleptic-resistant men in group A (F=17.0, df=1, 308, p<0.001) and group B (F=21.4, df=1, 308, p<0.001).

by-subtype cells are given in table 3. As can be seen, the onset for the female neuroleptic-responsive patients in group A was significantly later than the onset for their male counterparts and for the neuroleptic-resistant men in both group A and group B. None of the other response-by-subtype groups had a significant male-female difference.

The data collected in this study were used to determine the likelihood of being neuroleptic resistant as a function of age at onset by means of Bayesian computation, as described in the Method section. The results are given in table 4. It may be seen that if the age at onset for a male is 21 years or less, the probability of being neuroleptic resistant is more than 30% but less than 40%. With onset between ages 22 and 24, the probability of being neuroleptic resistant drops below 20%, increases to 25.4% between ages 25 and 27, and then decreases to 17.6% at and after age 28. For females, the probability of being neuroleptic resistant exceeds 30% with an age at onset of 18 years or less.

DISCUSSION

The major findings of this study are that neuroleptic-resistant patients had a significantly younger age at onset than neuroleptic-responsive patients and that the gender difference in age at onset in neuroleptic-resistant schizophrenic patients was not significant whereas the expected gender difference in age at onset was confirmed in neuroleptic-responsive patients. We also confirmed the previous finding that the gender difference in age at onset was significant in only some subgroups of schizophrenic patients, especially the paranoid subtype, but only in patients who were neuroleptic responsive. We confirmed an earlier onset in male schizophrenic patients as a group, even though the age at onset was not significantly different in neuroleptic-resistant men and women. The interaction of gender and neuroleptic

TABLE 4. Conditional Probability of Being Resistant to Neuroleptic Treatment as a Function of Age at Onset for 194 Male and 128 Female Patients With Schizophrenia or Schizoaffective Disorder

| | Conditional Probability[a] | |
Age at Onset (years)	Men	Women
≤15	0.324	0.359
16–18	0.389	0.345
19–21	0.343	0.282
22–24	0.177	0.265
25–27	0.254	0.284
≥28	0.176	0.239

[a]See text for method of computation.

responsivity did not reach statistical significance, because the age at onset for the men was less than that for the women, regardless of neuroleptic responsivity status. A power calculation (41) reported here indicated that a sample size of 151 cases per cell would provide a power of 0.8 to identify a significant interaction with alpha=0.05. Another power size calculation determined that 391 neuroleptic-resistant women and 391 neuroleptic-resistant men would be required with a power of 0.8 and alpha=0.05 to demonstrate that male neuroleptic-resistant patients had a younger age at onset than their female counterparts. Only 77 women and 119 men in this study were neuroleptic resistant.

The definition of age at onset of schizophrenia as the onset of positive psychotic symptoms is one of many that have been used for this purpose. The age at onset of psychosis is generally recalled with accuracy by family members and by patients, even if some patients are initially guarded about admitting delusions and hallucinations. The intraclass correlations for age at onset in the separate reliability study reported here were satisfactory. It seems unlikely that there was any systematic difference based on gender or neuroleptic resistance in the reliability of ascertaining age at time of first psychotic symptoms. It is unlikely that the neuroleptic-responsive schizophrenic women, on average, had psychotic episodes 3–4 years earlier than reported here.

We found no significant difference in the interval between age at onset and age at first hospitalization between the male and female schizophrenic patients. However, this interval was significantly shorter in the neuroleptic-resistant patients than in the neuroleptic-responsive patients. The latter finding might affect the earlier identification of schizophrenia in the neuroleptic-resistant patients, but this could not explain the gender effect noted here. Loebel et al. (16) reported that 18.9% of patients with first-episode schizophrenia or schizoaffective disorder failed to respond adequately to typical neuroleptics. There was no difference between the men and women in this study in this regard. Since neuroleptic resistance is relatively rare at the time of first admission, it is unlikely that neuroleptic resistance per se could influence the results on age at onset reported here.

The mean age at onset of the patients in this study was lower for both the neuroleptic-responsive and neuroleptic-resistant men and women than was reported in most of the literature reviewed by Angermeyer and Kuhn (21). However, we compared the results reported here to those reported in more-recent studies and found that the group of neuroleptic-responsive women was not significantly different in age at onset from the women in four of these studies (23–26) and that the male group did not differ in age at onset from those reported by Loranger (22) and Beratis et al. (24). Whelton et al. (42) reported age at first psychiatric contact as 21.4 years (SD=4.5) in 31 schizophrenic patients. These studies used a definition of age at onset that was similar to the one used here. Neuroleptic responders would be expected to predominate in most populations of schizophrenic patients, since about 70% of schizophrenic patients are believed to respond to neuroleptic treatment (18), if response is defined according to the criteria used here. If the results reported here are valid, studies that indicate a large difference in age at onset between males and females may include mainly neuroleptic-responsive patients.

The significant difference in age at onset as a function of gender and treatment resistance was found only for the neuroleptic-responsive subgroup with the paranoid, residual, and schizoaffective subtypes. For the patients with the undifferentiated and disorganized subtypes, the difference in age at onset as a function of gender was not significant in either the neuroleptic-responsive or neuroleptic-resistant patients. Other studies have shown similar gender differences in age at onset as a function of subtype (24, 32–35). The results for patients with the paranoid subtype are in close accord with those from the study of Beratis et al. (24). It thus appears that both neuroleptic responsivity and subtype of schizophrenia are important in the gender effect on age at onset, with neuroleptic-responsive females with the paranoid subtype having onsets 5 to 7 years later, on average, than their male counterparts.

The Bayesian computation indicated that an age at onset of ≤21 years for males and ≤18 years for females was associated with a slightly greater likelihood of being neuroleptic resistant. This method assumed that the overall incidence of neuroleptic resistance in a population of schizophrenic persons is 30%. If the true proportion of neuroleptic resistance differs from this, the probability of being neuroleptic resistant for a given age at onset is directly proportional to the difference between 30% and the observed proportion; e.g., if the proportion were 15%, the probability of a male with age at onset ≤15 being neuroleptic resistant would be 0.162 rather than 0.324.

The results of the current study suggest that younger age at onset, particularly for women, is associated with resistance to typical neuroleptic treatment. This finding is consistent with the results of Kolakowska et al. (13). In this regard, it should be noted that of 319 neuroleptic-resistant patients in the U.S. multicenter clozapine trial (18), 80% of whom were males, the average age at first hospitalization was 20.4 years (SD=4.6), which is similar to the average age at onset for neuroleptic-resistant men in this study (mean=19.4 years, SD=4.7). The modest difference between these two figures may be due to the tendency of the first hospitalization to be 1 to 3 years later than the appearance of first psychotic symptoms (22, 27, 43). Similarly, Miller et al. (43) reported a mean age at onset of 18.9 years (SD= 2.2) in 29 neuroleptic-resistant patients (20 male, nine female). The ages at onset of these neuroleptic-resistant patients are lower than those for unselected groups of schizophrenic patients (21, 23, 30).

Both environmental and biological factors may contribute to the relationships of gender, diagnostic subtype, and neuroleptic responsivity to age at onset. It is possible that differences in life events, e.g., stress and learned capacity to cope with stress, may contribute to the gender-related differences in age at onset. However, it is unlikely that such factors could be sufficiently different in neuroleptic-responsive and -resistant females to account for the 4.1-year difference in age at onset between these two groups.

Differences in biological factors seem more likely to account for the differences in age at onset among the four groups. It is possible that differences in neurotransmitters related to psychosis (e.g., dopamine, serotonin, glutamate), sex steroids (estrogens, progesterone, testosterone), glucocorticoids, or other complex processes related to psychosis (synaptic pruning) may operate differentially in neuroleptic-responsive female patients with the paranoid subtype of schizophrenia to provide for a later age at onset than in other patients with schizophrenia. Thus, sex differences in brain organization, vulnerability to birth trauma, rate of postnatal maturation, and effects of sex steroids on various biological processes during the premorbid period (see references 4 and 44–47 for review and further discussion) may contribute to the results reported here, which link these processes with the subsequent development or manifestation of neuroleptic resistance. The younger age at onset in male than in female schizophrenic patients has been attributed to the influence of estrogen on brain dopaminergic neurotransmission (45). Similarly, the differences in age at onset between neuroleptic-resistant and neuroleptic-responsive patients and between paranoid and nonparanoid patients might also be due to differences in dopaminergic mechanisms. Paranoid symptoms have been specifically related to increased dopaminergic activity on the basis of amphetamine-induced psychosis (48, 49). It has been suggested that disorganized and undifferentiated symptoms may be related to glutamatergic neurotransmission because of their similarity to behavioral changes induced by phencyclidine, a noncompetitive antagonist of glutamate receptors (50, 51). These abnormalities may also contribute to the earlier onset in neuroleptic-resistant patients who do not respond to neuroleptic drugs at first exposure. Differences in the responses of male and female schizophrenic patients to serotonergic challenge drugs have also been reported (52). Although males have been reported to have more structural brain abnormalities than females (53), this difference has not been found in most other studies (54). No relationship between ventricle-brain ratio or prefrontal sulcal prominence and age was found in the subjects in this study (data not presented).

Studies of a possible gender difference in age at onset for patients with bipolar affective disorder (35, 55–57) have shown no difference or an earlier onset among females. Thus, the specificity of the gender-related differences in age at onset in this study, which were much stronger in the neuroleptic-responsive than neuroleptic-resistant patients, provides further support for the importance of the neuroleptic-responsive versus -resistant distinction (58).

In conclusion, as in previous studies, the onset of neuroleptic-resistant schizophrenia was found to be earlier than that of neuroleptic-responsive schizophrenia. This relationship was most evident in the female patients but was also apparent in the men as well. A crucial interaction with diagnostic subtype, i.e., paranoid, schizoaffective, and residual subtypes compared to the undifferentiated and disorganized subtypes, was found. The small difference in age at onset between the male and female neuroleptic-resistant patients suggests that the onset of psychosis in this subgroup of patients is more related to gender-independent than gender-specific biological processes. We previously reported that premorbid function during childhood is also gender independent in neuroleptic-resistant patients but not in neuroleptic-responsive patients (58). Furthermore, these results suggest neuroleptic resistance may be a distinctive subtype of schizophrenia, as previously proposed on other grounds (59). The results reported here suggest that studies of the pathogenesis and pathophysiology of schizophrenia should examine gender, neuroleptic responsivity, subtype, and the interaction of these variables.

REFERENCES

1. Weinberger DR: Implications of normal brain development for the pathogenesis of schizophrenia. Arch Gen Psychiatry 1987; 44:660–669

2. Lewis SW, Murray RM: Obstetric complications, neurodevelopmental endurance, and risk of schizophrenia. Psychiatry Res 1987; 21:413–421

3. Bloom FE: Advancing a neurodevelopmental origin for schizophrenia. Arch Gen Psychiatry 1993; 50:224–227

4. Saugstad LF: Age at puberty and mental illness: towards a neurodevelopmental aetiology of Kraepelin's endogenous psychoses. Br J Psychiatry 1989; 155:536–544

5. Pearlson GD, Kreger L, Rabins P, Chase GA, Cohen B, Wirth JB, Schlaepfer TB, Tune LE: A chart review study of late-onset and early-onset schizophrenia. Am J Psychiatry 1989; 146:1568–1574

6. Howard R, Levy R: Late onset schizophrenia current status and future developments, in Schizophrenia: Exploring the Spectrum of Psychosis. Edited by Ancill RJ, Holliday S, Higgenbottam J. Chichester, England, John Wiley & Sons, 1994, pp 327–338

7. Andreasen NC, Flaum M, Swayze VW II, Tyrrell G, Arndt S: Positive and negative symptoms in schizophrenia: a critical reappraisal. Arch Gen Psychiatry 1990; 47:615–621

8. Kenny J, Meltzer HY: Attention and higher cortical functions in schizophrenia. J Neuropsychiatry Clin Neurosci 1991; 3:269–275

9. Haas GL, Sweeney JA: Premorbid and onset features of first-episode schizophrenia. Schizophr Bull 1992; 18:373–387

10. Bilder RM, Lipschutz-Broch L, Reiter G, Geisler SH, Mayerhoff DI, Lieberman JA: Intellectual deficits in first-episode schizophrenia: evidence for progressive deterioration. Schizophr Bull 1992; 18:437–448

11. De Lisi LE: The significance of age of onset for schizophrenia. Schizophr Bull 1992; 18:209–215

12. Johnstone EC, Owens DG, Bydder GM, Colter N, Crow TJ, Frith CD: The spectrum of structural brain changes in schizophrenia: age of onset as a predictor of cognitive and clinical impairments and their cerebral correlates. Psychol Med 1989; 19: 91–103

13. Kolakowska T, Williams AO, Ardern M, Reveley MA, Jambor K, Gelder MG, Mandelbrote BM: Schizophrenia with good and poor outcome, I: early clinical features, response to neuroleptics and signs of organic dysfunction. Br J Psychiatry 1985; 146:229–239

14. Nimgaonkar VL, Wesseley S, Tune LE, Murray RM: Response to drugs in schizophrenia: the influence of family history, obstetric complications and ventricular enlargement. Psychol Med 1988; 18:583–592

15. Eaton WW, Mortensen PB, Herrman H, Freeman H, Bilker W, Burgess P, Wooff K: Long-term course of hospitalization for schizophrenia, part I: risk for rehospitalization. Schizophr Bull 1992; 18:217–228

16. Loebel AD, Lieberman JA, Alvir JMJ, Mayerhoff DI, Geisler SH, Szymanski SR: Duration of psychosis and outcome in first-episode schizophrenia. Am J Psychiatry 1992; 149:1183–1188

17. Harvey PD, Putnam KM, Davidson M, Kahn RS, Powchik P, McQueeney R, Keefe RS, Davis KL: Brief neuroleptic discontinuation and clinical symptoms in Kraepelinian and non-Kraepelinian chronic schizophrenic patients. Psychiatry Res 1991; 38: 285–292

18. Kane J, Honigfeld G, Singer J, Meltzer H: Clozapine for the treatment-resistant schizophrenic: a double-blind comparison with chlorpromazine. Arch Gen Psychiatry 1988; 45:789–796

19. Carpenter WT, Buchanan RW: Domains of psychopathology relevant to the study of etiology and treatment in schizophrenia, in Schizophrenia: Scientific Progress. Edited by Schulz SC, Tamminga CA. New York, Oxford University Press, 1989, pp 13–22

20. Buchanan RW, Kirkpatrick B, Heinrichs DW, Carpenter WT Jr: Clinical correlates of the deficit syndrome of schizophrenia. Am J Psychiatry 1990; 147:290–294

21. Angermeyer MD, Kuhn L: Gender differences in age of onset of schizophrenia: an overview. Eur Arch Psychiatry Neurol Sci 1988; 237:351–364

22. Loranger AW: Sex difference in age of onset of schizophrenia. Arch Gen Psychiatry 1984; 41:157–161

23. Gureje O: Gender and schizophrenia: age of onset and sociodemographic attributes. Acta Psychiatr Scand 1991; 83:402–405

24. Beratis S, Gabriel J, Hoidas S: Age at onset in subtypes of schizophrenic disorders. Schizophr Bull 1994; 20:287–296

327

25. Goldstein JM, Tsuang MT, Faraone SV: Gender and schizophrenia: implications for understanding the heterogeneity of the illness. Psychiatry Res 1989; 28:243–253

26. Faraone SV, Chen WJ, Goldstein JM, Tsuang MT: Gender differences in age at onset of schizophrenia. Br J Psychiatry 1994; 164:625–629

27. Häfner H, Riecher-Rossler A, Maurer K, Fatkenheuer B, Loffler W: First onset and early symptomatology of schizophrenia: a chapter of epidemiological and neurobiological research into age and sex differences. Eur Arch Psychiatry Clin Neurosci 1992; 242:109–118

28. Hambrecht M, Maurer K, Hafner H, Sartorius N: Transnational stability of gender differences in schizophrenia? an analysis based on the WHO study on determinants of outcome of severe mental disorders. Eur Arch Psychiatry Clin Neurosci 1992; 242: 6–12

29. Shepherd M, Watt D, Falloon I, Smeeton N: The natural history of schizophrenia: a five-year follow-up study of outcome and prediction in a representative sample of schizophrenics. Psychol Med Monogr Suppl 1989; 15:1–46

30. Hafner H, Riecher A, Maurer K, Loffler W, Munk-Jorgensen P, Stromgren E: How does gender influence age at first hospitalization for schizophrenia? a transnational case register study. Psychol Med 1989; 19:903–918

31. Ganguli R, Brar JS: Generalizability of first-episode studies in schizophrenia. Schizophr Bull 1992; 18:463–470

32. Angst J, Baastrup P, Grof P, Hippius H, Pöldinger W, Varga E, Weiss P, Wyss F: Statistische Aspekte des Beginns und Verlaufs schizophrener Psychosen, in Verlauf und Augang schizophrener Erkrankungen. Edited by Huber G. New York, Schattauer, 1973

33. Diebold K, Engel T: Symptomatik, Syndromatik und Ersterkrankungsalter endogen depressiver und schizophrener Psychosen in Abhängigkeit von der Unter-bzw: Hauptdiagnose und dem Geschlecht. Nervenarzt 1977; 48:130–138

34. Bellodi L, Morabito A, Macciardi F, Gasperini M, Benvenuto MG, Grassi G, Marzorati-Spairani C, Smeraldi E: Analytic considerations about observed distribution of age of onset in schizophrenia. Neuropsychobiology 1982; 8:93–101

35. Rzewuska M, Angst J: Aspects of the course of bipolar manic-depressive, schizo-affective, and paranoid schizophrenic psychoses. Arch Psychiatr Nervenkr 1982; 231:487–501

36. Endicott J, Spitzer RL: A diagnostic interview: the Schedule for Affective Disorders and Schizophrenia. Arch Gen Psychiatry 1978; 35:837–844

37. Meltzer HY: Treatment of the neuroleptic-nonresponsive schizophrenic patient. Schizophr Bull 1992; 18:515–542

38. Winer BJ: Statistical Principles in Experimental Design. New York, McGraw-Hill, 1971

39. Hayes WL: Statistics for the Social Sciences, 2nd ed. New York, Holt, Rinehart & Winston, 1973

40. Davis JM, Schaffer CB, Killian GA, Kinard C, Chan C: Important issues in the drug treatment of schizophrenia. Schizophr Bull 1980; 6:70–87

41. Desu MM, Raghavarao D: Sample Size Methodology. Boston, Academic Press, 1990

42. Whelton CL, Cleghorn JM, Atley S, Durocher GJ, MacCrimmon D: Developmental and neurologic correlates of treatment response in schizophrenia. J Psychiatry Neurosci 1992; 7:15–22

43. Miller DD, Perry PJ, Cadoret RJ, Andreasen NC: Clozapine's effect on negative symptoms in treatment-refractory schizophrenics. Compr Psychiatry 1994; 35:8–15

44. Häfner H, Maurer K, Loffler W, Riecher-Rossler A: The influence of age and sex on the onset and early course of schizophrenia. Br J Psychiatry 1993; 162:80–86

45. Häfner H, Behrens S, De Vry J, Gattaz WF: An animal model for the effects of estradiol on dopamine-mediated behavior: implications for sex differences in schizophrenia. Psychiatry Res 1991; 38:125–134

46. Seeman MV, Lang M: The role of estrogens in schizophrenia gender differences. Schizophr Bull 1990; 16:185–194

47. Lewine RR, Gulley LR, Risch SC, Jewart R, Houpt JL: Sexual dimorphism, brain morphology, and schizophrenia. Schizophr Bull 1990; 16:195–203

48. Snyder S: Amphetamine psychosis: a "model" schizophrenia mediated by catecholamines. Am J Psychiatry 1973; 130:61–67

49. Ellenwood EH Jr, Sudilovsky A, Nelson LM: Evolving behavior in the clinical and experimental amphetamine (model) psychosis. Am J Psychiatry 1973; 130:1088–1093

50. Luby ED, Cohen BD, Rosenbaum G, Gottlieb JS, Kelley R: Study of a new schizophrenomimetic drug: sernyl. Arch Neurol Psychiatry 1959; 81:363–369

51. Tamminga CA, Thaker GK, Alphs LD, Chase TN: Limbic system: localization of PCP drug action in rat and schizophrenic manifestations in humans, in Schizophrenia: Scientific Progress. Edited by Schulz SC, Tamminga CA. New York, Oxford University Press, 1989, pp 163–172

52. Meltzer HY, Maes M, Lee MA: The cimetidine-induced increase in prolactin secretion in schizophrenia: effect of clozapine. Psychopharmacology (Berl) 1993; 112:S95–S104

53. Andreasen NC, Nasrallah HA, Dunn V, Olson SC, Grove WM, Ehrhardt JC, Coffman JA, Crossett JH: Structural abnormalities in the frontal system in schizophrenia: a magnetic resonance imaging study. Arch Gen Psychiatry 1986; 43:136–144

54. Nasrallah HA, Schwarzkopf SB, Olson SC, Coffman JA: Gender differences on CT and MRI brain scans. Schizophr Bull 1990; 16:205–210

55. Loranger AW, Levine PM: Age at onset of bipolar affective illness. Arch Gen Psychiatry 1978; 35:1345–1348

56. Peselow ED, Dunner DL, Fieve RR, Deutsch SI, Rubinstein ME: Age of onset of affective illness. Psychiatr Clin 1982; 15:124–132

57. Joyce PR: Age of onset in bipolar affective disorder and misdiagnosis as schizophrenia. Psychol Med 1984; 14:145–149

58. Findling R, Meltzer HY: Premorbid asociality in neuroleptic-resistant and -responsive schizophrenia. Psychol Med 1996; 26: 1033–1041

59. Brown WA, Herz LR: Neuroleptic response as a nosologic device, in Handbook of Schizophrenia, vol 3: Nosology, Epidemiology and Genetics. Edited by Tsuang MT, Simpson JG. New York, Elsevier, 1988, pp 139–149

328

Acknowledgments

Lewis, D.A., and Lieberman, J.A. "Catching up on Schizophrenia: Natural History and Neurobiology." *Neuron* 28 (2000): 325–334. Reprinted from *Neuron* 28 (2000): 325–334. Copyright 2000, with permission from Elsevier Science.

Andreasen, N.C. "A Unitary Model of Schizophrenia." *Arch Gen Psychiatry* 56 (1999): 781–787. Reprinted with the permission of American Medical Association.

Weinberger, D.R. "Implications of Normal Brain Development for the Pathogenesis of Schizophrenia." *Arch Gen Psychiatry* 44 (1987): 660–669. Reprinted with the permission of American Medical Association.

Kendler, K., Gallagher, T., Abelson, J., and Kessler, R.C. "Lifetime Prevalence, Demographic Risk Factors, and Diagnostic Validity of Nonaffective Psychosis as Assessed in a US Community Sample." *Arch Gen Psychiatry* 53 (1996): 1022–1031. Reprinted with the permission of American Medical Association.

Dalman, C., Allbeck, P., Cullberg, J., Grunewald, C., and Koster, M. "Obstetric Complications and the Risk of Schizophrenia." *Arch Gen Psychiatry* 56 (1996): 234–240. Reprinted with the permission of American Medical Association.

Mortensen, P.B., Pedersen, C.B., Westergaard, T., Wohlfahrt, J., Ewald, H., Mors, O., Andersen, P.K., and Melbye, M. "Effects of Family History and Place and Season of Birth on the Risk of Schizophrenia." *N Engl J Med* 340 (1999): 603–608. Copyright © 1999 Massachusetts Medical Society. All rights reserved.

Kety, S.S., Rosenthal, D., Wender, P.H., and Schulsinger, F. "The Types and Prevalence of Mental Illness in the Biological and Adoptive Families of Adopted Schizophrenics." *J Psychiatr Res* 6 (1968): 345–362. Reprinted with the permission of Elsevier Science Ireland Ltd.

Kendler, K.S., and Gruenberg, A.M. "An Independent Analysis of the Danish Adoption Study of Schizophrenia." *Arch Gen Psychiatry* 4 (1984): 555–564. Reprinted with the permission of American Medical Association.

Baron, M. "Genetics of Schizophrenia and the New Millennium: Progress and Pitfalls." *Am J Hum Genet* 68 (2001): 299–312. Reprinted with permission of the University of Chicago Press. Copyright 2001, American Society of Human Genetics.

Egan, M.F., Goldberg, T.E., Kolachana, B.S., et al. "Effect of COMT Val [108/158] Met Genotype on Frontal Lobe Function and Risk of Schizophrenia." *Proc Natl Acad Sci USA* 98 (2001): 6917–6922. National Academy of Sciences of the U.S.A., Proceed.

Bromet, E.J., and Fennig, S. "Epidemiology and Natural History of Schizophrenia." *Biol Psychiatry* 46 (1999): 871–881. Reprinted with the permission of Elsevier Science.

Heaton, R.K., Gladsjo, J.A., Palmer, B.W., Kuck, J., Marcotte, T.D., and Jeste, D.V. "Stability and Course of Neuropsychological Deficits in Schizophrenia." *Arch Gen Psychiatry* 58 (2001): 24–32. Reprinted with the permission of American Medical Association.

Robinson, D., Woerner, M.G., Alvir, J.M., Bilder, R., Goldman, R., Geisler, S., Koreen, A., Sheitman, B., Chakos, M., Mayerhoff, D., and Lieberman, J.A. "Predictors of Relapse following Response from a First Episode of Schizophrenia or Schizoaffective Disorder." *Arch Gen Psychiatry* 56 (1999): 241–247. Reprinted with the permission of American Medical Association.

Akil, M., Pierri, J.N., Whitehead, R.E., Edgar, C.L., Mohila, C., Sampson, A.R., and Lewis, D.A. "Lamina-Specific Alterations in the Dopamine Innervation of the Prefrontal Cortex in Schizophrenic Subjects." *Am J Psychiatry* 156 (1999): 1580–1589. Copyright 1999, the American Psychiatric Association. Reprinted by permission.

Arnold, S.E., Trojanowski, J.Q., Gur, R.E., Blackwell, P., Han, L.Y., and Choi, C. "Absence of Neurodegeneration and Neural Injury in the Cerebral Cortex in a Sample of Elderly Patients with Schizophrenia." *Arch Gen Psychiatry* 55 (1998): 225–232. Reprinted with the permission of American Medical Association.

Barch, D.M., Carter, C.S., Braver, T.S., et al. "Selective Deficits in Prefrontal Cortex Function in Medication-Naïve Patients with Schizophrenia." *Arch Gen Psychiatry* 58 (2001): 280–288. Reprinted with the permission of American Medical Association.

Gilbert, A.R., Rosenberg, D.R., Harenski, K., Spencer, S., Sweeney, J.A., and Keshavan, M.S. "Thalamic Volumes in Patients with First-Episode Schizophrenia." *Am J Psychiatry* 158 (2001): 618–624. Copyright 2001, the American Psychiatric Association. Reprinted by permission.

Glantz, L.A., and Lewis, D.A. "Decreased Dendritic Spine Density on Prefrontal Cortical Pyramidal Neurons in Schizophrenia." *Arch Gen Psychiatry* 57 (2000): 65–73. Reprinted with the permission of American Medical Association.

Goff, D.C., and Coyle, J.T. "The Emerging Role of Glutamate in the Pathophysiology and Treatment of Schizophrenia." *Am J Psychiatry* 158 (2001): 1367–1377. Copyright 2001, the American Psychiatric Association. Reprinted by permission.

Goldstein, J.M., Goodman, J.M., Seidman, L.J., et al. "Cortical Abnormalities in Schizophrenia Identified by Structural Magnetic Resonance Imaging." *Arch Gen Psychiatry* 56 (1999): 537–547. Reprinted with the permission of American Medical Association.

Harrison, P.J. "The Neuropathology of Schizophrenia: A Critical Review of the Data and Their Interpretation." *Brain* 122 (1999): 593–624. Reprinted with the permission of Oxford University Press.

Laruelle, M., Abi-Dargham, A., van Dyck, C.H., Gil, R., D'Souza, C.D., Erdos, J., McCance, E., Rosenblatt, W., Fingado, C., Zoghbi, S.S., Baldwin, R.M., Seibyl, J.P., Krystal, J.H., Charney, D.S., and Innis, R.B. "Single Photon Emission Computerized Tomography Imaging of Amphetamine-Induced Dopamine Release in Drug-Free Schizophrenic Subjects." *Proc Natl Acad Sci U.S.A.* 93 (1996): 9235–9240.

Lim, K.O., Hedehus, M., Moseley, M., et al. "Compromised White Matter Tract Integrity in Schizophrenia Inferred from Diffusion Tensor Imaging." *Arch Gen Psychiatry* 56 (1999): 367–374. Reprinted with the permission of American Medical Association.

Okubo, Y., Suhara, T., Suzuki, K., Kobayashi, K., Inoue, O., Terasaki, O., Someya, Y., Sassa, T., Sudo, Y., Matsushima, E., Iyo, M., Tateno, Y., and Toru, M. "Decreased Prefrontal Dopamine D1 Receptors in Schizophrenia Revealed by PET." *Nature* 385 (1997): 634–636. Reprinted by permission from Nature Vol. 385 pp. 634–636. Copyright © 1997 Macmillan Magazines Ltd.

Rajkowska, G., Selemon, L.D., and Goldman-Rakic, P.S. "Neuronal and Glial Somal Size in the Prefrontal Cortex: A Postmortem Morphometric Study of Schizophrenia and Huntington Disease." *Arch Gen Psychiatry* 55 (1998): 215–224. Reprinted with the permission of American Medical Association.

Selemon, L.D., and Goldman-Rakic, P.S. "The Reduced Neuropil Hypothesis: A Circuit Based Model of Schizophrenia." *Biol Psychiatry* 45 (1999): 17–25. Reprinted with the permission of Elsevier Science. Copyright 1999 by the Society of Biological Psychiatry.

Suddath, R.L., Christison, G.W., Torrey, E.F., Casanova, M.F., and Weinberger, D.R. "Anatomical Abnormalities in the Brains of Monozygotic Twins Discordant for Schizophrenia." *N Engl J Med* 322 (1990): 789–794. Copyright © 1990 Massachusetts Medical Society. All rights reserved.

Bustillo, J.R., Lauriello, J., Horan, W.P., and Keith, S.J. "The Psychosocial Treatment of Schizophrenia: An Update." *Am J Psychiatry* 158 (2001): 163–175. Copyright 2001, the American Psychiatric Association. Reprinted by permission.

Castner, S.A., Williams, G.V., and Goldman-Rakic, P.S. "Reversal of Antipsychotic Induced Working Memory Deficits by Short-Term Dopamine D1 Receptor Stimulation." *Science* 287 (2000): 2020–2022. Reprinted with permission from *Science* 287 (2000): 2020–2022. Copyright (2000) American Association for the Advancement of Science.

Kane, J., Honigfeld, G., Singer, J., and Meltzer, H. "Clozapine for the Treatment Resistant Schizophrenic: A Double-Blind Comparison with Chlorpromazine." *Arch Gen Psychiatry* 45, 9 (1988): 789–796. Reprinted with the permission of American Medical Association.

Kapur, S., Zipursky, R.B., and Remington, G. "Clinical and Theoretical Implications of 5 HT2 and D2 Receptor Occupancy of Clozapine, Risperidone, and Olanzapine in Schizophrenia." *Am J Psychiatry* 156 (1999): 286–293. Copyright 1999, the American Psychiatric Association. Reprinted by permission.

Lidow, M.S., Song, Z.-M., Castner, S.A., Allen, P.B., Greengard, P., and Goldman-Rakic, P.S. "Antipsychotic Treatment Induces Alterations in Dendrite- and Spine-Associated Proteins in Dopamine-Rich Areas of the Primate Cerebral Cortex." *Biol Psychiatry* 49 (2001): 1–12. Reprinted with the permission of Elsevier Science. Copyright 2001 by the Society of Biological Psychiatry.

Meltzer, H.Y., Rabinowitz, J., Lee, M.A., et al. "Age at Onset and Gender of Schizophrenic Patients in Relation to Neuroleptic Resistance." *Am J Psychiatry* 154 (1997): 475–482. Copyright 1997, the American Psychiatric Association. Reprinted by permission.

For Product Safety Concerns and Information please contact our EU
representative GPSR@taylorandfrancis.com
Taylor & Francis Verlag GmbH, Kaufingerstraße 24, 80331 München, Germany

www.ingramcontent.com/pod-product-compliance
Ingram Content Group UK Ltd.
Pitfield, Milton Keynes, MK11 3LW, UK
UKHW021113180425
457613UK00005B/72

*9 7 8 0 8 1 5 3 3 7 4 6 1 *